Guide to U.S.
HMOs & PPOs

2018

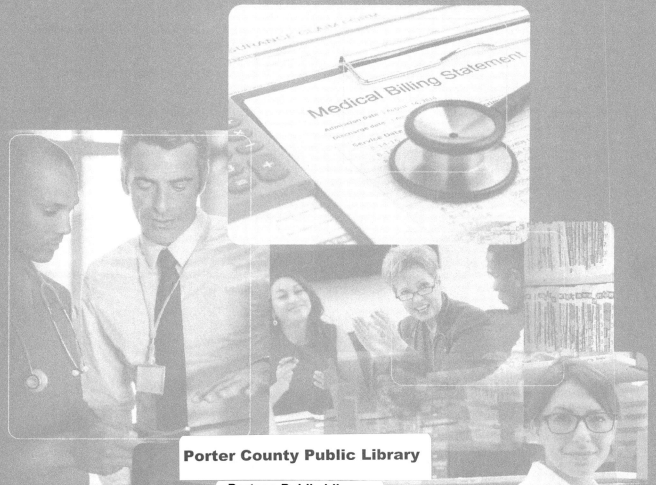

GREY HOUSE PUBLISHING

PUBLISHER: Leslie Mackenzie
EDITORIAL DIRECTOR: Laura Mars

PRODUCTION MANAGER: Kristen Thatcher
COMPOSITION: David Garoogian
MARKETING DIRECTOR: Jessica Moody

A Sedgwick Press Book
Grey House Publishing, Inc.
4919 Route 22
Amenia, NY 12501
518.789.8700
FAX 845.373.6390
www.greyhouse.com
e-mail: books @greyhouse.com

While every effort has been made to ensure the reliability of the information presented in this publication, Grey House Publishing neither guarantees the accuracy of the data contained herein nor assumes any responsibility for errors, omissions or discrepancies. Grey House accepts no payment for listing; inclusion in the publication of any organization, agency, institution, publication, service or individual does not imply endorsement of the editors or publisher.

Errors brought to the attention of the publisher and verified to the satisfaction of the publisher will be corrected in future editions.

First edition published 1987
Thirtieth edition published 2018
Printed in Canada

Guide to U.S. HMOs & PPOs — 1986–
    494 p. 28 cm.
    Annual
    Guide to U.S. HMOs & PPOs
    Includes index.
    ISSN: 0887-4484
1. Health maintenance organizations—United States—Directories. 2. Preferred provider organizations (Medical care)—United States—Directories. I. Title: Guide to U.S. HMOs & PPOs.

RA413.5.U5 H58
362.1'0425—dc21

ISBN: 978-1-68217-383-1 Softcover

Table of Contents

Introduction

This 30th edition of *Guide to U.S. HMOs & PPOs* profiles 859 managed care organizations in the United States. Formerly called *HMO/PPO Directory*, it lists current, comprehensive information for HMO, PPO, POS, and Vision & Dental Plans. Comprehensive coverage-from state listings to consolidations in the health insurance industry—is the cornerstone of this new edition. All entries have been reviewed and updated. This edition includes 66 brand new entries.

In addition to detailed profiles of Managed Healthcare Organizations, this edition includes:
- A 29-page report from the Census Bureau, "Health Insurance Coverage in the United States: 2016" with charts, tables and maps
- A full page chart showing population numbers without health insurance 2013-2016 by the top 25 populous metro areas, Boston being the most insured and Houston the least insured
- State Statistics and Rankings section with state-by-state numbers of individuals covered by type of health plans, and state ranking by number of individuals enrolled in health plans

Praise for *Guide to U.S. HMOs & PPOs:*

> "...of a topic that has grown exponentially more complex each year, this well-organized resource tries its best to keep it simple...The detailed user guide and five indexes enhance navigation...Written for both the consumer and the researcher, this work is a vital resource for public, academic and medical libraries."

> "...Information is clear, consistently presented, and easily located, making the guide extremely user friendly. Of particular note is the valuable...health care reform time line...A practical addition to public and medical library collections."
>
> —*Library Journal*

Arrangement

Plan profiles are arranged alphabetically by state. The first page of each state chapter is a State Summary chart of Health Insurance Coverage Status and Type of Coverage by Age. This chart includes a number of categories, from "Covered by some type of health insurance" to "Not covered at any time during the year."

Directly following the State Summary, plan listings provide crucial contact information, including key executives, often with direct phones and e-mails where available, fax numbers, web sites and hundreds of e-mail addresses. Each profile provides a detailed summary of the plan, including the following:
- Type of Plan, including Specialty and Benefits
- Type of Coverage
- Type of Payment Plan
- Subscriber Information
- Financial History
- Average Compensation Information
- Employer References
- Current Member Enrollment
- Hospital Affiliations
- Number of Primary Care and Specialty Physicians
- Federal Qualification Status
- For Profit Status
- Specialty Managed Care Partners
- Regional Business Coalitions
- Employer References
- Peer Review Information
- Accreditation Information

Additional Features

In addition to the detailed front matter, state statistics, and comprehensive plan profiles, *Guide to U.S. HMOs & PPOs* includes two Appendices and five Indexes.

- Appendix A: Glossary of Health Insurance Terms—Includes more than 150 terms such as Aggregate Indemnity, Diagnostic Related Groups, Non-participating Provider, and Waiting Period.
- Appendix B: Industry Web Sites—Contains dozens of the most valuable health care web sites and a detailed description, from Alliance of Community Health Plans to National Society of Certified Healthcare Business Consultants.
- Plan Index: Alphabetical list of insurance plans by seven plan types: HMO; PPO; HMO/PPO; Dental; Vision; Medicare; and Multiple.
- Personnel Index: Alphabetical list of all executives listed, with their affiliated organization.
- Membership Enrollment Index: List of organizations by member enrollment.
- Primary Care Physician Index: List of organizations by their number of primary care physicians.
- Referral/Specialty Care Physician Index: List of organizations by their number of referral and specialty care physicians.

To broaden its availability, the *Guide to U.S. HMOs & PPOs* is also available for subscription online at http://gold.greyhouse.com. Subscribers can search by plan details, geographic area, number of members, personnel name, title and much more. Users can print out prospect sheets or download data into their own spreadsheet or database. This database is a must for anyone in need of immediate access to contacts in the US managed care marketplace. Plus, buyers of the print directory get a free 30-day trial of the online database. Call (800) 562-2139 x118 for more information.

User Guide

Descriptive listings in the *HMO/PPO Directory* are organized by state, then alphabetically by health plan. Each numbered item is described in the User Key on the following pages. Terms are defined in the Glossary.

1. → **U Healthcare**
2. → **3000 Riverside Road**
   Sharon, CT 06069
3. → **Toll Free: 060-364-0000**
4. → **Phone: 060-364-0001**
5. → **Fax: 060-364-0002**
6. → Info@uhealth.com
7. → www.uhealth.com
8. → Mailing Address: PO Box 729 Sharon, CT 06069-0729
9. → Subsidiary of: USA Healthcare
10. → For Profit: Yes
11. → Year Founded: 1992
12. → Physician Owned: No
13. → Owned by an IDN: No
14. → Federally Qualified: Yes 08/01/82
15. → Number of Affiliated Hospitals: 2,649
16. → Number of Primary Physicians: 4,892
17. → Number of Referral/Specialty Physicians: 6,246
18. → Current Member Enrollment: 204,000 (as of 7/1/01)
19. → State Member Enrollment: 29,000

Healthplan and Services Defined
20. → Plan Type: HMO
21. → Model Type: Staff, IPA, Group, Network
22. → Plan Specialty: ASO, Chiropractic, Dental, Disease Management, Lab, Vision, Radiology
23. → Benefits Offered: Chiropractic, Dental, Disease Management, Vision, Wellness
24. → Offers a Demand Management Patient Information Service: Yes
    DMPI Services Offered: Vision Works, Medical Imaging Institute

25. → **Type of Coverage**
    Commercial, Medicare, Supplemental Medicare, Medicaid
    Catastrophic Illness Benefit: Varies by case

26. → **Type of Payment Plans Offered**
    POS, Capitated, FFS, Combination FFS & DFFS

27. → **Geographic Areas Served**
    Connecticut, Maryland, New Jersey, Vermont, New York

Subscriber Information
28. → Average Monthly Fee Per Subscriber (Employee & Employer Contribution):
    Employee Only (Self): $8.00
    Employee & 1 Family Member: $10.00
    Employee & 2 Family Members: $15.00
    Medicare: $ 10.00
29. → Average Annual Deductible Per Subscriber:
    Employee Only (Self): $200.00

              Employee & 1 Family Member: $250.00
              Employee & 2 Family Members: $500.00
              Medicare: $200.00

30.➤ Average Subscriber Co-Payment:
              Primary Care Physician: $8.00
              Non-Network Physician: $10.00
              Prescription Drugs: $5.00
              Hospital ER: $50.00
              Home Health Care: $25.00
              Home Health Care Max Days Covered/Visits: 30 days
              Nursing Home: $5.00
              Nursing Home Max Days/Visits Covered: 365 days

31.➤ **Network Qualifications**
              Minimum Years of Practice: 10
              Pre-Admission Certification: Yes

32.➤ **Peer Review Type**
              Utilization Review: Yes
              Second Surgical Opinion: No
              Case Management: Yes

33.➤ **Accreditation Certification**
              JCAHO, AAHC (formerly URAC), NCQA
              Publishes and Distributes a Report Card: Yes

34.➤ **Key Personnel**
              CFO...........................David Williams
              Marketing.....................Clarence J. Fist
              Medical Affairs..............Samantha Johnson, MD
              Provider Services............Laura Falk

              Average Claim Compensation
35.➤ Physician's Fee's Charged: 22%
36.➤ Hospital's Fee Charged: 34%

37.➤ **Specialty Managed Care Partners**
              AMBI, Pharmaceutical Treatment, OxiTherapy

38.➤ **Enters into Contracts with Regional Business Coalitions: Yes**
              New York Healthcare

39.➤ **Employer References**
              Life Science Corporation

User Key

1. → **Health Plan:** Formal name of health plan
2. → **Address:** Physical location
3. → **Toll Free:** Toll free number
4. → **Phone:** Main number of organization
5. → **Fax:** Fax number
6. → **E-mail:** Main e-mail address of health plan, if provided
7. → **Website:** Main website address of health plan, if provided
8. → **Mailing Address:** If different from physical address, above.
9. → **Subsidiary of:** Corporation the health plan is legally affiliated with
10. → **For Profit:** Indicates if the organization was formed to make a financial profit. Non-profit organizations can make a profit, but the profits must be used to benefit the organization or purpose the corporation was created to help
11. → **Year Founded:** The year the organization was recognized as a legal entity
12. → **Physician Owned:** Notes if the organization is owned by a group of physicians who are recognized as a legal entity
13. → **Owned by an IDN:** Notes if the organization is owned by an Integrated Delivery Network
14. → **Federally Qualified:** Shows if and when the plan received federally qualified status
15. → **Number of Affiliated Hospitals:** In-network hospitals contracted with the health plans
16. → **Number of Primary Physicians:** In-network primary physicians contracted with the health plan
17. → **Number of Referral/Specialty Physicians:** In-network referral/specialty physicians contracted with the health plan
18. → **Current Member Enrollment:** The number of health plan members or subscribers using health plan benefits, and date of last enrollment count
19. → **State Member Enrollment:** The number of health plan members or subscribers using health plan benefits in that state, and date of last enrollment count
20. → **Plan Type:** Identifies the health plan as an HMO, PPO, Other (neither an HMO or PPO) or Multiple (both an HMO and PPO, or an HMO and TPA or POS; see Glossary for definitions of terms). Note: If a plan is both an HMO and PPO with different product information, i.e. number of hospitals or physicians, the plan is listed as two separate entries
21. → **Model Type:** Describes the relationship between the health plan and its physicians
22. → **Plan Specialty:** Indicates specialized services provided by the plan
23. → **Benefits Offered:** Indicates specialized benefits offered in addition to standard coverage for physician services, hospitalization, diagnostic testing, and prescription drugs
24. → **Offers Demand Management Patient Information Services:** Notes if Triage and other services are offered to help plan members find the most appropriate type and level of care, and what those services are
25. → **Type of Coverage:** Lines of business offered
26. → **Type of Payment Plans Offered:** How the insuror pays its contracted providers
27. → **Geographical Areas Served:** Geographical areas the health plan services
28. → **Average Monthly Fee Per Subscriber:** Monthly premium due to the carrier for each member
29. → **Annual Average Deductible Per Subscriber:** The deductible each member must meet before expenses can be reimbursed
30. → **Average Subscriber Co-Payment:** The co-payment each member must pay at the time services are rendered
31. → **Network Qualifications:** Qualifications a physician must meet to contract with the plan
32. → **Peer Review Type:** The type of on-going peer review process used by the health plan

33. ➤**Accreditation Certification:** Specific certifications the health plan achieved after rigorous review of its policies, procedures, and clinical outcomes

34. ➤**Key Personnel:** Key Executives in the most frequently contacted departments within the plans, with phone and e-mails when provided

35. ➤**Physician's Fees Charged:** The percentage of physicians' billed charges that is actually paid out by the plan

36. ➤**Hospital's Fees Charged:** The percentage of hospitals' billed charges that is actually paid out by the plan

37. ➤**Specialty Managed Care Partners:** Specialty carve-out companies that are contracted with the health plan to offer a broader array of health services to members

38. ➤**Regional Business Coalitions:** Notes if physician or business entities have formed for the sole purpose of achieving economies of scale when purchasing supplies and services, and the names of those businesses

39. ➤**Employer References:** Large employers that have contracted with the health plan and are willing to serve as references for the health plan

Health Insurance Coverage in the United States: 2016

Current Population Reports

By Jessica C. Barnett and Edward R. Berchick
Issued September 2017
P60-260

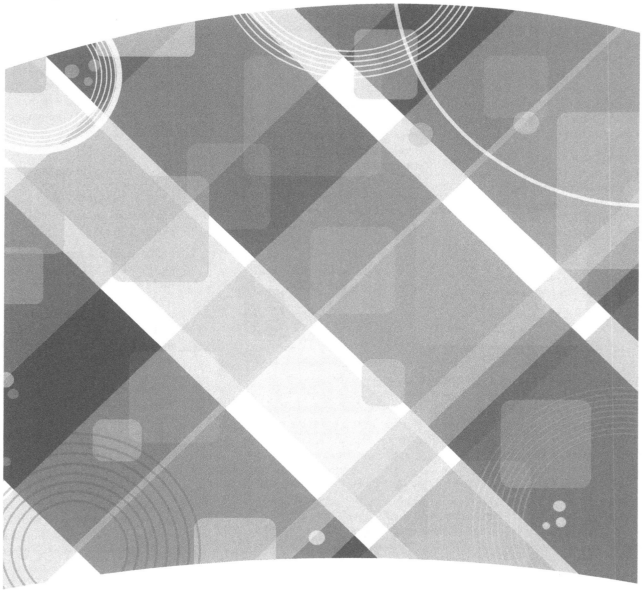

United States™ **Census** Bureau

U.S. Department of Commerce
Economics and Statistics Administration
U.S. CENSUS BUREAU
census.gov

Health Insurance Coverage in the United States: 2016

Introduction

Health insurance is a means for financing a person's health care expenses. While the majority of people have private health insurance, primarily through an employer, many others obtain coverage through programs offered by the government. Other individuals do not have health insurance at all (see the text box "What Is Health Insurance Coverage?").

Over time, changes in the rate of health insurance coverage and the distribution of coverage types may reflect economic trends, shifts in the demographic composition of the population, and policy changes that affect access to care. Several such policy changes occurred in 2014, when many provisions of the Patient Protection and Affordable Care Act

went into effect (see the text box "Health Insurance Coverage and the Affordable Care Act").

This report presents statistics on health insurance coverage in the United States in 2016, changes in health insurance coverage rates between 2015 and 2016, as well as changes in health insurance coverage rates between 2013 and 2016. The statistics in this report are based on information collected in two surveys conducted by the U.S. Census Bureau, the Current Population Survey Annual Social and Economic Supplement (CPS ASEC) and the American Community Survey (ACS) (see the text box "Two Measures of Health Insurance Coverage"). Throughout the report, unless otherwise noted, estimates come from the CPS ASEC.

Highlights

- The uninsured rate decreased between 2015 and 2016 by 0.3 percentage points as measured by the CPS ASEC. In 2016, the percentage of people without health insurance coverage for the entire calendar year was 8.8 percent, or 28.1 million, lower than the rate and number of uninsured in 2015 (9.1 percent or 29.0 million) (Figure 1 and Table 1).[1]

- The percentage of people with health insurance coverage for all or part of 2016 was 91.2 percent, higher than the rate in 2015 (90.9 percent) (Table 1).

- In 2016, private health insurance coverage continued to be more prevalent than government coverage, at 67.5 percent and 37.3 percent, respectively.[2] Of the subtypes of health insurance coverage, employer-based insurance covered 55.7 percent of the population for some or all of the calendar year, followed by Medicaid (19.4 percent), Medicare (16.7 percent), direct-purchase (16.2 percent), and military coverage (4.6 percent) (Table 1 and Figure 1).

- Between 2015 and 2016, the rate of Medicare coverage increased by 0.4 percentage points to cover 16.7 percent of people for part or all of 2016 (up from 16.3 percent

What Is Health Insurance Coverage?

Health insurance coverage in the Current Population Survey Annual Social and Economic Supplement (CPS ASEC) refers to comprehensive coverage during the calendar year.* For reporting purposes, the U.S. Census Bureau broadly classifies health insurance coverage as private insurance or government insurance. The CPS ASEC defines private health insurance as a plan provided through an employer or a union and coverage purchased directly by an individual from an insurance company or through an exchange. Government coverage includes federal programs, such as Medicare, Medicaid, the Children's Health Insurance Program (CHIP), individual state health plans, TRICARE, CHAMPVA (Civilian Health and Medical Program of the Department of Veterans Affairs), as well as care provided by the Department of Veterans Affairs and the military. In the CPS ASEC, people were considered "insured" if they were covered by any type of health insurance for part or all of the previous calendar year. They were considered uninsured if, for the entire year, they were not covered by any type of health insurance. Additionally, people were considered uninsured if they only had coverage through the Indian Health Service (IHS). For more information, see Appendix A, "Estimates of Health Insurance Coverage."

_____

* Comprehensive health insurance covers basic healthcare needs. This definition excludes single service plans, such as accident, disability, dental, vision, or prescription medicine plans.

_____

[1] For a discussion of the quality of the CPS ASEC health insurance coverage estimates, see Appendix B.

[2] Some people may have more than one coverage type during the calendar year.

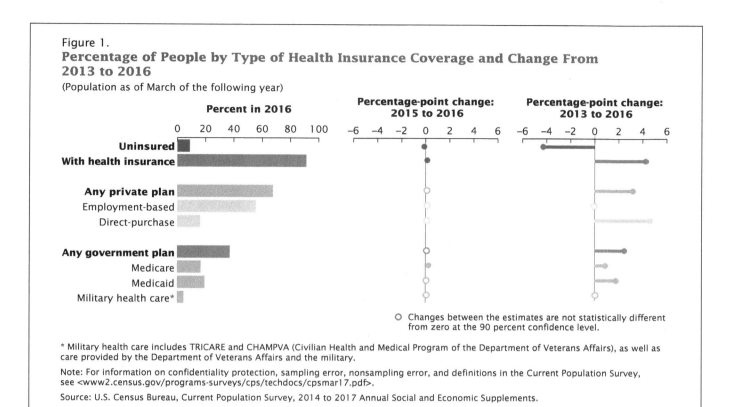

Figure 1.
Percentage of People by Type of Health Insurance Coverage and Change From 2013 to 2016
(Population as of March of the following year)

○ Changes between the estimates are not statistically different from zero at the 90 percent confidence level.

* Military health care includes TRICARE and CHAMPVA (Civilian Health and Medical Program of the Department of Veterans Affairs), as well as care provided by the Department of Veterans Affairs and the military.

Note: For information on confidentiality protection, sampling error, nonsampling error, and definitions in the Current Population Survey, see <www2.census.gov/programs-surveys/cps/techdocs/cpsmar17.pdf>.

Source: U.S. Census Bureau, Current Population Survey, 2014 to 2017 Annual Social and Economic Supplements.

in 2015) (Table 1 and Figure 1).[3] There was no statistically significant difference between 2015 and 2016 for any other subtype of health insurance.

- Between 2015 and 2016, the percentage of people without health insurance coverage dropped for most ages under 65, with generally larger decreases for working-age adults (aged 19 to 64) (Figure 4).[4, 5]

- The percentage of uninsured children under age 19, 5.4 percent,

did not significantly change between 2015 and 2016 (Table 2).

- In 2016, the uninsured rate for children under age 19 in poverty, 7.0 percent, was higher than the uninsured rate for children not in poverty, 5.0 percent (Figure 6).

- In 2016, non-Hispanic Whites had the lowest uninsured rate among race and Hispanic origin groups, at 6.3 percent. The uninsured rates for Blacks and Asians were higher than for non-Hispanic Whites, at 10.5 percent and 7.6 percent, respectively. Hispanics

had the highest uninsured rate, at 16.0 percent (Table 5).[6]

[6] Federal surveys give respondents the option of reporting more than one race. Therefore, two basic ways of defining a race group are possible. A group such as Asian may be defined as those who reported Asian and no other race (the race-alone or single-race concept) or as those who reported Asian regardless of whether they also reported another race (the race-alone-or-in-combination concept). The body of this report (text, figures, and tables) shows data using the first approach (race alone). Use of the single-race population does not imply that it is the preferred method of presenting or analyzing data. The Census Bureau uses a variety of approaches.
In this report, the term "non-Hispanic White" refers to people who are not Hispanic and who reported White and no other race. The Census Bureau uses non-Hispanic Whites as the comparison group for other race groups and Hispanics. Since Hispanics may be any race, data in this report for Hispanics overlap with data for race groups. Being Hispanic was reported by 15.1 percent of White householders who reported only one race, 4.8 percent of Black householders who reported only one race, and 2.3 percent of Asian householders who reported only one race.
Data users should exercise caution when interpreting aggregate results for the Hispanic population or for race groups because these populations consist of many distinct groups that differ in socioeconomic characteristics, culture, and recent immigration status. For further information, see <www.census.gov/cps>.

[3] This increase was likely due to growth in the number of people aged 65 and over. The population 65 years and older did not have a statistically significant change in the Medicare coverage rate between 2015 and 2016. However, the percentage of the U.S. population 65 years and older increased between 2015 and 2016.
[4] Estimates are from the 2015 and 2016 1-Year American Community Surveys.
[5] The change in the uninsured rate between 2015 and 2016 was not statistically significant for infants and for people aged 1, 3, 4, 6, 9, 37, 56, 57, 60, 61, and 63.

- Between 2015 and 2016, the percentage of people without health insurance at any time during the year fell 0.4 percentage points for non-Hispanic Whites, down to 6.3 percent. There was no statistical change in the uninsured rate for Blacks, Asians, or Hispanics during this period (Table 5).[7]

- Between 2015 and 2016, the percentage of people without health insurance coverage at the time of interview decreased in 39 states (Figure 8 and Table 6).[8] Eleven states and the District of Columbia did not have a statistically significant change in their uninsured rate.[9]

---

[7] The small sample size of the Asian population and the fact that the CPS does not use separate population controls for weighting the Asian sample to national totals contribute to the large variances surrounding estimates for this group. As a result, we are unable to detect statistically significant differences between some estimates for the Asian population. The ACS, based on a much larger sample size of the population, is a better source for estimating and identifying changes for small subgroups of the population.

[8] Estimates are from the 2015 and 2016 1-Year American Community Surveys.

[9] Alaska, Delaware, Hawaii, Kansas, Maine, Nebraska, New Hampshire, North Dakota, Oklahoma, Vermont, and Wyoming did not have a statistically significant change in their uninsured rates.

Estimates of Health Insurance Coverage

In 2016, 8.8 percent of people (or 28.1 million) were uninsured for the entire calendar year (Table 1 and Figure 1). This was a decrease of 0.3 percentage points from 2015, when 9.1 percent (or 29.0 million) were uninsured for the entire calendar year.

This report classifies health insurance coverage into three different groups: private coverage, government coverage, and the uninsured. Private coverage includes health insurance provided through an employer or union and coverage purchased directly by an individual from an insurance company or through an exchange.[10] Government coverage includes federal programs, such as Medicare, Medicaid, the Children's Health Insurance Program (CHIP), individual state health plans, TRICARE, CHAMPVA, as well as care provided by the Health and Medical Program of the Department of Veterans Affairs and the military (VA Care). Individuals are considered to be uninsured if they do not have health insurance coverage for the entire cal-

---

[10] Exchanges include coverage purchased through the federal Health Insurance Marketplace, as well as other state-based marketplaces, and include both subsidized and unsubsidized plans.

endar year. For more information, see the text box "What Is Health Insurance Coverage?"

In 2016, most people (91.2 percent) had health insurance coverage at some point during the calendar year, with more people having private health insurance (67.5 percent) than government coverage (37.3 percent). Employer-based insurance was the most common subtype of health insurance (55.7 percent of the civilian, noninstitutionalized population), followed by Medicaid (19.4 percent), Medicare (16.7 percent), direct-purchase (16.2 percent), and military health care (4.6 percent) (Table 1).

The percentage of people covered by any type of health insurance increased by 0.3 percentage points to 91.2 percent in 2016, up from 90.9 percent in 2015. Neither private coverage nor government coverage had a statistically significant increase during this period.

Medicare was the only subtype of health insurance that experienced a statistically significant change between 2015 and 2016. The rate of Medicare coverage increased by 0.4 percentage points, from 16.3 percent

---

Health Insurance Coverage and the Affordable Care Act

Since the passage of the Patient Protection and Affordable Care Act in 2010, several of its provisions have gone into effect at different times. For example, in 2010, the Young Adult Provision enabled adults under age 26 to remain as dependents on their parents' health insurance plans. Many more of the main provisions went into effect on January 1, 2014, including the expansion of Medicaid eligibility and the establishment of health insurance marketplaces (e.g., healthcare.gov).

In 2014, people under age 65, particularly adults aged 19 to 64, may have become eligible for coverage options under the Affordable Care Act. Based on family income, some people may have qualified for subsidies or tax credits to help pay for premiums associated with health insurance plans. In addition, the population with lower income may have become eligible for Medicaid coverage if they resided in one of the 30 states (or the District of Columbia) that expanded Medicaid eligibility on or before January 1, 2016. Twenty-four states and the District of Columbia expanded Medicaid eligibility by January 1, 2014. Between then and January 1, 2015, three additional states—Michigan, New Hampshire, and Pennsylvania—expanded Medicaid eligibility. By January 1, 2016, three more states—Alaska, Indiana, and Montana—expanded Medicaid eligibility.*

---

* For a list of the states and their Medicaid expansion status as of January 1, 2016, see Table 6: Percentage of People Without Health Insurance Coverage by State: 2013 to 2016.

Table 1.
Coverage Numbers and Rates by Type of Health Insurance: 2013 to 2016

(Numbers in thousands, margins of error in thousands or percentage points as appropriate. Population as of March of the following year. For information on confidentiality protection, sampling error, nonsampling error, and definitions, see www2.census.gov/programs-surveys/cps/techdocs/cpsmar17.pdf)

Coverage type	2013				2014				2015				2016				Change in number		Change in rate	
	Number	Margin of error[1] (±)	Rate	Margin of error[1] (±)	Number	Margin of error[1] (±)	Rate	Margin of error[1] (±)	Number	Margin of error[1] (±)	Rate	Margin of error[1] (±)	Number	Margin of error[1] (±)	Rate	Margin of error[1] (±)	2016 less 2015	2016 less 2013	2016 less 2015	2016 less 2013
Total................	313,401	109	X	X	316,168	92	X	X	318,868	95	X	X	320,372	96	X	X	X	X	X	X
Any health plan.........	271,606	636	86.7	0.2	283,200	568	89.6	0.2	289,903	650	90.9	0.2	292,320	541	91.2	0.2	*2,417	*20,714	*0.3	*4.6
Any private plan[2,3]......	201,038	1,140	64.1	0.4	208,600	1,221	66.0	0.4	214,238	1,118	67.2	0.4	216,203	1,145	67.5	0.4	*1,965	*15,165	0.3	*3.3
Employment-based[2]......	174,418	1,160	55.7	0.4	175,027	1,188	55.4	0.4	177,540	1,229	55.7	0.4	178,455	1,130	55.7	0.4	915	*4,037	Z	Z
Direct-purchase[2].......	35,755	615	11.4	0.2	46,165	798	14.6	0.3	52,057	916	16.3	0.3	51,961	874	16.2	0.3	-96	*16,206	-0.1	*4.8
Any government plan[2,4]...	108,287	1,115	34.6	0.4	115,470	1,035	36.5	0.3	118,395	1,067	37.1	0.3	119,361	1,018	37.3	0.3	966	*11,073	0.1	*2.7
Medicare[2]............	49,020	377	15.6	0.1	50,546	339	16.0	0.1	51,865	308	16.3	0.1	53,372	396	16.7	0.1	*1,507	*4,351	*0.4	*1.0
Medicaid[2]............	54,919	969	17.5	0.3	61,650	931	19.5	0.3	62,384	917	19.6	0.3	62,303	931	19.4	0.3	-81	*7,384	-0.1	*1.9
Military health care[2,5]...	14,016	595	4.5	0.2	14,143	568	4.5	0.2	14,849	626	4.7	0.2	14,638	575	4.6	0.2	-211	622	-0.1	0.1
Uninsured[6]............	41,795	614	13.3	0.2	32,968	561	10.4	0.2	28,966	634	9.1	0.2	28,052	519	8.8	0.2	*-914	*-13,743	*-0.3	*-4.6

* Changes between the estimates are statistically different from zero at the 90 percent confidence level.
X Not applicable.
Z Represents or rounds to zero.
[1] A margin of error is a measure of an estimate's variability. The larger the margin of error in relation to the size of the estimate, the less reliable the estimate. This number, when added to and subtracted from the estimate, forms the 90 percent confidence interval. Margins of error shown in this table are based on standard errors calculated using replicate weights. For more information, see "Standard Errors and Their Use" at <www2.census.gov/library/publications/2017/demo/p60-260sa.pdf>.
[2] The estimates by type of coverage are not mutually exclusive; people can be covered by more than one type of health insurance during the year.
[3] Private health insurance includes coverage provided through an employer or union, coverage purchased directly by an individual from an insurance company, or coverage through someone outside the household.
[4] Government health insurance coverage includes Medicaid, Medicare, TRICARE, CHAMPVA (Civilian Health and Medical Program of the Department of Veterans Affairs), and care provided by the Department of Veterans Affairs and the military.
[5] Military health care includes TRICARE and CHAMPVA, as well as care provided by the Department of Veterans Affairs and the military.
[6] Individuals are considered to be uninsured if they do not have health insurance coverage for the entire calendar year.
Source: U.S. Census Bureau, Current Population Survey, 2014 to 2017 Annual Social and Economic Supplements.

Two Measures of Health Insurance Coverage

This report includes two types of health insurance coverage measures: health insurance coverage during the entire calendar year and health insurance coverage at the time of the interview.

The first measure, health insurance coverage at any time during the calendar year, is collected with the Current Population Survey Annual Social and Economic Supplement (CPS ASEC). The CPS is the longest-running survey conducted by the U.S. Census Bureau. The key purpose of the CPS ASEC is to provide timely and detailed estimates of economic well-being, of which health insurance coverage is an important part. The Census Bureau conducts the CPS ASEC annually between February and April, and the resulting measure of health insurance coverage reflects an individual's coverage status during the entire previous calendar year.

The second measure, health insurance coverage at the time of the interview, is collected with the American Community Survey (ACS). The ACS is an ongoing survey that collects comprehensive information on social, economic, and housing topics. Due to its large sample size, the ACS provides estimates at many levels of geography and for smaller population groups. The Census Bureau conducts the ACS throughout the year, and the resulting measure of health coverage reflects an annual average of current health insurance coverage status.

As a result of the difference in the collection of health insurance coverage status, the resulting

uninsured rates measure different concepts. The CPS ASEC uninsured rate represents the percentage of people who had no health insurance coverage at any time during the previous calendar year. The ACS uninsured rate is a measure of the percentage of people who were uninsured at the time of the interview.

The two measures of health insurance coverage both point to a decrease in uninsured rates between 2015 and 2016 (Figure 2). For 2016, the uninsured rate was 8.8 percent as measured by the

CPS and 8.6 percent as measured by the ACS.

Over a longer period, as measured by the ACS, uninsured rates remained relatively stable between 2008 and 2013, but decreased sharply by 2.8 percentage points between 2013 and 2014. Uninsured rates then decreased by 2.3 percentage points between 2014 and 2015 and by 0.8 percentage points between 2015 and 2016. Overall, the uninsured rate decreased by 5.9 percentage points between 2013 and 2016.

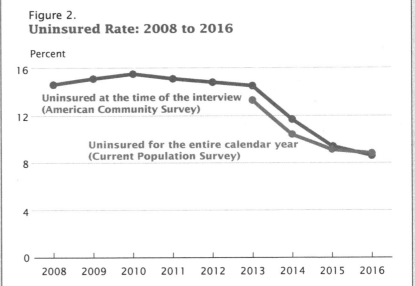

Figure 2.
Uninsured Rate: 2008 to 2016

Percent

Uninsured at the time of the interview
(American Community Survey)

Uninsured for the entire calendar year
(Current Population Survey)

Note: Estimates are for the civilian noninstitutionalized population. For the Current Population Survey, estimates reflect the population as of March of the following year. For information on confidentiality protection, sampling error, nonsampling error, and definitions in the Current Population Survey, see <www2.census.gov/programs-surveys/cps/techdocs/cpsmar17.pdf>. For the American Community Survey, estimates reflect the population as of July of the calendar year. For information on confidentiality protection, sampling error, nonsampling error, and definitions in the American Community Survey, see <www2.census.gov/programs-surveys/acs/tech_docs/accuracy/ACS_Accuracy_of_Data_2016.pdf>.

Source: U.S. Census Bureau, Current Population Survey, 2014 to 2017 Annual Social and Economic Supplements and 2008 to 2016 1-Year American Community Surveys.

in 2015 to 16.7 percent in 2016. This increase was likely due to growth in the number of people aged 65 and over and not to changes in Medicare coverage rates within any particular age group.

Multiple Coverage Types

While most people have a single type of insurance, some people may have more than one type of coverage during the calendar year. They may have multiple types of coverage at one time to supplement their primary insurance type, or they may switch coverage types over the course of the year. Of the population with health insurance coverage in 2016, 78.5 percent had one coverage type during the year and 21.5 percent had multiple coverage types over the course of the year (Figure 3).

Some types of health insurance were more likely to be held alone, while other types of health insurance

coverage were more likely to be held in combination with another type of insurance at some point during the year. Among people with employer-based health insurance coverage or Medicaid coverage, most had only one plan type during 2016 (78.5 percent and 66.4 percent, respectively).

People covered by direct-purchase insurance, Medicare, or military health care were more likely to have had more than one coverage type during the year. In 2016, 57.9 percent of people with direct-purchase health insurance, 60.7 percent of people with military health care, and 61.8 percent of people with Medicare had some other type of health insurance.[11]

---

[11] The percentage of people with Medicare coverage and another type of health insurance was not statistically different from the percentage of people with military health care and another type of health insurance.

Health Insurance Coverage by Selected Characteristics

Age

Age is strongly associated with the likelihood that a person has health insurance and the type of health insurance a person has. In 2016, adults aged 65 or over and children under 19 were more likely to have had health insurance coverage (98.8 percent and 94.6 percent, respectively) compared with working-age adults aged 19 to 64 (87.9 percent) (Table 2).

Adults aged 65 and over had the highest rate of health insurance coverage (98.8 percent) with 93.6 percent covered by a government plan (primarily Medicare) and 52.8 percent covered by a private plan, which may have supplemented their government coverage.

The rates of (overall) health insurance coverage, private coverage, and government coverage did not

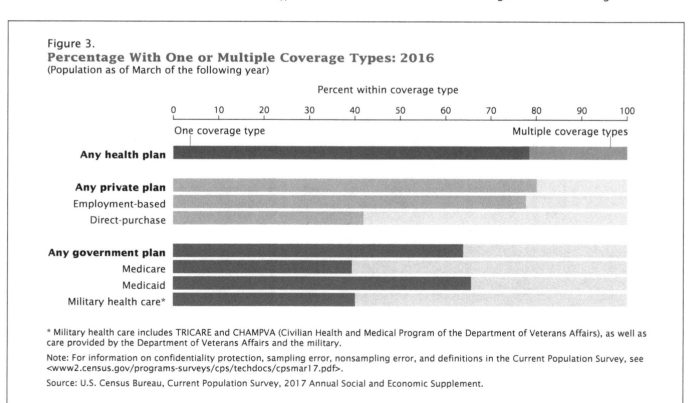

Figure 3.
Percentage With One or Multiple Coverage Types: 2016
(Population as of March of the following year)

* Military health care includes TRICARE and CHAMPVA (Civilian Health and Medical Program of the Department of Veterans Affairs), as well as care provided by the Department of Veterans Affairs and the military.

Note: For information on confidentiality protection, sampling error, nonsampling error, and definitions in the Current Population Survey, see <www2.census.gov/programs-surveys/cps/techdocs/cpsmar17.pdf>.

Source: U.S. Census Bureau, Current Population Survey, 2017 Annual Social and Economic Supplement.

Table 2.

Percentage of People by Type of Health Insurance Coverage by Age: 2015 and 2016

(Numbers in thousands, margins of error in percentage points. Population as of March of the following year. For information on confidentiality protection, sampling error, nonsampling error, and definitions, see www2.census.gov/programs-surveys/cps/techdocs/cpsmar17.pdf)

Characteristic	Number 2015	Number 2016	Any health insurance — Total 2015 Percent	Margin of error[2] (±)	2016 Percent	Margin of error[2] (±)	Change (2016 less 2015)[1,*]	Private health insurance[3] 2015 Percent	Margin of error[2] (±)	2016 Percent	Margin of error[2] (±)	Change (2016 less 2015)[1,*]	Government health insurance[4] 2015 Percent	Margin of error[2] (±)	2016 Percent	Margin of error[2] (±)	Change (2016 less 2015)[1,*]	Uninsured[5] 2015 Percent	Margin of error[2] (±)	2016 Percent	Margin of error[2] (±)	Change (2016 less 2015)[1,*]
Total	318,868	320,372	90.9	0.2	91.2	0.2	*0.3	67.2	0.4	67.5	0.4	0.3	37.1	0.3	37.3	0.3	0.1	9.1	0.2	8.8	0.2	*-0.3
Age																						
Under age 65...	271,322	271,098	89.5	0.2	89.9	0.2	*0.4	69.8	0.4	70.2	0.4	0.3	27.2	0.4	27.0	0.4	-0.2	10.5	0.2	10.1	0.2	*-0.4
Under age 18...	74,062	74,047	94.8	0.3	94.7	0.3	-0.1	62.3	0.6	62.7	0.6	0.4	43.0	0.7	41.9	0.6	*-1.1	5.2	0.3	5.3	0.3	0.1
Aged 18 to 64...	197,260	197,051	87.5	0.3	88.1	0.2	*0.5	72.7	0.4	73.0	0.4	0.3	21.3	0.3	21.4	0.3	0.2	12.5	0.3	11.9	0.2	*-0.5
Under age 19[6]...	78,182	78,150	94.7	0.3	94.6	0.3	-0.1	62.6	0.6	62.9	0.6	0.3	42.6	0.6	41.5	0.6	*-1.1	5.3	0.3	5.4	0.3	0.1
Aged 19 to 64...	193,140	192,948	87.4	0.3	87.9	0.2	*0.5	72.7	0.4	73.1	0.4	0.3	21.0	0.3	21.1	0.3	0.2	12.6	0.3	12.1	0.2	*-0.5
Aged 19 to 25[7]...	30,475	29,815	85.5	0.6	86.9	0.6	*1.4	69.9	0.9	71.3	0.8	*1.4	23.0	0.7	23.1	0.8	0.1	14.5	0.6	13.1	0.6	*-1.4
Aged 26 to 34...	38,960	39,736	83.7	0.6	84.3	0.6	0.6	69.6	0.7	69.7	0.7	0.1	20.1	0.7	20.4	0.6	0.3	16.3	0.6	15.7	0.6	-0.6
Aged 35 to 44...	40,005	40,046	86.3	0.5	86.9	0.5	0.6	72.7	0.6	73.3	0.7	0.6	19.3	0.6	19.3	0.6	Z	13.7	0.5	13.1	0.5	-0.6
Aged 45 to 64...	83,701	83,351	90.4	0.3	90.6	0.3	0.2	75.3	0.4	75.2	0.5	-0.1	21.4	0.5	21.7	0.5	0.3	9.6	0.3	9.4	0.3	-0.2
Aged 65 and older...	47,547	49,274	98.9	0.1	98.8	0.1	-0.2	52.1	0.8	52.8	0.8	0.7	93.8	0.3	93.6	0.3	-0.2	1.1	0.1	1.2	0.1	0.2

* Changes between the estimates are statistically different from zero at the 90 percent confidence level.

Z Represents or rounds to zero.

[1] Details may not sum to totals because of rounding.

[2] A margin of error is a measure of an estimate's variability. The larger the margin of error in relation to the size of the estimate, the less reliable the estimate. The margin of error shown in this table, when added to and subtracted from the estimate, forms the 90 percent confidence interval. Margins of error shown in this table are based on standard errors calculated using replicate weights. For more information, see "Standard Errors and Their Use" at <www2.census.gov/library/publications/2017/demo/p60-260sa.pdf>.

[3] Private health insurance includes coverage provided through an employer or union, coverage purchased directly by an individual from an insurance company, or coverage through someone outside the household.

[4] Government health insurance coverage includes Medicaid, Medicare, TRICARE, CHAMPVA (Civilian Health and Medical Program of the Department of Veterans Affairs), and care provided by the Department of Veterans Affairs and the military.

[5] Individuals are considered to be uninsured if they do not have health insurance coverage for the entire calendar year.

[6] Children under the age of 19 are eligible for Medicaid/CHIP.

[7] This age group is of special interest because of the Affordable Care Act's dependent coverage provision. Individuals aged 19 to 25 may be eligible to be a dependent on a parent's health insurance plan.

Note: The estimates by type of coverage are not mutually exclusive; people can be covered by more than one type of health insurance during the year.

Source: U.S. Census Bureau, Current Population Survey, 2016 and 2017 Annual Social and Economic Supplements.

demonstrate statistically significant change between 2015 and 2016 for adults aged 65 or over.

Children under age 19 were covered by health insurance at a higher rate than working-age adults in 2016. One reason for this difference could be that children from lower income families may be eligible for programs such as Medicaid or the Children's Health Insurance Program (CHIP).[12] In 2016, 62.9 percent of children under age 19 had private health insurance and 41.5 percent had government coverage. Some children were covered by both private and government coverage during the calendar year.

Between 2015 and 2016, neither the overall rate of health insurance coverage, nor the rate of private coverage, exhibited statistically significant change for children under 19. Children's rate of government coverage decreased by 1.1 percentage points to 41.5 percent in 2016, down from 42.6 percent in 2015.

Working-age adults (people aged 19 to 64) had a lower rate of health insurance coverage in 2016 (87.9 percent) than both children and older adults. Among working-age adults, the population aged 26 to 34 was the least likely to be insured, with a coverage rate of 84.3 percent. For adults aged 19 to 25, the health insurance coverage rate of 86.9 percent was higher than that for adults aged 26 to 34. For age groups between 26 and 64, the rate of health insurance coverage increased as age increased.

Working-age adults were more likely than other age groups to be covered by private health insurance, which provided coverage to 73.1 percent of the population aged 19 to 64 in 2016. They also had the lowest rate

of coverage through the government, at 21.1 percent.[13]

Between 2015 and 2016, the percentage of adults aged 19 to 64 with health insurance rose by 0.5 percentage points, driven by an increase in coverage for people aged 19 to 25. For this group of young adults, both the overall rate of health insurance coverage and the rate of private coverage increased by 1.4 percentage points in 2016, to 86.9 percent and 71.3 percent, respectively.[14, 15]

Between 2015 and 2016, the percentage of people without health insurance coverage dropped for most ages under 65, with generally larger decreases for working-age adults (aged 19 to 64) (Figure 4).[16, 17] Younger adults tended to experience a larger decline than older adults. For example, the uninsured rate decreased by 2.0 percentage points for 26-year-olds and 0.6 percentage points for 64-year-olds. These declines in the uninsured rate followed 2 years of decreases for all ages under 65.

The uneven downward shift in uninsured rates reduced some of the age-specific rate disparities. However, three notable sharp differences remained between single-year ages, specifically between

18- and 19-year-olds, between 25- and 26-year-olds, and between 64- and 65-year-olds. In 2016, the uninsured rate was about one-and-a-half times greater for 19-year-olds compared with 18-year-olds, almost one-and-a-quarter times greater for 26-year-olds compared with 25-year-olds, and the uninsured rate for 65-year-olds was about one-quarter of the rate of 64-year-olds.[18] Adults aged 26 continued to have the highest uninsured rate in 2016 (at 17.5 percent) (Figure 4).

Even within the broad age groups of children and working-age adults, uninsured rates for single years of age differed. In 2016, for children under age 19, uninsured rates generally increased with age, with rates of 3.2 percent for children under 1 year of age and 8.2 percent for 18-year-olds. Among young adults between the ages of 19 and 25, the uninsured rate was 12.5 percent for 19-year-olds and 14.7 percent for 25-year-olds. For adults between the ages 26 and 64, the uninsured rate declined generally across all ages from 17.5 percent for 26-year-olds to 6.3 percent for 64-year-olds. Among adults 65 years and over, the uninsured rate varied little by age.

Between 2013 and 2016, uninsured rates fell for all single-year ages under age 65, with the largest declines of about 11.5 or more percentage points for each age between 21 and 28.

Marital Status

Many adults obtain health insurance coverage through their spouse. In 2016, married adults aged 19 to 64 had the highest coverage rate, at 91.2 percent (Table 3).[19] The coverage rate

---

[12] The Children's Health Insurance Program is a government program that provides health insurance to children in families with income too high to qualify for Medicaid but who are unable to afford private health insurance.

[13] In 2016, the health insurance coverage rate for people aged 19 to 25 was not statistically different from the coverage rate for people aged 35 to 44.

[14] The percentage-point difference in the overall health insurance coverage rate between 2015 and 2016 for people aged 19 to 25 was not statistically different from the percentage-point difference in the private coverage rate for this age group.

[15] Between 2015 and 2016, there was no statistical difference in the government coverage rate for people aged 19 to 25.

[16] These estimates and estimates in the remainder of this section come from the 2013 through 2016 1-Year American Community Surveys (ACS). In the ACS, health insurance coverage status corresponds to coverage at the time of the interview (see the text box "Two Measures of Health Insurance Coverage").

[17] The change in the uninsured rate between 2015 and 2016 was not statistically significant for infants and for people aged 1, 3, 4, 6, 9, 37, 56, 57, 60, 61, and 63.

[18] In 2016, the uninsured rate was 1.53 times greater for 19-year-olds compared with 18-year-olds and 1.19 times greater for 26-year-olds compared with 25-year-olds. The uninsured rate for 65-year-olds was 0.25 times the rate of 64-year-olds.

[19] These estimates and estimates in the remainder of this section are for the population aged 19 to 64.

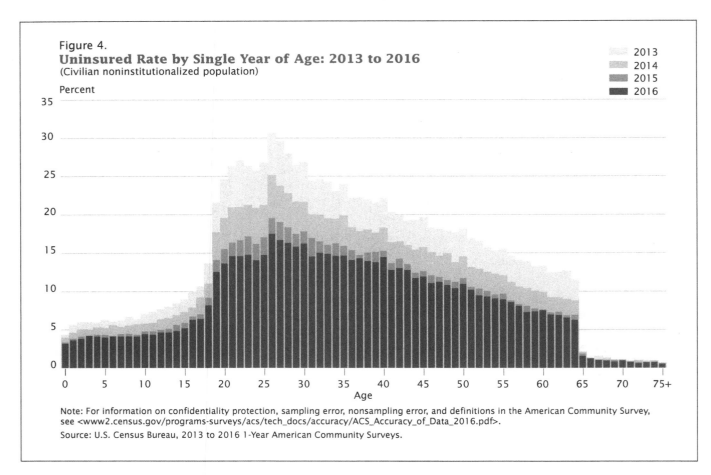

Figure 4.
Uninsured Rate by Single Year of Age: 2013 to 2016
(Civilian noninstitutionalized population)

Note: For information on confidentiality protection, sampling error, nonsampling error, and definitions in the American Community Survey, see <www2.census.gov/programs-surveys/acs/tech_docs/accuracy/ACS_Accuracy_of_Data_2016.pdf>.
Source: U.S. Census Bureau, 2013 to 2016 1-Year American Community Surveys.

was lowest for people who were separated (80.8 percent). Among people who were never married, 84.0 percent were covered by health insurance. The coverage rates for people who were widowed or divorced were both 86.1 percent.[20]

Between 2015 and 2016, the coverage rate for the divorced population increased by 1.0 percentage point, and the rate for people who were never married rose 0.8 percentage points.[21] People who were married, separated, or widowed did not have a statistically significant change in their coverage rates.

Disability Status

Adults aged 19 to 64 with a disability had a higher rate of health insurance coverage (91.2 percent) compared with adults with no disability (87.6 percent) in 2016 (Table 3).[22]

Adults with a disability were less likely to have private health insurance coverage and more likely to have government coverage compared with adults with no disability. In 2016, 43.5 percent of adults with a disability had private coverage compared with 75.9 percent of adults with no disability, a 32.4 percentage-point difference. At the same time, 58.6 percent of adults with a disability and 17.5 percent with no disability had government coverage, a 41.1 percentage-point difference.

Between 2015 and 2016, both the population with a disability and the population with no disability had statistically significant increases in their coverage rates. Coverage rates increased by 1.1 percentage points to 91.2 percent in 2016 for adults with a disability and by 0.5 percentage points to 87.6 percent in 2016 for adults with no disability.[23]

Work Experience

For many adults, health insurance coverage and type of coverage is related to work status, such as working full-time, year-round; working less than

[20] In 2016, the coverage rate of people who were widowed was not statistically different from the coverage rate of people who were divorced.

[21] The percentage-point change in the health insurance coverage rate between 2015 and 2016 for people who were divorced was not statistically different from the change for people who were never married.

[22] These estimates and estimates in the remainder of this section are for the population aged 19 to 64.

[23] The percentage-point change in the health insurance coverage rate between 2015 and 2016 for individuals with a disability was not statistically different from the change for people without a disability.

Table 3.

Percentage of People by Type of Health Insurance Coverage for Working-Age Adults Aged 19 to 64: 2015 and 2016

(Numbers in thousands, margins of error in percentage points. Population as of March of the following year. For information on confidentiality protection, sampling error, nonsampling error, and definitions, see www2.census.gov/programs-surveys/cps/techdocs/cpsmar17.pdf)

Characteristic	Number 2015	Number 2016	Any health insurance 2015 Per-cent	MOE (±)	2016 Per-cent	MOE (±)	Change (2016 less 2015)[1]*	Private health insurance[3] 2015 Per-cent	MOE (±)	2016 Per-cent	MOE (±)	Change (2016 less 2015)[1]*	Government health insurance[4] 2015 Per-cent	MOE (±)	2016 Per-cent	MOE (±)	Change (2016 less 2015)[1]*	Uninsured[5] 2015 Per-cent	MOE (±)	2016 Per-cent	MOE (±)	Change (2016 less 2015)[1]*
Total	318,868	320,372	90.9	0.2	91.2	0.2	*0.3	67.2	0.4	67.5	0.4	0.3	37.1	0.3	37.3	0.3	0.1	9.1	0.2	8.8	0.2	*–0.3
Total, 19 to 64 years old	193,140	192,948	87.4	0.3	87.9	0.2	*0.5	72.7	0.4	73.1	0.4	0.3	21.0	0.3	21.1	0.3	0.2	12.6	0.3	12.1	0.2	*–0.5
Marital Status																						
Married[6]	101,277	101,822	91.0	0.3	91.2	0.3	0.2	80.0	0.5	80.1	0.5	0.1	18.0	0.4	17.9	0.4	–0.1	9.0	0.3	8.8	0.3	–0.2
Widowed	3,451	3,633	85.8	1.6	86.1	1.6	0.2	59.1	2.2	58.7	2.0	–0.5	33.6	2.1	33.5	2.2	–0.1	14.2	1.6	13.9	1.6	–0.2
Divorced	19,817	19,460	85.1	0.7	86.1	0.6	*1.0	63.9	0.9	64.3	1.0	0.4	26.0	0.9	26.8	0.9	0.9	14.9	0.7	13.9	0.6	*–1.0
Separated	4,698	4,495	79.4	1.6	80.8	1.5	1.4	54.4	1.9	55.9	1.9	1.4	29.4	1.9	31.0	1.8	1.6	20.6	1.6	19.2	1.5	–1.4
Never married	63,896	63,537	83.2	0.5	84.0	0.5	*0.8	66.0	0.6	66.5	0.7	0.5	22.8	0.5	23.2	0.6	0.4	16.8	0.5	16.0	0.5	*–0.8
Disability Status[7]																						
With a disability	15,128	15,248	90.1	0.7	91.2	0.7	*1.1	43.4	1.2	43.5	1.2	0.1	58.3	1.2	58.6	1.1	0.3	9.9	0.7	8.8	0.7	*–1.1
With no disability	177,102	176,842	87.1	0.3	87.6	0.2	*0.5	75.5	0.4	75.9	0.4	0.4	17.4	0.3	17.5	0.3	0.2	12.9	0.3	12.4	0.2	*–0.5
Work Experience																						
All workers	148,503	149,105	88.4	0.3	88.8	0.3	*0.4	80.0	0.3	80.1	0.3	0.1	13.8	0.3	13.9	0.3	0.2	11.6	0.3	11.2	0.3	*–0.4
Worked full-time, year-round	105,533	107,577	90.1	0.3	90.2	0.3	0.1	84.5	0.4	84.5	0.3	Z	10.5	0.3	10.4	0.3	–0.1	9.9	0.3	9.8	0.3	–0.1
Less than full-time, year-round	42,970	41,528	84.2	0.5	85.2	0.5	*1.0	69.0	0.7	69.0	0.6	Z	21.7	0.6	23.1	0.6	*1.3	15.8	0.5	14.8	0.5	*–1.0
Did not work at least one week	44,637	43,843	84.2	0.5	85.0	0.5	*0.8	48.6	0.8	49.1	0.8	0.5	44.9	0.8	45.6	0.7	0.7	15.8	0.5	15.0	0.5	*–0.8
Educational Attainment																						
Total, 26 to 64 years old	162,665	163,133	87.8	0.3	88.1	0.2	0.4	73.3	0.4	73.4	0.4	0.1	20.6	0.4	20.8	0.3	0.2	12.2	0.3	11.9	0.2	–0.4
No high school diploma	16,079	15,389	72.4	1.1	72.7	1.1	0.3	43.1	1.2	40.9	1.1	*–2.2	35.4	1.1	37.7	1.1	*2.3	27.6	1.1	27.3	1.1	–0.3
High school graduate (includes equivalency)	44,925	45,401	84.4	0.5	84.8	0.5	0.5	65.2	0.7	65.0	0.7	–0.2	26.0	0.7	26.3	0.6	0.4	15.6	0.5	15.2	0.5	–0.5
Some college, no degree	27,246	26,594	88.1	0.6	88.4	0.5	0.3	71.7	0.8	71.8	0.8	0.1	23.7	0.7	23.8	0.7	0.1	11.9	0.6	11.6	0.5	–0.3
Associate degree	17,471	17,739	90.5	0.6	90.7	0.6	0.2	77.6	0.8	77.9	0.9	0.3	20.3	0.7	19.5	0.8	–0.9	9.5	0.6	9.3	0.6	–0.2
Bachelor's degree	35,870	36,528	93.0	0.4	93.2	0.4	0.2	86.2	0.5	86.8	0.5	0.6	11.6	0.5	11.6	0.4	Z	7.0	0.4	6.8	0.4	–0.2
Graduate or professional degree	21,075	21,482	95.2	0.5	95.2	0.4	Z	90.2	0.6	90.0	0.6	–0.2	9.1	0.6	9.8	0.6	0.7	4.8	0.5	4.8	0.4	Z

* Changes between the estimates are statistically different from zero at the 90 percent confidence level.
Z Represents or rounds to zero.
[1] Details may not sum to totals because of rounding.
[2] A margin of error is a measure of an estimate's variability. The larger the margin of error in relation to the size of the estimate, the less reliable the estimate. This number, when added to and subtracted from the estimate, forms the 90 percent confidence interval. Margins of error shown in this table are based on standard errors calculated using replicate weights. For more information, see "Standard Errors and Their Use" at <www2.census.gov/library/publications/2017/demo/p60-260sa.pdf>.
[3] Private health insurance includes coverage provided through an employer or union, coverage purchased directly by an individual from an insurance company, or coverage through someone outside the household.
[4] Government health insurance coverage includes Medicaid, Medicare, TRICARE, CHAMPVA (Civilian Health and Medical Program of the Department of Veterans Affairs), and care provided by the Department of Veterans Affairs and the military.
[5] Individuals are considered to be uninsured if they do not have health insurance coverage for the entire calendar year.
[6] The combined category "married" includes three individual categories: "married, civilian spouse present," "married, armed forces spouse present," and "married, spouse absent."
[7] The sum of those with and without a disability does not equal the total because disability status is not defined for individuals in the armed forces.
Note: The estimates by type of coverage are not mutually exclusive; people can be covered by more than one type of health insurance during the year.

full-time, year-round; or not working at all during the calendar year.[24, 25]

Among all workers, 88.8 percent had health insurance coverage in 2016. Full-time, year-round workers were more likely to be covered by health insurance (90.2 percent) than the population who worked less than full-time, year-round (85.2 percent) or nonworkers (85.0 percent) (Table 3).[26]

Workers were more likely to be covered by private health insurance coverage, compared with nonworkers. In 2016, 84.5 percent of full-time, year-round workers had private insurance coverage, compared with 69.0 percent of people who worked less than full-time, year-round and 49.1 percent of nonworkers.

In 2016, nonworkers were more than three times as likely to have government coverage (45.6 percent) than workers (13.9 percent). Among workers, 10.4 percent of people who worked full-time, year-round and 23.1 percent of people who worked less than full-time, year-round had government coverage in 2016.

Between 2015 and 2016, the health insurance coverage rate increased by 0.4 percentage points for people who worked at some point during the year. The coverage rate increased 1.0 percentage point for the population who worked less than full-time, year-round and 0.8 percentage points for the

population who did not work.[27] The health insurance coverage rate in 2016 was not statistically different from the rate in 2015 for the population who worked full-time, year-round.

Educational Attainment

People with higher levels of educational attainment were more likely to have health insurance coverage than people with lower levels of education. In 2016, 95.2 percent of the population aged 26 to 64 with a graduate or professional degree had health insurance coverage, compared with 93.2 percent of the population with a bachelor's degree, 84.8 percent of high school graduates, and 72.7 percent of the population with no high school diploma (Table 3).[28]

Between 2015 and 2016, no educational attainment group saw a statistically significant change in its overall rate of coverage.

People with no high school diploma were the only educational attainment group to have a statistically significant change for private coverage and government coverage. Their private coverage rate decreased by 2.2 percentage points to 40.9 percent in 2016, while their government coverage rate increased by 2.3 percentage points to 37.7 percent in 2016.

Household Income

In 2016, people with lower household income had lower overall health insurance coverage rates than people with higher income. During this time, 86.3 percent of people with an annual household income of less than

$25,000 had health insurance coverage, compared with 92.4 percent of people with household income of $75,000 to $99,999 and 95.8 percent of people with household income of $125,000 or more (Table 4).[29]

People with lower household income also had lower rates of private coverage than people with higher income. These differences varied more for lower income groups than for higher income groups. In 2016, the private health insurance coverage rate for people with household income between $25,000 and $49,999 (52.7 percent) was 22.3 percentage points higher than the rate for people with household income below $25,000 (30.4 percent). At the same time, the private health insurance coverage rate for people with household income at or above $125,000 (88.5 percent) was 4.8 percentage points higher than the rate for people with household income between $100,000 and $124,999 (83.8 percent).

Conversely, government coverage rates decreased as income increased, but as with private coverage, rates varied more at lower incomes than at higher incomes. In 2016, the government coverage rate for people with household income of less than $25,000 (68.0 percent) was 16.0 percentage points higher than the rate for people with household income between $25,000 and $49,999 (52.0 percent). For the two highest income groups, the difference was smaller. The government coverage rate for people with household income between $100,000 and $124,999 (21.8 percent) was 3.0 percentage points higher than the rate for people with household income at or above $125,000 (18.8 percent).

Only one income group saw a statistically significant change in its health insurance coverage rate between

---

[24] For this report, a full-time, year-round worker is a person who worked 35 or more hours per week (full-time) and 50 or more weeks during the previous calendar year (year-round). For school personnel, summer vacation is counted as weeks worked if they are scheduled to return to their job in the fall.

[25] These estimates and estimates in the remainder of this section are for the population aged 19 to 64.

[26] In 2016, the health insurance coverage rate for people who worked less than full-time, year-round was not statistically different from the coverage rate for nonworkers.

[27] The change between 2015 and 2016 in the health insurance coverage rate for people who worked at some point during the year was not statistically different from the change in the coverage rate for nonworkers.
The change between 2015 and 2016 in the health insurance coverage rate for people who worked less than full-time, year-round was not statistically different from the change in the coverage rate for nonworkers.

[28] These estimates and estimates in the remainder of this section are for the population aged 26 to 64.

[29] The 2015 income estimates are inflation-adjusted and presented in 2016 dollars.

2015 and 2016. The coverage rate increased by 1.1 percentage points to 86.3 percent for people with household income of less than $25,000.

Between 2015 and 2016, people with household income between $50,000 and $74,999 were the only income group to have a statistically significant change in the rate of private coverage. Their rate of private coverage decreased by 1.7 percentage points to 68.6 percent in 2016.

Most of the income groups showed a statistically significant change in their government coverage rates between 2015 and 2016. The rate of government coverage increased for three income groups: people with household income less than $25,000 (1.4 percentage-point increase), people with household income between $50,000 and $74,999 (2.2 percentage-point increase), and people with household income at or above $125,000 (0.8 percentage-point increase).[30] The government coverage rate decreased by 1.4 percentage points for people with household income between $75,000 and $99,999, down to 26.2 percent in 2016.

Income-to-Poverty Ratio

People and families are classified as being in poverty if their income is less than their poverty threshold.[31]

In 2016, the population living below 100 percent of poverty had the lowest health insurance coverage rate, at 83.7 percent, while people living at or above 400 percent of poverty had the highest coverage rate, at 95.6 percent (Table 4). The population with income between 100 percent and 399 percent of the poverty ratio had coverage rates that ranged from 87.4 percent for people with income between 100 and 199 percent of poverty to 92.5 percent for the population with income between 300 and 399 percent of poverty.

Government coverage continued to be most prevalent for the population in poverty (63.6 percent) and least prevalent for the population with income-to-poverty ratios at or above 400 percent of poverty (22.8 percent) in 2016.

Between 2015 and 2016, the health insurance coverage rate increased 1.1 percentage points for people with income below 100 percent of poverty (to 83.7 percent) and 0.9 percentage points for people with income between 100 and 199 percent of poverty (to 87.4 percent).[32] The coverage rate decreased 1.0 percentage point for people with income between 200 and 299 percent of poverty (89.2 percent).

In 2014, policy changes associated with the Affordable Care Act provided the option for states to expand Medicaid eligibility to people whose income-to-poverty ratio fell under a particular threshold (for more information, see the text box "Health Insurance and the Affordable Care

Act"). For adults aged 19 to 64, the relationship between poverty status and change in the uninsured rate between 2015 and 2016 may be related to the state of residence and whether or not that state expanded Medicaid eligibility (Figure 5).[33, 34] In states that expanded Medicaid eligibility on or before January 1, 2016, ("expansion states") and states that did not expand Medicaid eligibility ("non-expansion states"), the uninsured rate decreased as the income-to-poverty ratio increased for adults aged 19 to 64. However, in 2014, 2015, and 2016, the uninsured rate was higher in non-expansion states than in expansion states regardless of individuals' poverty status group. While the uninsured rate decreased for each income-to-poverty group between 2015 and 2016 (except for people living at or above 400 percent of poverty in non-expansion states), the overall decrease in the uninsured rate was greater in expansion states than in non-expansion states for all poverty status groups.

Family Status

Many people obtain health insurance coverage through a family member's plan. The Census Bureau classifies living arrangements into three types: families, unrelated subfamilies, and

---

[30] The percentage-point difference in the government coverage rate between 2015 and 2016 for people with household income below $25,000 was not statistically different from the percentage-point differences for people with household income between $50,000 and $74,999 and household income at or above $125,000.

[31] The Office of Management and Budget determined the official definition of poverty in Statistical Policy Directive 14. Appendix B of the report *Income and Poverty in the United States: 2016* provides a more detailed description of how the Census Bureau calculates poverty; see <www.census.gov/content/dam/Census/library/publications/2017/demo/p60-259.pdf>.

---

[32] The percentage-point difference in the health insurance coverage rate between 2015 and 2016 for people below 100 percent of poverty was not statistically different from the percentage-point difference for people between 100 and 199 percent of poverty.

---

[33] Estimates from Figure 5 are from the 2013 to 2016 1-Year American Community Surveys.

[34] Thirty states and the District of Columbia expanded Medicaid eligibility on or before January 1, 2016. For a list of the states and their Medicaid expansion status as of January 1, 2016, see Table 6: Percentage of People Without Health Insurance Coverage by State: 2013 to 2016.

Table 4.

Percentage of People by Type of Health Insurance Coverage by Household Income and Income-to-Poverty Ratio: 2015 and 2016

(Numbers in thousands, margins of error in percentage points. Population as of March of the following year. For information on confidentiality protection, sampling error, nonsampling error, and definitions, see www2.census.gov/programs-surveys/cps/techdocs/cpsmar17.pdf)

Characteristic	2015 Number	2016 Number	Any health insurance — Total 2015 Percent	MoE (±)	2016 Percent	MoE (±)	Change (2016 less 2015)[1],*	Private health insurance[3] 2015 Percent	MoE (±)	2016 Percent	MoE (±)	Change (2016 less 2015)[1],*	Government health insurance[4] 2015 Percent	MoE (±)	2016 Percent	MoE (±)	Change (2016 less 2015)[1],*	Uninsured[5] 2015 Percent	MoE (±)	2016 Percent	MoE (±)	Change (2016 less 2015)[1],*
Total	318,868	320,372	90.9	0.2	91.2	0.2	*-0.3	67.2	0.4	67.5	0.4	0.3	37.1	0.3	37.3	0.3	0.1	9.1	0.2	8.8	0.2	*-0.3
Household Income																						
Less than $25,000	51,526	48,346	85.2	0.5	86.3	0.6	*1.1	30.7	0.8	30.4	0.8	-0.3	66.6	0.8	68.0	0.8	*1.4	14.8	0.5	13.7	0.6	*-1.1
$25,000 to $49,999	64,874	63,644	87.5	0.5	88.1	0.4	0.6	52.9	0.8	52.7	0.8	-0.1	51.0	0.7	52.0	0.7	1.0	12.5	0.5	11.9	0.4	-0.6
$50,000 to $74,999	54,791	54,829	90.3	0.4	90.2	0.5	-0.1	70.3	0.8	68.6	0.8	*-1.7	34.7	0.8	36.9	0.7	*2.2	9.7	0.4	9.8	0.5	0.1
$75,000 to $99,999	42,794	44,225	92.6	0.4	92.4	0.4	-0.2	79.2	0.7	79.4	0.7	0.2	27.7	0.8	26.2	0.8	-1.4	7.4	0.4	7.6	0.4	0.2
$100,000 to $124,999	32,654	32,954	94.7	0.5	94.2	0.5	-0.5	84.7	0.8	83.8	0.8	-0.9	21.7	0.8	21.8	0.8	0.1	5.3	0.5	5.8	0.5	0.5
$125,000 or more	72,229	76,374	95.9	0.3	95.8	0.3	Z	88.6	0.5	88.5	0.5	-0.1	18.0	0.6	18.8	0.6	*0.8	4.1	0.3	4.2	0.3	Z
Income-to-Poverty Ratio																						
Below 100 percent of poverty	43,123	40,616	82.6	0.7	83.7	0.6	*1.1	28.6	0.9	28.6	0.9	Z	62.1	0.9	63.6	0.8	*1.5	17.4	0.7	16.3	0.6	*-1.1
Below 138 percent of poverty	64,711	61,039	83.6	0.5	84.7	0.5	*1.0	32.1	0.7	31.1	0.7	-0.9	61.4	0.7	63.1	0.6	*1.7	16.4	0.5	15.3	0.5	*-1.0
Between 100 and 199 percent of poverty	57,770	54,629	86.4	0.6	87.4	0.5	*0.9	46.5	0.9	45.4	0.9	-1.1	53.8	0.8	55.9	0.8	*2.0	13.6	0.6	12.6	0.5	*-0.9
Between 200 and 299 percent of poverty	49,668	51,705	90.2	0.4	89.2	0.5	*-1.0	66.9	0.8	66.2	0.8	-0.8	38.8	0.8	38.0	0.8	-0.8	9.8	0.4	10.8	0.5	*1.0
Between 300 and 399 percent of poverty	41,691	42,562	92.7	0.5	92.5	0.4	-0.2	78.3	0.7	76.4	0.7	*-1.9	29.8	0.7	31.1	0.7	*1.4	7.3	0.5	7.5	0.4	0.2
At or above 400 percent of poverty	126,202	130,398	95.5	0.2	95.6	0.2	0.1	86.4	0.4	86.6	0.4	0.2	22.6	0.4	22.8	0.4	0.2	4.5	0.2	4.4	0.2	-0.1

* Changes between the estimates are statistically different from zero at the 90 percent confidence level.

Z Represents or rounds to zero.

[1] Details may not sum to totals because of rounding.

[2] A margin of error is a measure of an estimate's variability. The larger the margin of error in relation to the size of the estimate, the less reliable the estimate. This number, when added to and subtracted from the estimate, forms the 90 percent confidence interval. Margins of error shown in this table are based on standard errors calculated using replicate weights. For more information, see "Standard Errors and Their Use" at <www2.census.gov/library/publications/2017/demo/p60-260sa.pdf>.

[3] Private health insurance includes coverage provided through an employer or union, coverage purchased directly by an individual from an insurance company, or coverage through someone outside the household.

[4] Government health insurance coverage includes Medicaid, Medicare, TRICARE, CHAMPVA (Civilian Health and Medical Program of the Department of Veterans Affairs), and care provided by the Department of Veterans Affairs and the military.

[5] Individuals are considered to be uninsured if they do not have health insurance coverage for the entire calendar year.

Note: The estimates by type of coverage are not mutually exclusive; people can be covered by more than one type of health insurance during the year.

Source: U.S. Census Bureau, Current Population Survey, 2016 and 2017 Annual Social and Economic Supplements.

Figure 5.
Uninsured Rate by Poverty Status and Medicaid Expansion of State for Adults Aged 19 to 64: 2013 to 2016
(Civilian noninstitutionalized population)

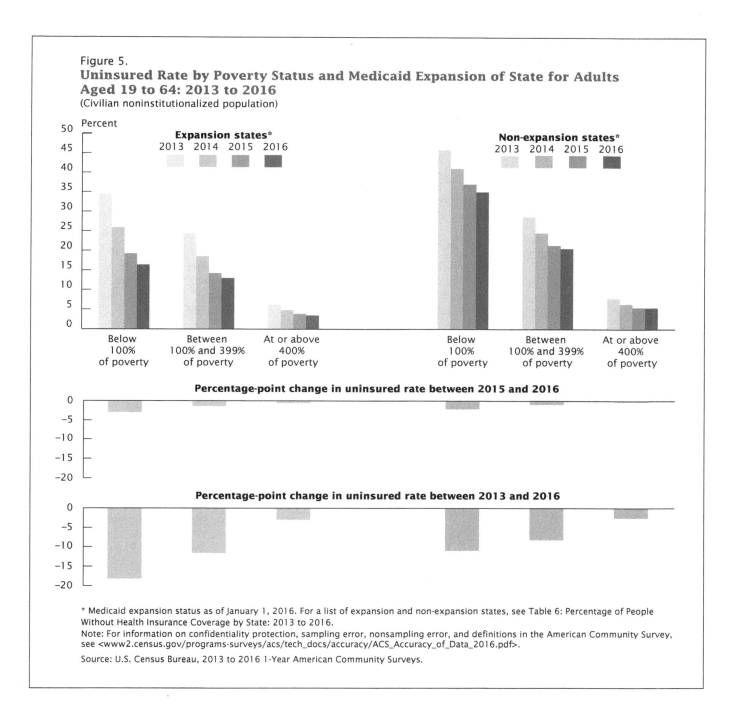

* Medicaid expansion status as of January 1, 2016. For a list of expansion and non-expansion states, see Table 6: Percentage of People Without Health Insurance Coverage by State: 2013 to 2016.

Note: For information on confidentiality protection, sampling error, nonsampling error, and definitions in the American Community Survey, see <www2.census.gov/programs-surveys/acs/tech_docs/accuracy/ACS_Accuracy_of_Data_2016.pdf>.

Source: U.S. Census Bureau, 2013 to 2016 1-Year American Community Surveys.

unrelated individuals.[35] Families are the largest of these categories (81.1 percent of the population in 2016), followed by unrelated individuals (18.5 percent), and unrelated subfamilies (0.4 percent).

In 2016, people living in families had a higher health insurance coverage rate (91.8 percent) than unrelated individuals (88.7 percent) and people living in unrelated subfamilies (86.5 percent) (Table 5).[36]

Between 2015 and 2016, the coverage rate increased by 1.0 percentage point for unrelated individuals to 88.7 percent in 2016. There was no statistically significant change in coverage rates between 2015 and 2016 for people with other types of living arrangements.

Residence

In 2016, the health insurance coverage rate was the highest for people living outside principal cities within metropolitan statistical areas, at 92.0 percent, and lowest for people living inside principal cities, at 90.3 percent (Table 5).[37, 38]

Between 2015 and 2016, the health insurance coverage rate increased by 0.8 percentage points for people living inside principal cities. There were no statistically significant changes between 2015 and 2016 for people living outside principal cities within metropolitan statistical areas and people living outside metropolitan statistical areas.

Race and Hispanic Origin

In 2016, 93.7 percent of non-Hispanic Whites had health insurance coverage. This rate was higher than the coverage rate for Blacks (89.5 percent), Asians (92.4 percent), and Hispanics (84.0 percent) (Table 5).

Non-Hispanic Whites and Asians were among the most likely to have private health insurance in 2016, at 73.9 percent and 74.2 percent, respectively.[39] Hispanics, who had the lowest rate of any health insurance coverage, also had the lowest rate of private coverage, at 52.4 percent. In 2016, 56.5 percent of Blacks had private health insurance coverage.

Rates of government health coverage followed a different pattern than private health insurance coverage. In 2016, the government coverage rate was the highest for Blacks, at 43.7 percent, followed by Hispanics (40.1 percent) and non-Hispanic Whites (35.9 percent). Asians had the lowest rate of health insurance coverage

through the government, at 27.1 percent in 2016.

Between 2015 and 2016, health insurance coverage rates increased 0.4 percentage points for non-Hispanic Whites. There were no statistically significant changes in the health insurance coverage rates for Blacks, Asians, or Hispanics between 2015 and 2016.

Nativity

In 2016, the overall health insurance coverage rate for the native-born population (92.7 percent) was larger than that of naturalized citizens (91.5 percent) and noncitizens (73.8 percent) (Table 5).

Between 2015 and 2016, the health insurance coverage rate increased by 0.4 percentage points for the native-born population to 92.7 percent. The foreign-born population did not have a statistically significant change in their health insurance coverage rate during this period.

Children and Adults Without Health Insurance Coverage

In 2016, for all selected characteristics, the uninsured rate for adults (aged 19 to 64) was significantly larger than for children (under 19 years of age) (Figure 6). Additionally, differences in the uninsured rates between demographic and socioeconomic groups were generally larger among adults than among children.[40]

---

[35] Families are defined as a group of two or more related people where one of them is the householder. Family members must be related by birth, marriage, or adoption and reside together. Unrelated subfamilies are family units that reside with, but are not related to, the primary householder. For example, unrelated subfamilies could include a married couple with or without children, or a single parent with one or more never-married children under 18 years old living in a household. An unrelated subfamily may also include people such as partners, roommates, or resident employees and their spouses and/ or children. The number of unrelated subfamily members is included in the total number of household members, but is not included in the count of family members. The remainder of the population is classified as unrelated individuals.

[36] In 2016, the health insurance coverage rate of unrelated individuals was not statistically different from the coverage rate of people living in unrelated subfamilies.

[37] The Census Bureau categorizes residency into two broad groups; individuals can either live inside a metropolitan statistical area or outside of one. People living inside metropolitan statistical areas include individuals living both inside and outside principal cities.

[38] In 2016, the health insurance coverage rate for people living inside principal cities within metropolitan statistical areas was not statistically different from the coverage rate for people living outside metropolitan statistical areas.

[39] In 2016, the private coverage rate for non-Hispanic Whites was not statistically different from the private coverage rate for Asians.

[40] In 2016, the percentage-point difference in the uninsured rate between children with household income between $100,000 and $124,999 and children with household income at or above $125,000 was not statistically different from the difference between adults with household income between $100,000 and $124,999 and adults with household income at or above $125,000. In 2016, the percentage-point difference in the uninsured rate between native-born children and naturalized children was not statistically different from the difference between native-born adults and naturalized adults.

Table 5.
Percentage of People by Type of Health Insurance Coverage by Selected Demographic Characteristics: 2015 and 2016

(Numbers in thousands, margins of errors in percentage points. Population as of March of the following year. For information on confidentiality protection, sampling error, nonsampling error, and definitions, see www2.census.gov/programs-surveys/cps/techdocs/cpsmar17.pdf)

Characteristic	Number 2015	Number 2016	Any health insurance — Percent 2015	MOE[2] 2015	Percent 2016	MOE[2] 2016	Change (2016 less 2015)[1]	Private health insurance[3] — Percent 2015	MOE[2] 2015	Percent 2016	MOE[2] 2016	Change (2016 less 2015)[1]	Government health insurance[4] — Percent 2015	MOE[2] 2015	Percent 2016	MOE[2] 2016	Change (2016 less 2015)[1]	Uninsured[5] — Percent 2015	MOE[2] 2015	Percent 2016	MOE[2] 2016	Change (2016 less 2015)[1]
Total	318,868	320,372	90.9	0.2	91.2	0.2	*0.3	67.2	0.4	67.5	0.4	0.3	37.1	0.3	37.3	0.3	0.1	9.1	0.2	8.8	0.2	*-0.3
Family Status																						
In families	258,121	259,863	91.7	0.2	91.8	0.2	0.2	68.3	0.4	68.7	0.4	0.3	36.6	0.4	36.4	0.4	-0.1	8.3	0.2	8.2	0.2	-0.2
Householder	82,199	82,854	91.3	0.3	91.6	0.3	0.3	70.5	0.5	71.2	0.5	*0.6	36.2	0.4	36.3	0.4	0.1	8.7	0.3	8.4	0.3	-0.3
Related children under age 18	72,558	72,674	94.8	0.3	94.8	0.3	-0.1	62.7	0.6	63.0	0.6	0.3	42.7	0.7	41.5	0.7	*-1.2	5.2	0.3	5.2	0.3	0.1
Related children under age 6	23,459	23,531	93.9	0.5	94.2	0.4	0.3	58.4	1.0	58.9	1.0	0.4	45.8	1.1	45.1	1.0	-0.7	6.1	0.5	5.8	0.4	-0.3
In unrelated subfamilies	1,344	1,208	87.9	2.7	86.5	2.9	-1.4	52.0	5.0	48.5	5.3	-3.5	47.1	4.5	48.6	4.9	1.5	12.1	2.7	13.5	2.9	1.4
Unrelated individuals	59,403	59,301	87.8	0.4	88.7	0.3	*1.0	62.7	0.6	62.8	0.6	0.1	39.4	0.6	40.6	0.5	*1.2	12.2	0.4	11.3	0.3	*-1.0
Residence																						
Inside metropolitan statistical areas	274,392	276,816	91.0	0.2	91.3	0.2	*0.3	68.0	0.4	68.5	0.4	0.3	35.9	0.4	35.9	0.4	Z	9.0	0.2	8.7	0.2	*-0.3
Inside principal cities	103,740	104,295	89.5	0.4	90.3	0.3	*0.8	63.6	0.7	64.1	0.7	0.6	37.6	0.6	37.8	0.7	0.2	10.5	0.4	9.7	0.3	*-0.8
Outside principal cities	170,652	172,521	91.9	0.3	92.0	0.3	0.1	70.7	0.5	71.1	0.5	0.4	34.9	0.4	34.8	0.4	-0.1	8.1	0.3	8.0	0.3	-0.1
Outside metropolitan statistical areas[6]	44,477	43,556	90.4	0.6	90.6	0.6	0.2	62.1	1.1	61.1	1.1	-1.0	44.4	1.0	45.7	1.1	*1.3	9.6	0.6	9.4	0.6	-0.2
Race[7] and Hispanic Origin																						
White	245,805	246,310	91.3	0.2	91.6	0.2	*0.3	69.0	0.4	69.4	0.4	0.4	36.5	0.4	36.6	0.3	0.2	8.7	0.2	8.4	0.2	*-0.3
White, not Hispanic	195,646	195,453	93.3	0.2	93.7	0.2	*0.4	73.6	0.4	73.9	0.4	0.3	35.3	0.4	35.9	0.4	*0.6	6.7	0.2	6.3	0.2	*-0.4
Black	41,703	42,040	88.9	0.5	89.5	0.5	0.6	55.9	1.0	56.5	1.0	0.5	44.1	0.9	43.7	0.9	-0.4	11.1	0.5	10.5	0.5	-0.6
Asian	18,249	18,897	92.5	0.6	92.4	0.7	-0.2	75.5	1.1	74.2	1.2	-1.3	27.1	1.1	27.1	1.2	0.1	7.5	0.6	7.6	0.7	0.2
Hispanic (any race)	56,873	57,670	83.8	0.5	84.0	0.5	0.2	51.6	1.0	52.4	1.0	0.7	41.2	0.8	40.1	0.8	-1.1	16.2	0.5	16.0	0.5	-0.2
Nativity																						
Native born	275,798	276,518	92.3	0.2	92.7	0.2	*0.4	68.4	0.3	68.7	0.4	0.3	38.0	0.3	38.1	0.3	0.2	7.7	0.2	7.3	0.2	*-0.4
Foreign born	43,070	43,854	81.9	0.6	82.0	0.6	0.2	59.4	0.9	59.9	0.7	0.4	31.8	0.8	31.7	0.7	Z	18.1	0.6	18.0	0.6	-0.2
Naturalized citizen	20,086	20,409	91.3	0.5	91.5	0.6	0.3	66.5	1.0	67.3	1.0	0.7	36.9	1.0	37.2	1.0	0.3	8.7	0.5	8.5	0.6	-0.3
Not a citizen	22,984	23,445	73.6	1.0	73.8	1.0	0.2	53.2	1.3	53.5	1.3	0.2	27.3	1.0	27.0	1.0	-0.2	26.4	1.0	26.2	1.0	-0.2

* Changes between the estimates are statistically different from zero at the 90 percent confidence level.

Z Represents or rounds to zero.

[1] Details may not sum to totals because of rounding.

[2] A margin of error is a measure of an estimate's variability. The larger the margin of error in relation to the size of the estimate, the less reliable the estimate. This number, when added to and subtracted from the estimate, forms the 90 percent confidence interval. Margins of error shown in this table are based on standard errors calculated using replicate weights. For more information, see "Standard Errors and Their Use" at <www2.census.gov/library/publications/2017/demo/p60-260sa.pdf>.

[3] Private health insurance includes coverage provided through an employer or union, coverage purchased directly by an individual from an insurance company, or coverage through someone outside the household.

[4] Government health insurance coverage includes Medicaid, Medicare, TRICARE, CHAMPVA (Civilian Health and Medical Program of the Department of Veterans Affairs) and care provided by the Department of Veterans Affairs and the military.

[5] Individuals are considered to be uninsured if they do not have health insurance coverage for the entire calendar year.

[6] The "Outside metropolitan statistical areas" category includes both micropolitan statistical areas and territory outside of metropolitan and micropolitan statistical areas. For more information, see <www.census.gov/programs-surveys/metro-micro/about/glossary.html>.

[7] Federal surveys now give respondents the option of reporting more than one race. Therefore, two basic ways of defining a race group are possible. A group such as Asian may be defined as those who reported Asian and no other race (the race-alone or single-race concept) or as those who reported Asian regardless of whether they also reported another race (the race-alone-or-in-combination concept). This table shows data using the first approach (race alone). The use of the single-race population does not imply that it is the preferred method of presenting or analyzing data. The Census Bureau uses a variety of approaches. Information on people who reported more than one race, such as White and American Indian and Alaska Native or Asian and Black or African American, is available from the 2010 Census through American FactFinder. About 2.9 percent of people reported more than one race in the 2010 Census. Data for American Indians and Alaska Natives, Native Hawaiians and Other Pacific Islanders, and those reporting two or more races are not shown separately.

Note: The estimates by type of coverage are not mutually exclusive; people can be covered by more than one type of health insurance during the year.

For both age groups, in 2016, uninsured rates were higher for people with household income below $25,000, compared with people with household income of $125,000 or more. Children with household income below $25,000 had an uninsured rate of 6.6 percent, while children with a household income at or above $125,000 had an uninsured rate of 2.9 percent. The uninsured rate for adults with household income of less than $25,000 was over four

times higher than it was for adults with household income of $125,000 or greater.

The overall percentage of children under the age of 19 without health insurance was 5.4 percent in 2016. Children in poverty were more likely to be uninsured (7.0 percent) than children not in poverty (5.0 percent).

The difference in the uninsured rate by poverty status was larger among adults than among children. The

uninsured rate for adults in poverty (24.7 percent) was over twice that for adults not in poverty (10.4 percent).

In 2016, non-Hispanic White children had an uninsured rate of 4.1 percent. Asian children had an uninsured rate of 5.0 percent, and Black children had an uninsured rate of 5.5 percent.[41] Hispanic children had the highest

[41] In 2016, the uninsured rate for Asian children was not statistically different from the uninsured rate for non-Hispanic White children or Black children.

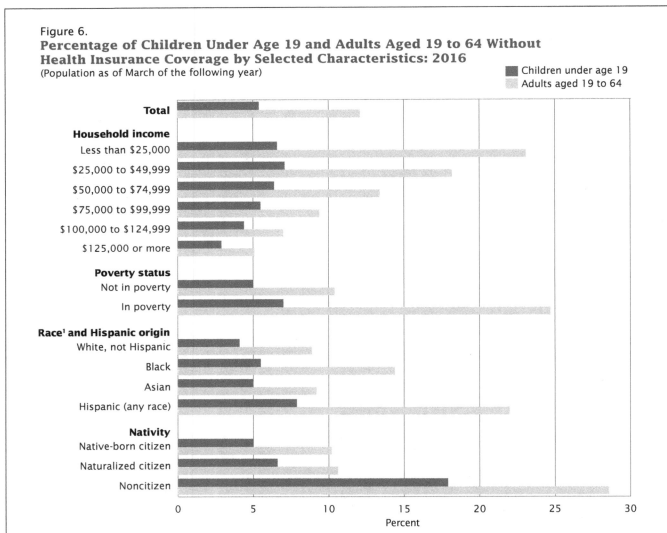

Figure 6.
Percentage of Children Under Age 19 and Adults Aged 19 to 64 Without Health Insurance Coverage by Selected Characteristics: 2016
(Population as of March of the following year)

■ Children under age 19
▨ Adults aged 19 to 64

[1] Federal surveys give respondents the option of reporting more than one race. This figure shows data using the race-alone concept. For example, Asian refers to people who reported Asian and no other race.

Note: For information on confidentiality protection, sampling error, nonsampling error, and definitions in the Current Population Survey, see <www2.census.gov/programs-surveys/cps/techdocs/cpsmar17.pdf>.

Source: U.S. Census Bureau, Current Population Survey, 2017 Annual Social and Economic Supplement.

uninsured rate, at 7.9 percent. For all race and Hispanic origin groups, the uninsured rate for adults was significantly larger than the uninsured rate for children.

The uninsured rate for noncitizen children in 2016 was 17.9 percent, over three-times greater than the uninsured rate for native-born citizen children (5.0 percent).

For adults in 2016, 28.6 percent of noncitizen adults were uninsured, which was over two-and-a-half times greater than the uninsured rate for native-born adults (10.2 percent).

State Estimates of Health Insurance Coverage

During 2016, the state with the lowest percentage of people without health insurance was Massachusetts (2.5 percent), while the state with the highest percentage was Texas (16.6 percent) (Figure 7 and Table 6).[42] Twenty-five states and the District of Columbia had an uninsured rate of 8.0 percent or less, and seven states (Connecticut, Hawaii, Iowa, Massachusetts, Minnesota, Rhode Island, and Vermont) and the District of Columbia had an uninsured rate of 5.0 percent or less.[43] Two states, Alaska and Texas, had an uninsured rate of 14.0 percent or more.

Between 2015 and 2016, the percentage of people without health insurance coverage decreased in 39 states (Figure 8 and Table 6). The decrease ranged from 0.3 percentage points (Massachusetts) to 3.5 percentage points (Montana).[44] Eleven states and the District of Columbia did not have a statistically significant change in their uninsured rates.[45]

In 2014, many provisions of the Patient Protection and Affordable Care Act went into effect. Since 2013, uninsured rates dropped in all 50 states and in the District of Columbia (Figure 8). However, the year-to-year changes in uninsured rates varied across states, as did uninsured rates in 2016.

Variation in both the uninsured rate in 2016 and change in the uninsured rate by state between 2013 and 2016 may be related to whether the state expanded Medicaid eligibility as part of the Affordable Care Act. Thirty states and the District of Columbia expanded Medicaid eligibility on or before January 1, 2016 (see the text box "Health Insurance Coverage and the Affordable Care Act").[46]

In general, in 2016, the uninsured rate in states that expanded Medicaid eligibility on or before January 1, 2016, was lower than in states that did not expand eligibility (Figure 7). In states that expanded Medicaid eligibility ("expansion states"), the uninsured rate in 2016 was 6.5 percent, compared with 11.7 percent in states that did not expand Medicaid eligibility ("non-expansion states"). Many Medicaid expansion states have uninsured rates near or lower than the national average, while many non-expansion states have uninsured rates near or above the national average (Figure 8). The uninsured rates by state ranged from 2.5 percent (Massachusetts) to 14.0 percent (Alaska) in expansion states, and from 5.3 percent (Wisconsin) to 16.6 percent (Texas) in non-expansion states.

Between 2015 and 2016, the overall decrease in the uninsured rate was 0.9 percentage points in expansion states, compared with 0.7 percentage points in non-expansion states. In general, decreases in the uninsured rate were greater in expansion states than in non-expansion states. Statistically significant decreases in the uninsured rate ranged from 3.5 percentage points to 0.3 percentage points in expansion states, and from 1.7 percentage points to 0.4 percentage points in non-expansion states.[47]

---

[42] These estimates and estimates in the remainder of this section come from the ACS, which measures insurance coverage at the time of survey. The ACS, which has a much larger sample size than the CPS, is also a useful source for estimating and identifying changes in the uninsured population at the state level. Estimates for Figure 7 come from the 2016 1-Year American Community Survey, and estimates for Figure 8 come from the 2008 to 2016 1-Year American Community Surveys.

[43] Consistent with Figure 7, classification into these categories is based on unrounded uninsured rates.

---

[44] The change in the uninsured rate between 2015 and 2016 in Massachusetts was not significantly different from the change in the uninsured rate in Arkansas, Colorado, Delaware, Hawaii, Idaho, Kansas, Maine, Maryland, Minnesota, Mississippi, Nebraska, Nevada, New Hampshire, North Dakota, Oklahoma, Texas, Vermont, Virginia, West Virginia, Wisconsin, Wyoming, and the District of Columbia.

[45] The states that did not have a significant change in the uninsured rate between 2015 and 2016 were Alaska, Delaware, Hawaii, Kansas, Maine, Nebraska, New Hampshire, North Dakota, Oklahoma, Vermont, and Wyoming.

[46] For a list of the states and their Medicaid expansion status as of January 1, 2016, see Table 6: Percentage of People Without Health Insurance Coverage by State: 2013 to 2016.

---

[47] The lower bound of the change in the uninsured rate between 2015 and 2016 for expansion states (0.3 percentage points) was not significantly different from the lower bound for non-expansion states (0.4 percentage points).

Table 6.

Percentage of People Without Health Insurance Coverage by State: 2013 to 2016

(Numbers in thousands. Civilian noninstitutionalized population. For information on confidentiality protection, sampling error, nonsampling error, and definitions, see www2.census.gov/programs-surveys/acs/tech_docs/accuracy/ACS_Accuracy_of_Data_2016.pdf)

State	Medicaid expansion state? Yes (Y) or No (N)[1]	2013 uninsured		2014 uninsured		2015 uninsured		2016 uninsured		Difference in uninsured			
										2016 less 2015		2016 less 2013	
		Percent	Margin of error[2] (±)	Percent	Margin of error[2] (±)	Percent	Margin of error[2] (±)	Percent	Margin of error[2] (±)	Percent	Margin of error[2] (±)	Percent	Margin of error[2] (±)
United States	X	14.5	0.1	11.7	0.1	9.4	0.1	8.6	0.1	*-0.8	0.1	*-5.9	0.1
Alabama	N	13.6	0.4	12.1	0.4	10.1	0.3	9.1	0.3	*-1.0	0.4	*-4.5	0.5
Alaska	+Y	18.5	1.0	17.2	0.9	14.9	0.7	14.0	0.9	-0.9	1.1	*-4.5	1.3
Arizona	Y	17.1	0.4	13.6	0.3	10.8	0.3	10.0	0.3	*-0.9	0.4	*-7.2	0.5
Arkansas	Y	16.0	0.5	11.8	0.4	9.5	0.4	7.9	0.4	*-1.6	0.6	*-8.1	0.6
California	Y	17.2	0.2	12.4	0.1	8.6	0.1	7.3	0.1	*-1.2	0.1	*-9.8	0.2
Colorado	Y	14.1	0.3	10.3	0.3	8.1	0.3	7.5	0.3	*-0.5	0.4	*-6.6	0.4
Connecticut	Y	9.4	0.4	6.9	0.3	6.0	0.4	4.9	0.3	*-1.1	0.5	*-4.5	0.5
Delaware	Y	9.1	0.7	7.8	0.7	5.9	0.6	5.7	0.5	-0.2	0.8	*-3.5	0.8
District of Columbia	Y	6.7	0.6	5.3	0.7	3.8	0.6	3.9	0.6	0.1	0.9	*-2.7	0.9
Florida	N	20.0	0.2	16.6	0.2	13.3	0.2	12.5	0.2	*-0.8	0.3	*-7.5	0.3
Georgia	N	18.8	0.3	15.8	0.3	13.9	0.3	12.9	0.3	*-0.9	0.4	*-5.9	0.4
Hawaii	Y	6.7	0.4	5.3	0.4	4.0	0.3	3.5	0.4	-0.4	0.5	*-3.2	0.6
Idaho	N	16.2	0.8	13.6	0.7	11.0	0.6	10.1	0.5	*-0.9	0.8	*-6.1	0.9
Illinois.............	Y	12.7	0.2	9.7	0.2	7.1	0.2	6.5	0.2	*-0.6	0.2	*-6.3	0.3
Indiana............	+Y	14.0	0.3	11.9	0.3	9.6	0.3	8.1	0.3	*-1.5	0.4	*-5.8	0.4
Iowa..............	Y	8.1	0.3	6.2	0.3	5.0	0.3	4.3	0.2	*-0.8	0.4	*-3.9	0.4
Kansas............	N	12.3	0.4	10.2	0.4	9.1	0.4	8.7	0.3	-0.4	0.5	*-3.5	0.5
Kentucky	Y	14.3	0.3	8.5	0.3	6.0	0.2	5.1	0.2	*-0.9	0.3	*-9.2	0.4
Louisiana..........	N	16.6	0.4	14.8	0.3	11.9	0.4	10.3	0.4	*-1.7	0.5	*-6.3	0.5
Maine.............	N	11.2	0.5	10.1	0.6	8.4	0.5	8.0	0.5	-0.4	0.7	*-3.1	0.7
Maryland	Y	10.2	0.3	7.9	0.3	6.6	0.2	6.1	0.3	*-0.5	0.3	*-4.0	0.4
Massachusetts........	Y	3.7	0.2	3.3	0.1	2.8	0.1	2.5	0.2	*-0.3	0.2	*-1.2	0.2
Michigan	^Y	11.0	0.2	8.5	0.2	6.1	0.1	5.4	0.1	*-0.7	0.2	*-5.6	0.2
Minnesota	Y	8.2	0.3	5.9	0.2	4.5	0.2	4.1	0.2	*-0.4	0.3	*-4.1	0.3
Mississippi..........	N	17.1	0.5	14.5	0.5	12.7	0.4	11.8	0.4	*-0.9	0.6	*-5.2	0.7
Missouri............	N	13.0	0.3	11.7	0.3	9.8	0.3	8.9	0.2	*-0.9	0.3	*-4.1	0.4
Montana...........	+Y	16.5	0.8	14.2	0.6	11.6	0.7	8.1	0.5	*-3.5	0.9	*-8.3	0.9
Nebraska..........	N	11.3	0.5	9.7	0.4	8.2	0.5	8.6	0.5	0.3	0.7	*-2.8	0.7
Nevada	Y	20.7	0.6	15.2	0.5	12.3	0.4	11.4	0.5	*-0.9	0.6	*-9.3	0.8
New Hampshire........	^Y	10.7	0.5	9.2	0.5	6.3	0.4	5.9	0.4	-0.4	0.6	*-4.8	0.7
New Jersey	Y	13.2	0.2	10.9	0.2	8.7	0.2	8.0	0.2	*-0.7	0.3	*-5.2	0.3
New Mexico.........	Y	18.6	0.6	14.5	0.5	10.9	0.5	9.2	0.5	*-1.8	0.7	*-9.5	0.8
New York	Y	10.7	0.2	8.7	0.1	7.1	0.1	6.1	0.1	*-1.0	0.2	*-4.6	0.2
North Carolina.........	N	15.6	0.3	13.1	0.3	11.2	0.2	10.4	0.2	*-0.8	0.3	*-5.2	0.3
North Dakota.........	Y	10.4	0.8	7.9	0.7	7.8	0.7	7.0	0.6	-0.7	0.9	*-3.3	1.0
Ohio..............	Y	11.0	0.2	8.4	0.2	6.5	0.2	5.6	0.2	*-0.9	0.2	*-5.4	0.2
Oklahoma	N	17.7	0.3	15.4	0.3	13.9	0.3	13.8	0.3	-0.1	0.4	*-3.9	0.5
Oregon............	Y	14.7	0.4	9.7	0.3	7.0	0.3	6.2	0.2	*-0.8	0.4	*-8.4	0.5
Pennsylvania	^Y	9.7	0.2	8.5	0.2	6.4	0.1	5.6	0.2	*-0.7	0.2	*-4.1	0.2
Rhode Island	Y	11.6	0.7	7.4	0.6	5.7	0.6	4.3	0.5	*-1.4	0.7	*-7.3	0.8
South Carolina........	N	15.8	0.4	13.6	0.4	10.9	0.3	10.0	0.3	*-0.9	0.4	*-5.8	0.5
South Dakota.........	N	11.3	0.7	9.8	0.5	10.2	0.6	8.7	0.5	*-1.5	0.8	*-2.5	0.8
Tennessee..........	N	13.9	0.3	12.0	0.3	10.3	0.3	9.0	0.2	*-1.2	0.4	*-4.8	0.4
Texas..............	N	22.1	0.2	19.1	0.2	17.1	0.2	16.6	0.2	*-0.5	0.3	*-5.5	0.3
Utah...............	N	14.0	0.5	12.5	0.5	10.5	0.5	8.8	0.4	*-1.7	0.6	*-5.2	0.6
Vermont...........	Y	7.2	0.6	5.0	0.4	3.8	0.4	3.7	0.4	-0.1	0.5	*-3.5	0.7
Virginia............	N	12.3	0.3	10.9	0.3	9.1	0.3	8.7	0.3	*-0.4	0.4	*-3.6	0.4
Washington	Y	14.0	0.3	9.2	0.2	6.6	0.2	6.0	0.2	*-0.7	0.3	*-8.0	0.4
West Virginia	Y	14.0	0.5	8.6	0.4	6.0	0.4	5.3	0.3	*-0.6	0.5	*-8.7	0.6
Wisconsin	N	9.1	0.2	7.3	0.2	5.7	0.2	5.3	0.2	*-0.4	0.2	*-3.9	0.3
Wyoming	N	13.4	0.9	12.0	0.8	11.5	1.0	11.5	1.0	Z	1.4	*-1.9	1.3

* Statistically different from zero at the 90 percent confidence level.

^ Expanded Medicaid eligibility after January 1, 2014, and on or before January 1, 2015.

\+ Expanded Medicaid eligibility after January 1, 2015, and on or before January 1, 2016.

X Not applicable.

Z Represents or rounds to zero.

[1] Medicaid expansion status as of January 1, 2016. For more information, see <www.medicaid.gov/medicaid/by-state/by-state.html>.

[2] Data are based on a sample and are subject to sampling variability. A margin of error is a measure of an estimate's variability. The larger the margin of error is in relation to the size of the estimate, the less reliable the estimate. This number, when added to and subtracted from the estimate, forms the 90 percent confidence interval.

Note: Differences are calculated with unrounded numbers, which may produce different results from using the rounded values in the table.

Source: U.S. Census Bureau, 2013 to 2016 1-Year American Community Surveys.

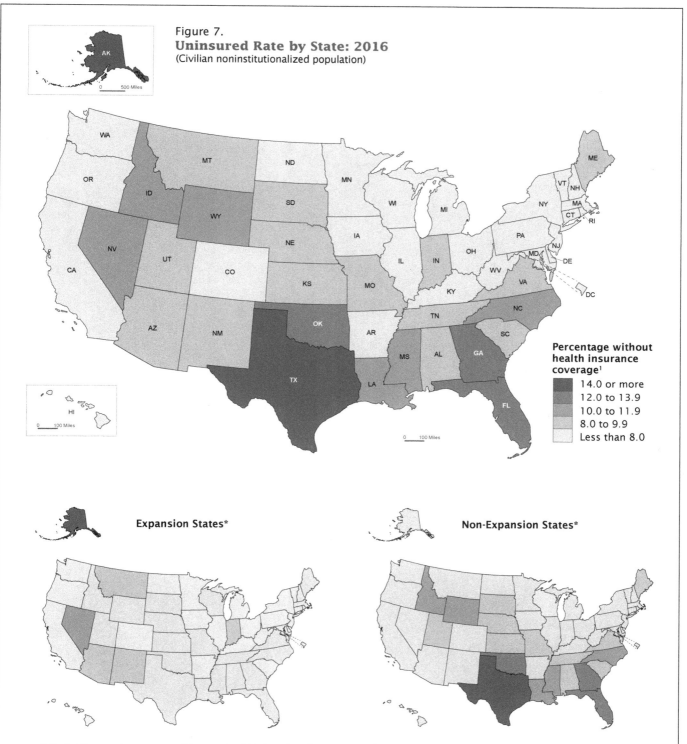

Figure 7.
Uninsured Rate by State: 2016
(Civilian noninstitutionalized population)

Percentage without health insurance coverage[1]

- 14.0 or more
- 12.0 to 13.9
- 10.0 to 11.9
- 8.0 to 9.9
- Less than 8.0

Expansion States*

Non-Expansion States*

* Medicaid expansion status as of January 1, 2016. For a list of expansion and non-expansion states, see Table 6: Percentage of People Without Health Insurance Coverage by State: 2013 to 2016.

[1] Classification is based on unrounded uninsured rates.

Note: For information on confidentiality protection, sampling error, nonsampling error, and definitions in the American Community Survey, see <www2.census.gov/programs-surveys/acs/tech_docs/accuracy/ACS_Accuracy_of_Data_2016.pdf>.

Source: U.S. Census Bureau, 2016 1-Year American Community Survey.

Figure 8.
Change in the Uninsured Rate by State: 2008 to 2016
(Civilian noninstitutionalized population)

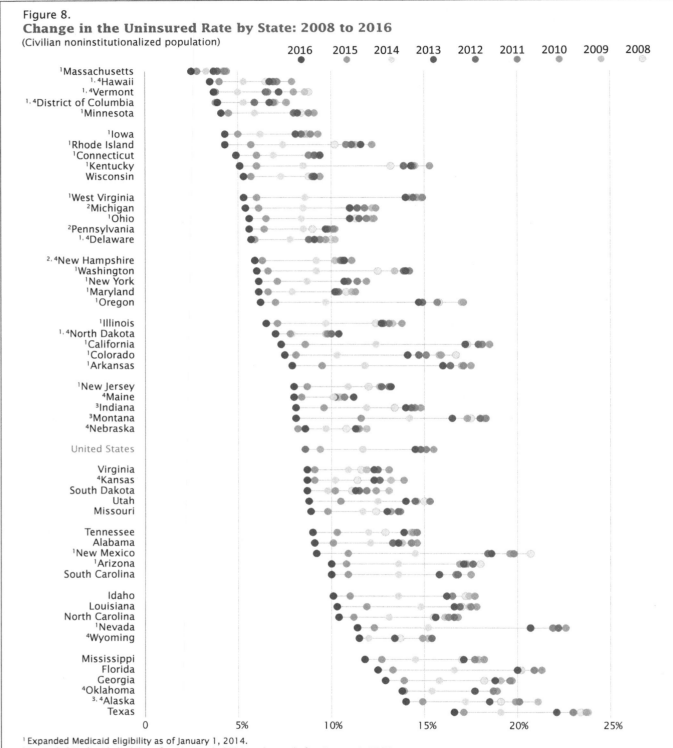

[1] Expanded Medicaid eligibility as of January 1, 2014.

[2] Expanded Medicaid eligibility after January 1, 2014, and on or before January 1, 2015.

[3] Expanded Medicaid eligibility after January 1, 2015, and on or before January 1, 2016.

[4] The change in the uninsured rate between 2015 and 2016 was not statistically different from zero at the 90 percent confidence level for Alaska, Delaware, Hawaii, Kansas, Maine, Nebraska, New Hampshire, North Dakota, Oklahoma, Vermont, Wyoming, and the District of Columbia.

Note: For information on confidentiality protection, sampling error, nonsampling error, and definitions in the American Community Survey, see <www2.census.gov/programs-surveys/acs/tech_docs/accuracy/ACS_Accuracy_of_Data_2016.pdf>.

Source: U.S. Census Bureau, 2008 to 2016 1-Year American Community Surveys.

More Information About Health Insurance Coverage

Additional Data and Contacts

Detailed tables, historical tables, press releases, and briefings are available electronically on the Census Bureau's Health Insurance Web site. The Web site may be accessed through the Census Bureau's home page at <www.census.gov> or directly at <www.census.gov/topics/health /health-insurance.html>.

Microdata are available for download by clicking on "Data Tools" on the Census Bureau's home page and then clicking the "DataFerrett" link. Technical methods have been applied to CPS microdata to avoid disclosing the identities of individuals from whom data were collected.

State and Local Estimates of Health Insurance Coverage

The Census Bureau publishes annual estimates of health insurance coverage by state and other smaller geographic units based on data collected in the ACS. Single-year estimates are available for geographic units with populations of 65,000 or more. Five-year estimates are available for all geographic units, including census tracts and block groups.

The Census Bureau's Small Area Health Insurance Estimates (SAHIE) program also produces single-year estimates of health insurance for states and all counties. These estimates are based on models using data from a variety of sources, including current surveys, administrative records, and intercensal population estimates. In general, SAHIE estimates have lower variances than ACS estimates but are released

later because they incorporate ACS data in the models.

Small Area Health Insurance Estimates are available at <www.census.gov /did/www/sahie/index.html>. The most recent estimates are for 2015.

Comments

The Census Bureau welcomes the comments and advice of data and report users. If you have suggestions or comments on the health insurance coverage report, please write to:

Jennifer Cheeseman Day
Assistant Division Chief, Employment
    Characteristics
Social, Economic, and Housing
    Statistics Division
U.S. Census Bureau
Washington, DC 20233-8500

or send e-mail to
<jennifer.cheeseman.day@census.gov>.

Sources of Estimates

The majority of the data in this report are from the 2014 to 2017 Current Population Survey Annual Social and Economic Supplements (CPS ASEC) and were collected in the 50 states and the District of Columbia. The data do not represent residents of Puerto Rico and the U.S. Island Areas.[48] The data are based on a sample of about 95,000 addresses. The estimates in this report are controlled to independent national population estimates by age, sex, race, and Hispanic origin for March of the year in which the data are collected. Beginning with 2010, estimates are based on 2010 Census population counts and are updated

[48] The U.S. Island Areas include American Samoa, Guam, the Commonwealth of the Northern Mariana Islands, and the Virgin Islands of the United States.

annually taking into account births, deaths, emigration, and immigration.

The CPS is a household survey primarily used to collect employment data. The sample universe for the basic CPS consists of the resident civilian, noninstitutionalized population of the United States. People in institutions, such as prisons, long-term care hospitals, and nursing homes, are not eligible to be interviewed in the CPS. Students living in dormitories are included in the estimates only if information about them is reported in an interview at their parents' home. Since the CPS is a household survey, people who are homeless and not living in shelters are not included in the sample. The sample universe for the CPS ASEC is slightly larger than that of the basic CPS since it includes military personnel who live in a household with at least one other civilian adult, regardless of whether they live off post or on post. All other armed forces are excluded. For further documentation about the CPS ASEC, see <www2.census.gov /programs-surveys/cps/techdocs /cpsmar17.pdf>.

Additional data in this report are from the American Community Survey (ACS) 1-year data, 2008 through 2016. The ACS is an ongoing, nationwide survey designed to provide demographic, social, economic, and housing data at different levels of geography. While the ACS includes Puerto Rico and the group quarters population, the ACS data in this report focus on the civilian noninstitutionalized population of the United States (excluding Puerto Rico and some people living in group quarters). It has an annual sample size of about 3.5 million addresses. For information on the ACS sample design and other top-ics, visit <www.census.gov/programs -surveys/acs/>.

Statistical Accuracy

The estimates in this report (which may be shown in text, figures, and tables) are based on responses from a sample of the population. Sampling error is the uncertainty between an estimate based on a sample and the corresponding value that would be obtained if the estimate were based on the entire population (as from a census). All comparative statements in this report have undergone sta-tistical testing, and comparisons are significant at the 90 percent level unless otherwise noted. Data are sub-ject to error arising from a variety of sources. Measures of sampling error are provided in the form of margins of error, or confidence intervals, for all estimates included in this report.

In addition to sampling error, non-sampling error may be introduced during any of the operations used to collect and process survey data, such as editing, reviewing, or keying data from questionnaires. In this report, the variances of estimates were calcu-lated using the Fay and Train (1995) Successive Difference Replication (SDR) method.

Most of the data from the 2017 CPS ASEC were collected in March (with some data collected in February and April). Each year, the CPS ASEC sample consists of approximately 100,000 addresses. In 2017, the CPS ASEC sample had 95,000 addresses, as approximately 5,000 randomly selected addresses were removed from the March sample. The 5,000 addresses were given the pre-2013 health insurance questions in order to fulfill budgetary requirements for

the 2017 fiscal year.[49, 50] Adjustments to the weights were made to account for the reduction in sample. Further information about the source and accuracy of the CPS ASEC estimates is available at <www2.census.gov /library/publications/2017/demo /p60-260sa.pdf>.

Most of the remaining data presented in this report are based on the ACS sample collected from January 2016 through December 2016. For more information on sampling and estima-tion methods, confidentiality protec-tion, and sampling and nonsampling errors, please see the 2016 ACS Accuracy of the Data document located at <www2.census.gov/programs -surveys/acs/tech_docs/accuracy/ACS _Accuracy_of_Data_2016.pdf>.

---

[49] Public Law 113-235, 2017.
[50] The series of questions asking about health insurance coverage in calendar year 2012 and earlier.

Table A-1.

Number of People by Type of Health Insurance Coverage by Age: 2015 and 2016

(Numbers in thousands, margins of error in thousands. Population as of March of the following year. For information on confidentiality protection, sampling error, nonsampling error, and definitions, see www2.census.gov/programs-surveys/cps/techdocs/cpsmar17.pdf)

Characteristic	Total 2015 Number	Total 2016 Number	Any health insurance 2015 Number	2015 Margin of error[2] (±)	2016 Number	2016 Margin of error[2] (±)	Change (2016 less 2015)[1,*]	Private health insurance[3] 2015 Number	2015 Margin of error[2] (±)	2016 Number	2016 Margin of error[2] (±)	Change (2016 less 2015)[1,*]	Government health insurance[4] 2015 Number	2015 Margin of error[2] (±)	2016 Number	2016 Margin of error[2] (±)	Change (2016 less 2015)[1,*]	Uninsured[5] 2015 Number	2015 Margin of error[2] (±)	2016 Number	2016 Margin of error[2] (±)	Change (2016 less 2015)[1,*]
Total	318,868	320,372	289,903	650	292,320	541	*2,417	214,238	1,118	216,203	1,145	*1,965	118,395	1,067	119,361	1,018	966	28,966	634	28,052	519	*–914
Age																						
Under age 65. . . .	271,322	271,098	242,862	639	243,645	582	783	189,467	1,050	190,198	1,051	730	73,786	1,015	73,220	991	–566	28,460	624	27,453	508	*–1,007
Under age 18. . . .	74,062	74,047	70,196	264	70,123	246	–72	46,138	482	46,393	438	255	31,853	486	31,020	481	*–833	3,866	218	3,924	192	58
Aged 18 to 64. . .	197,260	197,051	172,666	549	173,521	535	*855	143,330	739	143,805	772	475	41,933	692	42,200	689	267	24,594	521	23,530	438	*–1,064
Under age 19[6] . .	78,182	78,150	74,024	255	73,948	240	–76	48,959	496	49,185	452	226	33,320	505	32,439	505	*–880	4,158	225	4,203	205	44
Aged 19 to 64. . .	193,140	192,948	168,838	543	169,697	525	*859	140,509	717	141,013	750	504	40,466	668	40,781	662	314	24,302	513	23,251	435	*–1,051
Aged 19 to 25[7] .	30,475	29,815	26,060	298	25,917	274	–143	21,288	322	21,247	290	–41	7,019	232	6,898	263	–121	4,414	190	3,898	179	*–516
Aged 26 to 34 . .	38,960	39,736	32,622	293	33,499	267	*876	27,098	322	27,692	313	*594	7,814	259	8,097	258	283	6,337	235	6,237	224	–100
Aged 35 to 44 . .	40,005	40,046	34,517	226	34,794	197	277	29,099	253	29,373	270	274	7,737	235	7,728	228	–9	5,489	216	5,252	192	–236
Aged 45 to 64 . .	83,701	83,351	75,639	259	75,487	342	–151	63,025	368	62,702	449	–323	17,896	396	18,058	408	161	8,062	260	7,863	257	–199
Aged 65 and older	47,547	49,274	47,041	64	48,675	225	*1,635	24,771	383	26,005	378	*1,235	44,609	150	46,140	259	*1,532	506	62	598	69	93

* Changes between the estimates are statistically different from zero at the 90 percent confidence level.

[1] Details may not sum to totals because of rounding.

[2] A margin of error is a measure of an estimate's variability. The larger the margin of error in relation to the size of the estimate, the less reliable the estimate. This number, when added to and subtracted from the estimate, forms the 90 percent confidence interval. Margins of error shown in this table are based on standard errors calculated using replicate weights. For more information, see "Standard Errors and Their Use" at <www2.census.gov/library/publications/2017/demo/p60-260sa.pdf>.

[3] Private health insurance includes coverage provided through an employer or union, coverage purchased directly by an individual from an insurance company, or coverage through someone outside the household.

[4] Government health insurance coverage includes Medicaid, Medicare, TRICARE, CHAMPVA (Civilian Health and Medical Program of the Department of Veterans Affairs), and care provided by the Department of Veterans Affairs and the military.

[5] Individuals are considered to be uninsured if they do not have health insurance coverage for the entire calendar year.

[6] Children under the age of 19 are eligible for Medicaid/CHIP.

[7] This age group is of special interest because of the Affordable Care Act's dependent coverage provision. Individuals aged 19 to 25 may be eligible to be a dependent on a parent's health insurance plan.

Note: The estimates by type of coverage are not mutually exclusive; people can be covered by more than one type of health insurance during the year.

Source: U.S. Census Bureau, Current Population Survey, 2016 and 2017 Annual Social and Economic Supplements.

Table A-2.

Number of People by Type of Health Insurance Coverage for Working-Age Adults Aged 19 to 64: 2015 and 2016

(Numbers in thousands, margins of error in thousands. Population as of March of the following year. For information on confidentiality protection, sampling error, nonsampling error, and definitions, see www2.census.gov/programs-surveys/cps/techdocs/cpsmar17.pdf)

Characteristic	Total 2015 Number	Total 2016 Number	Any health insurance 2015 Number	2015 Margin of error (±)[2]	2016 Number	2016 Margin of error (±)[2]	Change (2016 less 2015)[1] *	Private health insurance[3] 2015 Number	2015 Margin of error (±)[2]	2016 Number	2016 Margin of error (±)[2]	Change (2016 less 2015)[1] *	Government health insurance[4] 2015 Number	2015 Margin of error (±)[2]	2016 Number	2016 Margin of error (±)[2]	Change (2016 less 2015)[1] *	Uninsured[5] 2015 Number	2015 Margin of error (±)[2]	2016 Number	2016 Margin of error (±)[2]	Change (2016 less 2015)[1] *
Total	318,868	320,372	289,903	650	292,320	541	*2,417	214,238	1,118	216,203	1,145	*1,965	118,395	1,067	119,361	1,018	966	28,966	634	28,052	519	*−914
Total, 19 to 64 years old	193,140	192,948	168,838	543	169,697	525	*859	140,509	717	141,013	750	504	40,466	668	40,781	662	314	24,302	513	23,251	435	*−1,051
Marital Status																						
Married[6]	101,277	101,822	92,147	686	92,821	670	674	81,072	699	81,594	666	522	18,204	478	18,230	447	27	9,131	325	9,001	333	−129
Widowed	3,451	3,633	2,962	142	3,127	158	165	2,041	117	2,131	117	90	1,160	87	1,218	101	59	489	61	506	61	17
Divorced	19,817	19,460	16,858	358	16,753	363	−105	12,655	310	12,503	317	−152	5,150	205	5,223	212	73	2,959	154	2,707	132	*−252
Separated	4,698	4,495	3,731	173	3,632	169	−99	2,558	135	2,512	144	−46	1,383	109	1,394	96	11	968	84	863	73	−105
Never married	63,896	63,537	53,140	566	53,364	547	224	42,182	552	42,272	552	90	14,570	334	14,716	392	145	10,756	297	10,174	320	*−582
Disability Status[7]																						
With a disability	15,128	15,248	13,627	300	13,899	358	272	6,559	224	6,633	231	74	8,820	271	8,933	287	114	1,501	106	1,349	109	−152
With no disability	177,102	176,842	154,301	578	154,940	572	639	133,713	695	134,162	765	449	30,737	547	30,989	558	252	22,801	516	21,902	417	*−899
Work Experience																						
All workers	148,503	149,105	131,240	655	132,422	587	*1,182	118,806	676	119,497	661	690	20,421	449	20,797	474	376	17,263	436	16,682	385	*−581
Worked full-time, year-round	105,533	107,577	95,059	671	97,049	652	*1,989	89,177	670	90,853	669	*1,677	11,078	303	11,224	313	146	10,474	322	10,528	292	54
Worked less than full-time, year-round	42,970	41,528	36,181	534	35,374	514	*−807	29,630	505	28,643	505	*−986	9,343	258	9,573	286	230	6,789	245	6,154	225	*−635
Did not work at least one week	44,637	43,843	37,598	491	37,275	507	−323	21,702	410	21,517	413	−186	20,045	444	19,984	395	−61	7,039	222	6,568	247	*−471
Educational Attainment																						
Total, 26 to 64 years old	162,665	163,133	142,778	495	143,780	473	*1,002	119,221	644	119,766	685	546	33,447	590	33,883	547	436	19,888	449	19,353	386	−535
No high school diploma	16,079	15,389	11,642	301	11,184	300	*−458	6,923	244	6,293	218	*−630	5,698	212	5,806	218	108	4,436	198	4,205	189	−231
High school graduate (includes equivalency)	44,925	45,401	37,894	572	38,511	605	617	29,277	508	29,512	541	235	11,676	354	11,961	328	285	7,031	248	6,890	232	−140
Some college, no degree	27,246	26,594	24,006	411	23,512	407	−494	19,536	398	19,102	383	−434	6,449	214	6,324	227	−126	3,240	167	3,082	147	−158
Associate degree	17,471	17,739	15,820	335	16,096	354	277	13,558	296	13,820	323	262	3,550	149	3,454	171	−96	1,652	110	1,642	110	−9
Bachelor's degree	35,870	36,528	33,354	518	34,032	503	678	30,919	517	31,698	498	*779	4,159	176	4,239	172	80	2,517	146	2,496	133	−21
Graduate or professional degree	21,075	21,482	20,062	432	20,444	437	383	19,009	429	19,342	432	333	1,914	131	2,098	122	*184	1,013	100	1,038	86	25

* Changes between the estimates are statistically different from zero at the 90 percent confidence level.

[1] Details may not sum to totals because of rounding.

[2] A margin of error is a measure of an estimate's variability. The larger the margin of error in relation to the size of the estimate, the less reliable the estimate. This number, when added to and subtracted from the estimate, forms the 90 percent confidence interval. Margins of error shown in this table are based on standard errors calculated using replicate weights. For more information, see "Standard Errors and Their Use" at <www2.census.gov/library/publications/2017/demo/p60-260sa.pdf>.

[3] Private health insurance includes coverage provided through an employer or union, coverage purchased directly by an individual from an insurance company, or coverage through someone outside the household.

[4] Government health insurance coverage includes Medicaid, Medicare, TRICARE, CHAMPVA (Civilian Health and Medical Program of the Department of Veterans Affairs), and care provided by the Department of Veterans Affairs and the military.

[5] Individuals are considered to be uninsured if they do not have health insurance coverage for the entire calendar year.

[6] The combined category "married" includes three individual categories: "married, civilian spouse present," "married, armed forces spouse present," and "married, spouse absent."

[7] The sum of those with and without a disability does not equal the total because disability status is not defined for individuals in the armed forces.

Note: The estimates by type of coverage are not mutually exclusive; people can be covered by more than one type of health insurance during the year.

Source: U.S. Census Bureau, Current Population Survey, 2016 and 2017 Annual Social and Economic Supplements.

Table A-3.
Number of People by Type of Health Insurance Coverage by Household Income and Income-to-Poverty Ratio: 2015 and 2016

(Numbers in thousands, margins of error in thousands. Population as of March of the following year. For information on confidentiality protection, sampling error, nonsampling error, and definitions, see www2.census.gov/programs-surveys/cps/techdocs/cpsmar17.pdf)

Characteristic	Total 2015 Number	Total 2016 Number	Any health insurance 2015 Number	Any health insurance 2015 MOE[2] (±)	Any health insurance 2016 Number	Any health insurance 2016 MOE[2] (±)	Any health insurance Change (2016 less 2015)[1],*	Private health insurance[3] 2015 Number	Private 2015 MOE[2] (±)	Private 2016 Number	Private 2016 MOE[2] (±)	Private Change (2016 less 2015)[1],*	Government health insurance[4] 2015 Number	Gov 2015 MOE[2] (±)	Gov 2016 Number	Gov 2016 MOE[2] (±)	Gov Change (2016 less 2015)[1],*	Uninsured[5] 2015 Number	Unins 2015 MOE[2] (±)	Uninsured 2016 Number	Unins 2016 MOE[2] (±)	Unins Change (2016 less 2015)[1],*
Total	318,868	320,372	289,903	650	292,320	541	*2,417	214,238	1,118	216,203	1,145	*1,965	118,395	1,067	119,361	1,018	966	28,966	634	28,052	519	*-914
Household Income																						
Less than $25,000	51,526	48,346	43,878	783	41,724	776	*-2,153	15,829	478	14,699	465	*-1,130	34,309	685	32,887	674	*-1,422	7,649	322	6,622	290	*-1,027
$25,000 to $49,999	64,874	63,644	56,744	944	56,046	936	-698	34,293	681	33,558	675	-735	33,092	770	33,080	709	-12	8,130	321	7,598	290	*-532
$50,000 to $74,999	54,791	54,829	49,472	968	49,446	927	-25	38,538	839	37,618	813	-920	19,032	571	20,236	525	*1,204	5,319	247	5,383	262	64
$75,000 to $99,999	42,794	44,225	39,646	829	40,881	835	*1,235	33,906	741	35,112	776	*1,206	11,848	420	11,607	396	-241	3,148	199	3,344	214	196
$100,000 to $124,999	32,654	32,954	30,915	763	31,037	753	122	27,659	721	27,606	683	-53	7,082	296	7,181	327	99	1,739	160	1,917	166	178
$125,000 or more	72,229	76,374	69,248	1,128	73,186	1,025	*3,937	64,014	1,087	67,610	1,028	*3,596	13,033	465	14,371	463	*1,337	2,980	223	3,188	222	208
Income-to-Poverty Ratio																						
Below 100 percent of poverty	43,123	40,616	35,634	853	34,004	683	*-1,630	12,352	470	11,620	420	*-732	26,772	713	25,826	585	*-945	7,489	317	6,612	261	*-877
Below 138 percent of poverty	64,711	61,039	54,124	971	51,681	820	*-2,443	20,744	583	19,001	537	*-1,743	39,732	814	38,522	692	*-1,210	10,586	368	9,357	316	*-1,229
Between 100 and 199 percent of poverty	57,770	54,629	49,932	829	47,735	876	*-2,198	26,853	664	24,786	671	*-2,067	31,096	670	30,518	651	-578	7,838	341	6,894	309	*-944
Between 200 and 299 percent of poverty	49,668	51,705	44,788	798	46,131	825	*1,343	33,251	681	34,216	742	965	19,275	535	19,631	478	356	4,880	232	5,574	258	*694
Between 300 and 399 percent of poverty	41,691	42,562	38,629	783	39,359	753	730	32,659	694	32,525	640	-134	12,411	386	13,258	448	*847	3,062	200	3,204	192	142
At or above 400 percent of poverty	126,202	130,398	120,539	1,178	124,665	1,256	*4,126	109,014	1,143	112,884	1,217	*3,870	28,524	596	29,793	575	*1,269	5,662	285	5,733	272	71

* Changes between the estimates are statistically different from zero at the 90 percent confidence level.

[1] Details may not sum to totals because of rounding.

[2] A margin of error is a measure of an estimate's variability. The larger the margin of error in relation to the size of the estimate, the less reliable the estimate. This number, when added to and subtracted from the estimate, forms the 90 percent confidence interval. Margins of error shown in this table are based on standard errors calculated using replicate weights. For more information, see "Standard Errors and Their Use" at <www2.census.gov/library/publications/2017/demo/p60-260sa.pdf>.

[3] Private health insurance includes coverage provided through an employer or union, coverage purchased directly by an individual from an insurance company, or coverage through someone outside the household.

[4] Government health insurance coverage includes Medicaid, Medicare, TRICARE, CHAMPVA (Civilian Health and Medical Program of the Department of Veterans Affairs), and care provided by the Department of Veterans Affairs and the military.

[5] Individuals are considered to be uninsured if they do not have health insurance coverage for the entire calendar year.

Note: The estimates by type of coverage are not mutually exclusive; people can be covered by more than one type of health insurance during the year.

Source: U.S. Census Bureau, Current Population Survey, 2016 and 2017 Annual Social and Economic Supplements.

Table A-4.

Number of People by Type of Health Insurance Coverage by Selected Demographic Characteristics: 2015 and 2016

(Numbers in thousands, margins of errors in thousands. Population as of March of the following year. For information on confidentiality protection, sampling error, nonsampling error, and definitions, see www2.census.gov/programs-surveys/cps/techdocs/cpsmar17.pdf)

Characteristic	Total 2015 Number	Total 2016 Number	Any health insurance — Total 2015 Number	2015 Margin of error[2] (±)	2016 Number	2016 Margin of error[2] (±)	Change (2016 less 2015)[1],*	Private health insurance[3] 2015 Number	2015 Margin of error[2] (±)	2016 Number	2016 Margin of error[2] (±)	Change (2016 less 2015)[1],*	Government health insurance[4] 2015 Number	2015 Margin of error[2] (±)	2016 Number	2016 Margin of error[2] (±)	Change (2016 less 2015)[1],*	Uninsured[5] 2015 Number	2015 Margin of error[2] (±)	2016 Number	2016 Margin of error[2] (±)	Change (2016 less 2015)[1],*
Total	318,868	320,372	289,903	650	292,320	541	*2,417	214,238	1,118	216,203	1,145	*1,965	118,395	1,067	119,361	1,018	966	28,966	634	28,052	519	*–914
Family Status																						
In families	258,121	259,863	236,575	997	238,655	883	*2,080	176,318	1,242	178,401	1,203	*2,084	94,366	1,075	94,707	936	341	21,546	563	21,208	504	–338
Householder	82,199	82,854	75,058	413	75,899	437	*840	57,981	466	58,954	458	*973	29,794	389	30,074	335	280	7,141	221	6,956	217	–185
Related children under 18	72,558	72,674	68,817	270	68,867	261	51	45,477	483	45,793	440	316	30,968	478	30,180	481	*–788	3,741	214	3,807	194	66
Related children under 6	23,459	23,531	22,175	138	22,037	128	139	13,708	226	13,848	224	140	10,743	255	10,603	238	–140	1,422	115	1,355	105	–67
In unrelated subfamilies	1,344	1,208	1,181	115	1,045	135	–137	699	97	585	102	–113	633	82	587	89	–46	163	40	163	37	Z
Unrelated individuals	59,403	59,301	52,146	813	52,621	729	475	37,222	691	37,217	645	–5	23,396	429	24,067	437	*671	7,257	284	6,680	227	*–576
Residence																						
Inside metropolitan statistical areas	274,392	276,816	249,708	2,748	252,854	2,596	*3,146	186,619	2,184	189,594	2,012	*2,975	98,627	1,565	99,455	1,589	828	24,684	664	23,961	579	–722
Inside principal cities	103,740	104,295	92,845	1,740	94,153	1,917	1,308	65,930	1,380	66,859	1,350	930	39,050	990	39,431	1,121	381	10,895	452	10,142	404	*–753
Outside principal cities	170,652	172,521	156,863	2,402	158,701	2,449	1,839	120,689	1,987	122,735	1,910	*2,045	59,577	1,187	60,024	1,274	447	13,789	512	13,820	490	31
Outside metropolitan statistical areas[6]	44,477	43,556	40,194	2,694	39,466	2,528	–729	27,620	1,886	26,609	1,720	*–1,010	19,768	1,403	19,905	1,397	138	4,282	373	4,091	373	–192
Race[7] and Hispanic Origin																						
White	245,805	246,310	224,351	539	225,497	491	*1,146	169,565	947	170,839	949	*1,274	89,598	911	90,220	847	622	21,454	529	20,813	455	–642
White, not Hispanic	195,646	195,453	182,546	442	183,139	422	*592	143,922	785	144,398	839	475	69,065	739	70,136	701	*1,071	13,100	411	12,314	360	*–785
Black	41,703	42,040	37,076	213	37,612	227	*536	23,330	430	23,739	415	409	18,387	381	18,377	378	–11	4,627	210	4,428	223	–200
Asian	18,249	18,897	16,889	193	17,455	208	*566	13,775	237	14,013	260	238	4,937	202	5,124	237	186	1,360	120	1,442	134	82
Hispanic (any race)	56,873	57,670	47,637	315	48,433	319	*796	29,352	554	30,192	453	*840	23,447	446	23,125	419	–322	9,235	309	9,237	316	2
Nativity																						
Native born	275,798	276,518	254,648	843	256,338	767	*1,691	188,639	1,103	189,946	1,126	1,307	104,719	976	105,440	982	721	21,150	513	20,180	438	*–971
Foreign born	43,070	43,854	35,255	591	35,982	538	727	25,600	521	26,258	469	658	13,676	399	13,921	389	245	7,815	313	7,872	312	57
Naturalized citizen	20,086	20,409	18,336	364	18,684	405	347	13,366	327	13,726	346	359	7,413	245	7,591	259	178	1,750	112	1,726	125	–24
Not a citizen	22,984	23,445	16,919	498	17,298	380	380	12,233	419	12,532	346	299	6,263	288	6,330	262	67	6,066	288	6,147	269	81

* Changes between the estimates are statistically different from zero at the 90 percent confidence level.

Z Represents or rounds to zero.

[1] Details may not sum to totals because of rounding.

[2] A margin of error is a measure of an estimate's variability. The larger the margin of error in relation to the size of the estimate, the less reliable the estimate. This number, when added to and subtracted from the estimate, forms the 90 percent confidence interval. Margins of error shown in this table are based on standard errors calculated using replicate weights. For more information, see "Standard Errors and Their Use" at <www2.census.gov/library/publications/2017/demo/p60-260sa.pdf>.

[3] Private health insurance includes coverage provided through an employer or union, coverage purchased directly by an individual from an insurance company, or coverage through someone outside the household.

[4] Government health insurance coverage includes Medicaid, Medicare, TRICARE, CHAMPVA (Civilian Health and Medical Program of the Department of Veterans Affairs), and care provided by the Department of Veterans Affairs and the military.

[5] Individuals are considered to be uninsured if they do not have health insurance coverage for the entire calendar year.

[6] The "Outside metropolitan statistical areas" category includes both micropolitan statistical areas and territory outside of metropolitan and micropolitan statistical areas. For more information, see <www.census.gov/programs-surveys/metro-micro/about/glossary.html>.

[7] Federal surveys now give respondents the option of reporting more than one race. Therefore, two basic ways of defining a race group are possible. A group such as Asian may be defined as those who reported Asian and no other race (the race-alone or single-race concept) or as those who reported Asian regardless of whether they also reported another race (the race-alone-or-in-combination concept). This table shows data using the first approach (race alone). The use of the single-race population does not imply that it is the preferred method of presenting or analyzing data. The Census Bureau uses a variety of approaches. Information on people who reported more than one race, such as White and American Indian and Alaska Native or Asian and Black or African American, is available from the 2010 Census through American FactFinder. About 2.9 percent of people reported more than one race in the 2010 Census. Data for American Indians and Alaska Natives, Native Hawaiians and Other Pacific Islanders, and those reporting two or more races are not shown separately.

Note: The estimates by type of coverage are not mutually exclusive; people can be covered by more than one type of health insurance during the year.

Source: U.S. Census Bureau, Current Population Survey, 2016 and 2017 Annual Social and Economic Supplements.

Table A-5.
Number of People Without Health Insurance Coverage by State: 2013 to 2016

(Numbers in thousands. Civilian noninstitutionalized population. For information on confidentiality protection, sampling error, nonsampling error, and definitions, see *www2.census.gov/programs-surveys/acs/tech_docs/accuracy/ACS_Accuracy_of_Data_2016.pdf*)

State	Medicaid expansion state? Yes (Y) or No (N)[1]	2013 uninsured Number	2013 uninsured Margin of error[2] (±)	2014 uninsured Number	2014 uninsured Margin of error[2] (±)	2015 uninsured Number	2015 uninsured Margin of error[2] (±)	2016 uninsured Number	2016 uninsured Margin of error[2] (±)	Difference in uninsured 2016 less 2015 Number	Difference 2016 less 2015 Margin of error[2] (±)	Difference 2016 less 2013 Number	Difference 2016 less 2013 Margin of error[2] (±)
United States	X	45,181	200	36,670	190	29,758	179	27,304	162	*–2,453	242	*–17,876	257
Alabama	N	645	17	579	17	484	16	435	14	*–49	21	*–210	22
Alaska	+Y	132	7	122	6	106	5	101	6	–5	8	*–31	10
Arizona	Y	1,118	24	903	18	728	21	681	21	*–47	30	*–437	32
Arkansas	Y	465	14	343	13	278	12	232	12	*–46	17	*–233	18
California	Y	6,500	57	4,767	47	3,317	34	2,844	41	*–473	53	*–3,656	70
Colorado	Y	729	18	543	16	433	15	410	14	*–23	21	*–319	23
Connecticut	Y	333	14	245	11	211	13	172	11	*–38	17	*–160	18
Delaware	Y	83	6	72	6	54	6	53	5	–1	7	*–30	7
District of Columbia	Y	42	4	34	4	25	4	26	4	1	6	*–16	6
Florida	N	3,853	43	3,245	43	2,662	40	2,544	47	*–117	62	*–1,309	64
Georgia	N	1,846	30	1,568	28	1,388	26	1,310	30	*–79	40	*–537	42
Hawaii	Y	91	6	72	5	55	4	49	5	–6	7	*–42	8
Idaho	N	257	12	219	11	180	10	168	8	–12	13	*–89	15
Illinois	Y	1,618	27	1,238	22	900	22	817	20	*–84	30	*–802	33
Indiana	+Y	903	19	776	22	628	17	530	17	*–97	24	*–373	25
Iowa	Y	248	9	189	8	155	8	132	8	*–23	11	*–116	11
Kansas	N	348	12	291	11	261	12	249	9	–12	15	*–99	15
Kentucky	Y	616	14	366	11	261	11	223	10	*–38	14	*–393	17
Louisiana	N	751	17	672	16	546	17	470	17	*–76	24	*–281	24
Maine	N	147	7	134	8	111	7	106	7	–5	10	*–41	10
Maryland	Y	593	17	463	16	389	11	363	16	*–26	19	*–230	23
Massachusetts	Y	247	10	219	8	189	9	171	10	*–18	14	*–76	15
Michigan	^Y	1,072	19	837	18	597	14	527	14	*–70	20	*–545	24
Minnesota	Y	440	14	317	12	245	11	225	10	*–20	15	*–215	17
Mississippi	N	500	16	424	14	372	12	346	12	*–25	17	*–154	20
Missouri	N	773	18	694	19	583	15	532	14	*–51	21	*–241	23
Montana	+Y	165	8	143	6	119	7	83	6	*–35	9	*–81	10
Nebraska	N	209	9	179	7	154	9	161	9	7	13	*–48	13
Nevada	Y	570	17	427	15	351	12	330	13	*–20	18	*–240	21
New Hampshire	^Y	140	7	120	7	83	6	78	6	–6	8	*–63	9
New Jersey	Y	1,160	22	965	19	771	22	705	19	*–66	29	*–455	29
New Mexico	Y	382	13	298	10	224	9	188	10	*–36	14	*–195	17
New York	Y	2,070	30	1,697	28	1,381	25	1,183	26	*–198	36	*–887	40
North Carolina	N	1,509	26	1,276	25	1,103	23	1,038	21	*–64	31	*–471	34
North Dakota	Y	73	6	57	5	57	5	52	5	–5	7	*–21	7
Ohio	Y	1,258	21	955	20	746	19	644	18	*–103	26	*–614	27
Oklahoma	N	666	13	584	11	533	12	530	13	–3	17	*–136	18
Oregon	Y	571	15	383	13	280	12	253	10	*–27	16	*–318	18
Pennsylvania	^Y	1,222	22	1,065	21	802	17	708	21	*–93	27	*–514	31
Rhode Island	Y	120	7	77	6	59	6	45	5	*–14	7	*–75	8
South Carolina	N	739	18	642	17	523	14	486	14	*–37	20	*–253	23
South Dakota	N	93	5	82	4	86	5	74	4	*–12	7	*–19	7
Tennessee	N	887	20	776	19	667	19	592	16	*–75	25	*–294	25
Texas	N	5,748	55	5,047	43	4,615	55	4,545	55	–70	78	*–1,203	78
Utah	N	402	13	366	13	311	14	265	12	*–47	18	*–137	18
Vermont	Y	45	4	31	3	24	2	23	2	–1	3	*–22	5
Virginia	N	991	22	884	22	746	23	715	21	*–31	31	*–276	31
Washington	Y	960	22	643	17	468	13	428	15	*–40	19	*–532	26
West Virginia	Y	255	10	156	8	108	6	96	6	*–12	9	*–159	12
Wisconsin	N	518	14	418	12	323	10	300	10	*–22	14	*–218	17
Wyoming	N	77	5	69	5	66	6	67	6	Z	8	*–11	8

* Statistically different from zero at the 90 percent confidence level.
^ Expanded Medicaid eligibility after January 1, 2014, and on or before January 1, 2015.
+ Expanded Medicaid eligibility after January 1, 2015, and on or before January 1, 2016.
X Not applicable.
Z Represents or rounds to zero.
[1] Medicaid expansion status as of January 1, 2016. For more information, see <www.medicaid.gov/medicaid/by-state/by-state.html>.
[2] Data are based on a sample and are subject to sampling variability. A margin of error is a measure of an estimate's variability. The larger the margin of error is in relation to the size of the estimate, the less reliable the estimate. This number, when added to and subtracted from the estimate, forms the 90 percent confidence interval.
Note: Differences are calculated with unrounded numbers, which may produce different results from using the rounded values in the table.
Source: U.S. Census Bureau, 2013 to 2016 1-Year American Community Surveys.

Population Without Health Insurance Coverage
The 25 Most Populous Metro Areas

2016　2015　2014　2013

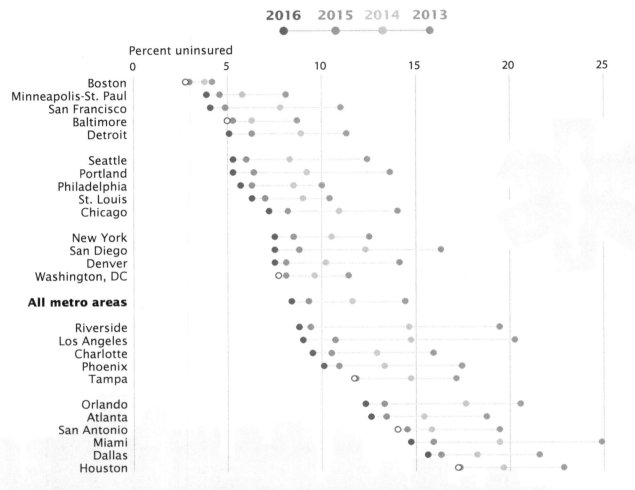

O Year-to-year change is not statistically different from zero at the 90 percent confidence level.

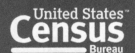

U.S. Department of Commerce
Economics and Statistics Administration
U.S. CENSUS BUREAU
census.gov

Source: 2013 to 2016 American Community Survey
www.census.gov/acs

State Statistics & Rankings

Covered by Some Type of Health Insurance

All Persons		Under 18 Years		Under 65 Years	
State	Percent	State	Percent	State	Percent
Massachusetts	97.5 (0.2)	Massachusetts	99.0 (0.2)	Massachusetts	97.1 (0.2)
Hawaii	96.5 (0.4)	Vermont	98.5 (0.4)	Hawaii	95.8 (0.5)
Vermont	96.3 (0.4)	Rhode Island	97.8 (0.6)	District of Columbia	95.7 (0.7)
District of Columbia	96.1 (0.6)	West Virginia	97.7 (0.5)	Vermont	95.5 (0.5)
Minnesota	95.9 (0.2)	Hawaii	97.5 (0.7)	Minnesota	95.2 (0.2)
Iowa	95.7 (0.2)	New York	97.5 (0.2)	Iowa	95.0 (0.3)
Rhode Island	95.7 (0.5)	Illinois	97.4 (0.2)	Rhode Island	94.9 (0.5)
Connecticut	95.1 (0.3)	Iowa	97.4 (0.4)	Connecticut	94.3 (0.4)
Kentucky	94.9 (0.2)	Alabama	97.3 (0.3)	Kentucky	94.0 (0.3)
West Virginia	94.7 (0.3)	New Hampshire	97.3 (0.6)	Wisconsin	93.8 (0.2)
Wisconsin	94.7 (0.2)	Washington	97.3 (0.3)	Michigan	93.7 (0.2)
Michigan	94.6 (0.1)	Connecticut	97.2 (0.5)	West Virginia	93.5 (0.4)
Ohio	94.4 (0.2)	California	96.9 (0.1)	Delaware	93.4 (0.6)
Pennsylvania	94.4 (0.2)	Delaware	96.9 (0.8)	Ohio	93.4 (0.2)
Delaware	94.3 (0.5)	District of Columbia	96.9 (1.3)	Pennsylvania	93.3 (0.2)
New Hampshire	94.1 (0.4)	Michigan	96.9 (0.2)	Washington	93.1 (0.2)
Washington	94.0 (0.2)	Kentucky	96.7 (0.4)	Maryland	93.0 (0.3)
Maryland	93.9 (0.3)	Louisiana	96.7 (0.4)	New York	93.0 (0.2)
New York	93.9 (0.1)	Maryland	96.6 (0.4)	New Hampshire	92.9 (0.5)
Oregon	93.8 (0.2)	Minnesota	96.6 (0.4)	Oregon	92.7 (0.3)
Illinois	93.5 (0.2)	Oregon	96.6 (0.5)	Illinois	92.6 (0.2)
North Dakota	93.0 (0.6)	New Jersey	96.3 (0.3)	North Dakota	91.9 (0.7)
California	92.7 (0.1)	Tennessee	96.3 (0.4)	California	91.7 (0.1)
Colorado	92.5 (0.3)	Wisconsin	96.3 (0.3)	Colorado	91.4 (0.3)
Arkansas	92.1 (0.4)	Ohio	96.2 (0.3)	New Jersey	90.8 (0.2)
Maine	92.0 (0.5)	Arkansas	96.0 (0.5)	Arkansas	90.7 (0.5)
New Jersey	92.0 (0.2)	Colorado	95.7 (0.4)	Indiana	90.6 (0.3)
Indiana	91.9 (0.3)	South Carolina	95.7 (0.4)	Utah	90.3 (0.4)
Montana	91.9 (0.5)	Pennsylvania	95.6 (0.3)	Montana	90.2 (0.7)
Nebraska	91.4 (0.5)	Kansas	95.5 (0.4)	Maine	90.1 (0.6)
United States	91.4 (0.1)	North Carolina	95.3 (0.3)	Nebraska	90.1 (0.6)
Kansas	91.3 (0.3)	South Dakota	95.3 (0.8)	United States	90.0 (0.1)
South Dakota	91.3 (0.5)	United States	95.3 (0.1)	Kansas	89.9 (0.4)
Virginia	91.3 (0.3)	Maine	95.2 (0.9)	Virginia	89.9 (0.3)
Utah	91.2 (0.4)	Mississippi	95.2 (0.6)	South Dakota	89.7 (0.6)
Missouri	91.1 (0.2)	Missouri	95.2 (0.4)	Missouri	89.5 (0.3)
Tennessee	91.0 (0.2)	Idaho	95.1 (0.8)	Tennessee	89.4 (0.3)
Alabama	90.9 (0.3)	Montana	95.1 (0.9)	Alabama	89.3 (0.4)
New Mexico	90.8 (0.5)	Virginia	95.0 (0.4)	New Mexico	89.2 (0.6)
Arizona	90.0 (0.3)	Nebraska	94.9 (0.7)	Idaho	88.2 (0.6)
South Carolina	90.0 (0.3)	New Mexico	94.7 (0.7)	Arizona	88.1 (0.4)
Idaho	89.9 (0.5)	Indiana	94.1 (0.5)	Louisiana	88.1 (0.4)
Louisiana	89.7 (0.4)	Utah	94.0 (0.6)	South Carolina	88.1 (0.3)
North Carolina	89.6 (0.2)	Florida	93.4 (0.4)	North Carolina	87.8 (0.2)
Nevada	88.6 (0.5)	Georgia	93.3 (0.5)	Nevada	86.9 (0.5)
Wyoming	88.5 (1.0)	Nevada	93.0 (0.7)	Wyoming	86.6 (1.2)
Mississippi	88.2 (0.4)	Arizona	92.4 (0.5)	Mississippi	86.1 (0.5)
Florida	87.5 (0.2)	Oklahoma	92.3 (0.5)	Georgia	85.2 (0.3)
Georgia	87.1 (0.3)	North Dakota	92.0 (1.2)	Florida	84.7 (0.3)
Oklahoma	86.2 (0.3)	Wyoming	91.2 (1.9)	Alaska	84.5 (1.0)
Alaska	86.0 (0.9)	Texas	90.2 (0.3)	Oklahoma	83.9 (0.4)
Texas	83.4 (0.2)	Alaska	89.7 (1.5)	Texas	81.4 (0.2)

Note: Numbers in thousands; Figures cover civilian noninstitutionalized population in 2016; N/A indicates that data was not available; Z represents or rounds to zero; Margin of error appears in parenthesis and is calculated using replicate weights.
Source: U.S. Census Bureau, American Community Survey, Table HIC-4_ACS. Health Insurance Coverage Status and Type of Coverage by State—All People: 2008 to 2016, Table HIC-5_ACS. Health Insurance Coverage Status and Type of Coverage by State—Children Under 18: 2008 to 2016, Table HIC-6_ACS. Health Insurance Coverage Status and Type of Coverage by State—Persons Under 65: 2008 to 2016

Covered by Private Health Insurance

All Persons		Under 18 Years		Under 65 Years	
State	**Percent**	**State**	**Percent**	**State**	**Percent**
North Dakota	80.5 *(1.0)*	Utah	77.6 *(1.0)*	North Dakota	81.3 *(1.1)*
Utah	78.7 *(0.6)*	North Dakota	75.6 *(1.7)*	Utah	80.5 *(0.6)*
Hawaii	77.2 *(0.7)*	Minnesota	71.6 *(0.7)*	Hawaii	78.8 *(0.9)*
Minnesota	76.8 *(0.4)*	New Hampshire	71.5 *(1.8)*	New Hampshire	78.0 *(1.0)*
Virginia	76.6 *(0.4)*	Virginia	71.1 *(0.7)*	Virginia	77.8 *(0.4)*
New Hampshire	76.5 *(0.9)*	Hawaii	70.9 *(1.6)*	Minnesota	77.6 *(0.4)*
Nebraska	76.0 *(0.8)*	Wyoming	70.9 *(3.2)*	Nebraska	77.6 *(0.9)*
Iowa	75.3 *(0.6)*	Massachusetts	69.8 *(0.8)*	Wisconsin	77.1 *(0.4)*
Wisconsin	75.2 *(0.4)*	Nebraska	69.1 *(1.4)*	Iowa	76.9 *(0.6)*
Kansas	75.1 *(0.6)*	Wisconsin	69.1 *(0.8)*	Kansas	76.5 *(0.7)*
Maryland	74.5 *(0.5)*	Kansas	68.7 *(1.1)*	Wyoming	75.4 *(1.6)*
Wyoming	74.1 *(1.4)*	Iowa	68.0 *(1.2)*	Massachusetts	75.2 *(0.5)*
Massachusetts	73.9 *(0.5)*	Rhode Island	67.6 *(2.3)*	Maryland	75.1 *(0.5)*
South Dakota	73.5 *(0.9)*	New Jersey	67.4 *(0.7)*	South Dakota	75.1 *(1.1)*
Pennsylvania	72.9 *(0.3)*	Maryland	66.7 *(1.1)*	New Jersey	73.9 *(0.4)*
New Jersey	72.3 *(0.4)*	Connecticut	66.0 *(1.2)*	Pennsylvania	73.8 *(0.4)*
Connecticut	71.9 *(0.5)*	South Dakota	65.8 *(2.0)*	Connecticut	73.7 *(0.6)*
Rhode Island	71.7 *(1.1)*	Maine	65.7 *(2.0)*	Rhode Island	73.6 *(1.2)*
Delaware	71.4 *(1.0)*	Missouri	65.2 *(0.9)*	Missouri	73.4 *(0.5)*
Washington	71.4 *(0.4)*	Delaware	64.5 *(2.0)*	Washington	72.4 *(0.4)*
Missouri	71.3 *(0.4)*	Pennsylvania	64.2 *(0.7)*	Delaware	72.1 *(1.1)*
Michigan	71.2 *(0.3)*	Colorado	63.8 *(0.9)*	Colorado	71.9 *(0.5)*
Indiana	70.8 *(0.4)*	Michigan	63.2 *(0.6)*	Indiana	71.8 *(0.5)*
Illinois	70.4 *(0.3)*	Washington	63.2 *(0.9)*	Illinois	71.7 *(0.3)*
Maine	70.3 *(0.9)*	Ohio	63.1 *(0.7)*	Maine	71.6 *(1.0)*
Colorado	70.2 *(0.4)*	Indiana	62.7 *(0.9)*	Idaho	71.5 *(1.0)*
Idaho	70.1 *(0.9)*	Illinois	62.4 *(0.7)*	Michigan	70.8 *(0.4)*
Ohio	69.5 *(0.4)*	Idaho	61.7 *(1.7)*	Ohio	70.8 *(0.4)*
District of Columbia	68.4 *(1.3)*	Oregon	61.5 *(1.2)*	Montana	69.9 *(1.0)*
Montana	68.4 *(0.9)*	New York	61.3 *(0.5)*	Oregon	69.3 *(0.6)*
Oregon	68.3 *(0.5)*	Alaska	61.1 *(2.2)*	United States	69.1 *(0.1)*
Vermont	68.2 *(1.4)*	Nevada	59.8 *(1.4)*	District of Columbia	68.9 *(1.4)*
Alabama	67.9 *(0.5)*	United States	59.8 *(0.2)*	Alabama	68.8 *(0.6)*
United States	67.8 *(0.1)*	Montana	59.5 *(1.9)*	Vermont	68.8 *(1.6)*
North Carolina	67.6 *(0.4)*	Vermont	57.8 *(2.9)*	North Carolina	68.4 *(0.4)*
Alaska	67.3 *(1.2)*	Tennessee	57.7 *(1.0)*	New York	68.0 *(0.3)*
South Carolina	66.7 *(0.5)*	Kentucky	57.3 *(1.2)*	Alaska	67.8 *(1.3)*
New York	66.6 *(0.3)*	North Carolina	56.0 *(0.8)*	Tennessee	67.6 *(0.5)*
Georgia	66.3 *(0.4)*	Georgia	55.9 *(0.8)*	South Carolina	67.5 *(0.6)*
Tennessee	66.3 *(0.5)*	South Carolina	55.9 *(1.1)*	Georgia	67.3 *(0.4)*
Kentucky	65.3 *(0.6)*	Alabama	55.8 *(1.1)*	Nevada	66.9 *(0.9)*
Nevada	64.7 *(0.8)*	Arizona	55.7 *(0.8)*	Kentucky	65.7 *(0.7)*
Oklahoma	64.0 *(0.5)*	California	55.5 *(0.4)*	Florida	65.0 *(0.4)*
California	63.0 *(0.2)*	West Virginia	53.4 *(1.9)*	California	64.9 *(0.2)*
Texas	62.8 *(0.3)*	Florida	53.3 *(0.6)*	Oklahoma	64.3 *(0.5)*
Florida	62.4 *(0.3)*	District of Columbia	52.9 *(3.1)*	Texas	63.9 *(0.3)*
West Virginia	62.3 *(0.9)*	Texas	52.3 *(0.6)*	Arizona	63.6 *(0.5)*
Arizona	62.2 *(0.4)*	Oklahoma	52.1 *(1.0)*	Arkansas	62.7 *(0.8)*
Arkansas	62.0 *(0.7)*	Louisiana	49.4 *(1.3)*	Louisiana	62.2 *(0.7)*
Louisiana	61.4 *(0.6)*	Arkansas	48.3 *(1.4)*	West Virginia	62.0 *(1.0)*
Mississippi	60.2 *(0.6)*	Mississippi	46.9 *(1.2)*	Mississippi	61.3 *(0.7)*
New Mexico	55.1 *(0.9)*	New Mexico	42.2 *(1.6)*	New Mexico	55.0 *(1.0)*

Note: Numbers in thousands; Figures cover civilian noninstitutionalized population in 2016; N/A indicates that data was not available; Z represents or rounds to zero; Margin of error appears in parenthesis and is calculated using replicate weights.
Source: U.S. Census Bureau, American Community Survey, Table HIC-4_ACS. Health Insurance Coverage Status and Type of Coverage by State—All People: 2008 to 2016, Table HIC-5_ACS. Health Insurance Coverage Status and Type of Coverage by State—Children Under 18: 2008 to 2016, Table HIC-6_ACS. Health Insurance Coverage Status and Type of Coverage by State—Persons Under 65: 2008 to 2016

Covered by Private Health Insurance: Employer-based

All Persons		Under 18 Years		Under 65 Years	
State	**Percent**	**State**	**Percent**	**State**	**Percent**
Utah	65.0 *(0.7)*	Utah	66.6 *(1.1)*	New Hampshire	69.0 *(1.1)*
New Hampshire	64.0 *(1.0)*	New Hampshire	66.2 *(1.8)*	Utah	68.5 *(0.7)*
Hawaii	63.8 *(0.9)*	Minnesota	64.3 *(0.8)*	Wisconsin	68.2 *(0.5)*
Massachusetts	63.0 *(0.5)*	Wisconsin	63.5 *(0.9)*	Minnesota	67.8 *(0.5)*
Maryland	62.8 *(0.5)*	Massachusetts	63.4 *(0.9)*	Iowa	67.0 *(0.7)*
New Jersey	62.0 *(0.4)*	North Dakota	61.7 *(2.2)*	Massachusetts	67.0 *(0.6)*
Minnesota	61.8 *(0.5)*	Iowa	61.1 *(1.3)*	North Dakota	66.9 *(1.4)*
Wisconsin	61.7 *(0.4)*	New Jersey	61.1 *(0.8)*	Hawaii	66.2 *(1.0)*
North Dakota	61.5 *(1.3)*	Wyoming	60.4 *(3.3)*	New Jersey	66.0 *(0.4)*
Connecticut	60.4 *(0.6)*	Rhode Island	60.2 *(2.4)*	Maryland	65.0 *(0.5)*
Delaware	60.3 *(1.2)*	Connecticut	59.5 *(1.3)*	Nebraska	64.8 *(1.0)*
Iowa	60.1 *(0.6)*	Nebraska	59.1 *(1.4)*	Connecticut	64.7 *(0.7)*
Michigan	59.9 *(0.3)*	Maryland	58.5 *(1.1)*	Pennsylvania	64.1 *(0.4)*
Virginia	59.7 *(0.5)*	Maine	58.0 *(2.2)*	Kansas	63.6 *(0.8)*
Ohio	59.2 *(0.4)*	Ohio	57.7 *(0.8)*	Ohio	63.5 *(0.4)*
Nebraska	58.9 *(0.8)*	Michigan	57.3 *(0.6)*	Delaware	63.4 *(1.4)*
Pennsylvania	58.7 *(0.4)*	Pennsylvania	57.3 *(0.7)*	Indiana	63.4 *(0.5)*
Indiana	58.6 *(0.5)*	Virginia	57.3 *(0.8)*	Virginia	63.4 *(0.5)*
Illinois	58.5 *(0.3)*	Kansas	57.2 *(1.3)*	Wyoming	63.4 *(1.9)*
Wyoming	58.5 *(1.5)*	Indiana	57.0 *(0.9)*	Rhode Island	63.1 *(1.5)*
Kansas	58.0 *(0.7)*	Delaware	56.9 *(2.3)*	Illinois	62.7 *(0.3)*
Rhode Island	57.5 *(1.3)*	Missouri	56.2 *(1.0)*	Missouri	62.4 *(0.5)*
District of Columbia	57.3 *(1.4)*	Illinois	55.8 *(0.6)*	Michigan	62.2 *(0.4)*
Missouri	57.2 *(0.5)*	Hawaii	55.6 *(1.9)*	Washington	61.2 *(0.5)*
Washington	57.2 *(0.4)*	South Dakota	54.1 *(2.3)*	South Dakota	60.9 *(1.4)*
New York	55.8 *(0.2)*	Oregon	53.3 *(1.3)*	Maine	60.4 *(1.1)*
Colorado	55.3 *(0.5)*	Washington	53.2 *(0.9)*	Colorado	59.2 *(0.5)*
Alaska	55.0 *(1.2)*	Colorado	52.4 *(0.9)*	Vermont	59.2 *(1.5)*
Maine	54.7 *(0.9)*	Nevada	51.7 *(1.5)*	New York	58.7 *(0.3)*
United States	54.7 *(0.1)*	New York	51.7 *(0.5)*	Oregon	58.6 *(0.7)*
South Dakota	54.4 *(1.2)*	Vermont	51.7 *(2.9)*	United States	58.6 *(0.1)*
Vermont	54.4 *(1.4)*	United States	51.4 *(0.2)*	District of Columbia	58.4 *(1.5)*
Alabama	53.5 *(0.5)*	Idaho	50.3 *(1.9)*	Alabama	57.2 *(0.6)*
Oregon	53.5 *(0.6)*	Kentucky	49.5 *(1.1)*	Nevada	57.1 *(0.9)*
Kentucky	53.4 *(0.6)*	Tennessee	48.9 *(0.9)*	Idaho	56.8 *(1.2)*
Georgia	52.7 *(0.4)*	West Virginia	48.9 *(1.8)*	Kentucky	56.8 *(0.6)*
West Virginia	52.7 *(0.8)*	Montana	48.8 *(1.8)*	Tennessee	56.7 *(0.5)*
Nevada	52.6 *(0.8)*	Alaska	48.0 *(2.5)*	West Virginia	55.8 *(0.9)*
Tennessee	52.2 *(0.4)*	California	47.6 *(0.4)*	Alaska	55.7 *(1.3)*
Idaho	51.7 *(1.0)*	Alabama	47.5 *(1.1)*	Georgia	55.7 *(0.4)*
South Carolina	51.6 *(0.6)*	Arizona	47.0 *(0.8)*	South Carolina	55.6 *(0.6)*
North Carolina	51.3 *(0.4)*	South Carolina	46.7 *(1.1)*	Montana	55.1 *(1.1)*
California	51.2 *(0.2)*	Georgia	46.6 *(0.8)*	North Carolina	54.9 *(0.4)*
Texas	50.9 *(0.3)*	North Carolina	44.9 *(0.8)*	California	54.4 *(0.2)*
Oklahoma	49.8 *(0.5)*	District of Columbia	44.7 *(3.4)*	Texas	53.7 *(0.3)*
Montana	49.4 *(0.9)*	Texas	44.3 *(0.5)*	Arizona	53.2 *(0.5)*
Louisiana	48.8 *(0.7)*	Oklahoma	42.9 *(1.0)*	Oklahoma	53.1 *(0.5)*
Arizona	48.7 *(0.4)*	Florida	41.9 *(0.5)*	Arkansas	52.0 *(0.8)*
Arkansas	47.6 *(0.7)*	Louisiana	41.5 *(1.4)*	Louisiana	51.6 *(0.8)*
Mississippi	46.8 *(0.6)*	Arkansas	41.4 *(1.4)*	Mississippi	51.1 *(0.7)*
Florida	44.9 *(0.3)*	Mississippi	38.9 *(1.0)*	Florida	49.7 *(0.3)*
New Mexico	43.7 *(1.0)*	New Mexico	35.7 *(1.7)*	New Mexico	45.9 *(1.1)*

Note: Numbers in thousands; Figures cover civilian noninstitutionalized population in 2016; N/A indicates that data was not available; Z represents or rounds to zero; Margin of error appears in parenthesis and is calculated using replicate weights.
Source: U.S. Census Bureau, American Community Survey, Table HIC-4_ACS. Health Insurance Coverage Status and Type of Coverage by State—All People: 2008 to 2016, Table HIC-5_ACS. Health Insurance Coverage Status and Type of Coverage by State—Children Under 18: 2008 to 2016, Table HIC-6_ACS. Health Insurance Coverage Status and Type of Coverage by State—Persons Under 65: 2008 to 2016

Covered by Private Health Insurance: Direct Purchase

All Persons		Under 18 Years		Under 65 Years	
State	**Percent**	**State**	**Percent**	**State**	**Percent**
North Dakota	20.4 *(0.8)*	North Dakota	12.9 *(1.5)*	Idaho	15.3 *(0.7)*
South Dakota	19.6 *(0.9)*	South Dakota	11.7 *(1.4)*	North Dakota	15.3 *(0.8)*
Idaho	19.2 *(0.6)*	Idaho	10.9 *(1.2)*	Florida	14.9 *(0.2)*
Montana	19.0 *(0.7)*	Utah	10.9 *(0.8)*	South Dakota	14.6 *(1.0)*
Nebraska	18.1 *(0.5)*	New York	10.4 *(0.3)*	Montana	14.4 *(0.7)*
Florida	17.6 *(0.2)*	Florida	10.0 *(0.3)*	Nebraska	13.5 *(0.5)*
Kansas	17.5 *(0.5)*	Nebraska	10.0 *(0.8)*	Kansas	12.6 *(0.6)*
Iowa	17.1 *(0.4)*	Kansas	9.7 *(0.9)*	Utah	12.6 *(0.5)*
Minnesota	17.0 *(0.3)*	Wyoming	9.5 *(2.0)*	North Carolina	12.5 *(0.2)*
Rhode Island	16.4 *(0.8)*	Colorado	9.0 *(0.5)*	Virginia	12.5 *(0.3)*
Maine	16.3 *(0.6)*	Virginia	9.0 *(0.4)*	Rhode Island	12.1 *(0.8)*
Oregon	16.3 *(0.3)*	Oregon	8.9 *(0.6)*	Wyoming	12.0 *(1.2)*
Wyoming	16.3 *(1.0)*	Montana	8.8 *(1.1)*	Colorado	11.7 *(0.3)*
Pennsylvania	16.2 *(0.2)*	Missouri	8.4 *(0.5)*	Oregon	11.7 *(0.4)*
North Carolina	16.1 *(0.2)*	Arizona	8.2 *(0.5)*	Alabama	11.5 *(0.4)*
Virginia	15.7 *(0.3)*	North Carolina	8.0 *(0.4)*	Maine	11.5 *(0.6)*
Vermont	15.5 *(0.8)*	Rhode Island	8.0 *(1.3)*	Missouri	11.5 *(0.4)*
Missouri	15.2 *(0.3)*	Minnesota	7.8 *(0.4)*	Iowa	11.4 *(0.4)*
Wisconsin	15.2 *(0.3)*	Hawaii	7.7 *(0.8)*	District of Columbia	11.3 *(0.8)*
Alabama	14.9 *(0.3)*	Tennessee	7.7 *(0.5)*	Georgia	11.1 *(0.3)*
South Carolina	14.8 *(0.3)*	United States	7.7 *(0.1)*	Minnesota	11.1 *(0.3)*
Arkansas	14.7 *(0.4)*	California	7.6 *(0.2)*	South Carolina	11.1 *(0.3)*
Tennessee	14.6 *(0.3)*	Oklahoma	7.6 *(0.4)*	California	11.0 *(0.1)*
Utah	14.5 *(0.5)*	Washington	7.6 *(0.5)*	Pennsylvania	11.0 *(0.2)*
Colorado	14.2 *(0.3)*	Pennsylvania	7.5 *(0.3)*	Tennessee	10.9 *(0.3)*
United States	14.1 *(0.1)*	Iowa	7.4 *(0.5)*	United States	10.9 *(0.1)*
Washington	14.1 *(0.2)*	Massachusetts	7.4 *(0.4)*	New York	10.8 *(0.2)*
Indiana	14.0 *(0.3)*	Georgia	7.3 *(0.4)*	Vermont	10.8 *(0.8)*
Oklahoma	14.0 *(0.3)*	Maine	7.3 *(0.9)*	Arkansas	10.7 *(0.4)*
Arizona	13.9 *(0.3)*	Nevada	7.3 *(0.8)*	Louisiana	10.7 *(0.4)*
Illinois	13.9 *(0.2)*	Maryland	7.2 *(0.5)*	Oklahoma	10.6 *(0.3)*
Michigan	13.7 *(0.2)*	District of Columbia	7.0 *(1.5)*	Arizona	10.4 *(0.3)*
New Hampshire	13.7 *(0.6)*	Texas	7.0 *(0.2)*	Washington	10.4 *(0.3)*
Georgia	13.5 *(0.3)*	New Jersey	6.9 *(0.4)*	Illinois	10.3 *(0.2)*
Massachusetts	13.5 *(0.3)*	Alabama	6.8 *(0.5)*	Maryland	10.2 *(0.3)*
Connecticut	13.2 *(0.3)*	Illinois	6.8 *(0.3)*	Texas	10.2 *(0.2)*
Louisiana	13.2 *(0.4)*	Louisiana	6.8 *(0.6)*	Massachusetts	10.1 *(0.3)*
Mississippi	13.0 *(0.4)*	Delaware	6.6 *(1.4)*	Wisconsin	10.0 *(0.3)*
New York	13.0 *(0.2)*	Mississippi	6.6 *(0.7)*	Connecticut	9.8 *(0.3)*
Maryland	12.9 *(0.3)*	Connecticut	6.4 *(0.5)*	Mississippi	9.8 *(0.4)*
Delaware	12.8 *(0.7)*	Kentucky	6.3 *(0.5)*	New Hampshire	9.8 *(0.6)*
California	12.7 *(0.1)*	Michigan	6.3 *(0.4)*	Hawaii	9.7 *(0.6)*
District of Columbia	12.6 *(0.7)*	South Carolina	6.3 *(0.5)*	Michigan	9.7 *(0.2)*
Kentucky	12.4 *(0.3)*	Indiana	6.2 *(0.4)*	Indiana	9.6 *(0.3)*
New Jersey	12.4 *(0.2)*	Arkansas	6.1 *(0.6)*	Nevada	9.6 *(0.5)*
Hawaii	12.2 *(0.6)*	Vermont	6.0 *(1.1)*	Delaware	9.2 *(0.8)*
Ohio	12.1 *(0.2)*	Wisconsin	5.7 *(0.4)*	New Jersey	9.2 *(0.2)*
Texas	12.1 *(0.2)*	New Hampshire	5.6 *(0.8)*	Kentucky	8.6 *(0.3)*
Nevada	11.9 *(0.5)*	Ohio	5.4 *(0.3)*	New Mexico	8.3 *(0.5)*
West Virginia	10.9 *(0.5)*	New Mexico	4.8 *(0.6)*	Ohio	8.2 *(0.2)*
New Mexico	10.8 *(0.4)*	West Virginia	4.7 *(0.7)*	Alaska	7.0 *(0.7)*
Alaska	7.8 *(0.7)*	Alaska	4.4 *(0.9)*	West Virginia	6.9 *(0.5)*

Note: Numbers in thousands; Figures cover civilian noninstitutionalized population in 2016; N/A indicates that data was not available; Z represents or rounds to zero; Margin of error appears in parenthesis and is calculated using replicate weights.
Source: U.S. Census Bureau, American Community Survey, Table HIC-4_ACS. Health Insurance Coverage Status and Type of Coverage by State—All People: 2008 to 2016, Table HIC-5_ACS. Health Insurance Coverage Status and Type of Coverage by State—Children Under 18: 2008 to 2016, Table HIC-6_ACS. Health Insurance Coverage Status and Type of Coverage by State—Persons Under 65: 2008 to 2016

Covered by Private Health Insurance: TRICARE

All Persons		Under 18 Years		Under 65 Years	
State	Percent	State	Percent	State	Percent
Alaska	9.8 *(0.9)*	Hawaii	13.9 *(1.2)*	Alaska	9.7 *(1.0)*
Hawaii	9.1 *(0.5)*	Alaska	12.4 *(1.8)*	Hawaii	9.2 *(0.6)*
Virginia	7.8 *(0.2)*	Virginia	8.5 *(0.4)*	Virginia	7.0 *(0.2)*
South Carolina	5.3 *(0.3)*	South Carolina	5.0 *(0.5)*	South Carolina	4.1 *(0.3)*
North Carolina	4.6 *(0.1)*	North Carolina	4.9 *(0.3)*	North Carolina	3.9 *(0.2)*
Alabama	4.5 *(0.2)*	Washington	4.6 *(0.4)*	South Dakota	3.8 *(0.5)*
Washington	4.4 *(0.2)*	Kansas	4.4 *(0.4)*	Washington	3.8 *(0.2)*
South Dakota	4.2 *(0.4)*	North Dakota	4.2 *(1.1)*	Kansas	3.6 *(0.2)*
Colorado	4.1 *(0.2)*	South Dakota	4.2 *(0.8)*	Georgia	3.5 *(0.2)*
Kansas	4.1 *(0.2)*	Colorado	4.1 *(0.3)*	Alabama	3.4 *(0.3)*
New Mexico	4.1 *(0.4)*	Georgia	3.9 *(0.3)*	Colorado	3.4 *(0.2)*
Georgia	4.0 *(0.1)*	Alabama	3.5 *(0.4)*	North Dakota	3.4 *(0.6)*
Mississippi	3.9 *(0.3)*	Maryland	3.4 *(0.4)*	Montana	3.2 *(0.4)*
Montana	3.9 *(0.4)*	Montana	3.4 *(0.7)*	New Mexico	3.2 *(0.4)*
Oklahoma	3.9 *(0.2)*	New Mexico	3.3 *(0.6)*	Maryland	3.1 *(0.2)*
Nevada	3.7 *(0.2)*	Oklahoma	3.3 *(0.4)*	Oklahoma	3.1 *(0.2)*
North Dakota	3.7 *(0.6)*	Wyoming	3.2 *(1.0)*	Mississippi	2.9 *(0.3)*
Maryland	3.6 *(0.2)*	Florida	3.0 *(0.2)*	Wyoming	2.8 *(0.5)*
Florida	3.5 *(0.1)*	Mississippi	3.0 *(0.5)*	Florida	2.7 *(0.1)*
Arkansas	3.4 *(0.2)*	Tennessee	2.9 *(0.3)*	Nevada	2.7 *(0.2)*
Maine	3.4 *(0.3)*	Kentucky	2.7 *(0.3)*	Tennessee	2.6 *(0.2)*
Tennessee	3.4 *(0.1)*	Nebraska	2.7 *(0.4)*	Nebraska	2.5 *(0.3)*
Wyoming	3.3 *(0.5)*	Idaho	2.6 *(0.5)*	Kentucky	2.4 *(0.2)*
Idaho	3.2 *(0.3)*	Nevada	2.6 *(0.4)*	Arkansas	2.3 *(0.2)*
Arizona	3.1 *(0.1)*	Delaware	2.5 *(0.9)*	Delaware	2.3 *(0.5)*
Delaware	3.1 *(0.4)*	Texas	2.5 *(0.1)*	Idaho	2.3 *(0.3)*
Nebraska	3.1 *(0.2)*	Maine	2.4 *(0.6)*	Texas	2.3 *(0.1)*
Kentucky	3.0 *(0.2)*	United States	2.4 *(Z)*	Arizona	2.2 *(0.1)*
Texas	3.0 *(0.1)*	Louisiana	2.3 *(0.3)*	Maine	2.1 *(0.4)*
United States	2.7 *(Z)*	Arizona	2.2 *(0.2)*	United States	2.1 *(Z)*
Louisiana	2.6 *(0.1)*	District of Columbia	2.2 *(0.7)*	Louisiana	2.0 *(0.1)*
Missouri	2.5 *(0.1)*	Arkansas	2.1 *(0.4)*	Missouri	1.9 *(0.1)*
New Hampshire	2.4 *(0.3)*	Missouri	2.0 *(0.2)*	Utah	1.8 *(0.2)*
Utah	2.4 *(0.2)*	Utah	2.0 *(0.3)*	District of Columbia	1.7 *(0.3)*
West Virginia	2.3 *(0.2)*	California	1.7 *(0.1)*	West Virginia	1.6 *(0.2)*
District of Columbia	2.0 *(0.3)*	Vermont	1.6 *(0.6)*	California	1.4 *(0.1)*
Oregon	2.0 *(0.1)*	Ohio	1.4 *(0.2)*	New Hampshire	1.4 *(0.3)*
California	1.8 *(0.1)*	West Virginia	1.4 *(0.4)*	Vermont	1.4 *(0.3)*
Vermont	1.8 *(0.3)*	Iowa	1.3 *(0.3)*	Iowa	1.3 *(0.2)*
Iowa	1.7 *(0.2)*	Rhode Island	1.3 *(0.5)*	Rhode Island	1.3 *(0.3)*
Rhode Island	1.7 *(0.3)*	Wisconsin	1.3 *(0.2)*	Ohio	1.2 *(0.1)*
Ohio	1.6 *(0.1)*	Connecticut	1.2 *(0.3)*	Oregon	1.2 *(0.1)*
Indiana	1.5 *(0.1)*	New Hampshire	1.2 *(0.4)*	Indiana	1.1 *(0.1)*
Minnesota	1.5 *(0.1)*	Indiana	1.1 *(0.2)*	Wisconsin	1.1 *(0.1)*
Pennsylvania	1.5 *(0.1)*	Oregon	1.1 *(0.3)*	Connecticut	1.0 *(0.1)*
Wisconsin	1.5 *(0.1)*	Minnesota	1.0 *(0.2)*	Minnesota	1.0 *(0.1)*
Connecticut	1.3 *(0.1)*	Pennsylvania	1.0 *(0.1)*	Pennsylvania	1.0 *(0.1)*
Michigan	1.3 *(0.1)*	Illinois	0.9 *(0.1)*	Michigan	0.9 *(0.1)*
Massachusetts	1.2 *(0.1)*	Massachusetts	0.9 *(0.2)*	Illinois	0.8 *(0.1)*
Illinois	1.1 *(0.1)*	New Jersey	0.9 *(0.1)*	Massachusetts	0.8 *(0.1)*
New Jersey	1.0 *(0.1)*	Michigan	0.8 *(0.1)*	New Jersey	0.7 *(0.1)*
New York	0.9 *(Z)*	New York	0.8 *(0.1)*	New York	0.7 *(Z)*

Note: Numbers in thousands; Figures cover civilian noninstitutionalized population in 2016; N/A indicates that data was not available; Z represents or rounds to zero; Margin of error appears in parenthesis and is calculated using replicate weights.
Source: U.S. Census Bureau, American Community Survey, Table HIC-4_ACS. Health Insurance Coverage Status and Type of Coverage by State—All People: 2008 to 2016, Table HIC-5_ACS. Health Insurance Coverage Status and Type of Coverage by State—Children Under 18: 2008 to 2016, Table HIC-6_ACS. Health Insurance Coverage Status and Type of Coverage by State—Persons Under 65: 2008 to 2016

Covered by Public Health Insurance

All Persons		Under 18 Years		Under 65 Years	
State	**Percent**	**State**	**Percent**	**State**	**Percent**
West Virginia	48.4 (0.7)	New Mexico	56.8 (1.5)	New Mexico	38.7 (1.0)
New Mexico	48.2 (0.9)	Arkansas	52.0 (1.3)	West Virginia	37.0 (0.9)
Arkansas	43.2 (0.5)	Mississippi	52.0 (1.2)	Kentucky	33.2 (0.7)
Kentucky	43.0 (0.5)	Louisiana	51.6 (1.3)	Arkansas	32.8 (0.6)
Vermont	42.7 (1.2)	West Virginia	50.0 (2.0)	Vermont	30.9 (1.5)
Oregon	39.8 (0.5)	District of Columbia	48.2 (3.4)	California	30.1 (0.2)
Arizona	39.7 (0.4)	Vermont	45.8 (2.9)	Louisiana	30.1 (0.6)
Louisiana	39.6 (0.5)	California	45.3 (0.4)	District of Columbia	30.0 (1.4)
Mississippi	39.4 (0.5)	Alabama	44.8 (1.1)	New York	29.3 (0.3)
New York	39.2 (0.2)	Oklahoma	44.8 (0.9)	Mississippi	29.2 (0.6)
California	38.9 (0.2)	South Carolina	44.1 (1.1)	Oregon	28.4 (0.6)
Michigan	38.7 (0.3)	Kentucky	43.8 (1.2)	Arizona	28.1 (0.5)
Montana	37.8 (0.8)	Florida	43.5 (0.6)	Michigan	27.4 (0.3)
Florida	37.6 (0.2)	Tennessee	43.2 (0.9)	Ohio	26.4 (0.4)
Ohio	37.6 (0.3)	North Carolina	42.8 (0.8)	Tennessee	26.3 (0.5)
Rhode Island	37.4 (1.0)	New York	41.8 (0.5)	Rhode Island	26.0 (1.2)
Tennessee	37.3 (0.4)	Georgia	40.8 (0.8)	Massachusetts	25.9 (0.5)
South Carolina	37.2 (0.4)	Oregon	40.6 (1.2)	Alabama	25.3 (0.5)
Delaware	37.1 (1.0)	Arizona	40.5 (1.0)	Washington	25.3 (0.4)
District of Columbia	37.1 (1.2)	Texas	40.5 (0.5)	South Carolina	25.1 (0.5)
Alabama	36.9 (0.4)	Montana	39.6 (2.0)	Montana	24.9 (0.9)
Massachusetts	36.5 (0.4)	United States	39.6 (0.2)	Delaware	24.6 (1.2)
Maine	36.4 (0.7)	Washington	39.3 (0.9)	United States	24.6 (0.1)
Pennsylvania	36.4 (0.3)	Michigan	38.9 (0.6)	Pennsylvania	24.0 (0.3)
Washington	35.8 (0.3)	Illinois	38.2 (0.7)	Nevada	23.8 (0.8)
United States	35.4 (0.1)	Idaho	38.0 (2.1)	Connecticut	23.7 (0.6)
Connecticut	35.0 (0.5)	Ohio	38.0 (0.7)	Illinois	23.7 (0.3)
North Carolina	34.7 (0.3)	Pennsylvania	37.1 (0.7)	Oklahoma	23.7 (0.4)
Iowa	34.6 (0.5)	Delaware	36.7 (2.2)	North Carolina	23.4 (0.3)
Oklahoma	34.6 (0.4)	Nevada	36.7 (1.5)	Florida	23.2 (0.3)
Nevada	34.5 (0.7)	Rhode Island	36.7 (2.1)	Colorado	23.1 (0.4)
Hawaii	34.1 (0.7)	Colorado	35.6 (0.9)	Iowa	22.7 (0.6)
Illinois	34.0 (0.3)	Iowa	35.5 (1.3)	Indiana	22.4 (0.4)
Indiana	33.3 (0.3)	Indiana	35.3 (0.8)	Maine	22.4 (0.9)
Wisconsin	33.0 (0.3)	Connecticut	35.1 (1.3)	Alaska	21.8 (0.9)
Colorado	32.8 (0.4)	Massachusetts	34.3 (0.9)	Minnesota	21.7 (0.3)
Minnesota	32.8 (0.3)	Alaska	33.9 (2.0)	Georgia	21.6 (0.3)
Idaho	32.6 (0.8)	Maine	33.8 (1.9)	Hawaii	21.4 (0.8)
Maryland	31.9 (0.4)	South Dakota	33.5 (2.0)	Maryland	21.4 (0.5)
Missouri	31.5 (0.3)	Maryland	33.3 (1.0)	Idaho	21.1 (0.9)
Georgia	31.3 (0.3)	Wisconsin	32.8 (0.9)	Wisconsin	20.9 (0.4)
New Hampshire	31.3 (0.7)	Missouri	32.7 (0.9)	Texas	20.3 (0.2)
New Jersey	31.1 (0.3)	New Jersey	32.0 (0.7)	New Jersey	19.7 (0.3)
South Dakota	31.0 (0.8)	Kansas	31.5 (1.2)	Missouri	19.3 (0.3)
Alaska	29.4 (0.9)	Hawaii	31.4 (1.6)	South Dakota	18.8 (1.0)
Kansas	29.2 (0.5)	Minnesota	30.4 (0.6)	New Hampshire	18.2 (0.8)
Texas	29.2 (0.2)	New Hampshire	28.9 (1.6)	Kansas	17.4 (0.5)
Virginia	27.5 (0.3)	Nebraska	28.5 (1.3)	Virginia	15.7 (0.3)
Nebraska	27.3 (0.5)	Virginia	26.8 (0.7)	Nebraska	15.4 (0.6)
Wyoming	27.3 (0.9)	Wyoming	24.4 (2.3)	Wyoming	15.1 (1.1)
North Dakota	26.0 (0.8)	North Dakota	21.2 (1.8)	North Dakota	14.3 (0.9)
Utah	21.5 (0.4)	Utah	19.6 (0.9)	Utah	12.9 (0.5)

Note: Numbers in thousands; Figures cover civilian noninstitutionalized population in 2016; N/A indicates that data was not available; Z represents or rounds to zero; Margin of error appears in parenthesis and is calculated using replicate weights.

Source: U.S. Census Bureau, American Community Survey, Table HIC-4_ACS. Health Insurance Coverage Status and Type of Coverage by State—All People: 2008 to 2016, Table HIC-5_ACS. Health Insurance Coverage Status and Type of Coverage by State—Children Under 18: 2008 to 2016, Table HIC-6_ACS. Health Insurance Coverage Status and Type of Coverage by State—Persons Under 65: 2008 to 2016

Covered by Public Health Insurance: Medicaid

All Persons		Under 18 Years		Under 65 Years	
State	Percent	State	Percent	State	Percent
New Mexico	32.5 (0.8)	New Mexico	56.6 (1.5)	New Mexico	35.8 (0.9)
West Virginia	28.8 (0.8)	Arkansas	51.6 (1.3)	West Virginia	32.6 (0.9)
District of Columbia	28.3 (1.3)	Mississippi	51.5 (1.2)	Kentucky	29.3 (0.6)
California	27.3 (0.2)	Louisiana	51.1 (1.3)	Arkansas	28.9 (0.6)
Kentucky	26.7 (0.5)	West Virginia	49.6 (2.0)	Vermont	28.7 (1.5)
Arkansas	26.6 (0.5)	District of Columbia	47.9 (3.4)	District of Columbia	28.5 (1.4)
New York	26.3 (0.2)	Vermont	45.7 (2.9)	California	28.3 (0.2)
Vermont	26.2 (1.2)	California	44.7 (0.4)	New York	27.5 (0.3)
Louisiana	25.5 (0.5)	Alabama	44.3 (1.1)	Louisiana	27.1 (0.5)
Mississippi	24.6 (0.5)	South Carolina	43.7 (1.1)	Oregon	25.7 (0.7)
Massachusetts	23.5 (0.4)	Kentucky	43.2 (1.2)	Arizona	25.6 (0.5)
Arizona	23.3 (0.4)	Florida	43.0 (0.6)	Mississippi	25.6 (0.6)
Oregon	23.3 (0.6)	Oklahoma	42.9 (1.0)	Michigan	24.9 (0.3)
Michigan	22.8 (0.3)	Tennessee	42.9 (0.9)	Massachusetts	24.6 (0.5)
Rhode Island	22.1 (1.1)	North Carolina	42.2 (0.8)	Ohio	23.6 (0.4)
Tennessee	21.6 (0.4)	New York	41.5 (0.5)	Rhode Island	23.4 (1.2)
Ohio	21.4 (0.3)	Arizona	40.3 (1.0)	Tennessee	23.1 (0.4)
Washington	21.1 (0.4)	Oregon	40.3 (1.2)	Washington	22.7 (0.4)
United States	20.9 (0.1)	Texas	40.2 (0.5)	Delaware	22.1 (1.1)
Connecticut	20.5 (0.5)	Georgia	39.9 (0.8)	United States	22.1 (0.1)
Delaware	20.3 (1.0)	Montana	39.3 (2.0)	Connecticut	21.8 (0.6)
Illinois	20.2 (0.3)	United States	39.1 (0.2)	Illinois	21.7 (0.3)
Alabama	20.1 (0.4)	Washington	39.0 (0.9)	Montana	21.5 (0.8)
Pennsylvania	19.9 (0.3)	Michigan	38.7 (0.6)	Pennsylvania	21.5 (0.3)
South Carolina	19.9 (0.4)	Illinois	37.9 (0.7)	South Carolina	21.3 (0.5)
Montana	19.8 (0.7)	Idaho	37.8 (2.0)	Alabama	21.0 (0.4)
Nevada	19.6 (0.6)	Ohio	37.6 (0.8)	Nevada	21.0 (0.8)
Colorado	19.4 (0.4)	Pennsylvania	36.8 (0.7)	Colorado	20.7 (0.4)
Maine	19.2 (0.7)	Nevada	36.5 (1.5)	Iowa	20.7 (0.6)
Iowa	19.1 (0.5)	Delaware	36.4 (2.2)	Florida	20.2 (0.3)
Florida	19.0 (0.2)	Rhode Island	36.2 (2.1)	North Carolina	19.8 (0.3)
North Carolina	18.7 (0.3)	Colorado	35.2 (0.9)	Maine	19.7 (0.9)
Alaska	18.3 (0.9)	Iowa	35.2 (1.3)	Minnesota	19.7 (0.3)
Oklahoma	18.2 (0.4)	Connecticut	35.0 (1.3)	Indiana	19.6 (0.4)
Indiana	18.1 (0.3)	Indiana	35.0 (0.8)	Oklahoma	19.3 (0.4)
Minnesota	18.1 (0.3)	Massachusetts	34.2 (0.8)	Maryland	19.1 (0.5)
Georgia	18.0 (0.3)	Alaska	33.7 (2.1)	Hawaii	18.8 (0.8)
Maryland	18.0 (0.4)	Maine	33.5 (1.9)	Wisconsin	18.8 (0.4)
Wisconsin	17.8 (0.3)	South Dakota	33.0 (2.0)	Alaska	18.6 (0.9)
Hawaii	17.7 (0.7)	Maryland	32.7 (1.0)	Idaho	18.5 (0.9)
Idaho	17.6 (0.8)	Wisconsin	32.6 (0.9)	Georgia	18.4 (0.3)
Texas	17.5 (0.2)	Missouri	32.2 (0.8)	New Jersey	18.0 (0.3)
New Jersey	17.2 (0.3)	New Jersey	31.7 (0.7)	Texas	17.9 (0.2)
South Dakota	14.8 (0.8)	Hawaii	31.1 (1.6)	Missouri	15.7 (0.4)
Missouri	14.7 (0.3)	Kansas	31.1 (1.2)	South Dakota	15.6 (0.9)
Kansas	14.1 (0.4)	Minnesota	30.3 (0.6)	New Hampshire	15.0 (0.7)
New Hampshire	13.8 (0.6)	New Hampshire	28.5 (1.5)	Kansas	14.8 (0.5)
Nebraska	13.0 (0.5)	Nebraska	28.2 (1.3)	Nebraska	13.3 (0.6)
Wyoming	12.1 (0.9)	Virginia	25.9 (0.7)	Wyoming	12.4 (1.0)
North Dakota	11.6 (0.7)	Wyoming	24.3 (2.3)	Virginia	12.1 (0.3)
Virginia	11.6 (0.3)	North Dakota	20.8 (1.8)	North Dakota	12.0 (0.9)
Utah	11.3 (0.4)	Utah	19.5 (0.9)	Utah	11.4 (0.4)

Note: Numbers in thousands; Figures cover civilian noninstitutionalized population in 2016; N/A indicates that data was not available; Z represents or rounds to zero; Margin of error appears in parenthesis and is calculated using replicate weights.
Source: U.S. Census Bureau, American Community Survey, Table HIC-4_ACS. Health Insurance Coverage Status and Type of Coverage by State—All People: 2008 to 2016, Table HIC-5_ACS. Health Insurance Coverage Status and Type of Coverage by State—Children Under 18: 2008 to 2016, Table HIC-6_ACS. Health Insurance Coverage Status and Type of Coverage by State—Persons Under 65: 2008 to 2016

Covered by Public Health Insurance: Medicare

All Persons		Under 18 Years		Under 65 Years	
State	**Percent**	**State**	**Percent**	**State**	**Percent**
West Virginia	22.9 (0.3)	Oklahoma	2.2 (0.3)	West Virginia	5.8 (0.4)
Maine	22.1 (0.4)	Georgia	1.1 (0.2)	Alabama	5.1 (0.2)
Florida	21.6 (0.1)	California	1.0 (0.1)	Kentucky	5.0 (0.2)
Vermont	20.5 (0.4)	Kentucky	1.0 (0.2)	Arkansas	4.8 (0.2)
Montana	20.0 (0.3)	Rhode Island	0.9 (0.4)	Maine	4.7 (0.4)
Alabama	19.8 (0.2)	Louisiana	0.8 (0.2)	Mississippi	4.7 (0.2)
Arkansas	19.8 (0.2)	Maryland	0.8 (0.2)	Louisiana	4.2 (0.2)
South Carolina	19.6 (0.2)	North Dakota	0.8 (0.4)	Oklahoma	4.1 (0.1)
Delaware	19.3 (0.4)	Delaware	0.7 (0.4)	Rhode Island	4.1 (0.4)
Kentucky	19.2 (0.2)	Maine	0.7 (0.3)	Missouri	4.0 (0.2)
Pennsylvania	19.2 (0.1)	New York	0.7 (0.1)	South Carolina	4.0 (0.2)
Rhode Island	19.0 (0.3)	Ohio	0.7 (0.1)	Tennessee	3.9 (0.1)
New Hampshire	18.9 (0.3)	Virginia	0.7 (0.2)	Michigan	3.8 (0.1)
Michigan	18.8 (0.1)	Alabama	0.6 (0.2)	Vermont	3.8 (0.4)
Missouri	18.7 (0.1)	Arkansas	0.6 (0.2)	North Carolina	3.7 (0.1)
New Mexico	18.7 (0.3)	Florida	0.6 (0.1)	New Mexico	3.6 (0.3)
Mississippi	18.6 (0.2)	Indiana	0.6 (0.1)	Indiana	3.5 (0.1)
Oregon	18.6 (0.2)	Mississippi	0.6 (0.2)	Montana	3.5 (0.4)
Arizona	18.5 (0.1)	Missouri	0.6 (0.2)	New Hampshire	3.4 (0.3)
Tennessee	18.4 (0.1)	North Carolina	0.6 (0.1)	Ohio	3.4 (0.1)
Ohio	18.3 (0.1)	United States	0.6 (Z)	Florida	3.3 (0.1)
North Carolina	18.1 (0.1)	West Virginia	0.6 (0.3)	Pennsylvania	3.3 (0.1)
Hawaii	17.9 (0.3)	Colorado	0.5 (0.1)	Georgia	3.2 (0.1)
Oklahoma	17.8 (0.1)	District of Columbia	0.5 (0.4)	Delaware	3.0 (0.3)
Wisconsin	17.8 (0.1)	Idaho	0.5 (0.2)	United States	3.0 (Z)
Iowa	17.6 (0.2)	Illinois	0.5 (0.1)	Oregon	2.9 (0.2)
Louisiana	17.3 (0.2)	Michigan	0.5 (0.1)	Idaho	2.8 (0.3)
South Dakota	17.3 (0.4)	New Hampshire	0.5 (0.2)	Kansas	2.8 (0.2)
Connecticut	17.2 (0.1)	New Jersey	0.5 (0.1)	New York	2.8 (0.1)
Indiana	17.2 (0.1)	New Mexico	0.5 (0.2)	Wisconsin	2.8 (0.1)
Idaho	17.0 (0.2)	Pennsylvania	0.5 (0.1)	South Dakota	2.7 (0.4)
United States	17.0 (Z)	South Dakota	0.5 (0.3)	Virginia	2.7 (0.1)
New York	16.8 (0.1)	Tennessee	0.5 (0.1)	District of Columbia	2.6 (0.3)
Kansas	16.7 (0.2)	Alaska	0.4 (0.2)	Maryland	2.6 (0.1)
Massachusetts	16.7 (0.1)	Arizona	0.4 (0.1)	Washington	2.6 (0.1)
Nevada	16.4 (0.2)	Iowa	0.4 (0.1)	Arizona	2.5 (0.1)
New Jersey	16.4 (0.1)	Kansas	0.4 (0.2)	Connecticut	2.5 (0.2)
Washington	16.4 (0.1)	Montana	0.4 (0.2)	Illinois	2.5 (0.1)
Virginia	16.3 (0.1)	Nebraska	0.4 (0.2)	Iowa	2.5 (0.2)
Wyoming	16.3 (0.4)	Nevada	0.4 (0.2)	Massachusetts	2.5 (0.1)
Minnesota	16.2 (0.1)	South Carolina	0.4 (0.1)	Nevada	2.5 (0.2)
Nebraska	15.9 (0.2)	Texas	0.4 (Z)	California	2.4 (Z)
Illinois	15.8 (0.1)	Washington	0.4 (0.2)	New Jersey	2.4 (0.1)
Maryland	15.8 (0.1)	Wisconsin	0.4 (0.1)	Colorado	2.3 (0.1)
North Dakota	15.6 (0.3)	Massachusetts	0.3 (0.1)	North Dakota	2.3 (0.3)
Georgia	15.4 (0.1)	Minnesota	0.3 (0.1)	Minnesota	2.2 (0.1)
California	14.9 (Z)	Oregon	0.3 (0.1)	Texas	2.2 (0.1)
Colorado	14.8 (0.1)	Vermont	0.3 (0.2)	Wyoming	2.2 (0.4)
Texas	13.2 (0.1)	Connecticut	0.2 (0.1)	Nebraska	2.1 (0.2)
District of Columbia	12.8 (0.3)	Hawaii	0.2 (0.1)	Hawaii	1.9 (0.2)
Utah	11.4 (0.1)	Utah	0.2 (0.1)	Alaska	1.7 (0.4)
Alaska	11.3 (0.4)	Wyoming	0.1 (0.1)	Utah	1.6 (0.1)

Note: Numbers in thousands; Figures cover civilian noninstitutionalized population in 2016; N/A indicates that data was not available; Z represents or rounds to zero; Margin of error appears in parenthesis and is calculated using replicate weights.
Source: U.S. Census Bureau, American Community Survey, Table HIC-4_ACS. Health Insurance Coverage Status and Type of Coverage by State—All People: 2008 to 2016, Table HIC-5_ACS. Health Insurance Coverage Status and Type of Coverage by State—Children Under 18: 2008 to 2016, Table HIC-6_ACS. Health Insurance Coverage Status and Type of Coverage by State—Persons Under 65: 2008 to 2016

Covered by Public Health Insurance: VA Care

All Persons		Under 18 Years		Under 65 Years	
State	**Percent**	**State**	**Percent**	**State**	**Percent**
Montana	4.2 *(0.3)*	Virginia	0.5 *(0.1)*	Alaska	2.7 *(0.4)*
Alaska	3.9 *(0.4)*	Mississippi	0.4 *(0.2)*	Montana	2.4 *(0.3)*
South Dakota	3.8 *(0.3)*	Georgia	0.3 *(0.1)*	South Dakota	2.1 *(0.2)*
Wyoming	3.8 *(0.4)*	North Carolina	0.3 *(0.1)*	Virginia	2.1 *(0.1)*
West Virginia	3.6 *(0.2)*	Oregon	0.3 *(0.1)*	Wyoming	2.0 *(0.3)*
Arkansas	3.3 *(0.1)*	Alabama	0.2 *(0.1)*	Oklahoma	1.9 *(0.1)*
Nevada	3.3 *(0.1)*	Arkansas	0.2 *(0.1)*	South Carolina	1.9 *(0.1)*
Oklahoma	3.3 *(0.1)*	District of Columbia	0.2 *(0.2)*	West Virginia	1.9 *(0.2)*
South Carolina	3.3 *(0.1)*	Florida	0.2 *(Z)*	Nevada	1.8 *(0.1)*
Oregon	3.2 *(0.1)*	Hawaii	0.2 *(0.2)*	Alabama	1.7 *(0.1)*
Idaho	3.1 *(0.2)*	Iowa	0.2 *(0.1)*	Arkansas	1.7 *(0.1)*
Maine	3.1 *(0.2)*	Kentucky	0.2 *(0.1)*	Georgia	1.7 *(0.1)*
Florida	3.0 *(0.1)*	Montana	0.2 *(0.2)*	North Carolina	1.7 *(0.1)*
New Hampshire	3.0 *(0.2)*	Nebraska	0.2 *(0.1)*	Oregon	1.7 *(0.1)*
New Mexico	3.0 *(0.2)*	New Hampshire	0.2 *(0.2)*	Washington	1.7 *(0.1)*
Alabama	2.9 *(0.1)*	New Mexico	0.2 *(0.1)*	Florida	1.6 *(0.1)*
Arizona	2.9 *(0.1)*	North Dakota	0.2 *(0.2)*	Hawaii	1.6 *(0.2)*
Nebraska	2.9 *(0.1)*	Oklahoma	0.2 *(0.1)*	Idaho	1.6 *(0.2)*
North Carolina	2.9 *(0.1)*	South Carolina	0.2 *(0.1)*	Mississippi	1.6 *(0.2)*
Virginia	2.9 *(0.1)*	South Dakota	0.2 *(0.2)*	New Mexico	1.6 *(0.2)*
Kentucky	2.8 *(0.1)*	Washington	0.2 *(0.1)*	Colorado	1.5 *(0.1)*
Mississippi	2.8 *(0.2)*	Wisconsin	0.2 *(0.1)*	Kentucky	1.5 *(0.1)*
Missouri	2.8 *(0.1)*	Arizona	0.1 *(Z)*	Maine	1.5 *(0.2)*
North Dakota	2.8 *(0.2)*	California	0.1 *(Z)*	New Hampshire	1.5 *(0.2)*
Washington	2.7 *(0.1)*	Colorado	0.1 *(0.1)*	Tennessee	1.5 *(0.1)*
Tennessee	2.6 *(0.1)*	Idaho	0.1 *(0.1)*	Arizona	1.4 *(0.1)*
Georgia	2.5 *(0.1)*	Illinois	0.1 *(Z)*	Missouri	1.4 *(0.1)*
Hawaii	2.5 *(0.2)*	Indiana	0.1 *(Z)*	Nebraska	1.4 *(0.1)*
Iowa	2.5 *(0.1)*	Kansas	0.1 *(0.1)*	North Dakota	1.4 *(0.2)*
Kansas	2.5 *(0.1)*	Louisiana	0.1 *(0.1)*	Kansas	1.3 *(0.1)*
Minnesota	2.5 *(0.1)*	Maine	0.1 *(0.1)*	Texas	1.3 *(Z)*
Colorado	2.4 *(0.1)*	Maryland	0.1 *(Z)*	Louisiana	1.2 *(0.1)*
Vermont	2.4 *(0.2)*	Massachusetts	0.1 *(Z)*	Ohio	1.2 *(0.1)*
Wisconsin	2.4 *(0.1)*	Michigan	0.1 *(Z)*	United States	1.2 *(Z)*
Indiana	2.3 *(0.1)*	Minnesota	0.1 *(Z)*	Vermont	1.2 *(0.2)*
Ohio	2.3 *(0.1)*	Missouri	0.1 *(0.1)*	Wisconsin	1.2 *(0.1)*
United States	2.3 *(Z)*	Nevada	0.1 *(0.1)*	Indiana	1.1 *(0.1)*
Pennsylvania	2.2 *(0.1)*	New Jersey	0.1 *(0.1)*	Iowa	1.1 *(0.1)*
Rhode Island	2.2 *(0.2)*	New York	0.1 *(Z)*	Maryland	1.1 *(0.1)*
Texas	2.2 *(Z)*	Ohio	0.1 *(Z)*	Rhode Island	1.1 *(0.2)*
Louisiana	2.1 *(0.1)*	Pennsylvania	0.1 *(Z)*	District of Columbia	1.0 *(0.2)*
Michigan	2.1 *(0.1)*	Tennessee	0.1 *(0.1)*	Michigan	1.0 *(0.1)*
Maryland	1.9 *(0.1)*	Texas	0.1 *(Z)*	Minnesota	1.0 *(0.1)*
Delaware	1.8 *(0.2)*	United States	0.1 *(Z)*	Pennsylvania	1.0 *(0.1)*
District of Columbia	1.7 *(0.3)*	Vermont	0.1 *(0.1)*	California	0.9 *(Z)*
Illinois	1.7 *(0.1)*	West Virginia	0.1 *(0.1)*	Delaware	0.9 *(0.2)*
California	1.6 *(Z)*	Wyoming	0.1 *(0.1)*	Illinois	0.8 *(Z)*
Connecticut	1.5 *(0.1)*	Alaska	Z *(Z)*	Connecticut	0.7 *(0.1)*
Massachusetts	1.5 *(0.1)*	Connecticut	Z *(Z)*	New York	0.7 *(Z)*
Utah	1.5 *(0.1)*	Delaware	Z *(Z)*	Utah	0.7 *(0.1)*
New York	1.4 *(Z)*	Rhode Island	Z *(Z)*	Massachusetts	0.6 *(0.1)*
New Jersey	1.1 *(0.1)*	Utah	Z *(Z)*	New Jersey	0.4 *(Z)*

Note: Numbers in thousands; Figures cover civilian noninstitutionalized population in 2016; N/A indicates that data was not available; Z represents or rounds to zero; Margin of error appears in parenthesis and is calculated using replicate weights.

Source: U.S. Census Bureau, American Community Survey, Table HIC-4_ACS. Health Insurance Coverage Status and Type of Coverage by State—All People: 2008 to 2016, Table HIC-5_ACS. Health Insurance Coverage Status and Type of Coverage by State—Children Under 18: 2008 to 2016, Table HIC-6_ACS. Health Insurance Coverage Status and Type of Coverage by State—Persons Under 65: 2008 to 2016

Not Covered by Health Insurance at any Time During the Year

All Persons		Under 18 Years		Under 65 Years	
State	**Percent**	**State**	**Percent**	**State**	**Percent**
Texas	16.6 *(0.2)*	Alaska	10.3 *(1.5)*	Texas	18.6 *(0.2)*
Alaska	14.0 *(0.9)*	Texas	9.8 *(0.3)*	Oklahoma	16.1 *(0.4)*
Oklahoma	13.8 *(0.3)*	Wyoming	8.8 *(1.9)*	Alaska	15.5 *(1.0)*
Georgia	12.9 *(0.3)*	North Dakota	8.0 *(1.2)*	Florida	15.3 *(0.3)*
Florida	12.5 *(0.2)*	Oklahoma	7.7 *(0.5)*	Georgia	14.8 *(0.3)*
Mississippi	11.8 *(0.4)*	Arizona	7.6 *(0.5)*	Mississippi	13.9 *(0.5)*
Wyoming	11.5 *(1.0)*	Nevada	7.0 *(0.7)*	Wyoming	13.4 *(1.2)*
Nevada	11.4 *(0.5)*	Georgia	6.7 *(0.5)*	Nevada	13.1 *(0.5)*
North Carolina	10.4 *(0.2)*	Florida	6.6 *(0.4)*	North Carolina	12.2 *(0.2)*
Louisiana	10.3 *(0.4)*	Utah	6.0 *(0.6)*	Arizona	11.9 *(0.4)*
Idaho	10.1 *(0.5)*	Indiana	5.9 *(0.5)*	Louisiana	11.9 *(0.4)*
Arizona	10.0 *(0.3)*	New Mexico	5.3 *(0.7)*	South Carolina	11.9 *(0.3)*
South Carolina	10.0 *(0.3)*	Nebraska	5.1 *(0.7)*	Idaho	11.8 *(0.6)*
New Mexico	9.2 *(0.5)*	Virginia	5.0 *(0.4)*	New Mexico	10.8 *(0.6)*
Alabama	9.1 *(0.3)*	Idaho	4.9 *(0.8)*	Alabama	10.7 *(0.4)*
Tennessee	9.0 *(0.2)*	Montana	4.9 *(0.9)*	Tennessee	10.6 *(0.3)*
Missouri	8.9 *(0.2)*	Maine	4.8 *(0.9)*	Missouri	10.5 *(0.3)*
Utah	8.8 *(0.4)*	Mississippi	4.8 *(0.6)*	South Dakota	10.3 *(0.6)*
Kansas	8.7 *(0.3)*	Missouri	4.8 *(0.4)*	Kansas	10.1 *(0.4)*
South Dakota	8.7 *(0.5)*	North Carolina	4.7 *(0.3)*	Virginia	10.1 *(0.3)*
Virginia	8.7 *(0.3)*	South Dakota	4.7 *(0.8)*	United States	10.0 *(0.1)*
Nebraska	8.6 *(0.5)*	United States	4.7 *(0.1)*	Maine	9.9 *(0.6)*
United States	8.6 *(0.1)*	Kansas	4.5 *(0.4)*	Nebraska	9.9 *(0.6)*
Indiana	8.1 *(0.3)*	Pennsylvania	4.4 *(0.3)*	Montana	9.8 *(0.7)*
Montana	8.1 *(0.5)*	Colorado	4.3 *(0.4)*	Utah	9.7 *(0.4)*
Maine	8.0 *(0.5)*	South Carolina	4.3 *(0.4)*	Indiana	9.4 *(0.3)*
New Jersey	8.0 *(0.2)*	Arkansas	4.0 *(0.5)*	Arkansas	9.3 *(0.5)*
Arkansas	7.9 *(0.4)*	Ohio	3.8 *(0.3)*	New Jersey	9.2 *(0.2)*
Colorado	7.5 *(0.3)*	New Jersey	3.7 *(0.3)*	Colorado	8.6 *(0.3)*
California	7.3 *(0.1)*	Tennessee	3.7 *(0.4)*	California	8.3 *(0.1)*
North Dakota	7.0 *(0.6)*	Wisconsin	3.7 *(0.3)*	North Dakota	8.1 *(0.7)*
Illinois	6.5 *(0.2)*	Maryland	3.4 *(0.4)*	Illinois	7.4 *(0.2)*
Oregon	6.2 *(0.2)*	Minnesota	3.4 *(0.4)*	Oregon	7.3 *(0.3)*
Maryland	6.1 *(0.3)*	Oregon	3.4 *(0.5)*	New Hampshire	7.1 *(0.5)*
New York	6.1 *(0.1)*	Kentucky	3.3 *(0.4)*	Maryland	7.0 *(0.3)*
Washington	6.0 *(0.2)*	Louisiana	3.3 *(0.4)*	New York	7.0 *(0.2)*
New Hampshire	5.9 *(0.4)*	California	3.1 *(0.1)*	Washington	6.9 *(0.2)*
Delaware	5.7 *(0.5)*	Delaware	3.1 *(0.8)*	Pennsylvania	6.7 *(0.2)*
Ohio	5.6 *(0.2)*	District of Columbia	3.1 *(1.3)*	Delaware	6.6 *(0.6)*
Pennsylvania	5.6 *(0.2)*	Michigan	3.1 *(0.2)*	Ohio	6.6 *(0.2)*
Michigan	5.4 *(0.1)*	Connecticut	2.8 *(0.5)*	West Virginia	6.5 *(0.4)*
West Virginia	5.3 *(0.3)*	Alabama	2.7 *(0.3)*	Michigan	6.3 *(0.2)*
Wisconsin	5.3 *(0.2)*	New Hampshire	2.7 *(0.6)*	Wisconsin	6.2 *(0.2)*
Kentucky	5.1 *(0.2)*	Washington	2.7 *(0.3)*	Kentucky	6.0 *(0.3)*
Connecticut	4.9 *(0.3)*	Illinois	2.6 *(0.2)*	Connecticut	5.7 *(0.4)*
Iowa	4.3 *(0.2)*	Iowa	2.6 *(0.4)*	Rhode Island	5.1 *(0.5)*
Rhode Island	4.3 *(0.5)*	Hawaii	2.5 *(0.7)*	Iowa	5.0 *(0.3)*
Minnesota	4.1 *(0.2)*	New York	2.5 *(0.2)*	Minnesota	4.8 *(0.2)*
District of Columbia	3.9 *(0.6)*	West Virginia	2.3 *(0.5)*	Vermont	4.5 *(0.5)*
Vermont	3.7 *(0.4)*	Rhode Island	2.2 *(0.6)*	District of Columbia	4.3 *(0.7)*
Hawaii	3.5 *(0.4)*	Vermont	1.5 *(0.4)*	Hawaii	4.2 *(0.5)*
Massachusetts	2.5 *(0.2)*	Massachusetts	1.0 *(0.2)*	Massachusetts	2.9 *(0.2)*

Note: Numbers in thousands; Figures cover civilian noninstitutionalized population in 2016; N/A indicates that data was not available; Z represents or rounds to zero; Margin of error appears in parenthesis and is calculated using replicate weights.

Source: U.S. Census Bureau, American Community Survey, Table HIC-4_ACS. Health Insurance Coverage Status and Type of Coverage by State—All People: 2008 to 2016, Table HIC-5_ACS. Health Insurance Coverage Status and Type of Coverage by State—Children Under 18: 2008 to 2016, Table HIC-6_ACS. Health Insurance Coverage Status and Type of Coverage by State—Persons Under 65: 2008 to 2016

Managed Care Organizations Ranked by Total Enrollment

State	Total Enrollment	Organization	Plan Type
Alabama	30,000,000	Trinity Health of Alabama	Other
Alabama	502,000	Behavioral Health Systems	PPO
Alabama	90,000	VIVA Health	HMO
Alabama	66,000	North Alabama Managed Care Inc	PPO
Alabama	45,000	Health Choice of Alabama	PPO
Alaska	800,000	Moda Health Alaska	Multiple
Arizona	7,800,000	United Concordia of Arizona	Dental
Arizona	3,500,000	Avesis: Arizona	Multiple
Arizona	1,500,000	Blue Cross & Blue Shield of Arizona	HMO/PPO
Arizona	325,000	Mercy Care Plan/Mercy Care Advantage	Multiple
Arizona	175,000	Arizona Foundation for Medical Care	Multiple
Arizona	130,000	Employers Dental Services	Dental
Arizona	115,000	Health Choice Arizona	HMO
Arizona	50,715	Maricopa Health Plan	HMO
Arizona	50,000	Care1st Health Plan Arizona	HMO
Arkansas	2,000,000	Delta Dental of Arkansas	Dental
Arkansas	500,000	HealthSCOPE Benefits	Other
California	118,000,000	Kaiser Permanente Northern California	HMO/PPO
California	30,000,000	Trinity Health of California	Other
California	25,900,000	American Specialty Health	HMO
California	11,800,000	Kaiser Permanente	HMO/PPO
California	11,800,000	Kaiser Permanente Southern California	Multiple
California	7,800,000	United Concordia of California	Dental
California	7,300,000	Managed Health Network, Inc.	Other
California	6,600,000	Dental Benefit Providers: California	Dental
California	6,100,000	Health Net, Inc.	HMO
California	4,000,000	eHealthInsurance Services, Inc.	Multiple
California	3,000,000	Liberty Dental Plan of California	Dental
California	2,900,000	Health Net Federal Services	Multiple
California	2,000,000	First Health	PPO
California	2,000,000	L.A. Care Health Plan	HMO
California	560,000	Partnership HealthPlan of California	Other
California	413,795	CalOptima	HMO
California	390,000	Dental Alternatives Insurance Services	Dental
California	338,000	Pacific Health Alliance	PPO
California	320,000	Care1st Health Plan California	HMO
California	315,440	Western Dental Services	Dental
California	250,000	Lakeside Community Healthcare Network	HMO
California	250,000	Santa Clara Family Health Foundations Inc	HMO
California	210,000	Central California Alliance for Health	HMO
California	175,000	CenCal Health	HMO
California	150,000	Landmark Healthplan of California	HMO/PPO
California	146,000	Community Health Group	HMO
California	140,000	Alameda Alliance for Health	HMO
California	140,000	Contra Costa Health Services	HMO
California	128,272	SCAN Health Plan	HMO
California	125,000	Premier Access Insurance/Access Dental	PPO
California	123,880	Access Dental Services	Dental
California	120,000	Sant, Community Physicians	HMO/PPO
California	109,000	Health Plan of San Joaquin	HMO

State	Total Enrollment	Organization	Plan Type
California	97,000	Kern Family Health Care	HMO
California	92,000	Western Health Advantage	HMO
California	90,000	BEST Life and Health Insurance Co.	PPO
California	90,000	Dental Health Services of California	Dental
California	87,740	Health Plan of San Mateo	HMO
California	55,000	San Francisco Health Plan	HMO
California	49,000	Sharp Health Plan	HMO
California	17,000	Primecare Dental Plan	Dental
California	14,600	Inter Valley Health Plan	Medicare
California	13,582	Chinese Community Health Plan	HMO
California	12,000	Medica HealthCare Plans, Inc	Medicare
California	8,000	Easy Choice Health Plan	Medicare
California	1,000	On Lok Lifeways	HMO
Colorado	11,800,000	Kaiser Permanente Northern Colorado	HMO
Colorado	11,800,000	Kaiser Permanente Southern Colorado	HMO/PPO
Colorado	326,000	Colorado Health Partnerships	HMO
Colorado	236,962	Rocky Mountain Health Plans	HMO/PPO
Colorado	60,000	Boulder Valley Individual Practice Association	PPO
Colorado	15,000	Denver Health Medical Plan	HMO
Colorado	5,000	Colorado Choice Health Plans	HMO
Connecticut	46,700,000	Aetna Inc.	Multiple
Connecticut	30,000,000	Trinity Health of Connecticut	Other
Delaware	30,000,000	Trinity Health of Delaware	Other
District of Columbia	90,000	Quality Plan Administrators	HMO/PPO
Florida	30,000,000	Trinity Health of Florida	Other
Florida	7,800,000	United Concordia of Florida	Dental
Florida	5,000,000	Coventry Health Care of Florida	HMO/PPO
Florida	3,700,000	WellCare Health Plans	Medicare
Florida	2,000,000	Liberty Dental Plan of Florida	Dental
Florida	340,000	AvMed	Medicare
Florida	340,000	AvMed Ft. Lauderdale	Medicare
Florida	340,000	AvMed Gainesville	HMO
Florida	340,000	AvMed Jacksonville	HMO
Florida	340,000	AvMed Orlando	HMO
Florida	340,000	AvMed Pembroke Pines	Medicare
Florida	340,000	AvMed Tampa Bay	HMO
Florida	125,000	Capital Health Plan	HMO
Florida	111,000	CarePlus Health Plans	Medicare
Florida	108,000	Neighborhood Health Partnership	HMO
Florida	45,000	Preferred Care Partners	Multiple
Florida	27,000	Leon Medical Centers Health Plan	HMO
Georgia	30,000,000	Trinity Health of Georgia	Other
Georgia	7,800,000	United Concordia of Georgia	Dental
Georgia	5,000,000	Coventry Health Care of Georgia	HMO/PPO
Georgia	68,000	Secure Health PPO Newtork	PPO
Georgia	15,000	Alliant Health Plans	HMO/PPO
Hawaii	70,000	AlohaCare	HMO
Idaho	30,000,000	Trinity Health of Idaho	Other

State	Total Enrollment	Organization	Plan Type
Idaho	2,400,000	Regence BlueShield of Idaho	Multiple
Idaho	563,000	Blue Cross of Idaho Health Service, Inc.	HMO/PPO
Illinois	105,000,000	BlueCross BlueShield Association	Medicare
Illinois	30,000,000	Trinity Health of Illinois	Other
Illinois	15,000,000	Health Care Service Corporation	HMO/PPO
Illinois	8,100,000	Blue Cross & Blue Shield of Illinois	HMO/PPO
Illinois	6,200,000	Dental Network of America	Dental
Illinois	2,000,000	Liberty Dental Plan of Illinois	Dental
Illinois	1,500,000	OSF Healthcare	HMO
Illinois	1,100,000	CoreSource	PPO
Illinois	750,000	Meridian Health Plan of Illinois	Medicare
Illinois	475,000	Trustmark Companies	PPO
Illinois	316,000	Preferred Network Access	PPO
Illinois	255,494	Health Alliance Medicare	Medicare
Illinois	13,000	Cigna HealthSpring CarePlan of Illinois	Medicare
Indiana	30,000,000	Trinity Health of Indiana	Other
Indiana	1,000,000	CareSource Indiana	Medicare
Indiana	900,000	Anthem Blue Cross & Blue Shield of Indiana	HMO/PPO
Iowa	50,000	Sanford Health Plan	HMO
Iowa	45,000	Medical Associates	HMO
Kansas	5,000,000	PCC Preferred Chiropractic Care	PPO
Kansas	400,000	Preferred Mental Health Management	Multiple
Kansas	152,000	ProviDRs Care Network	PPO
Kansas	134,000	Advance Insurance Company of Kansas	Multiple
Kansas	95,000	Health Partners of Kansas	PPO
Kentucky	1,000,000	CareSource Kentucky	Medicare
Kentucky	170,000	Passport Health Plan	HMO
Kentucky	136,472	Baptist Health Plan	HMO/PPO
Kentucky	110,000	Preferred Health Plan, Inc.	PPO
Louisiana	1,300,000	Blue Cross and Blue Shield of Louisiana	HMO/PPO
Louisiana	50,000	Peoples Health	HMO
Louisiana	50,000	Vantage Health Plan	HMO
Louisiana	14,000	Vantage Medicare Advantage	Medicare
Maine	70,000	Martin's Point HealthCare	Multiple
Maryland	30,000,000	Trinity Health of Maryland	Other
Maryland	17,000,000	Spectera Eyecare Networks	Multiple
Maryland	7,800,000	United Concordia of Maryland	Dental
Maryland	6,600,000	Dental Benefit Providers	Dental
Maryland	3,500,000	Avesis: Maryland	PPO
Maryland	3,200,000	CareFirst BlueCross BlueShield	HMO/PPO
Maryland	614,350	Kaiser Permanente Mid-Atlantic	Multiple
Maryland	205,000	American Postal Workers Union (APWU) Health Plan	PPO
Maryland	185,000	Priority Partners Health Plans	HMO
Maryland	10,000	Denta-Chek of Maryland	Dental
Massachusetts	30,000,000	Trinity Health of Massachusetts	Other
Massachusetts	14,000,000	Dentaquest	Dental
Massachusetts	3,500,000	Avesis: Massachusetts	PPO

State	Total Enrollment	Organization	Plan Type
Massachusetts	3,000,000	Blue Cross & Blue Shield of Massachusetts	HMO
Massachusetts	737,411	Tufts Health Plan	Multiple
Massachusetts	430,000	Neighborhood Health Plan	HMO
Massachusetts	250,000	Araz Group	PPO
Massachusetts	240,890	Medical Center Healthnet Plan	HMO
Massachusetts	200,000	Health New England	HMO/PPO
Michigan	30,000,000	Trinity Health	Other
Michigan	30,000,000	Trinity Health of Michigan	Other
Michigan	14,100,000	Delta Dental of Michigan	Dental
Michigan	7,800,000	United Concordia of Michigan	Dental
Michigan	5,800,000	Blue Cross Blue Shield of Michigan	Multiple
Michigan	4,500,000	DenteMax	Dental
Michigan	2,500,000	Cofinity	PPO
Michigan	807,000	Blue Care Network of Michigan	HMO
Michigan	750,000	Meridian Health Plan	HMO
Michigan	650,000	HAP-Health Alliance Plan: Flint	HMO/PPO
Michigan	650,000	Health Alliance Plan	HMO/PPO
Michigan	596,220	Priority Health	HMO
Michigan	390,000	SVS Vision	Vision
Michigan	383,000	Health Alliance Medicare	Medicare
Michigan	187,000	Paramount Care of Michigan	HMO/PPO
Michigan	130,000	Golden Dental Plans	Dental
Michigan	90,000	Total Health Care	HMO
Michigan	68,942	Physicians Health Plan of Mid-Michigan	HMO/PPO
Michigan	47,000	Upper Peninsula Health Plan	HMO
Michigan	17,000	ConnectCare	PPO
Michigan	14,000	HAP-Health Alliance Plan: Senior Medicare Plan	Medicare
Minnesota	70,000,000	UnitedHealth Group	Medicare
Minnesota	3,500,000	Avesis: Minnesota	PPO
Minnesota	2,700,000	Blue Cross & Blue Shield of Minnesota	HMO
Minnesota	1,700,000	Medica	HMO
Minnesota	147,000	UCare	Multiple
Minnesota	10,500	Hennepin Health	HMO
Mississippi	155,070	Health Link PPO	PPO
Missouri	11,000,000	Centene Corporation	HMO/PPO
Missouri	3,000,000	Liberty Dental Plan of Missouri	Dental
Missouri	1,700,000	Dental Health Alliance	Dental
Missouri	942,000	American Health Care Alliance	PPO
Missouri	60,000	Essence Healthcare	Medicare
Missouri	49,976	Children's Mercy Integrated Care Solutions	HMO
Missouri	5,000	Cox Healthplans	HMO/PPO
Montana	250,000	Blue Cross & Blue Shield of Montana	HMO
Montana	80,000	First Choice Health	PPO
Nebraska	5,000,000	Coventry Health Care of Nebraska	HMO/PPO
Nebraska	717,000	Blue Cross & Blue Shield of Nebraska	PPO
Nebraska	615,000	Midlands Choice	PPO
Nebraska	54,418	Mutual of Omaha Health Plans	HMO/PPO
Nevada	2,000,000	Liberty Dental Plan of Nevada	Dental
Nevada	418,000	Health Plan of Nevada	HMO

State	Total Enrollment	Organization	Plan Type
Nevada	150,000	Nevada Preferred Healthcare Providers	PPO
Nevada	32,000	Hometown Health Plan	Multiple
New Jersey	30,000,000	Trinity Health of New Jersey	Other
New Jersey	3,000,000	Liberty Dental Plan of New Jersey	Dental
New Jersey	975,000	CHN PPO	PPO
New Jersey	750,000	QualCare	Multiple
New Jersey	467,000	Horizon NJ Health	PPO
New Jersey	265,000	AmeriHealth New Jersey	HMO/PPO
New Jersey	150,000	Atlanticare Health Plans	HMO/PPO
New Mexico	7,800,000	United Concordia of New Mexico	Dental
New Mexico	400,000	Presbyterian Health Plan	HMO
New Mexico	367,000	Blue Cross & Blue Shield of New Mexico	HMO/PPO
New York	55,000,000	Davis Vision	Vision
New York	30,000,000	Trinity Health of New York	Other
New York	7,800,000	United Concordia of New York	Dental
New York	3,500,000	Healthplex	Dental
New York	3,100,000	Group Health Insurance	HMO/PPO
New York	2,000,000	Liberty Dental Plan of New York	Dental
New York	2,000,000	Universal American Medicare Plans	Medicare
New York	1,500,000	Excellus BlueCross BlueShield	HMO
New York	1,500,000	Univera Healthcare	HMO
New York	1,326,000	MagnaCare	PPO
New York	700,000	MVP Health Care	Multiple
New York	625,000	Fidelis Care	Multiple
New York	555,405	BlueCross BlueShield of Western New York	HMO/PPO
New York	400,000	CDPHP Medicare Plan	Medicare
New York	365,000	Independent Health	HMO/PPO
New York	350,000	CDPHP: Capital District Physicians' Health Plan	HMO/PPO
New York	332,128	MetroPlus Health Plan	Medicare
New York	210,000	Nova Healthcare Administrators	Multiple
New York	205,677	Guardian Life Insurance Company of America	HMO/PPO
New York	193,498	BlueShield of Northeastern New York	HMO/PPO
New York	154,162	Aetna Health of New York	HMO/PPO
New York	134,837	Affinity Health Plan	HMO
New York	53,000	GHI Medicare Plan	Medicare
New York	52,000	Island Group Administration, Inc.	PPO
New York	19,000	Quality Health Plans of New York	Medicare
New York	16,000	Elderplan	Medicare
North Carolina	7,800,000	United Concordia of North Carolina	Dental
North Carolina	5,000,000	Coventry Health Care of the Carolinas	HMO/PPO
North Carolina	3,890,000	Blue Cross Blue Shield of North Carolina	HMO/PPO
North Carolina	670,000	MedCost	PPO
North Carolina	40,000	Crescent Health Solutions	PPO
North Carolina	13,000	FirstCarolinaCare	HMO
North Dakota	1,600,000	Medica: North Dakota	HMO
North Dakota	1,000	Heart of America Health Plan	HMO
Ohio	43,000,000	EyeMed Vision Care	Vision
Ohio	30,000,000	Trinity Health of Ohio	Other
Ohio	1,000,000	CareSource Ohio	Medicare
Ohio	500,000	Aultcare Corporation	HMO/PPO

State	Total Enrollment	Organization	Plan Type
Ohio	380,000	The Health Plan of the Ohio Valley/Mountaineer Region	HMO/PPO
Ohio	370,000	Ohio Health Choice	PPO
Ohio	300,000	The Dental Care Plus Group	Multiple
Ohio	187,000	Paramount Elite Medicare Plan	Medicare
Ohio	187,000	Paramount Health Care	HMO/PPO
Ohio	144,000	Medical Mutual Services	PPO
Ohio	100,000	OhioHealth Group	PPO
Ohio	55,000	MediGold	Medicare
Ohio	52,000	Ohio State University Health Plan Inc.	Multiple
Ohio	26,000	SummaCare Medicare Advantage Plan	Medicare
Ohio	20,000	Prime Time Health Medicare Plan	Medicare
Oklahoma	1,000,000	Delta Dental of Oklahoma	Dental
Oklahoma	600,000	Blue Cross & Blue Shield of Oklahoma	HMO/PPO
Oklahoma	500,000	CommunityCare	Multiple
Oregon	7,800,000	United Concordia of Oregon	Dental
Oregon	2,400,000	Regence BlueCross BlueShield of Oregon	Multiple
Oregon	275,000	PacificSource Health Plans	HMO/PPO
Oregon	275,000	PacificSource Health Plans	Multiple
Oregon	250,000	CareOregon Health Plan	Medicare
Oregon	125,000	Managed HealthCare Northwest	PPO
Oregon	54,000	AllCare Health	Medicare
Pennsylvania	30,000,000	Trinity Health of Pennsylvania	Other
Pennsylvania	22,000,000	Value Behavioral Health of Pennsylvania	PPO
Pennsylvania	7,800,000	United Concordia Dental	Dental
Pennsylvania	7,800,000	United Concordia of Pennsylvania	Dental
Pennsylvania	5,300,000	Highmark Blue Shield	PPO
Pennsylvania	540,000	Geisinger Health Plan	HMO/PPO
Pennsylvania	265,000	AmeriHealth Pennsylvania	HMO/PPO
Pennsylvania	263,200	Health Partners Plans	Medicare
Pennsylvania	174,309	Valley Preferred	Multiple
Pennsylvania	101,000	UPMC Health Plan	Multiple
Pennsylvania	33,000	South Central Preferred Health Network	PPO
Pennsylvania	2,375	Vale-U-Health	PPO
Puerto Rico	300,000	Medical Card System (MCS)	Multiple
Puerto Rico	180,000	First Medical Health Plan	Multiple
Puerto Rico	126,000	MMM Holdings	Multiple
Puerto Rico	53,000	PMC Medicare Choice	Medicare
Rhode Island	70,000,000	CVS CareMark	Other
Rhode Island	1,018,589	Tufts Health Plan: Rhode Island	Multiple
Rhode Island	600,000	Blue Cross & Blue Shield of Rhode Island	HMO
Rhode Island	190,000	Neighborhood Health Plan of Rhode Island	HMO
South Carolina	950,000	Blue Cross & Blue Shield of South Carolina	HMO/PPO
South Carolina	330,000	Select Health of South Carolina	HMO
South Carolina	205,000	BlueChoice Health Plan of South Carolina	Multiple
South Carolina	30,000	InStil Health	Medicare
South Dakota	60,000,000	Delta Dental of South Dakota	Dental
South Dakota	1,800,000	Wellmark Blue Cross & Blue Shield of South Dakota	Multiple
South Dakota	118,600	DakotaCare	HMO
South Dakota	87,000	First Choice of the Midwest	PPO

State	Total Enrollment	Organization	Plan Type
South Dakota	63,000	Avera Health Plans	HMO
Tennessee	3,000,000	Blue Cross & Blue Shield of Tennessee	Multiple
Tennessee	518,000	Health Choice LLC	PPO
Tennessee	423,244	Baptist Health Services Group	Other
Tennessee	200,000	Initial Group	PPO
Tennessee	48,477	HealthPartners	PPO
Texas	7,800,000	United Concordia of Texas	Dental
Texas	5,427,579	USA Managed Care Organization	PPO
Texas	5,000,000	American National Insurance Company	PPO
Texas	3,500,000	Avesis: Texas	PPO
Texas	3,500,000	Galaxy Health Network	PPO
Texas	3,000,000	Liberty Dental Plan of Texas	Dental
Texas	2,000,000	MHNet Behavioral Health	Multiple
Texas	1,000,000	HealthSmart	PPO
Texas	200,000	Scott & White Health Plan	Multiple
Texas	120,000	Horizon Health Corporation	PPO
Texas	110,000	Community First Health Plans	HMO/PPO
Texas	80,000	Alliance Regional Health Network	PPO
Texas	44,000	Sterling Insurance	Medicare
Texas	42,000	TexanPlus Medicare Advantage HMO	Multiple
Texas	22,000	Valley Baptist Health Plan	HMO
Texas	15,000	Seton Healthcare Family	HMO
Texas	1,000	UTMB HealthCare Systems	HMO
Utah	2,400,000	Regence BlueCross BlueShield of Utah	Multiple
Utah	750,000	Intermountain Healthcare	HMO
Utah	177,854	Public Employees Health Program	PPO
Utah	150,000	Opticare of Utah	Vision
Utah	148,000	Altius Health Plans	Multiple
Utah	86,000	University Health Plans	HMO/PPO
Utah	6,000	Emi Health	HMO/PPO
Vermont	180,000	Blue Cross & Blue Shield of Vermont	PPO
Virginia	68,000,000	Delta Dental of Virginia	Dental
Virginia	24,000,000	Dominion Dental Services	Dental
Virginia	7,800,000	United Concordia of Virginia	Dental
Virginia	3,400,000	CareFirst Blue Cross & Blue Shield of Virginia	HMO/PPO
Virginia	2,800,000	Anthem Blue Cross & Blue Shield of Virginia	HMO
Virginia	430,000	Optima Health Plan	HMO/PPO
Virginia	88,366	Virginia Health Network	PPO
Virginia	30,000	Piedmont Community Health Plan	Multiple
Washington	7,800,000	United Concordia of Washington	Dental
Washington	1,900,000	LifeWise	PPO
Washington	300,000	Community Health Plan of Washington	Multiple
Washington	71,000	Asuris Northwest Health	Multiple
Washington	17,000	Soundpath Health	Medicare
West Virginia	5,300,000	Highmark BCBS West Virginia	PPO
West Virginia	1,000,000	CareSource West Virginia	Medicare
West Virginia	80,000	UniCare West Virginia	Multiple
Wisconsin	247,881	Dean Health Plan	Multiple

State	Total Enrollment	Organization	Plan Type
Wisconsin	200,000	Care Plus Dental Plans	Dental
Wisconsin	187,000	Security Health Plan of Wisconsin	Multiple
Wisconsin	175,000	Wisconsin Physician's Service	Multiple
Wisconsin	150,000	ChiroCare of Wisconsin	PPO
Wisconsin	130,000	Managed Health Services	HMO
Wisconsin	119,712	Prevea Health Network	PPO
Wisconsin	118,000	Network Health Plan of Wisconsin	HMO
Wisconsin	112,000	Physicians Plus Insurance Corporation	HMO/PPO
Wisconsin	90,000	Gundersen Lutheran Health Plan	HMO
Wisconsin	90,000	Unity Health Insurance	Multiple
Wisconsin	80,000	Group Health Cooperative of South Central Wisconsin	HMO
Wisconsin	75,000	Group Health Cooperative of Eau Claire	HMO
Wisconsin	34,000	Health Tradition	HMO
Wisconsin	5,000	Trilogy Health Insurance	PPO
Wyoming	100,000	Blue Cross & Blue Shield of Wyoming	HMO

Managed Care Organizations Ranked by State Enrollment

State	State Enrollment	Organization	Plan Type
Alabama	3,000,000	Blue Cross and Blue Shield of Alabama	HMO/PPO
Alabama	90,000	VIVA Health	HMO
Alabama	45,000	Health Choice of Alabama	PPO
Arizona	1,500,000	Blue Cross & Blue Shield of Arizona	HMO/PPO
Arizona	892,000	Delta Dental of Arizona	Dental
Arizona	325,000	Mercy Care Plan/Mercy Care Advantage	Multiple
Arizona	130,000	Employers Dental Services	Dental
Arizona	39,997	Maricopa Health Plan	HMO
California	8,521,345	Kaiser Permanente	HMO/PPO
California	4,390,019	Kaiser Permanente Southern California	Multiple
California	4,131,326	Kaiser Permanente Northern California	HMO/PPO
California	3,000,000	Blue Shield of California	HMO/PPO
California	585,000	First Health	PPO
California	402,000	CalOptima	HMO
California	250,000	Lakeside Community Healthcare Network	HMO
California	250,000	Santa Clara Family Health Foundations Inc	HMO
California	197,000	Pacific Health Alliance	PPO
California	190,000	Central California Alliance for Health	HMO
California	146,000	Community Health Group	HMO
California	110,000	Alameda Alliance for Health	HMO
California	109,000	Health Plan of San Joaquin	HMO
California	92,000	Western Health Advantage	HMO
California	90,074	Kern Family Health Care	HMO
California	87,740	Health Plan of San Mateo	HMO
California	55,000	San Francisco Health Plan	HMO
California	49,000	Sharp Health Plan	HMO
California	12,283	SCAN Health Plan	HMO
California	8,000	Easy Choice Health Plan	Medicare
California	6,336	Chinese Community Health Plan	HMO
California	942	On Lok Lifeways	HMO
Colorado	1,000,000	Delta Dental of Colorado	Dental
Colorado	675,279	Kaiser Permanente Northern Colorado	HMO
Colorado	675,279	Kaiser Permanente Southern Colorado	HMO/PPO
Colorado	236,962	Rocky Mountain Health Plans	HMO/PPO
Delaware	27,179	Aetna Health of Delaware	HMO/PPO
Florida	375,000	Coventry Health Care of Florida	HMO/PPO
Florida	340,000	AvMed	Medicare
Florida	340,000	AvMed Ft. Lauderdale	Medicare
Florida	340,000	AvMed Gainesville	HMO
Florida	340,000	AvMed Jacksonville	HMO
Florida	340,000	AvMed Orlando	HMO
Florida	340,000	AvMed Pembroke Pines	Medicare
Florida	340,000	AvMed Tampa Bay	HMO
Florida	141,178	Neighborhood Health Partnership	HMO
Florida	125,000	Capital Health Plan	HMO
Florida	111,000	CarePlus Health Plans	Medicare
Georgia	269,962	Kaiser Permanente Georgia	HMO
Georgia	200,000	Coventry Health Care of Georgia	HMO/PPO

State	State Enrollment	Organization	Plan Type
Georgia	68,000	Secure Health PPO Newtork	PPO
Georgia	15,000	Alliant Health Plans	HMO/PPO
Hawaii	700,000	Hawaii Medical Service Association	HMO/PPO
Hawaii	242,978	Kaiser Permanente Hawaii	HMO
Idaho	700,000	Trinity Health of Idaho	Other
Idaho	563,000	Blue Cross of Idaho Health Service, Inc.	HMO/PPO
Idaho	160,000	Regence BlueShield of Idaho	Multiple
Illinois	15,000,000	Health Care Service Corporation	HMO/PPO
Illinois	8,100,000	Blue Cross & Blue Shield of Illinois	HMO/PPO
Illinois	2,000,000	Delta Dental of Illinois	Dental
Illinois	316,000	Preferred Network Access	PPO
Illinois	240,000	Meridian Health Plan of Illinois	Medicare
Illinois	13,000	Cigna HealthSpring CarePlan of Illinois	Medicare
Kansas	880,000	Blue Cross and Blue Shield of Kansas	HMO
Kansas	95,000	Health Partners of Kansas	PPO
Kentucky	170,000	Passport Health Plan	HMO
Kentucky	110,000	Preferred Health Plan, Inc.	PPO
Kentucky	65,428	Baptist Health Plan	HMO/PPO
Louisiana	1,300,000	Blue Cross and Blue Shield of Louisiana	HMO/PPO
Louisiana	50,000	Vantage Health Plan	HMO
Louisiana	4,707	Peoples Health	HMO
Maryland	205,000	American Postal Workers Union (APWU) Health Plan	PPO
Maryland	185,000	Priority Partners Health Plans	HMO
Massachusetts	3,000,000	Blue Cross & Blue Shield of Massachusetts	HMO
Massachusetts	430,000	Neighborhood Health Plan	HMO
Massachusetts	240,890	Medical Center Healthnet Plan	HMO
Massachusetts	200,000	Health New England	HMO/PPO
Massachusetts	160,000	Araz Group	PPO
Michigan	4,500,000	Blue Cross Blue Shield of Michigan	Multiple
Michigan	650,000	HAP-Health Alliance Plan: Flint	HMO/PPO
Michigan	650,000	Health Alliance Plan	HMO/PPO
Michigan	235,000	UnitedHealthcare Great Lakes Health Plan	HMO
Michigan	90,000	Total Health Care	HMO
Michigan	68,942	Physicians Health Plan of Mid-Michigan	HMO/PPO
Michigan	47,000	Upper Peninsula Health Plan	HMO
Michigan	36,000	ConnectCare	PPO
Michigan	20,000	Dencap Dental Plans	Dental
Michigan	14,000	HAP-Health Alliance Plan: Senior Medicare Plan	Medicare
Minnesota	2,700,000	Blue Cross & Blue Shield of Minnesota	HMO
Minnesota	245,000	Americas PPO	PPO
Missouri	1,700,000	Delta Dental of Missouri	Dental
Missouri	860,000	American Health Care Alliance	PPO
Missouri	49,976	Children's Mercy Integrated Care Solutions	HMO
Missouri	26,000	Med-Pay	Other
Missouri	1,964	Cox Healthplans	HMO/PPO

State	State Enrollment	Organization	Plan Type
Montana	250,000	Blue Cross & Blue Shield of Montana	HMO
Montana	56,000	First Choice Health	PPO
Nebraska	717,000	Blue Cross & Blue Shield of Nebraska	PPO
Nebraska	28,978	Mutual of Omaha Health Plans	HMO/PPO
Nevada	150,000	Nevada Preferred Healthcare Providers	PPO
Nevada	25,576	Health Plan of Nevada	HMO
Nevada	10,000	Hometown Health Plan	Multiple
New Jersey	3,800,000	Horizon Blue Cross Blue Shield of New Jersey	HMO/PPO
New Jersey	750,000	QualCare	Multiple
New Jersey	467,000	Horizon NJ Health	PPO
New Jersey	150,000	Atlanticare Health Plans	HMO/PPO
New Mexico	400,000	Presbyterian Health Plan	HMO
New Mexico	390,000	Delta Dental of New Mexico	Dental
New Mexico	367,000	Blue Cross & Blue Shield of New Mexico	HMO/PPO
New York	3,100,000	Group Health Insurance	HMO/PPO
New York	1,500,000	Univera Healthcare	HMO
New York	928,200	MagnaCare	PPO
New York	625,000	Fidelis Care	Multiple
New York	365,000	Independent Health	HMO/PPO
New York	350,000	CDPHP: Capital District Physicians' Health Plan	HMO/PPO
New York	332,128	MetroPlus Health Plan	Medicare
New York	197,194	BlueCross BlueShield of Western New York	HMO/PPO
New York	154,162	Aetna Health of New York	HMO/PPO
New York	134,837	Affinity Health Plan	HMO
New York	72,563	BlueShield of Northeastern New York	HMO/PPO
New York	15,000	Elderplan	Medicare
North Carolina	670,000	MedCost	PPO
North Carolina	187,000	Coventry Health Care of the Carolinas	HMO/PPO
North Carolina	40,000	Crescent Health Solutions	PPO
North Carolina	13,000	FirstCarolinaCare	HMO
North Dakota	2,049	Heart of America Health Plan	HMO
Ohio	380,000	The Health Plan of the Ohio Valley/Mountaineer Region	HMO/PPO
Ohio	370,000	Ohio Health Choice	PPO
Ohio	100,000	OhioHealth Group	PPO
Ohio	73,724	SummaCare Medicare Advantage Plan	Medicare
Ohio	55,000	MediGold	Medicare
Ohio	52,000	Ohio State University Health Plan Inc.	Multiple
Ohio	20,000	Prime Time Health Medicare Plan	Medicare
Ohio	5,151	Aultcare Corporation	HMO/PPO
Oklahoma	600,000	Blue Cross & Blue Shield of Oklahoma	HMO/PPO
Oregon	730,000	Regence BlueCross BlueShield of Oregon	Multiple
Oregon	523,967	Kaiser Permanente Northwest	HMO
Oregon	250,000	CareOregon Health Plan	Medicare
Oregon	54,000	AllCare Health	Medicare

State	State Enrollment	Organization	Plan Type
Pennsylvania	300,000	Gateway Health	HMO
Pennsylvania	209,211	UPMC Health Plan	Multiple
Pennsylvania	174,209	Valley Preferred	Multiple
Pennsylvania	33,000	South Central Preferred Health Network	PPO
Puerto Rico	180,000	First Medical Health Plan	Multiple
Rhode Island	190,000	Neighborhood Health Plan of Rhode Island	HMO
South Carolina	950,000	Blue Cross & Blue Shield of South Carolina	HMO/PPO
South Carolina	330,000	Select Health of South Carolina	HMO
South Carolina	205,000	BlueChoice Health Plan of South Carolina	Multiple
South Dakota	340,000	Delta Dental of South Dakota	Dental
South Dakota	300,000	Wellmark Blue Cross & Blue Shield of South Dakota	Multiple
South Dakota	63,000	Avera Health Plans	HMO
South Dakota	25,000	First Choice of the Midwest	PPO
South Dakota	24,310	DakotaCare	HMO
Tennessee	3,000,000	Blue Cross & Blue Shield of Tennessee	Multiple
Tennessee	1,500,000	Delta Dental of Tennessee	Dental
Tennessee	518,000	Health Choice LLC	PPO
Tennessee	106,364	Initial Group	PPO
Tennessee	48,477	HealthPartners	PPO
Texas	4,700,000	Blue Cross & Blue Shield of Texas	HMO/PPO
Texas	3,200,000	Galaxy Health Network	PPO
Texas	1,118,582	USA Managed Care Organization	PPO
Texas	200,000	Scott & White Health Plan	Multiple
Texas	110,000	Community First Health Plans	HMO/PPO
Texas	79,500	Alliance Regional Health Network	PPO
Texas	44,000	Sterling Insurance	Medicare
Texas	12,004	Valley Baptist Health Plan	HMO
Texas	1,500	Dental Source: Dental Health Care Plans	Dental
Utah	330,000	Regence BlueCross BlueShield of Utah	Multiple
Utah	177,854	Public Employees Health Program	PPO
Utah	150,000	Opticare of Utah	Vision
Utah	84,000	Altius Health Plans	Multiple
Utah	65,000	Emi Health	HMO/PPO
Utah	50,000	University Health Plans	HMO/PPO
Vermont	54,023	Blue Cross & Blue Shield of Vermont	PPO
Virginia	2,800,000	Anthem Blue Cross & Blue Shield of Virginia	HMO
Virginia	2,000,000	Delta Dental of Virginia	Dental
Virginia	490,000	Dominion Dental Services	Dental
Virginia	430,000	Optima Health Plan	HMO/PPO
Virginia	88,366	Virginia Health Network	PPO
Virginia	30,000	Piedmont Community Health Plan	Multiple
Washington	300,000	Community Health Plan of Washington	Multiple
Washington	17,000	Soundpath Health	Medicare
West Virginia	500,000	Highmark BCBS West Virginia	PPO

State	State Enrollment	Organization	Plan Type
Wisconsin	223,000	Wisconsin Physician's Service	Multiple
Wisconsin	187,000	Security Health Plan of Wisconsin	Multiple
Wisconsin	164,700	Managed Health Services	HMO
Wisconsin	112,000	Physicians Plus Insurance Corporation	HMO/PPO
Wisconsin	90,000	Gundersen Lutheran Health Plan	HMO
Wisconsin	75,000	Unity Health Insurance	Multiple
Wisconsin	67,812	Network Health Plan of Wisconsin	HMO
Wisconsin	40,000	Health Tradition	HMO
Wisconsin	15,706	Prevea Health Network	PPO
Wyoming	100,000	Blue Cross & Blue Shield of Wyoming	HMO

HMO/PPO Profiles

HMO/PPO DIRECTORY

Health Insurance Coverage Status and Type of Coverage by Age

Category	All Persons		Under 18 years		Under 65 years	
	Number	%	Number	%	Number	%
Total population	4,783	-	1,170	-	4,020	-
Covered by some type of health insurance	4,348 (14)	90.9 (0.3)	1,138 (6)	97.3 (0.3)	3,588 (14)	89.3 (0.4)
Covered by private health insurance	3,249 (24)	67.9 (0.5)	653 (14)	55.8 (1.1)	2,764 (24)	68.8 (0.6)
Employer-based	2,560 (26)	53.5 (0.5)	556 (13)	47.5 (1.1)	2,301 (26)	57.2 (0.6)
Direct purchase	712 (16)	14.9 (0.3)	80 (6)	6.8 (0.5)	461 (15)	11.5 (0.4)
TRICARE	215 (10)	4.5 (0.2)	41 (5)	3.5 (0.4)	136 (10)	3.4 (0.3)
Covered by public health insurance	1,762 (19)	36.9 (0.4)	525 (13)	44.8 (1.1)	1,017 (18)	25.3 (0.5)
Medicaid	962 (18)	20.1 (0.4)	519 (13)	44.3 (1.1)	846 (18)	21.0 (0.4)
Medicare	948 (9)	19.8 (0.2)	7 (2)	0.6 (0.2)	204 (8)	5.1 (0.2)
VA Care	137 (5)	2.9 (0.1)	2 (1)	0.2 (0.1)	67 (4)	1.7 (0.1)
Not covered at any time during the year	435 (14)	9.1 (0.3)	32 (4)	2.7 (0.3)	432 (14)	10.7 (0.4)

Note: Numbers in thousands; Figures cover civilian noninstitutionalized population in 2016; N/A indicates that data was not available; Z represents or rounds to zero; Margin of error appears in parenthesis and is calculated using replicate weights.

Source: U.S. Census Bureau, American Community Survey, Table HIC-4_ACS. Health Insurance Coverage Status and Type of Coverage by State—All People: 2008 to 2016, Table HIC-5_ACS. Health Insurance Coverage Status and Type of Coverage by State—Children Under 18: 2008 to 2016, Table HIC-6_ACS. Health Insurance Coverage Status and Type of Coverage by State—Persons Under 65: 2008 to 2016

Alabama

1 Aetna Health of Alabama

151 Farmington Avenue
Hartford, CT 06156
Toll-Free: 800-872-3862
Phone: 860-273-0123
www.aetna.com
Subsidiary of: Aetna Inc.
For Profit Organization: Yes

Healthplan and Services Defined
PLAN TYPE: PPO
Model Type: Network
Plan Specialty: Behavioral Health, Lab, PBM, Radiology
Benefits Offered: Behavioral Health, Dental, Disease
   Management, Long-Term Care, Physical Therapy,
   Podiatry, Prescription, Psychiatric, Vision, Wellness, Life,
   LTD, STD

Type of Coverage
Commercial, Supplemental Medicare, Student health

Type of Payment Plans Offered
POS, FFS

Geographic Areas Served
Statewide

Key Personnel
CEO. . . . . Mark Bertolini

2 Ascension At Home

St Vincent's Home Health & Hospice
1400 Urban Center Drive, Suite 240
Birmingham, AL 35242
Phone: 205-313-2800
ascensionathome.com
Subsidiary of: Ascension
Non-Profit Organization: Yes

Healthplan and Services Defined
PLAN TYPE: Other
Plan Specialty: Disease Management
Benefits Offered: Dental, Disease Management, Home Care,
   Wellness, Ambulance & Transportation; Nursing Service;
   Short-and-long-term care management planning; Hospice

Geographic Areas Served
Texas, Alabama, Indiana, Kansas, Michigan, Mississippi,
Oklahoma, Wisconsin

Key Personnel
President. . . . . Kirk Allen
Dir., Home Health Service . . . . Darcy Burthay

3 Behavioral Health Systems

2 Metroplex Drive
Suite 500
Birmingham, AL 35209
Toll-Free: 800-245-1150
Phone: 205-879-1150
www.behavioralhealthsystems.com

For Profit Organization: Yes
Year Founded: 1989
Total Enrollment: 502,000

Healthplan and Services Defined
PLAN TYPE: PPO
Plan Specialty: Behavioral Health
Benefits Offered: Behavioral Health, Psychiatric, Wellness,
   Worker's Compensation, EAP, Drug Testing

Geographic Areas Served
Nationwide

Network Qualifications
Minimum Years of Practice: 5
Pre-Admission Certification: Yes

Peer Review Type
Utilization Review: Yes
Case Management: Yes

Publishes and Distributes Report Card: Yes

Accreditation Certification
AAAHC, TJC, URAC, CARF
Utilization Review, Pre-Admission Certification, Quality
   Assurance Program

Key Personnel
Founder, Chairman & CEO . . . . Deborah L Stephens
President, Safety First . . . . Danny Cooner
Executive Vice President . . . . Kyle Strange
Chief Financial Officer . . . . Mark Gordon
Medical Director . . . . William M. Patterson, MD
Chief Information Officer . . . . Richard Convington
Vice President, Business . . . . Judi Braswell
Public & Corp. Relations . . . . Shannon Flanagan
   205-443-5483

Specialty Managed Care Partners
State of Alabama, Drummond Co, MTD Products
Enters into Contracts with Regional Business Coalitions: Yes
Employers Coalition on Healthcare Options (ECHO),
   Louisiana Business Group on Health (LBGH), Louisiana
   Health Care Alliance (LHCA)

4 Blue Cross and Blue Shield of Alabama

450 Riverchase Parkway East
Birmingham, AL 35244
Toll-Free: 888-267-2955
www.bcbsal.org
Year Founded: 1936
State Enrollment: 3,000,000

Healthplan and Services Defined
PLAN TYPE: HMO/PPO
Model Type: IPA
Plan Specialty: Behavioral Health, Dental, Lab
Benefits Offered: Behavioral Health, Dental, Physical
   Therapy, Prescription, Wellness

Type of Coverage
Commercial, Individual, Medicare, Supplemental Medicare

Geographic Areas Served
Statewide

Accreditation Certification
URAC

Key Personnel
President & CEO . . . . Terry Kellogg

5 Bright Health Alabama
219 N 2nd Street
Suite 310
Minneapolis, MN 55401
Phone: 844-426-4086
brighthealthplan.com
Year Founded: 2016
Number of Primary Care Physicians: 1,500

Healthplan and Services Defined
PLAN TYPE: HMO
Benefits Offered: Wellness

Key Personnel
Chief Executive Officer . . . . Bob Sheehy
Chief Medical Officer . . . . Tom Valdivia
President . . . . Kyle Rolfing

6 Health Choice of Alabama
2800 University Boulevard
Suite 304
Birmingham, AL 35233
Toll-Free: 866-508-4800
Phone: 205-939-7030
Fax: 205-930-2349
www.healthchoiceofalabama.com
Subsidiary of: Alabama Premier Network (APN)
Non-Profit Organization: Yes
Year Founded: 1984
Number of Affiliated Hospitals: 90
Number of Primary Care Physicians: 4,600
Total Enrollment: 45,000
State Enrollment: 45,000

Healthplan and Services Defined
PLAN TYPE: PPO
Model Type: Group, Network
Plan Specialty: Chiropractic
Benefits Offered: Chiropractic

Type of Coverage
Commercial

Type of Payment Plans Offered
POS, DFFS, FFS

Geographic Areas Served
Statewide

Specialty Managed Care Partners
Aetna, Superien, MNHO

7 Humana Health Insurance of Alabama
600 Blvd South SW
Suite 104
Huntsville, AL 35802
Toll-Free: 800-942-0605
Phone: 256-705-3551
Fax: 904-876-8791
www.humana.com
Secondary Address: 2204 Lakeshore Drive, Suite 100,
Birmingham, AL 35209, 205-879-7374
Subsidiary of: Humana
For Profit Organization: Yes

Healthplan and Services Defined
PLAN TYPE: HMO/PPO
Model Type: Network
Plan Specialty: Dental, Vision
Benefits Offered: Dental, Vision, Life, LTD, STD

Type of Coverage
Commercial, Medicare, Medicaid

Accreditation Certification
URAC, NCQA, CORE

Key Personnel
President/CEO . . . . Bruce Broussard
SVP/CFO . . . . Brian Kane
SVP/General Counsel . . . . Christopher M. Todoroff
SVP/Chief Medical Officer . . . . Roy A. Beveridge, MD
SVP/Chief, Human Resource . . . . Tim Huval
SVP/Chief Info Officer . . . . Brian LeClaire

8 North Alabama Managed Care Inc
699-A Gallatin Street
Huntsville, AL 35801
Toll-Free: 800-636-2624
Phone: 256-532-2755
lori.farlinger@namci.com
www.namci.com
Non-Profit Organization: Yes
Year Founded: 1991
Number of Affiliated Hospitals: 100
Number of Primary Care Physicians: 13,000
Total Enrollment: 66,000

Healthplan and Services Defined
PLAN TYPE: PPO
Model Type: Network
Plan Specialty: Group Health
Benefits Offered: Behavioral Health, Chiropractic, Physical
Therapy, Podiatry, Psychiatric, Vision, PPO Network;
Radiology; Durable Medical Equipment; Chemical
Dependency Recovery Facilities; Kidney Dialysis Centers

Type of Coverage
Commercial, Individual

Type of Payment Plans Offered
Combination FFS & DFFS

Geographic Areas Served
North Alabama: Colbert, Cullman, Franklin, Jackson, Lauderdale, Lawrence, Limestone, Madison, Marshall, Morgan and Winston

Subscriber Information
Average Subscriber Co-Payment:
Primary Care Physician: Varies by plan
Nursing Home: Varies

Network Qualifications
Pre-Admission Certification: Yes

Key Personnel
Executive Director . . . . Sherree Clark
sherree.clark@namci.com
Operations Manager . . . . Brenda Willoughby
brenda.willoughby@namci.com
Services Coordinator . . . . Judy Marks
judy.marks@namci.com

Specialty Managed Care Partners
Enters into Contracts with Regional Business Coalitions: Yes
ECHO

Employer References
Huntsville HospitalSunshine Homes

9   Trinity Health of Alabama
Mercy LIFE
2900 Springhill Avenue
Mobile, AL 36607
Phone: 251-284-8420
www.trinity-health.org
Secondary Address: 20555 Victor Parkway, Livonia, MI 48152-7018, 734-343-1000
Subsidiary of: Trinity Health
Non-Profit Organization: Yes
Year Founded: 2013
Number of Affiliated Hospitals: 93
Total Enrollment: 30,000,000

Healthplan and Services Defined
PLAN TYPE: Other
Benefits Offered: Disease Management, Home Care, Long-Term Care, Psychiatric, Hospice programs, PACE (Program of All Inclusive Care for the Elderly)

Geographic Areas Served
Gulf Coast region

Key Personnel
Executive Director . . . . Diane Brown
251-287-8420
dianeb@mercymedical.com
Sales/Marketing Manager . . . . Gemma Campbell
251-287-8427
gemmac@mercymedical.com

10   UnitedHealthcare of Alabama
33 Inverness Center Parkway
Suite 350
Birmingham, AL 35242
Toll-Free: 800-345-1520
www.uhc.com/contact-us/alabama
Subsidiary of: UnitedHealth Group
For Profit Organization: Yes
Year Founded: 1991

Healthplan and Services Defined
PLAN TYPE: HMO/PPO
Model Type: Network
Plan Specialty: Behavioral Health, Dental, Disease Management, PBM, Vision
Benefits Offered: Behavioral Health, Dental, Disease Management, Long-Term Care, Prescription, Vision, Wellness, AD&D, Life, LTD, STD

Type of Coverage
Commercial, Individual, Medicare, Supplemental Medicare, Medicaid, Family, Military, Veterans, Group,

Geographic Areas Served
Statewide

Accreditation Certification
NCQA

11   VIVA Health
417 20th Street N
Suite 100
Birmingham, AL 35203
Toll-Free: 888-830-8482
Phone: 205-558-7466
www.vivahealth.com
Secondary Address: Viva Medicare Member Services, Birmingham, AL , 800-633-1542
Year Founded: 1995
Number of Affiliated Hospitals: 70
Total Enrollment: 90,000
State Enrollment: 90,000

Healthplan and Services Defined
PLAN TYPE: HMO
Other Type: Medicare
Plan Specialty: Medicare
Benefits Offered: Prescription, Medicare

Type of Coverage
Medicare, Supplemental Medicare

Geographic Areas Served
Statewide

Key Personnel
CEO/President . . . . Brad Rollow
Chief Operating Officer . . . . Cardwell Feagin
VP of Provider Services . . . . Terry Knight
Provider Network Dev. . . . . Megan Schrimsher

Health Insurance Coverage Status and Type of Coverage by Age

Category	All Persons		Under 18 years		Under 65 years	
	Number	%	Number	%	Number	%
Total population	718	-	197	-	644	-
Covered by some type of health insurance	618 *(6)*	86.0 *(0.9)*	176 *(3)*	89.7 *(1.5)*	544 *(7)*	84.5 *(1.0)*
Covered by private health insurance	483 *(9)*	67.3 *(1.2)*	120 *(4)*	61.1 *(2.2)*	437 *(9)*	67.8 *(1.3)*
Employer-based	395 *(9)*	55.0 *(1.2)*	94 *(5)*	48.0 *(2.5)*	359 *(9)*	55.7 *(1.3)*
Direct purchase	56 *(5)*	7.8 *(0.7)*	9 *(2)*	4.4 *(0.9)*	45 *(4)*	7.0 *(0.7)*
TRICARE	71 *(6)*	9.8 *(0.9)*	24 *(4)*	12.4 *(1.8)*	63 *(6)*	9.7 *(1.0)*
Covered by public health insurance	211 *(6)*	29.4 *(0.9)*	67 *(4)*	33.9 *(2.0)*	140 *(6)*	21.8 *(0.9)*
Medicaid	131 *(6)*	18.3 *(0.9)*	66 *(4)*	33.7 *(2.1)*	120 *(6)*	18.6 *(0.9)*
Medicare	81 *(3)*	11.3 *(0.4)*	1 *(Z)*	0.4 *(0.2)*	11 *(2)*	1.7 *(0.4)*
VA Care	28 *(3)*	3.9 *(0.4)*	Z *(Z)*	Z *(Z)*	18 *(2)*	2.7 *(0.4)*
Not covered at any time during the year	101 *(6)*	14.0 *(0.9)*	20 *(3)*	10.3 *(1.5)*	100 *(6)*	15.5 *(1.0)*

Note: Numbers in thousands; Figures cover civilian noninstitutionalized population in 2016; N/A indicates that data was not available; Z represents or rounds to zero; Margin of error appears in parenthesis and is calculated using replicate weights.
Source: U.S. Census Bureau, American Community Survey, Table HIC-4_ACS. Health Insurance Coverage Status and Type of Coverage by State—All People: 2008 to 2016, Table HIC-5_ACS. Health Insurance Coverage Status and Type of Coverage by State—Children Under 18: 2008 to 2016, Table HIC-6_ACS. Health Insurance Coverage Status and Type of Coverage by State—Persons Under 65: 2008 to 2016

Alaska

12 Aetna Health of Alaska

151 Farmington Avenue
Hartford, CT 06156
Toll-Free: 800-872-3862
Phone: 860-273-0123
www.aetna.com
Subsidiary of: Aetna Inc.
For Profit Organization: Yes

Healthplan and Services Defined
  PLAN TYPE: PPO
  Other Type: POS
  Model Type: Network
  Plan Specialty: Behavioral Health, EPO, Lab, PBM,
    Radiology
  Benefits Offered: Behavioral Health, Dental, Disease
    Management, Long-Term Care, Physical Therapy,
    Podiatry, Prescription, Psychiatric, Vision, Wellness, Life,
    LTD, STD

Type of Coverage
  Commercial, Supplemental Medicare, Student health

Type of Payment Plans Offered
  POS, FFS

Geographic Areas Served
  Statewide

Subscriber Information
  Average Monthly Fee Per Subscriber
    (Employee + Employer Contribution):
      Employee Only (Self): Varies
      Employee & 2 Family Members: Varies
  Average Annual Deductible Per Subscriber:
      Employee Only (Self): Varies
      Employee & 2 Family Members: Varies
  Average Subscriber Co-Payment:
      Primary Care Physician: Varies
      Prescription Drugs: Varies

Key Personnel
  CEO . . . . Mark Bertolini

13 Coventry Health Care of Alaska

6720-B Rockledge Drive
Suite 700
Bethesda, MD 20817
Phone: 301-581-0600
www.coventryhealthcare.com
Subsidiary of: Aetna Inc.
For Profit Organization: Yes

Healthplan and Services Defined
  PLAN TYPE: HMO/PPO
  Model Type: Network
  Plan Specialty: Behavioral Health, Dental, Worker's
    Compensation
  Benefits Offered: Behavioral Health, Dental, Prescription,
    Wellness, Worker's Compensation

Type of Coverage
  Commercial, Medicare, Medicaid

Geographic Areas Served
  Statewide

Key Personnel
  Chief Executive Officer . . . . Mark T. Bertolini
  President . . . . Karen S. Lynch
  Chief Financial Officer . . . . Shawn M. Guertin
  Operations & Technology . . . . Meg McCarthy
  General Counsel . . . . Thomas Banatino Jr.
  Chief Medical Officer . . . . Harold L. Paz
  Government Services . . . . Fran S. Soistman

14 Humana Health Insurance of Alaska

1498 SE Tech Center Place
Suite 300
Vancouver, WA 98683
Toll-Free: 800-781-4203
Phone: 360-253-7523
Fax: 360-253-7524
www.humana.com
For Profit Organization: Yes
Year Founded: 1961
Federally Qualified: Yes

Healthplan and Services Defined
  PLAN TYPE: HMO/PPO
  Model Type: IPA
  Benefits Offered: Behavioral Health, Chiropractic, Dental,
    Prescription, Psychiatric, Transplant, Vision, Worker's
    Compensation

Type of Coverage
  Commercial, Individual

Geographic Areas Served
  Statewide

Accreditation Certification
  TJC, URAC, NCQA, CORE

Key Personnel
  President & CEO . . . . Bruce D. Broussard
  Chief Medical Officer . . . . Roy A. Beveridge
  Chief Consumer Officer . . . . Jody L. Bilney
  Human Resources . . . . Tim Huval
  Chief Financial Officer . . . . Brian Kane
  Chief Information Officer . . . . Brian LeClaire
  General Counsel . . . . Christopher M. Todoroff

15 Moda Health Alaska

510 L Street
Suite 270
Anchorage, AK 99501-6303
Toll-Free: 877-605-3229
www.modahealth.com
Year Founded: 1955
Total Enrollment: 800,000

Healthplan and Services Defined
  PLAN TYPE: Multiple
  Other Type: PPO, POS, Dental

Plan Specialty: Dental
Benefits Offered: Chiropractic, Dental, Disease Management, Home Care, Inpatient SNF, Physical Therapy, Podiatry, Prescription, Psychiatric, Vision, Wellness

Type of Coverage
Commercial, Individual, Medicare

Subscriber Information
Average Monthly Fee Per Subscriber
(Employee + Employer Contribution):
Employee Only (Self): Varies
Medicare: Varies
Average Annual Deductible Per Subscriber:
Employee Only (Self): Varies
Medicare: Varies
Average Subscriber Co-Payment:
Primary Care Physician: Varies
Non-Network Physician: Varies
Prescription Drugs: Varies
Hospital ER: Varies
Home Health Care: Varies
Home Health Care Max. Days/Visits Covered: Varies
Nursing Home: Varies
Nursing Home Max. Days/Visits Covered: Varies

Accreditation Certification
URAC

Key Personnel
Chief Executive Officer . . . . Robert Gootee
President . . . . William Johnson
Executive Vice President . . . . Steve Wynee
Senior Vice President . . . . Robin Richardson
Senior Vice President . . . . Tracie Murphy
Senior Vice President . . . . Dave Evans
Senior Vice President . . . . Kraig Anderson
Senior Vice President . . . . Jay Lamb
Strategic Communications . . . . Jonathan Nicholas
503-219-3673
jonathan.nicholas@modahealth.com

---

16 Premera Blue Cross Blue Shield of Alaska
3800 Centerpoint Drive
Suite 940
Anchorage, AK 99503
Toll-Free: 800-508-4722
www.premera.com/ak/visitor
Subsidiary of: Premera
For Profit Organization: Yes
Year Founded: 1952
Number of Primary Care Physicians: 3,300

Healthplan and Services Defined
PLAN TYPE: PPO
Other Type: EPO
Model Type: Network
Plan Specialty: Dental, Vision
Benefits Offered: Behavioral Health, Dental, Home Care, Inpatient SNF, Long-Term Care, Prescription, Vision, Life, LTD, STD

Type of Coverage
Commercial, Individual, Medicare, Supplemental Medicare

Geographic Areas Served
Alaska and Washington, excluding Clark County

Accreditation Certification
AAAHC, URAC, TJC

Key Personnel
President & CEO . . . . Jim Grazko
VP, Sales and Service . . . . Lynn Rust

---

17 UnitedHealthcare of Alaska
5757 Plaza Drive
Cypress, CA 90630
Toll-Free: 800-343-2608
www.uhc.com/contact-us/alaska
Subsidiary of: UnitedHealth Group
For Profit Organization: Yes

Healthplan and Services Defined
PLAN TYPE: HMO/PPO
Model Type: Network
Plan Specialty: Behavioral Health, Dental, Disease Management, PBM, Vision
Benefits Offered: Behavioral Health, Dental, Disease Management, Long-Term Care, Prescription, Vision, Wellness, Life, LTD, STD

Type of Coverage
Commercial, Individual, Medicare, Supplemental Medicare, Medicaid, Family, Group

Geographic Areas Served
Statewide. Alaska is covered by the California branch

Health Insurance Coverage Status and Type of Coverage by Age

Category	All Persons		Under 18 years		Under 65 years	
	Number	%	Number	%	Number	%
Total population	6,825	-	1,732	-	5,665	-
Covered by some type of health insurance	6,143 *(21)*	90.0 *(0.3)*	1,601 *(10)*	92.4 *(0.5)*	4,992 *(21)*	88.1 *(0.4)*
Covered by private health insurance	4,246 *(29)*	62.2 *(0.4)*	965 *(14)*	55.7 *(0.8)*	3,601 *(28)*	63.6 *(0.5)*
Employer-based	3,323 *(30)*	48.7 *(0.4)*	814 *(15)*	47.0 *(0.8)*	3,015 *(29)*	53.2 *(0.5)*
Direct purchase	946 *(19)*	13.9 *(0.3)*	142 *(8)*	8.2 *(0.5)*	587 *(17)*	10.4 *(0.3)*
TRICARE	212 *(10)*	3.1 *(0.1)*	38 *(3)*	2.2 *(0.2)*	124 *(8)*	2.2 *(0.1)*
Covered by public health insurance	2,711 *(30)*	39.7 *(0.4)*	702 *(16)*	40.5 *(1.0)*	1,590 *(30)*	28.1 *(0.5)*
Medicaid	1,592 *(30)*	23.3 *(0.4)*	698 *(17)*	40.3 *(1.0)*	1,451 *(29)*	25.6 *(0.5)*
Medicare	1,261 *(8)*	18.5 *(0.1)*	7 *(1)*	0.4 *(0.1)*	143 *(7)*	2.5 *(0.1)*
VA Care	195 *(7)*	2.9 *(0.1)*	1 *(1)*	0.1 *(Z)*	81 *(5)*	1.4 *(0.1)*
Not covered at any time during the year	681 *(21)*	10.0 *(0.3)*	132 *(9)*	7.6 *(0.5)*	674 *(21)*	11.9 *(0.4)*

Note: Numbers in thousands; Figures cover civilian noninstitutionalized population in 2016; N/A indicates that data was not available; Z represents or rounds to zero; Margin of error appears in parenthesis and is calculated using replicate weights.
Source: U.S. Census Bureau, American Community Survey, Table HIC-4_ACS. Health Insurance Coverage Status and Type of Coverage by State—All People: 2008 to 2016, Table HIC-5_ACS. Health Insurance Coverage Status and Type of Coverage by State—Children Under 18: 2008 to 2016, Table HIC-6_ACS. Health Insurance Coverage Status and Type of Coverage by State—Persons Under 65: 2008 to 2016

Arizona

18 Aetna Health of Arizona

151 Farmington Avenue
Hartford, CT 06156
Toll-Free: 800-872-3862
Phone: 860-273-0123
www.aetna.com
Subsidiary of: Aetna Inc.
For Profit Organization: Yes
Year Founded: 1988

Healthplan and Services Defined
PLAN TYPE: HMO
Other Type: POS
Model Type: Network
Plan Specialty: Behavioral Health, Dental, Lab, PBM, Vision, Radiology
Benefits Offered: Behavioral Health, Dental, Disease Management, Long-Term Care, Physical Therapy, Podiatry, Prescription, Psychiatric, Vision, Wellness, Life, LTD, STD

Type of Coverage
Commercial, Supplemental Medicare, Catastrophic

Type of Payment Plans Offered
POS, Capitated, Combination FFS & DFFS

Geographic Areas Served
Statewide

Network Qualifications
Minimum Years of Practice: 2
Pre-Admission Certification: Yes

Peer Review Type
Utilization Review: Yes

Publishes and Distributes Report Card: Yes

Accreditation Certification
NCQA

Key Personnel
CEO . . . . Mark Bertolini

Specialty Managed Care Partners
Behavioral Health, Prescription, Dental, Vision

19 AHCCS/Medicaid

1 East Washington Street
Suite 1700
Phoenix, AZ 85004
Toll-Free: 800-985-2356
Phone: 800-348-4058
www.uhc.com/contact-us/arizona
Subsidiary of: UnitedHealth Group
For Profit Organization: Yes

Healthplan and Services Defined
PLAN TYPE: Other
Other Type: Medicaid
Model Type: Network
Benefits Offered: Dental, Disease Management, Prescription, Vision, Wellness

Type of Coverage
Medicaid

Geographic Areas Served
Available in Apache, Cochise, Coconino, Graham, Greenlee, La Paz, Maricopa, Mohave, Navajo, Pima, Santa Cruz, Yavapai, Yuma

20 Arizona Foundation for Medical Care

2700 N Central Avenue
Suite 810
Phoenix, AZ 85004-1163
Toll-Free: 800-624-4277
Phone: 602-252-4042
Fax: 602-254-3086
marketing@azfmc.com
www.azfmc.com
Non-Profit Organization: Yes
Year Founded: 1969
Number of Affiliated Hospitals: 77
Total Enrollment: 175,000

Healthplan and Services Defined
PLAN TYPE: Multiple
Other Type: HMO, PPO, POS, EPO
Model Type: Group, Network
Plan Specialty: Chiropractic, Disease Management, EPO, Worker's Compensation, PPO, POS, Medical Management, Case Management, Utilization Management, Wellness Services, 24/7 Nurse Line
Benefits Offered: Disease Management, Wellness, Maternity Management
Offers Demand Management Patient Information Service: Yes
DMPI Services Offered: 24-Hour Nurse Care Line

Type of Coverage
Commercial, Individual, Indemnity

Type of Payment Plans Offered
POS

Geographic Areas Served
Statewide

Network Qualifications
Pre-Admission Certification: Yes

Peer Review Type
Utilization Review: Yes
Case Management: Yes

Accreditation Certification
TJC, URAC, NCQA

Key Personnel
President . . . . Stanley A. Gering
Vice President . . . . Thomas F. Moore
Treasurer . . . . Sebastian B. Ruggeri
Secretary . . . . Nandini Kanagal

Specialty Managed Care Partners
American Health Holding

21   Avesis: Arizona

10400 N 25th Avenue
Suite 200
Phoenix, AZ 85012
Toll-Free: 800-522-0258
www.avesis.com
Secondary Address: Executive Offic, 10324 S Dilfield Road,
    Owings Mills, MD 21117, 800-643-1132
Subsidiary of: Guardian Life Insurance Company
Year Founded: 1978
Number of Primary Care Physicians: 25,000
Total Enrollment: 3,500,000

Healthplan and Services Defined
    PLAN TYPE: Multiple
    Model Type: Network
    Plan Specialty: Dental, Vision, Hearing, Medicare/Medicaid
    Benefits Offered: Dental, Vision

Type of Coverage
    Commercial, Medicare, Supplemental Medicare, Medicaid

Type of Payment Plans Offered
    POS, Capitated, Combination FFS & DFFS

Geographic Areas Served
    Statewide

Publishes and Distributes Report Card: Yes

Accreditation Certification
    AAAHC
    TJC Accreditation

Key Personnel
    Chief Executive Officer . . . . Chris Swanker
    VP of Finance. . . . . Amy Jackson
    Business Development . . . . Alan Cohn
    Chief Information Officer . . . . Laura Gill

22   Blue Cross & Blue Shield of Arizona

2444 West Las Palmaritas Drive
Phoenix, AZ 85021
Phone: 602-864-4100
www.azblue.com
Secondary Address: Flagstaff Customer Service Officer, 1500
    E Cedar Avenue, Suite 56, Flagstaff, AZ 86004
Non-Profit Organization: Yes
Year Founded: 1939
Number of Affiliated Hospitals: 65
Number of Primary Care Physicians: 1,611
Total Enrollment: 1,500,000
State Enrollment: 1,500,000

Healthplan and Services Defined
    PLAN TYPE: HMO/PPO
    Model Type: Network
    Benefits Offered: Behavioral Health, Chiropractic, Dental,
        Prescription, Wellness, STD

Type of Coverage
    Commercial, Individual, Indemnity, Supplemental Medicare

Geographic Areas Served
    Statewide

Accreditation Certification
    URAC
    TJC Accreditation, Medicare Approved, Utilization Review,
        Pre-Admission Certification, State Licensure, Quality
        Assurance Program

Key Personnel
    Chief Operating Officer . . . . Sandy Gibson
    SVP, Service Officer . . . . H. Jody Chandler
    SVP, Financial Officer . . . . Karen Abraham
    SVP, General Counsel. . . . . Deanna Salazar
    SVP, Sales/Marketing . . . . Jeff Stelnik
    Chief Medical Officer . . . . Vishu J. Jhaveri, MD
    Chief Information Officer . . . . Elizabeth A. Messina
    Media Contact . . . . Jeremy Adler
        310-360-5782
        jeremy.adler@dpnww.com

23   Care1st Health Plan Arizona

2355 E Camelback Road
Suite 300
Phoenix, AZ 85016
Toll-Free: 866-560-4042
Phone: 602-778-1800
az.care1st.com/az
Subsidiary of: Care1st Health Plan
For Profit Organization: Yes
Year Founded: 1994
Total Enrollment: 50,000

Healthplan and Services Defined
    PLAN TYPE: HMO
    Benefits Offered: Disease Management, Wellness

Type of Coverage
    Medicare

Geographic Areas Served
    Maricopa County and Pima County

Accreditation Certification
    NCQA

Key Personnel
    Administrative Officer . . . . Scott Cummings
    Chief Operating Officer . . . . Susan Cordier
    Chief Financial Officer. . . . . Deena Sigel
    Chief Medical Officer . . . . Satya Sarma
    Dir., Sales & Marketing. . . . . Anna Maria Maldonado
    Dir., Quality Improvement. . . . . Nancy DeRosa
    Value Based Partnerships . . . . Kathy Thurman
    Dir., Member Services. . . . . Mike Ferguson
    Dir., Provider Network . . . . Jessica Sedita-Igneri

24   CareCentrix: Arizona

7740 N 16th Street
Suite 100
Phoenix, AZ 85020
Toll-Free: 800-808-1902
carecentrix.com
Year Founded: 1996
Number of Primary Care Physicians: 8,000

Healthplan and Services Defined
　PLAN TYPE: HMO
　Benefits Offered: Home Care, Physical Therapy, Durable
　　Medical Equipment; Occupational & Respiratory Therapy;
　　Orthotics; Prosthetics

Key Personnel
　Chief Executive Officer . . . . John Driscoll
　Chief Data Officer. . . . . Tej Anand
　Chief Medical Officer. . . . . Michael Cantor
　Chief Operating Officer . . . . Mary Daschner
　Chief Customer Officer . . . . Tom Gaffney

25　Cigna HealthCare of Arizona

900 Cottage Grove Road
Bloomfield, CT 06002
Toll-Free: 800-997-1654
www.cigna.com
For Profit Organization: Yes

Healthplan and Services Defined
　PLAN TYPE: HMO/PPO
　Other Type: POS
　Model Type: IPA, Network
　Benefits Offered: Behavioral Health, Chiropractic,
　　Complementary Medicine, Disease Management, Home
　　Care, Inpatient SNF, Long-Term Care, Physical Therapy,
　　Podiatry, Prescription, Psychiatric, Transplant, Vision,
　　Wellness

Type of Coverage
　Commercial, Individual, Medicare

Type of Payment Plans Offered
　POS

Accreditation Certification
　NCQA

Key Personnel
　Chairman & CEO . . . . David M. Cordani

26　Cigna Medical Group

25500 N Norterra Drive
Phoenix, AZ 85085
Phone: 480-987-6917
CMGservice@cigna.com
www.cigna.com/cmgaz
Subsidiary of: Cigna Corporation
For Profit Organization: Yes

Healthplan and Services Defined
　PLAN TYPE: HMO
　Model Type: Staff
　Plan Specialty: Primary care, pediatrics
　Benefits Offered: Podiatry, Prescription, Vision, After-Hours
　　Nurseline, General Surgery, Hearing, Ophthalmology,
　　Outpatient Surgery,

Key Personnel
　President & CEO . . . . David Cordani
　EVP, Marketing . . . . Lisa Bacus
　EVP, General Counsel. . . . . Nicole Jones
　Chief Financial Officer. . . . . Eric Palmer

Chief Medical Officer . . . . Alan Muney
Human Resources. . . . . John Murabito

27　Delta Dental of Arizona

5656 West Talavi Boulevard
Glendale, AZ 85306
Toll-Free: 800-352-6132
Phone: 602-938-3131
www.deltadentalaz.com
Mailing Address: P.O. Box 43000, Phoenix, AZ 85080-3000
Non-Profit Organization: Yes
Year Founded: 1972
State Enrollment: 892,000

Healthplan and Services Defined
　PLAN TYPE: Dental
　Other Type: Vision
　Model Type: Network
　Plan Specialty: Dental, Vision
　Benefits Offered: Dental, Vision

Type of Coverage
　Commercial, Individual, Indemnity

Type of Payment Plans Offered
　FFS

Geographic Areas Served
　Statewide

Accreditation Certification
　NCQA

Key Personnel
　President & CEO . . . . Allan Allford
　VP, Financial Officer . . . . Mark Anderson
　VP, Business Development . . . . Brad Clothier
　VP of Operations. . . . . Craig Livesay
　VP of Marketing & Comm. . . . . Scott Pederson

28　Employers Dental Services

3430 E Sunrise
Suite 160
Tuscon, AZ 85718
Toll-Free: 800-722-9772
Phone: 520-696-4343
edscs@exchange.principal.com
www.employersdental.com
Subsidiary of: Principal Financial Group
Year Founded: 1974
Owned by an Integrated Delivery Network (IDN): Yes
Number of Primary Care Physicians: 1,340
Total Enrollment: 130,000
State Enrollment: 130,000

Healthplan and Services Defined
　PLAN TYPE: Dental
　Model Type: Group, Individual
　Plan Specialty: Dental, Vision
　Benefits Offered: Dental, Prescription, Vision, Prepaid

Type of Coverage
　DHMO, Orthodontic

Geographic Areas Served
Arizona Statewide

Peer Review Type
Utilization Review: Yes
Case Management: Yes

Accreditation Certification
Utilization Review, Quality Assurance Program

Key Personnel
Chairman, President & CEO . . . . Daniel J. Houston

Specialty Managed Care Partners
Enters into Contracts with Regional Business Coalitions: Yes

29   Health Choice Arizona

410 N 44th Street
Suite 900
Phoenix, AZ 85008
Toll-Free: 800-322-8670
Phone: 480-968-6866
comments@healthchoiceaz.com
www.healthchoiceaz.com
Subsidiary of: IASIS Healthcare
For Profit Organization: Yes
Year Founded: 1990
Number of Affiliated Hospitals: 4
Number of Primary Care Physicians: 132
Total Enrollment: 115,000

Healthplan and Services Defined
PLAN TYPE: HMO
Model Type: IPA
Plan Specialty: Services to AHCCCS members
Benefits Offered: Behavioral Health, Dental, Disease
Management, Prescription, Wellness, Care Coordination,
Maternal Child Health

Type of Coverage
Medicaid, Managed Medicaid

Geographic Areas Served
Apache, Coconino, Gila, Maricopa, Mohave, Navajo, Pima,
Pinal counties

Network Qualifications
Pre-Admission Certification: Yes

Peer Review Type
Utilization Review: Yes
Second Surgical Opinion: Yes
Case Management: Yes

Accreditation Certification
URAC
Utilization Review

Key Personnel
President & CEO . . . . Mike Uchrin
Chief Financial Officer . . . . Jeff Butcher
Chief Compliance Officer . . . . Phil Nieri
Chief Operating Officer. . . . . Troy Smith
Chief Medical Officer. . . . . Richard Sanchez
Media Relations . . . . Diana Alvarez
   480-397-3881
   dalvarez@dalvarez@iasishealthcare.com

30   Humana Health Insurance of Arizona

2231 E Camelback Road
Suite 400
Phoenix, AZ 85016
Toll-Free: 800-889-0301
Phone: 602-760-1700
www.humana.com
Secondary Address: 5210 E Williams Circle, Suite 200,
   Tucson, AZ 85711, 520-571-6548
For Profit Organization: Yes
Year Founded: 1984

Healthplan and Services Defined
PLAN TYPE: HMO/PPO
Model Type: IPA
Benefits Offered: Dental, Disease Management, Prescription,
Transplant, Vision, Wellness, Life, LTD, STD

Type of Coverage
Commercial, Individual, Medicare, Medicaid

Type of Payment Plans Offered
POS, Combination FFS & DFFS

Geographic Areas Served
Apache, Cochise, Coconino, Gila, Graham, Greenlee, La Paz,
Maricipa, Mohave, Navajo, Pima, Pinal, Santa Cruz, Yavapai,
Yuma counties

Peer Review Type
Utilization Review: Yes
Second Surgical Opinion: Yes
Case Management: Yes

Publishes and Distributes Report Card: Yes

Accreditation Certification
URAC, NCQA, CORE
TJC Accreditation

Key Personnel
President & CEO . . . . Bruce D. Broussard
Chief Medical Officer. . . . . Roy A. Beverdige
Chief Consumer Officer. . . . . Jody L. Bilney
Human Resources. . . . . Tim Huval
Chief Financial Officer . . . . Brian Kane
Chief Information Officer . . . . Brian LeClaire
SVP, General Counsel . . . . Christopher M. Todoroff

Specialty Managed Care Partners
Enters into Contracts with Regional Business Coalitions: Yes

31   Magellan Health

4800 N Schottsdale Road
Suite 4400
Scottsdale, AZ 85251
MagellanHealthComInquiries@magellanhealth.com
www.magellanhealth.com
For Profit Organization: Yes

Healthplan and Services Defined
PLAN TYPE: Other
Plan Specialty: ASO, Behavioral Health, Diagnostic imaging
   & specialty pharma services
Benefits Offered: Behavioral Health, Long-Term Care,
   Prescription

Type of Coverage
Medicare, Medicaid

Key Personnel
Chairman & CEO . . . . Barry M. Smith
Chief Financial Officer . . . . Jonathan N. Rubin
General Counsel . . . . Daniel N. Gregoire
Human Resources. . . . . Caskie Lewis-Clapper
Chief Medical Officer . . . . Karen Amstutz
Chief Information Officer . . . . Srini Koushik

32 Magellan Healthcare

4800 N Scottsdale Road
Suite 4400
Scottsdale, AZ 85251
MagellanHealthComInquiries@magellanhealth.com
www.magellanhealthcare.com
Subsidiary of: Magellan Health
For Profit Organization: Yes

Healthplan and Services Defined
PLAN TYPE: Other
Plan Specialty: Behavioral Health
Benefits Offered: Behavioral Health, Prescription,
Diagnostics

Type of Coverage
Commercial, Medicare, Medicaid, Public sector, Federal,
military

Key Personnel
Chairman & CEO . . . . Barry M. Smith
Chief Financial Officer . . . . Jonathan N. Rubin
General Counsel . . . . Daniel N. Gregoire
Human Resources. . . . . Caskie Lewis-Clapper
Chief Medical Officer . . . . Karen Amstutz
Chief Information Officer . . . . Srini Koushik

33 Magellan Rx Management

101 Billerica Avenue
Building 4
North Billeria, MA 01862
Toll-Free: 978-856-2345
Fax: 978-856-2335
info@magellandx.com
www.magellanrx.com
Subsidiary of: Magellan Health
For Profit Organization: Yes

Healthplan and Services Defined
PLAN TYPE: Other
Other Type: PBM
Plan Specialty: PBM

Key Personnel
President & CEO . . . . Amy Winslow
Chief Operating Officer . . . . Hossein Maleknia
Director of Sales . . . . Jennifer Zonderman
Director of Finance . . . . Janine LeBlanc

34 Maricopa Health Plan

2701 E Elvira Road
Tucson, AZ 85756
Toll-Free: 800-582-8686
Phone: 520-874-5290
Fax: 866-465-8340
www.mhpaz.com
Subsidiary of: University of Arizona Health Network
Non-Profit Organization: Yes
Year Founded: 1981
Number of Affiliated Hospitals: 10
Number of Primary Care Physicians: 124
Number of Referral/Specialty Physicians: 317
Total Enrollment: 50,715
State Enrollment: 39,997

Healthplan and Services Defined
PLAN TYPE: HMO
Model Type: Network
Plan Specialty: Behavioral Health, Lab, Radiology
Benefits Offered: Behavioral Health, Dental, Physical
Therapy, Prescription, Wellness

Type of Coverage
Individual, Medicare, Medicaid

Type of Payment Plans Offered
Capitated, FFS

Geographic Areas Served
Maricopa County

Network Qualifications
Pre-Admission Certification: Yes

Peer Review Type
Utilization Review: Yes
Second Surgical Opinion: No
Case Management: Yes

Publishes and Distributes Report Card: Yes

Accreditation Certification
TJC Accreditation, Medicare Approved, Utilization Review,
Pre-Admission Certification, State Licensure, Quality
Assurance Program

Specialty Managed Care Partners
Enters into Contracts with Regional Business Coalitions: Yes

35 Mercy Care Plan/Mercy Care Advantage

4350 East Cotton Center Boulevard
Building D
Phoenix, AZ 85040
Toll-Free: 800-624-3879
Phone: 602-263-3000
www.mercycareplan.com
Subsidiary of: Southwest Catholic Health Network
Non-Profit Organization: Yes
Year Founded: 1985
Total Enrollment: 325,000
State Enrollment: 325,000

Healthplan and Services Defined
PLAN TYPE: Multiple
Other Type: HMO, Medicare

Model Type: Group
Benefits Offered: Disease Management, Long-Term Care,
   Prescription, Wellness

Type of Coverage
Medicare, Medicaid

Geographic Areas Served
Cochise, Gila, Graham, Greenlee, La Paz, Maricopa, Pima,
Pinal, Santa Cruz, Yavapai, Yuma counties

Key Personnel
Chief Operating Officer . . . . Lorry Bottrill
VP, Health Operations . . . . John Monte
Chief Medical Officer . . . . Charlton Wilson

---

36   NIA Magellan
4800 N Scottsdale Road
Suite 4400
Scottsdale, AZ 85251
Toll-Free: 877-NIA-9762
www.niahealthcare.com
Subsidiary of: Magellan Health
For Profit Organization: Yes
Year Founded: 1995

Healthplan and Services Defined
   PLAN TYPE: Other
   Plan Specialty: Radiology, Radiology benefits management

Key Personnel
Chief Medical Officer . . . . Michael J. Pentecost
SVP, Sales . . . . Edie Jardine
VP, Finance . . . . William F. Henderson
VP, Client Services . . . . Annalisa Cooper

---

37   Outlook Benefit Solutions
1550 E McKellips Road
Suite 112
Mesa, AZ 85203
Toll-Free: 800-342-7188
Phone: 480-461-9001
Fax: 480-461-9021
customerservice@outlookvision.com
www.outlookvision.com
Year Founded: 1990
Federally Qualified: Yes

Healthplan and Services Defined
   PLAN TYPE: Vision
   Plan Specialty: Vision
   Benefits Offered: Prescription, Vision, Hearing

Type of Coverage
Commercial, Individual

Geographic Areas Served
Available nationwide, except for AK, CT, MT, RI, VT and
WA

---

38   Phoenix Health Plan
7878 North 16th Street
Suite 105
Phoenix, AZ 85020
Toll-Free: 800-747-7997
Phone: 602-824-3700
www.phoenixhealthplan.com
Non-Profit Organization: Yes
Year Founded: 1983
Number of Affiliated Hospitals: 28
Number of Primary Care Physicians: 3,780

Healthplan and Services Defined
   PLAN TYPE: HMO
   Model Type: IPA
   Benefits Offered: Behavioral Health, Dental, Disease
      Management, Prescription, Wellness, Nurse Advice Line;
      Transportation

Type of Coverage
Medicaid

Type of Payment Plans Offered
POS, Combination FFS & DFFS

Geographic Areas Served
Maricopa County

Publishes and Distributes Report Card: Yes

Accreditation Certification
NCQA
TJC Accreditation, Medicare Approved, Utilization Review,
   Pre-Admission Certification, State Licensure, Quality
   Assurance Program

Specialty Managed Care Partners
Enters into Contracts with Regional Business Coalitions: Yes

---

39   Pivot Health
29308 N 108th Place
Scottdales, AZ 85262
Toll-Free: 866-566-2707
pivothealth.com
Year Founded: 2015

Healthplan and Services Defined
   PLAN TYPE: Other
   Other Type: Supplemental

Type of Coverage
Short-term; Supplemental; Zero Dedu

Geographic Areas Served
Alabama, Arizona, Arkansas, the District of Columbia,
   Florida, Georgia, Illinois, Indiana, Iowa, Kentucky, Michigan,
   Mississippi, Nebraska, Ohio, Oklahoma, Pennsylvania,
   Tennessee, Texas, Virginia, West Virginia, and Wisconsin

Key Personnel
Chief Executive Officer . . . . Jeff Smedsrud
VP of Sales & Marketing . . . . Kyle Dietz

40   **Preferred Therapy Providers**
23460 North 19th Avenue
Suite 250
Phoenix, Z 85027
Toll-Free: 800-664-5240
Phone: 623-869-9101
www.preferredtherapy.com
For Profit Organization: Yes
Year Founded: 1992
Physician Owned Organization: No
Federally Qualified: No
Number of Referral/Specialty Physicians: 3,000

Healthplan and Services Defined
PLAN TYPE: HMO/PPO
Model Type: Network
Plan Specialty: Physical, Occupational, Speech Therapies
Benefits Offered: Physical Therapy, Ocupational Therapy,
    Speech Therapy
Offers Demand Management Patient Information Service: No

Type of Coverage
Commercial

Geographic Areas Served
35 states

Network Qualifications
Pre-Admission Certification: No

Publishes and Distributes Report Card: No

Accreditation Certification
NCQA, AAPPO

Specialty Managed Care Partners
Enters into Contracts with Regional Business Coalitions: No

41   **Premier Access Insurance/Access Dental**
P.O. Box 659010
Sacramento, CA 95865-9010
Toll-Free: 888-634-6074
Phone: 916-920-2500
Fax: 916-563-9000
info@premierlife.com
www.premierppo.com
Subsidiary of: Guardian Life Insurance Co.
For Profit Organization: Yes
Year Founded: 1989
Number of Primary Care Physicians: 1,000

Healthplan and Services Defined
PLAN TYPE: PPO
Other Type: Dental
Plan Specialty: Dental
Benefits Offered: Dental

Key Personnel
President & CEO . . . . Deanna M. Mulligan

42   **SilverScript**
P.O. Box 52067
Phoenix, AZ 85072-2067
Toll-Free: 866-362-6212
silverscript.com
Subsidiary of: CVS Health
Year Founded: 2006

Healthplan and Services Defined
PLAN TYPE: Medicare
Plan Specialty: Medicare Part D
Benefits Offered: Prescription

Type of Coverage
Medicare

Geographic Areas Served
SilverScript Choice: Nationwide and the District of Columbia;
SilverScript Plus: Nationwide and the District of Columbia,
except Alaska

Key Personnel
President & CEO . . . . Larry J. Merlo

43   **Total Dental Administrators**
2111 E Highland Avenue
Suite 250
Phoenix, AZ 85016-4735
Toll-Free: 888-422-1995
Phone: 602-266-1995
Fax: 602-266-1948
www.tdadental.com
Secondary Address: 6985 Union Park Center, Suite 675,
    Cottonwood Heights, UT 84047, 800-880-3536
Subsidiary of: Companion Life Insurance Co.

Healthplan and Services Defined
PLAN TYPE: Dental
Plan Specialty: PPO, Prepaid
Benefits Offered: Dental

Type of Coverage
Indemnity

Key Personnel
President/CEO . . . . Jeremy Spencer
Provider Relations Mgr. . . . . Meg Pipkin
Director of Operations . . . . Jeff Wilkinson
Digital Marketing Manager . . . . Brent Singleton
Director of Information . . . . Chris Parrott

44   **United Concordia of Arizona**
2198 E Camelback Road
Suite 260
Phoenix, AZ 85016
Phone: 602-667-2200
www.unitedconcordia.com
For Profit Organization: Yes
Year Founded: 1971
Number of Primary Care Physicians: 97,300
Total Enrollment: 7,800,000

Healthplan and Services Defined
PLAN TYPE: Dental

Model Type: Network
Plan Specialty: Dental
Benefits Offered: Dental

Type of Coverage
Commercial, Individual, Military personnel & families

Geographic Areas Served
Nationwide

Accreditation Certification
URAC

Key Personnel
President & COO. . . . . F.G. (Chip) Merkel

45   UnitedHealthcare of Arizona

1 East Washington Street
Suite 1700
Phoenix, AZ 85004
Toll-Free: 800-985-2356
www.uhc.com/contact-us/arizona
Subsidiary of: UnitedHealth Group
For Profit Organization: Yes

Healthplan and Services Defined
PLAN TYPE: HMO/PPO
Model Type: Network
Plan Specialty: Behavioral Health, Dental, Vision
Benefits Offered: Behavioral Health, Dental, Disease
   Management, Prescription, Vision, Wellness, AD&D, Life

Type of Coverage
Commercial, Individual, Medicare, Supplemental Medicare,
   Medicaid

Geographic Areas Served
Statewide

46   University Care Advantage

2701 E Elvira Road
Tuscon, AZ 85756
Toll-Free: 877-874-3930
universitycareadvantage.com
Subsidiary of: University of Arizona Health Plans

Healthplan and Services Defined
PLAN TYPE: HMO
Benefits Offered: Chiropractic, Dental, Podiatry, Prescription,
   Vision

Geographic Areas Served
Cochise, Gila, Graham, Greenlee, La Paz, Pima, Pinal, Santa
   Cruz, Yavapai, Yuma counties

Key Personnel
Chief Executive Officer . . . . Kathleen Oestreich

47   University Family Care Health Plan

2701 E Elvira Road
Tucson, AZ 85756
Toll-Free: 800-582-8686
Phone: 520-874-5290
www.ufcaz.com
Subsidiary of: University Physicians Health Plans

Non-Profit Organization: Yes

Healthplan and Services Defined
PLAN TYPE: HMO

Type of Coverage
Individual

Geographic Areas Served
Cochise, Gila, Graham, Greenlee, La Paz, Pima, Pinal, Santa
   Cruz, Yavapai, and Yuma counties

Key Personnel
CEO . . . . Kathleen Oestreich

Health Insurance Coverage Status and Type of Coverage by Age

Category	All Persons		Under 18 years		Under 65 years	
	Number	%	Number	%	Number	%
Total population	2,934	-	754	-	2,463	-
Covered by some type of health insurance	2,702 *(12)*	92.1 *(0.4)*	724 *(5)*	96.0 *(0.5)*	2,233 *(13)*	90.7 *(0.5)*
Covered by private health insurance	1,820 *(20)*	62.0 *(0.7)*	364 *(10)*	48.3 *(1.4)*	1,543 *(20)*	62.7 *(0.8)*
Employer-based	1,398 *(20)*	47.6 *(0.7)*	312 *(10)*	41.4 *(1.4)*	1,281 *(19)*	52.0 *(0.8)*
Direct purchase	430 *(12)*	14.7 *(0.4)*	46 *(4)*	6.1 *(0.6)*	263 *(10)*	10.7 *(0.4)*
TRICARE	100 *(6)*	3.4 *(0.2)*	16 *(3)*	2.1 *(0.4)*	56 *(6)*	2.3 *(0.2)*
Covered by public health insurance	1,269 *(15)*	43.2 *(0.5)*	392 *(10)*	52.0 *(1.3)*	807 *(15)*	32.8 *(0.6)*
Medicaid	780 *(16)*	26.6 *(0.5)*	389 *(10)*	51.6 *(1.3)*	712 *(15)*	28.9 *(0.6)*
Medicare	580 *(6)*	19.8 *(0.2)*	4 *(1)*	0.6 *(0.2)*	119 *(6)*	4.8 *(0.2)*
VA Care	98 *(4)*	3.3 *(0.1)*	2 *(1)*	0.2 *(0.1)*	42 *(3)*	1.7 *(0.1)*
Not covered at any time during the year	232 *(12)*	7.9 *(0.4)*	30 *(4)*	4.0 *(0.5)*	230 *(12)*	9.3 *(0.5)*

Note: Numbers in thousands; Figures cover civilian noninstitutionalized population in 2016; N/A indicates that data was not available; Z represents or rounds to zero; Margin of error appears in parenthesis and is calculated using replicate weights.
Source: U.S. Census Bureau, American Community Survey, Table HIC-4_ACS. Health Insurance Coverage Status and Type of Coverage by State—All People: 2008 to 2016, Table HIC-5_ACS. Health Insurance Coverage Status and Type of Coverage by State—Children Under 18: 2008 to 2016, Table HIC-6_ACS. Health Insurance Coverage Status and Type of Coverage by State—Persons Under 65: 2008 to 2016

Arkansas

48 Aetna Health of Arkansas

151 Farmington Avenue
Hartford, CT 06156
Toll-Free: 800-872-3862
Phone: 860-273-0123
www.aetna.com
Secondary Address: 6730-B Rockledge Drive, Suite 700,
Bethesda, MD 20817, 301-581-0600
Subsidiary of: Aetna Inc.
For Profit Organization: Yes

Healthplan and Services Defined
PLAN TYPE: PPO
Other Type: POS
Model Type: Network
Plan Specialty: Behavioral Health, Dental, EPO, Lab, PBM,
Vision, Radiology
Benefits Offered: Behavioral Health, Dental, Disease
Management, Long-Term Care, Physical Therapy,
Podiatry, Prescription, Psychiatric, Vision, Wellness, Life,
LTD, STD

Type of Coverage
Commercial, Supplemental Medicare, Student health

Type of Payment Plans Offered
POS, FFS

Geographic Areas Served
Statewide

Key Personnel
CEO . . . . Mark Bertolini

49 Arkansas Blue Cross Blue Shield

P.O. Box 2181
Little Rock, AR 72203-2181
Toll-Free: 800-238-8379
www.arkansasbluecross.com
Non-Profit Organization: Yes
Year Founded: 1948

Healthplan and Services Defined
PLAN TYPE: Multiple
Other Type: HMO, Medicare
Model Type: Network
Plan Specialty: Dental, Vision
Benefits Offered: Chiropractic, Dental, Home Care, Inpatient
SNF, Physical Therapy, Podiatry, Prescription, Vision,
Worker's Compensation, Life, Mental Health, Substance
Abuse, Emergency, Short-Term, Federal Employees

Type of Coverage
Commercial, Individual, Medicare, Supplemental Medicare
Catastrophic Illness Benefit: Varies per case

Geographic Areas Served
Statewide

Subscriber Information
Average Subscriber Co-Payment:
Home Health Care: Varies
Nursing Home: Varies

Accreditation Certification
TJC, URAC, NCQA

Key Personnel
President/CEO . . . . Curtis Barnett
EVP/Chief Admin Officer . . . . David Bridges
EVP/CFO . . . . Gray Dillard
VP, Claims Administration . . . . Marcus James
SVP/Chief Legal Officer . . . . Lee Douglas
VP/Chief Medical Officer . . . . Connie Meeks, MD
VP, Human Resources . . . . Richard Cooper
VP, Info Technology . . . . Melvin Hardy

50 Delta Dental of Arkansas

1513 Country Club Road
Sherwood, AR 72120
Toll-Free: 800-462-5410
Phone: 501-835-3400
www.deltadentalar.com
Mailing Address: P.O. Box 15965, Little Rock, AR 72231
Non-Profit Organization: Yes
Year Founded: 1982
Total Enrollment: 2,000,000

Healthplan and Services Defined
PLAN TYPE: Dental
Other Type: Vision
Model Type: Network
Plan Specialty: Dental, Vision
Benefits Offered: Dental, Vision

Type of Coverage
Commercial, Individual, Group

Type of Payment Plans Offered
DFFS

Geographic Areas Served
Statewide

Publishes and Distributes Report Card: Yes

Key Personnel
President & CEO . . . . Ed Choate
Senior VP & CFO . . . . Phyllis Rogers
Vice President, Sales . . . . Jay Reavis

51 Frazier Insurance Agency

808 Reservoir Road
Suite B
Little Rock, AR 72227
Phone: 501-225-1818
Fax: 501-223-8682
frazieragency.com

Healthplan and Services Defined
PLAN TYPE: HMO/PPO
Benefits Offered: Wellness, AD&D, Life

Type of Coverage
Medicare

Geographic Areas Served
Statewide

52   HealthSCOPE Benefits

27 Corporate Hill Drive
Little Rock, AR 72205
Toll-Free: 800-972-3025
customerservice.ar@healthscopebenefits.com
www.healthscopebenefits.com
For Profit Organization: Yes
Year Founded: 1985
Total Enrollment: 500,000

Healthplan and Services Defined
   PLAN TYPE: Other
   Plan Specialty: Healthcare management services

Type of Coverage
   Catastrophic Illness Benefit: Maximum $1M

Type of Payment Plans Offered
   POS, DFFS, FFS, Combination FFS & DFFS

Geographic Areas Served
   Nationwide

Network Qualifications
   Minimum Years of Practice: 3
   Pre-Admission Certification: Yes

Peer Review Type
   Utilization Review: Yes
   Second Surgical Opinion: Yes
   Case Management: Yes

Accreditation Certification
   TJC, URAC
   Utilization Review, State Licensure

Key Personnel
   Chief Executive Officer. . . . . Joe Edwards
   President . . . . Mary Catherine Person
   VP, Business Development . . . . Tom Bartlett
   VP, Quality/Assurance . . . . Cathleen Armstrong
   SVP, Legal & Compliance . . . . Brett Edwards
   VP of Sales . . . . Pepper Schafer
   Chief Information Officer . . . . Tim Beasley

Specialty Managed Care Partners
   American Health Holdings, PHCS, Advance PCS, Caremark, CCN
   Enters into Contracts with Regional Business Coalitions: Yes
   Alaska Business Coalition

Employer References
   American Greetings, Alcoa, MedCath, Whirlpool

53   Humana Health Insurance of Arkansas

425 West Capitol Avenue
Little Rock, AR 72201
Toll-Free: 800-941-4951
Fax: 501-223-2094
www.humana.com
Secondary Address: 5206 Village Parkway, Suite 4, Rogers, AR 72758, 479-418-7140
Subsidiary of: Humana
For Profit Organization: Yes

Healthplan and Services Defined
   PLAN TYPE: HMO/PPO
   Model Type: Network
   Plan Specialty: Dental, Vision
   Benefits Offered: Dental, Prescription, Vision, Life, LTD, STD

Type of Coverage
   Commercial, Medicare

Accreditation Certification
   URAC, NCQA, CORE

54   Mercy Clinic Arkansas

214 Carter Street
Berryville, AR 72616
Phone: 870-423-3355
mercy.net
Subsidiary of: IBM Watson Health
Non-Profit Organization: Yes
Number of Affiliated Hospitals: 44
Number of Primary Care Physicians: 700
Number of Referral/Specialty Physicians: 2,000

Healthplan and Services Defined
   PLAN TYPE: HMO
   Benefits Offered: Behavioral Health, Disease Management, Home Care, Inpatient SNF, Physical Therapy, Podiatry, Vision, Wellness, Non-Surgical Weight Loss; Urgent Care; Dermatology; Rehabilitation; Breast Cancer; Orthopedics; Ostoclerosis; Pediatrics

Geographic Areas Served
   Arkansas, Kansas, Missouri, and Oklahoma

Key Personnel
   General Manager . . . . Deborah DiSanzo

55   NovaSys Health

10801 Executive Center Drive
Little Rock, AR 72221
Toll-Free: 800-294-3557
Phone: 501-219-4444
novasyshealth.com
Year Founded: 1996
Number of Affiliated Hospitals: 67
Number of Primary Care Physicians: 4,000

Healthplan and Services Defined
   PLAN TYPE: PPO
   Model Type: Network
   Plan Specialty: Integrated provider network & administrative services

Geographic Areas Served
   Statewide

Key Personnel
   Chief Executive Officer . . . . John P. Ryan

56   **UnitedHealthcare of Arkansas**
1401 West Capital Avenue
Suite 375
Little Rock, AR 72201
Toll-Free: 877-842-3210
Fax: 615-372-3564
www.uhc.com/contact-us/arkansas
Subsidiary of: UnitedHealth Group
For Profit Organization: Yes

Healthplan and Services Defined
  PLAN TYPE: HMO/PPO
  Model Type: Network
  Plan Specialty: Behavioral Health, Dental, Disease
    Management, PBM, Vision
  Benefits Offered: Behavioral Health, Dental, Disease
    Management, Long-Term Care, Prescription, Vision,
    Wellness, Life, LTD, STD

Type of Coverage
  Commercial, Individual, Medicare, Supplemental Medicare,
    Medicaid, Family

Type of Payment Plans Offered
  POS, FFS

Geographic Areas Served
  Statewide

Network Qualifications
  Pre-Admission Certification: Yes

Peer Review Type
  Utilization Review: Yes

Publishes and Distributes Report Card: Yes

Accreditation Certification
  URAC, NCQA
  TJC Accreditation, Medicare Approved, Utilization Review,
    Pre-Admission Certification, State Licensure, Quality
    Assurance Program

Specialty Managed Care Partners
  Enters into Contracts with Regional Business Coalitions: Yes

Health Insurance Coverage Status and Type of Coverage by Age

Category	All Persons		Under 18 years		Under 65 years	
	Number	%	Number	%	Number	%
Total population	38,764	-	9,603	-	33,512	-
Covered by some type of health insurance	35,920 *(41)*	92.7 *(0.1)*	9,304 *(18)*	96.9 *(0.1)*	30,723 *(39)*	91.7 *(0.1)*
Covered by private health insurance	24,428 *(79)*	63.0 *(0.2)*	5,334 *(38)*	55.5 *(0.4)*	21,736 *(71)*	64.9 *(0.2)*
Employer-based	19,862 *(79)*	51.2 *(0.2)*	4,572 *(39)*	47.6 *(0.4)*	18,231 *(76)*	54.4 *(0.2)*
Direct purchase	4,927 *(47)*	12.7 *(0.1)*	728 *(21)*	7.6 *(0.2)*	3,692 *(42)*	11.0 *(0.1)*
TRICARE	685 *(22)*	1.8 *(0.1)*	163 *(11)*	1.7 *(0.1)*	470 *(20)*	1.4 *(0.1)*
Covered by public health insurance	15,077 *(72)*	38.9 *(0.2)*	4,354 *(40)*	45.3 *(0.4)*	10,098 *(71)*	30.1 *(0.2)*
Medicaid	10,576 *(75)*	27.3 *(0.2)*	4,289 *(41)*	44.7 *(0.4)*	9,473 *(72)*	28.3 *(0.2)*
Medicare	5,778 *(19)*	14.9 *(Z)*	100 *(9)*	1.0 *(0.1)*	809 *(17)*	2.4 *(Z)*
VA Care	609 *(13)*	1.6 *(Z)*	5 *(1)*	0.1 *(Z)*	288 *(10)*	0.9 *(Z)*
Not covered at any time during the year	2,844 *(41)*	7.3 *(0.1)*	300 *(14)*	3.1 *(0.1)*	2,789 *(39)*	8.3 *(0.1)*

Note: Numbers in thousands; Figures cover civilian noninstitutionalized population in 2016; N/A indicates that data was not available; Z represents or rounds to zero; Margin of error appears in parenthesis and is calculated using replicate weights.
Source: U.S. Census Bureau, American Community Survey, Table HIC-4_ACS. Health Insurance Coverage Status and Type of Coverage by State—All People: 2008 to 2016, Table HIC-5_ACS. Health Insurance Coverage Status and Type of Coverage by State—Children Under 18: 2008 to 2016, Table HIC-6_ACS. Health Insurance Coverage Status and Type of Coverage by State—Persons Under 65: 2008 to 2016

California

57 Access Dental Services

2693 Florin Road
Sacramento, CA 95822
Toll-Free: 866-682-9904
Phone: 916-424-5500
Fax: 916-646-9000
info@accessdental.com
www.accessdental.com
Mailing Address: P.O. Box 659005, Sacramento, CA 95865
For Profit Organization: Yes
Year Founded: 1989
Number of Primary Care Physicians: 2,000
Total Enrollment: 123,880

Healthplan and Services Defined
PLAN TYPE: Dental
Model Type: Staff
Plan Specialty: Dental
Benefits Offered: Dental

Type of Coverage
Commercial, Individual, Medicare, Supplemental Medicare, Medicaid

Geographic Areas Served
Statewide

Key Personnel
Chief Executive Officer. . . . . George Neal
Chief Clinical Officer . . . . Cherag Sarkari
Human Resources . . . . Laura Shively
VP, Operations. . . . . Payam Pardis

58 Aetna Health of California

151 Farmington Avenue
Hartford, CT 06156
Toll-Free: 800-872-3862
Phone: 860-273-0123
www.aetna.com
Subsidiary of: Aetna Inc.
For Profit Organization: Yes

Healthplan and Services Defined
PLAN TYPE: HMO/PPO
Other Type: POS
Model Type: Network
Plan Specialty: Behavioral Health, EPO, Lab, PBM, Radiology
Benefits Offered: Behavioral Health, Dental, Disease Management, Long-Term Care, Physical Therapy, Podiatry, Prescription, Psychiatric, Vision, Wellness, Life, LTD, STD

Type of Coverage
Commercial, Supplemental Medicare, Catastrophic, Student health

Geographic Areas Served
Statewide

Key Personnel
CEO. . . . . Mark Bertolini

59 Alameda Alliance for Health

1240 South Loop Road
Alameda, CA 94502
Phone: 510-747-4500
www.alamedaalliance.org
Secondary Address: 3075 Adeline Street, Suite 160, Berkeley, CA 94703, 510-747-6100
Non-Profit Organization: Yes
Year Founded: 1996
Federally Qualified: Yes
Number of Affiliated Hospitals: 15
Number of Primary Care Physicians: 4,000
Total Enrollment: 140,000
State Enrollment: 110,000

Healthplan and Services Defined
PLAN TYPE: HMO
Model Type: Network
Plan Specialty: Dental
Benefits Offered: Dental, Prescription, Vision, Medi-Cal, Healthy Families, Alliance Group Care

Type of Coverage
Individual, Government Sponsored Programs

Type of Payment Plans Offered
POS

Geographic Areas Served
Alameda County

Peer Review Type
Second Surgical Opinion: Yes

Accreditation Certification
NCQA
State Licensure

Key Personnel
Chief Executive Officer . . . . Scott Coffin
Chief Operations Officer. . . . . Matthew Woodruff
Chief Financial Officer . . . . Gil Riojas
General Counsel . . . . Matthew Levin
Chief Information Officer . . . . Aman Bahsin

60 Alameda Medi-Cal Plan

1240 South Loop Road
Alameda, CA 94502
Toll-Free: 800-698-1118
Phone: 510-777-2300
www.alamedaalliance.org
Subsidiary of: Alameda Alliance for Health
Non-Profit Organization: Yes
Federally Qualified: Yes
Number of Affiliated Hospitals: 15
Number of Primary Care Physicians: 4,000

Healthplan and Services Defined
PLAN TYPE: Other
Plan Specialty: Serving families and children, people with disabilities, and seniors
Benefits Offered: Dental, Inpatient SNF, Vision, Wellness

Geographic Areas Served
Alameda County

Key Personnel
Chief Executive Officer . . . . Scott Coffin
Chief Operations Officer . . . . Matthew Woodruff
Chief Financial Officer . . . . Gil Riojas
General Counsel . . . . Matthew Levin
Chief Information Officer . . . . Aman Bahsin

61 Alignment Health Plan

1100 W Town and Country Road
Suite 1600
Orange, CA 92868
Toll-Free: 866-634-2247
Phone: 323-728-7232
Fax: 323-728-8494
www.alignmenthealthplan.com

Healthplan and Services Defined
PLAN TYPE: Medicare

Type of Coverage
Medicare, Supplemental Medicare

Geographic Areas Served
Los Angeles, Northern Orange County, San Bernardino, Riverside, Stanislaus, San Joaquin and Santa Clara

Key Personnel
President & CEO . . . . John Kao

62 Allied Pacific IPA

1668 S. Garfield Avenue
2nd Floor
Alhambra, CA 91801
Toll-Free: 877-282-8272
Phone: 626-282-0288
CustomerService.Dept@nmm.cc
www.alliedipa.com
Secondary Address: 568 W. Garvey Avenue, Monterey Park, CA 91754, 888-888-7424
Year Founded: 1992
Physician Owned Organization: Yes
Number of Primary Care Physicians: 800

Healthplan and Services Defined
PLAN TYPE: HMO
Other Type: IPA
Model Type: IPA
Benefits Offered: Disease Management, Wellness

Type of Coverage
Commercial, Individual

63 American Specialty Health

10221 Wateridge Circle
San Diego, CA 92121
Toll-Free: 800-848-3555
Fax: 619-237-3859
www.ashcompanies.com
Secondary Address: Corporate Headquarters, 12800 N Meridian Street, Carmel, IN 46032
For Profit Organization: Yes
Year Founded: 1987

Total Enrollment: 25,900,000

Healthplan and Services Defined
PLAN TYPE: HMO
Model Type: Network
Plan Specialty: Chiropractic
Benefits Offered: Chiropractic, Complementary Medicine, Acupuncture

Type of Coverage
Commercial, Supplemental Medicare

Type of Payment Plans Offered
POS, Capitated

Geographic Areas Served
Nationwide - ASH Network, California - ASH Plans

Network Qualifications
Pre-Admission Certification: Yes

Peer Review Type
Utilization Review: Yes
Case Management: Yes

Accreditation Certification
URAC, NCQA, HITRUST

Key Personnel
CEO . . . . George T. DeVries, III
President/COO . . . . Robert White
President/COO HealthyRoad . . . . Julie Jennings
Chief Health Officer . . . . Douglas Metz
Chief Financial Officer . . . . William Comer
Chief Technology Officer . . . . Jerome Bonhomme

Specialty Managed Care Partners
Enters into Contracts with Regional Business Coalitions: Yes

64 Anthem Blue Cross of California

P.O. Box 60007
Los Angeles, CA 90060-0007
Toll-Free: 855-715-5316
Phone: 844-285-5159
www.anthem.com
Subsidiary of: Anthem, Inc.
For Profit Organization: Yes

Healthplan and Services Defined
PLAN TYPE: HMO/PPO
Model Type: Network
Plan Specialty: Behavioral Health, Dental, Disease Management, Lab, PBM, Vision, Radiology
Benefits Offered: Behavioral Health, Dental, Disease Management, Inpatient SNF, Physical Therapy, Prescription, Psychiatric, Transplant, Vision, Wellness, Life

Type of Coverage
Commercial, Individual, Medicare, Supplemental Medicare, Minimum coverage

Geographic Areas Served
Santa Clara, San Joaquin, Stanislaus, Merced, and Tulare

Accreditation Certification
URAC

Key Personnel
President/CEO . . . . Brian Ternan

65   **BEST Life and Health Insurance Co.**
17701 Mitchell N
Irvine, CA 92614-6028
Toll-Free: 800-433-0088
Fax: 208-893-5040
cs@bestlife.com
www.bestlife.com
Mailing Address: P.O. Box 890, Meridian, ID 83680-0890
For Profit Organization: Yes
Year Founded: 1970
Number of Affiliated Hospitals: 5,005
Number of Primary Care Physicians: 772,292
Total Enrollment: 90,000

Healthplan and Services Defined
  PLAN TYPE: PPO
  Model Type: PPO/Indemnity
  Benefits Offered: Dental, Disease Management, Vision,
    Wellness, Life, STD

Type of Coverage
  Commercial

Geographic Areas Served
  AK, AL, AR, AZ, CA, CO, DC, FL, GA, HI, ID, IL, IN, KS,
  KY, LA, MD, MI, MS, MO, MT, NC, ND, NE, NM, NV, OH,
  OK, OR, PA, SC, SD, TN, TX, UT, VA, WA, WY

Network Qualifications
  Pre-Admission Certification: Yes

Peer Review Type
  Case Management: Yes

Accreditation Certification
  URAC, NCQA
  Quality Assurance Program

Key Personnel
  President . . . . Paul Peatross

66   **Blue Shield of California**
50 Beale Street
San Francisco, CA 94105-1808
Toll-Free: 800-393-6130
Phone: 415-229-5000
www.blueshieldca.com
Mailing Address: P.O. Box 272540, Chico, CA 95927-2540
Non-Profit Organization: Yes
Year Founded: 1939
State Enrollment: 3,000,000

Healthplan and Services Defined
  PLAN TYPE: HMO/PPO
  Plan Specialty: Dental, Vision
  Benefits Offered: Behavioral Health, Chiropractic, Dental,
    Home Care, Inpatient SNF, Podiatry, Prescription, Vision,
    Life, Benefits vary depending on the plan

Type of Coverage
  Commercial, Individual, Medicare, Supplemental Medicare,
    Medicaid

Geographic Areas Served
  Statewide

Accreditation Certification
  NCQA

Key Personnel
  President/CEO . . . . Paul Markovich
  SVP/CFO . . . . Michael Murray
  SVP/General Counsel . . . . Seth Jacobs, Esq
  SVP/Chief Info Officer . . . . Michael Mathias

67   **Brand New Day HMO**
5455 Garden Grove Boulevard
Suite 500
Westminster, CA 92683
Toll-Free: 866-255-4795
Fax: 657-400-1208
bndhmo.com
For Profit Organization: Yes
Year Founded: 1985

Healthplan and Services Defined
  PLAN TYPE: HMO
  Plan Specialty: Behavioral Health
  Benefits Offered: Behavioral Health, Dental, Disease
    Management, Prescription, Psychiatric, Vision, Wellness

Type of Coverage
  Individual, Medicare, Medicaid

Geographic Areas Served
  Statewide

Key Personnel
  CEO . . . . Jeff Davis

68   **Bright Now! Dental**
3358 South Bristol Street
Santa Ana, CA 92704
Toll-Free: 844-400-7645
Phone: 714-361-2141
www.brightnow.com
Secondary Address: 1601 W 17th Street, Suite G, Santa Ana,
  CA 92706, 714-567-9255
Subsidiary of: Smile Brands Inc.
Year Founded: 1998
Number of Primary Care Physicians: 300
Number of Referral/Specialty Physicians: 416

Healthplan and Services Defined
  PLAN TYPE: Dental
  Model Type: Staff, Network
  Plan Specialty: Dental
  Benefits Offered: Dental

Type of Payment Plans Offered
  Capitated

Geographic Areas Served
  AZ, CA, CO, FL, IN, MD, OH, OR, PA, TN, TX, UT, VA,
  WA

Subscriber Information
  Average Monthly Fee Per Subscriber
    (Employee + Employer Contribution):
      Employee Only (Self): $40.00
      Employee & 1 Family Member: $75.00

Employee & 2 Family Members: $110.00

Network Qualifications
Pre-Admission Certification: Yes

Key Personnel
President/CEO . . . . Steven Bilt
CFO . . . . Brad Schmidt
CIO . . . . George Suda

Specialty Managed Care Partners
Enters into Contracts with Regional Business Coalitions: No

---

69 California Dental Network

23291 Mill Creek Drive
Suite 100
Laguna Hills, CA 92653
Toll-Free: 877-433-6825
Fax: 949-830-1655
www.caldental.net

Healthplan and Services Defined
PLAN TYPE: Dental
Plan Specialty: Dental
Benefits Offered: Dental

Type of Coverage
Individual

Geographic Areas Served
Statewide

Key Personnel
CEO . . . . Brian Watts
President, DentaQuest . . . . Steve Pollock

---

70 California Foundation for Medical Care

3993 Jurupa Avenue
Riverside, CA 92506
Toll-Free: 800-334-7341
Fax: 951-686-1692
www.cfmcnet.org
For Profit Organization: Yes
Number of Affiliated Hospitals: 250
Number of Primary Care Physicians: 30,000
Number of Referral/Specialty Physicians: 5,000

Healthplan and Services Defined
PLAN TYPE: PPO
Plan Specialty: Behavioral Health, EPO, Lab, Worker's
Compensation, UR, Chemical Dependency Centers.
Surgical Centers
Benefits Offered: Worker's Compensation

Geographic Areas Served
Statewide

Key Personnel
President . . . . Debi Hardwick
831-754-3800
dhardwick@costalmgmt.com
Vice President . . . . Carolyn Temple
661-616-4814
ctemple@kernfmc.com

Chief Executive Officer . . . . Dolores L. Green
951-686-9049
dgreen@rcmanet.com
Administration Director . . . . Ester M. Sanchez
800-334-7341
esanchez@rfasi.com

---

71 CalOptima

505 City Parkway W
Orange, CA 92868
Toll-Free: 888-587-8088
Phone: 714-246-8500
www.caloptima.org
For Profit Organization: Yes
Year Founded: 1993
Owned by an Integrated Delivery Network (IDN): Yes
Number of Primary Care Physicians: 3,500
Total Enrollment: 413,795
State Enrollment: 402,000

Healthplan and Services Defined
PLAN TYPE: HMO
Model Type: Group
Plan Specialty: ASO, Behavioral Health, Chiropractic, Dental,
Disease Management, EPO, Lab, MSO, PBM, Vision,
Radiology, Worker's Compensation
Benefits Offered: Behavioral Health, Chiropractic, Dental,
Disease Management, Home Care, Prescription, Vision,
Wellness

Type of Coverage
Individual, Supplemental Medicare, Medicaid, Medi-Cal

Geographic Areas Served
Orange County

Key Personnel
Chief Executive Officer . . . . Michael Schrader
Chief Counsel . . . . Gary Crockett
Chief Information Officer . . . . Len Rosignoli
Chief Operating Officer . . . . Ladan Khamseh
Chief Medical Officer . . . . Richard Helmer, MD

---

72 Care1st Cal MediConnect Plan

601 Potrero Grande Drive
Montery Park, CA 91755
Toll-Free: 800-544-0088
Fax: 323-889-2101
care1st.com
Subsidiary of: Care1st Health Plan

Healthplan and Services Defined
PLAN TYPE: Other
Plan Specialty: Combines Medicare and Medi-Cal benefits
into a single plan.
Benefits Offered: Behavioral Health, Long-Term Care,
Prescription

Geographic Areas Served
Los Angeles and San Diego counties

Key Personnel
President . . . . Greg Buchert

Chief Operating Officer . . . . Amanda Flaum
Chief Medical Officer. . . . . Tanya Dansky
Chief Financial Officer . . . . Michael Engelhard
DVP, Legal Counsel. Alan Bloom
Information Technology . . . . Herbert Woo

73   Care1st Health Plan California

601 Potrero Grande Drive
Monterey Park, CA 91755
Toll-Free: 800-544-0088
Phone: 323-889-6638
Fax: 323-889-2101
www.care1st.com
Secondary Address: 3131 Camino del Rio North, Suite 1300,
   San Diego, CA 92108, 619-528-4800
For Profit Organization: Yes
Year Founded: 1994
Total Enrollment: 320,000

Healthplan and Services Defined
   PLAN TYPE: HMO
   Benefits Offered: Dental, Disease Management, Wellness,
      Medi-Cal Health, Medi-Cal Dental, Healthy Families

Type of Coverage
   Commercial, Medicare, Supplemental Medicare, Medicaid

Geographic Areas Served
   Los Angeles, Orange, San Bernardino, Riverside and San
   Diego counties

Accreditation Certification
   NCQA

Key Personnel
   President. . . . . Greg Buchert
   Chief Financial Officer . . . . Michael Engelhard
   Chief Medical Officer. . . . . Tanya Dansky
   DVP, Legal Counsel. Alan Bloom
   Chief Operating Officer . . . . Amanda Flaum
   Information Technology . . . . Herbert Woo

74   Care1st Medicare

601 Potrero Grande Drive
Monterey Park, CA 91755
Toll-Free: 800-544-0088
Fax: 323-889-2101
www.care1st.com
Year Founded: 1994

Healthplan and Services Defined
   PLAN TYPE: Medicare
   Benefits Offered: Disease Management, Wellness

Type of Coverage
   Medicare, Supplemental Medicare

Geographic Areas Served
   California, Texas

Accreditation Certification
   NCQA

Key Personnel
   President. . . . . Greg Buchert

Chief Operating Officer . . . . Amanda Flaum
Chief Medical Officer. . . . . Tanya Dansky
Chief Financial Officer . . . . Michael Engelhard
DVP, Legal Counsel. Alan Bloom
Information Technology . . . . Herbert Woo

75   CareMore Health Plan

12900 Park Plaza Drive
Suite 150, MS-6150
Cerritos, CA 90703
Toll-Free: 800-499-2793
Fax: 562-741-4406
www.caremore.com

Healthplan and Services Defined
   PLAN TYPE: Medicare
   Plan Specialty: Seniors healthcare
   Benefits Offered: Home Care

Type of Coverage
   Medicare

Geographic Areas Served
   Arizona, California, Iowa, Nevada, Ohio, Tennessee, Virginia

Key Personnel
   President & CEO . . . . Sachin H. Jain
   Chief Operations Officer. . . . . Karen Sugano
   Chief Financial Officer . . . . Michael Plumb
   Chief Medical Officer . . . . Zubin Eapen
   Chief Quality Officer. . . . . David Ramirez

76   CenCal Health

4050 Calle Real
Santa Barbara, CA 93110
Toll-Free: 800-421-2560
Phone: 805-685-9525
www.cencalhealth.org
Secondary Address: 1288 Morro Street, Suite 100, San Luis
   Obispo, CA 93401
Non-Profit Organization: Yes
Year Founded: 1983
Number of Primary Care Physicians: 260
Number of Referral/Specialty Physicians: 1,300
Total Enrollment: 175,000

Healthplan and Services Defined
   PLAN TYPE: HMO
   Benefits Offered: Complementary Medicine, Disease
      Management, Prescription, Wellness

Type of Coverage
   Individual, Medicare, Medicaid, Medi-Cal, Healthy Families

Geographic Areas Served
   Santa Barbara and San Luis Obispo counties

Key Personnel
   Chief Executive Officer . . . . Bob Freeman
   Chief Operating Officer . . . . Paul Jaconette
   Chief Financial Officer. . . . . David Ambrose
   Chief Information Officer . . . . Barrie Parker
   Human Resources . . . . Karyn Fish
   Chief Medical Officer . . . . Darryl Leong

Director of Pharmacy . . . . Jeff Januska

77 Central California Alliance for Health

1600 Green Hills Road
Suite 101
Scotts Valley, CA 95066-4981
Toll-Free: 800-700-3874
Phone: 831-430-5500
www.ccah-alliance.org
Secondary Address: 950 East Blanco Road, Suite 101, Salinas, CA 93901-3400, 831-755-6000
Non-Profit Organization: Yes
Year Founded: 1996
Physician Owned Organization: No
Federally Qualified: No
Number of Primary Care Physicians: 1,590
Total Enrollment: 210,000
State Enrollment: 190,000

Healthplan and Services Defined
PLAN TYPE: HMO
Model Type: County Org Health System
Benefits Offered: Chiropractic, Long-Term Care, Vision, Medi-Cal, Healthy Families, Healthy Kids, Alliance Care Access for Infants and Mothers, Alliance Care IHSS
Offers Demand Management Patient Information Service: No

Geographic Areas Served
Santa Cruz, Monterey and Merced counties

Network Qualifications
Pre-Admission Certification: No

Publishes and Distributes Report Card: No

Key Personnel
Executive Director . . . . Alan McCay
Chief Information Officer . . . . Dory Hicks
Chief Operating Officer . . . . Stephanie Sonnenshine
Claims Director . . . . Frank Souza
Utilization Management . . . . Mary Brusuelas, RN, BSN
Gov. Relations Director . . . . Danita Carlson
Quality Improvement Dir . . . . Michelle N. Stott, RN
Reg Dir, Monterey County . . . . Lilia Chagolla
Medical Director. . . . . Elizabeth Murphy, MD
Reg Dir, Merced County . . . . Jennifer Mockus, RN
Operations Director. . . . . Traci Webb
Member Services Director. . . . . Jan Wolf

Specialty Managed Care Partners
Enters into Contracts with Regional Business Coalitions: No

78 Central Health Medicare Plan

1540 Bridgegate Drive
Diamond Bar, CA 91765
Toll-Free: 866-314-2427
mbrsvcs@centralhealthplan.com
www.centralhealthplan.com
Year Founded: 2004

Healthplan and Services Defined
PLAN TYPE: Medicare
Other Type: HMO

Benefits Offered: Chiropractic, Dental, Home Care, Inpatient SNF, Physical Therapy, Podiatry, Vision, Wellness, Diagnostics/Labs/Imaging; Rehabilitation; Medical Equipment

Type of Coverage
Medicare, Supplemental Medicare

Geographic Areas Served
Los Angeles, Orange, San Bernardino and Ventura counties

Key Personnel
Chief Executive Officer . . . . Lee Suyenaga

79 Chinese Community Health Plan

445 Grant Avenue
Suite 700
San Francisco, CA 94108
Toll-Free: 888-775-7888
Phone: 415-955-8800
Fax: 415-955-8818
www.cchphmo.com
Secondary Address: 827 Pacific Ave, San Francisco, CA 94133, 415-834-2118
For Profit Organization: Yes
Year Founded: 1986
Owned by an Integrated Delivery Network (IDN): Yes
Number of Affiliated Hospitals: 5
Number of Primary Care Physicians: 160
Number of Referral/Specialty Physicians: 144
Total Enrollment: 13,582
State Enrollment: 6,336

Healthplan and Services Defined
PLAN TYPE: HMO
Model Type: IPA
Benefits Offered: Prescription, Vision, Wellness, Acupuncture Services, Worldwide Emergency

Type of Coverage
Medicare

Geographic Areas Served
San Francisco, Northern San Mateo

Subscriber Information
Average Monthly Fee Per Subscriber
(Employee + Employer Contribution):
Employee Only (Self): $218.00
Employee & 1 Family Member: $419.00
Employee & 2 Family Members: $384.53
Average Subscriber Co-Payment:
Primary Care Physician: $10.00
Non-Network Physician: Not covered
Prescription Drugs: $6.00
Hospital ER: $25.00
Home Health Care Max. Days/Visits Covered: None except mental
Nursing Home Max. Days/Visits Covered: 10 days

Network Qualifications
Pre-Admission Certification: Yes

Peer Review Type
Utilization Review: Yes

Second Surgical Opinion: Yes
Case Management: Yes

Accreditation Certification
TJC Accreditation, Medicare Approved, Utilization Review,
Pre-Admission Certification, State Licensure, Quality
Assurance Program

Key Personnel
Sales Representative . . . . Yolanda Lee
415-955-8000
Yolanda.Lee@CCHPHealthPlan.com
President/CEO . . . . Brenda Yee, RN

Specialty Managed Care Partners
Enters into Contracts with Regional Business Coalitions: No

---

80   ChiroSource, Inc.
PO Box 130
Clayton, CA 94517
Toll-Free: 800-680-9997
Fax: 925-844-3124
info@chirosource.com
www.chpc.com
For Profit Organization: Yes
Year Founded: 1997

Healthplan and Services Defined
PLAN TYPE: Multiple
Model Type: Network
Plan Specialty: Chiropractic, Physical Medicine,
Accupuncture, Massage
Benefits Offered: Worker's Compensation, Health-Group &
Individual, Medicare Advantage, IME Networks

Type of Coverage
PPO, EPO, POS, MPN, HCN, IME

Type of Payment Plans Offered
FFS

Geographic Areas Served
National

Network Qualifications
Pre-Admission Certification: Yes

Peer Review Type
Utilization Review: Yes

Publishes and Distributes Report Card: No

Specialty Managed Care Partners
Enters into Contracts with Regional Business Coalitions: Yes

---

81   Cigna HealthCare of California
900 Cottage Grove Road
Bloomfield, CT 06002
Toll-Free: 800-997-1654
www.cigna.com
For Profit Organization: Yes

Healthplan and Services Defined
PLAN TYPE: Multiple
Other Type: POS
Plan Specialty: Behavioral Health, Dental, Substance Abuse
Centers

Benefits Offered: Behavioral Health, Dental, Life

Type of Coverage
Commercial, Individual

Key Personnel
Chairman & CEO . . . . David M. Cordani

---

82   Coastal TPA, Inc.
928 East Blanco Road
Suite 235
Salinas, CA 93901
Toll-Free: 800-564-7475
Phone: 831-754-3800
Fax: 831-754-3830
info@coastalmgmt.com
www.coastalmgmt.com
For Profit Organization: Yes
Year Founded: 1961

Healthplan and Services Defined
PLAN TYPE: PPO
Plan Specialty: Third party claims administration and
proprietary regional PPO.
Benefits Offered: Dental, Disease Management, Prescription,
Vision, PPO Network

Type of Coverage
Commercial
Catastrophic Illness Benefit: Unlimited

Type of Payment Plans Offered
FFS

Geographic Areas Served
Monterey, Santa Cruz, San Benito, San Luis Obispo and Santa
Clara counties

Peer Review Type
Utilization Review: No
Second Surgical Opinion: Yes
Case Management: No

Accreditation Certification
NCQA

Average Claim Compensation
Physician's Fees Charged: 70%
Hospital's Fees Charged: 85%

---

83   Community Health Group
2420 Fenton St
Suite 100
Chula Vista, CA 91914
Toll-Free: 800-224-7766
Phone: 619-422-0422
Fax: 619-422-5930
info@chgsd.com
www.chgsd.com
Non-Profit Organization: Yes
Year Founded: 1982
Number of Affiliated Hospitals: 28
Number of Primary Care Physicians: 488
Number of Referral/Specialty Physicians: 1,820
Total Enrollment: 146,000

State Enrollment: 146,000

Healthplan and Services Defined
PLAN TYPE: HMO
Model Type: Network
Plan Specialty: Behavioral Health, Disease Management,
Lab, Vision, Radiology, UR
Benefits Offered: Behavioral Health, Disease Management,
Home Care, Inpatient SNF, Physical Therapy, Podiatry,
Prescription, Psychiatric, Transplant, Wellness
Offers Demand Management Patient Information Service:
Yes

Type of Coverage
Medi-Cal, CommuniCare Advantage
Catastrophic Illness Benefit: None

Type of Payment Plans Offered
Capitated, FFS

Geographic Areas Served
San Diego county

Network Qualifications
Pre-Admission Certification: Yes

Peer Review Type
Utilization Review: Yes
Second Surgical Opinion: Yes
Case Management: Yes

Publishes and Distributes Report Card: Yes

Accreditation Certification
NCQA
Utilization Review, Pre-Admission Certification, State
Licensure, Quality Assurance Program

Key Personnel
CEO . . . . Norma Diaz

Specialty Managed Care Partners
Enters into Contracts with Regional Business Coalitions: No

---

84 **CONCERN: Employee Assistance Program**
1503 Grant Road
Suite 120
Mountain View, CA 94040
Toll-Free: 800-344-4222
info@concern-eap.com
www.concern-eap.com
Non-Profit Organization: Yes

Healthplan and Services Defined
PLAN TYPE: Other
Other Type: EAP
Benefits Offered: Behavioral Health, Psychiatric, Wellness

Type of Coverage
Commercial, EAP

Geographic Areas Served
Silicon Valley

Key Personnel
Chief Executive Officer . . . . Cecile Currier

---

85 **Contra Costa Health Services**
50 Douglas Drive
Suite 310
Martinez, CA 94553
Toll-Free: 800-232-4636
cchealth.org
Non-Profit Organization: Yes
Year Founded: 1973
Federally Qualified: Yes
Number of Affiliated Hospitals: 1
Total Enrollment: 140,000

Healthplan and Services Defined
PLAN TYPE: HMO
Model Type: Staff, Network
Benefits Offered: Behavioral Health, Disease Management,
Wellness, 24-hour psychiatric emergency services

Geographic Areas Served
Contra Costa County

Peer Review Type
Utilization Review: Yes
Second Surgical Opinion: Yes
Case Management: Yes

Publishes and Distributes Report Card: Yes

Accreditation Certification
URAC Accredition
TJC Accreditation, Medicare Approved, Utilization Review,
State Licensure, Quality Assurance Program

Key Personnel
Director & Health Officer . . . . William Walker, MD
925-957-5403
COO & CFO . . . . Patrick Godley
925-957-5405
Communications Officer . . . . Victoria Balladares
925-313-6268

Specialty Managed Care Partners
Enters into Contracts with Regional Business Coalitions: Yes

---

86 **Coventry Health Care of California**
2200 W Orangewood Avenue
Suite 120
Orange, CA 92868
Phone: 714-450-4463
www.coventryhealthcare.com
Subsidiary of: Aetna Inc.
For Profit Organization: Yes

Healthplan and Services Defined
PLAN TYPE: HMO/PPO
Model Type: Network
Plan Specialty: Behavioral Health, Dental, Worker's
Compensation
Benefits Offered: Behavioral Health, Dental, Prescription,
Wellness, Worker's Compensation

Type of Coverage
Commercial, Individual, Medicare, Medicaid

Geographic Areas Served
Statewide

87   Delta Dental of California

P.O. Box 997330
Sacramento, CA 95899-7330
Toll-Free: 800-765-6003
www.deltadentalins.com
Secondary Address: DeltaCare USA Customer Service, P.O.
    Box 1803, Alpharetta, GA 30023, 800-422-4234
Non-Profit Organization: Yes
Year Founded: 1955

Healthplan and Services Defined
    PLAN TYPE: Dental
    Other Type: Dental PPO
    Model Type: Network
    Plan Specialty: Dental
    Benefits Offered: Dental

Type of Coverage
    Commercial, Individual

Type of Payment Plans Offered
    DFFS, Capitated, FFS

Geographic Areas Served
    Statewide

Network Qualifications
    Pre-Admission Certification: No

Peer Review Type
    Utilization Review: Yes
    Second Surgical Opinion: Yes
    Case Management: Yes

Publishes and Distributes Report Card: Yes

Key Personnel
    President & CEO . . . . Anthony S. Barth
    Chief Financial Officer . . . . Michael Castro
    Chief Operating Officer . . . . Nilesh Patel
    Chief Marketing Officer . . . . Belinda Martinez
    Chief Legal Officer . . . . Michael Hankinson

Specialty Managed Care Partners
    PMI Dental Health Plan
    Enters into Contracts with Regional Business Coalitions: Yes

88   Dental Alternatives Insurance Services

Toll-Free: 800-445-8119
Fax: 714-429-1261
info@gotodais.com
www.gotodais.com
Subsidiary of: SafeGuard Health Plans, Inc.
For Profit Organization: Yes
Year Founded: 1977
Total Enrollment: 390,000

Healthplan and Services Defined
    PLAN TYPE: Dental
    Model Type: IPA
    Plan Specialty: Dental
    Benefits Offered: Dental
    Offers Demand Management Patient Information Service:
        Yes

Network Qualifications
    Pre-Admission Certification: Yes

Peer Review Type
    Utilization Review: Yes
    Second Surgical Opinion: Yes
    Case Management: Yes

Publishes and Distributes Report Card: Yes

Accreditation Certification
    NCQA

Specialty Managed Care Partners
    Enters into Contracts with Regional Business Coalitions: Yes

89   Dental Benefit Providers: California

425 Market Street
14th Floor
San Francisco, CA 94105
Phone: 415-778-3800
www.dbp.com
Secondary Address: 9700 Health Care Lane, Minnetonka, MN
    55343, 800-842-3585
Subsidiary of: UnitedHealth Group
For Profit Organization: Yes
Year Founded: 1984
Number of Primary Care Physicians: 125,000
Total Enrollment: 6,600,000

Healthplan and Services Defined
    PLAN TYPE: Dental
    Model Type: IPA
    Plan Specialty: ASO, Dental, EPO, DHMO, PPO, CSO,
        Preventive, Claims Repricing and Network Access
    Benefits Offered: Dental

Type of Coverage
    Indemnity, Medicare, Medicaid

Type of Payment Plans Offered
    POS, DFFS, Capitated, FFS

Geographic Areas Served
    48 states including District of Columbia, Puerto Rico and
    Virgin Islands

Accreditation Certification
    NCQA

Key Personnel
    President, UH Dental . . . . Paul Hebert
    Vice President . . . . Scott Murphy

90   Dental Health Services of California

3833 Atlantic Avenue
Long Beach, CA 90807
Toll-Free: 800-637-6453
Phone: 562-595-6000
Fax: 562-424-0150
www.dentalhealthservices.com
For Profit Organization: Yes
Year Founded: 1974
Physician Owned Organization: Yes
Federally Qualified: Yes

Number of Primary Care Physicians: 1,000
Number of Referral/Specialty Physicians: 400
Total Enrollment: 90,000

Healthplan and Services Defined
PLAN TYPE: Dental
Model Type: Network
Plan Specialty: Dental
Benefits Offered: Dental

Type of Coverage
Commercial, Individual
Catastrophic Illness Benefit: None

Type of Payment Plans Offered
DFFS

Geographic Areas Served
California, Washington, and Oregon

Subscriber Information
Average Monthly Fee Per Subscriber
(Employee + Employer Contribution):
Employee Only (Self): Varies
Employee & 1 Family Member: Varies
Employee & 2 Family Members: Varies

Network Qualifications
Pre-Admission Certification: Yes

Peer Review Type
Second Surgical Opinion: Yes
Case Management: Yes

Publishes and Distributes Report Card: Yes

Accreditation Certification
Dhm
TJC Accreditation, Utilization Review, State Licensure,
Quality Assurance Program

Key Personnel
Founder . . . . Godfrey Pernell

Specialty Managed Care Partners
United Association, 7up
Enters into Contracts with Regional Business Coalitions: No

---

91 **Dentistat**
1688 Dell Avenue
Suite 210
Campbell, CA 95008
Toll-Free: 800-336-8250
Phone: 408-376-0336
Fax: 408-376-0736
info@dentistat.com
www.dentistat.com
For Profit Organization: Yes
Year Founded: 1968
Number of Primary Care Physicians: 80,000

Healthplan and Services Defined
PLAN TYPE: Dental
Model Type: Network
Plan Specialty: Dental
Benefits Offered: Dental

Type of Payment Plans Offered
DFFS, Capitated, FFS, Combination FFS & DFFS

Geographic Areas Served
Nationwide

Accreditation Certification
NCQA
Utilization Review, Quality Assurance Program

Key Personnel
President . . . . Bret Guenther
Chief Information Officer . . . . Sondra Zambino

Specialty Managed Care Partners
Enters into Contracts with Regional Business Coalitions: Yes

---

92 **Easy Choice Health Plan**
10803 Hope Street
Suite B
Cypress, CA 90630
Toll-Free: 866-999-3945
Fax: 877-999-3945
info@easychoicehealthplan.com
www.easychoicehealthplan.com
Mailing Address: P.O. Box 260519, Plano, TX 75026
Subsidary of: WellCare
Total Enrollment: 8,000
State Enrollment: 8,000

Healthplan and Services Defined
PLAN TYPE: Medicare
Benefits Offered: Dental, Disease Management, Prescription,
Vision, Wellness

Type of Coverage
Medicare

Geographic Areas Served
Los Angeles, Orange, Riverside, and San Bernardino counties

Key Personnel
CEO, WellCare . . . . Ken Burdick
COO . . . . Karen M. Johnson
Senior Director . . . . Rachael Rudd
Director, Net. Management . . . . Daniel Dugger
Medical Director . . . . Richard Garcia

---

93 **eHealthInsurance Services, Inc.**
440 E Middlefield Road
Mountain View, CA 94043
Toll-Free: 877-456-7180
headquarters@ehealth.com
www.ehealthinsurance.com
Subsidiary of: eHealth, Inc.
Year Founded: 1997
Total Enrollment: 4,000,000

Healthplan and Services Defined
PLAN TYPE: Multiple
Plan Specialty: Dental, Vision
Benefits Offered: Behavioral Health, Chiropractic, Dental,
Disease Management, Home Care, Inpatient SNF, Podiatry,
Prescription, Vision, Wellness, Life, STD, Benefits vary
according to plan

Type of Coverage
Commercial, Individual, Medicare, Supplemental Medicare

Geographic Areas Served
Nationwide, including the District of Columbia

Key Personnel
Chief Executive Officer . . . . Scott N. Flanders
CFO/COO. . . . . Dave Francis
SVP/General Counsel . . . . Scott Giesler
Chief Marketing Manager . . . . Tim Hannan
SVP of Sales & Operations . . . . Dave Nicklaus

---

94 First Health

Coventry Health Care, Inc.
6730-B Rockledge Drive, Suite 700
Bethesda, MD 20817
Toll-Free: 800-226-5116
www.firsthealth.com
Subsidiary of: Coventry Health Care
For Profit Organization: Yes
Year Founded: 1984
Number of Affiliated Hospitals: 134
Number of Primary Care Physicians: 1,923
Number of Referral/Specialty Physicians: 5,744
Total Enrollment: 2,000,000
State Enrollment: 585,000

Healthplan and Services Defined
PLAN TYPE: PPO
Model Type: Network
Benefits Offered: Disease Management, Wellness

Type of Payment Plans Offered
DFFS

Geographic Areas Served
State of Oklahoma and contiguous border cities of Missouri, Arkansas, Kansas and Texas

Key Personnel
President & CEO . . . . Blaine Faulkner
VP, Business Development . . . . Kara Dornig
VP, Account Management . . . . Susan Korth
VP, Operations . . . . Kelly Wright
Sales Director . . . . John Bryan

Average Claim Compensation
Physician's Fees Charged: 72%
Hospital's Fees Charged: 62%

---

95 Foundation f. Medical Care f. Kern & Santa Barbara Counties

5701 Truxtun Avenue
Suite 100
Bakersfield, CA 93309
Phone: 661-327-7581
Fax: 661-327-5129
www.kernfmc.com
Number of Affiliated Hospitals: 400
Number of Primary Care Physicians: 30,000
Number of Referral/Specialty Physicians: 7,000

Healthplan and Services Defined
PLAN TYPE: PPO
Model Type: IPA, Group, Network
Benefits Offered: Dental, Disease Management, Prescription, Wellness
Offers Demand Management Patient Information Service: Yes

Type of Payment Plans Offered
POS, DFFS, FFS, Combination FFS & DFFS

Geographic Areas Served
Kern and Santa Barbara counties

Network Qualifications
Pre-Admission Certification: Yes

Peer Review Type
Utilization Review: Yes
Second Surgical Opinion: Yes
Case Management: Yes

Accreditation Certification
TJC Accreditation, Medicare Approved, Utilization Review, Pre-Admission Certification, State Licensure

Key Personnel
Chief Executive Officer. . . . . Carolyn J Temple
ctemple@kernfmc.com
Chief Operating Officer . . . . Deborah Hankins
dhankinskernfmc.com
Executive Assistant. Lisa Garzelli
lgarzelli@kernfmc.com
Manager, Customer Service . . . . Annette Charlton
acharlton@kernfmc.com
Provider Relations . . . . Kelly Swartz
kswartz@kernfmc.com
Exec Admin Supervisor . . . . Lisa Garzelli
lgarzelli@kernfmc.com

Specialty Managed Care Partners
Enters into Contracts with Regional Business Coalitions: No

---

96 GEMCare Health Plan

4550 California Avenue
Suite 500
Bakersfield, CA 93309
Phone: 661-716-7100
Fax: 661-716-9200
gemcare.com
Year Founded: 1992
Number of Primary Care Physicians: 120

Healthplan and Services Defined
PLAN TYPE: Medicare
Model Type: IPA

Type of Coverage
Medicare, Supplemental Medicare

Geographic Areas Served
Kern County, including Bakersfield and the outlying communities of Arvin, Delano, Lake Isabella, Shafter, Taft, Tehachapi and Wasco

Key Personnel
President & CEO . . . . Michael R Myers
Chief Operating Officer . . . . Tonya Rhoades

Chief Financial Officer . . . . Jeff Mihal

Chief Medical Officer . . . . Stephan Bass, MD

97 Golden West Dental & Vision

5171 Verdugo Way
Camarillo, CA 93012
Toll-Free: 800-219-9216
www.goldenwestdental.com
Subsidiary of: Anthem
For Profit Organization: Yes
Year Founded: 1974

Healthplan and Services Defined
PLAN TYPE: Multiple
Plan Specialty: Dental, Vision
Benefits Offered: Dental, Vision
Offers Demand Management Patient Information Service:
Yes

Type of Payment Plans Offered
Capitated, Combination FFS & DFFS

Geographic Areas Served
Statewide

Peer Review Type
Second Surgical Opinion: Yes

Publishes and Distributes Report Card: Yes

Key Personnel
CFO . . . . Steve Sheehan
CIO. . . . . Shenoy Manju
Marketing . . . . Chris McConathy
Dental Director . . . . Karen Feldman

Average Claim Compensation
Physician's Fees Charged: 80%

Specialty Managed Care Partners
Enters into Contracts with Regional Business Coalitions: Yes

98 Health Net Dental

340 Commerce
Suite 100
Irvine, CA 92602
Toll-Free: 800-977-7307
www.hndental.com
For Profit Organization: Yes

Healthplan and Services Defined
PLAN TYPE: Dental
Model Type: Network
Plan Specialty: Dental
Benefits Offered: Dental

Type of Coverage
Individual, Dental coverage for Healthy Familie

Geographic Areas Served
Los Angeles and Sacramento County

99 Health Net Federal Services

2025 Aerojet Road
Mail Code CA-169-01-27
Rancho Cordova, CA 95742
Toll-Free: 877-874-2273
www.hnfs.com
Subsidiary of: Centene Corporation
For Profit Organization: Yes
Total Enrollment: 2,900,000

Healthplan and Services Defined
PLAN TYPE: Multiple
Model Type: Network
Plan Specialty: Behavioral Health
Benefits Offered: Behavioral Health, Anger management;
DUI program; alcohol & drug assessments

Type of Coverage
Commercial, Individual, Medicare, Supplemental Medicare

Geographic Areas Served
Alaska, Arizona, California, Colorado, Hawaii, Idaho, Iowa
(except the Rock Island Arsenal area), Kansas, Minnesota,
Missouri, (except the St. Louis area), Montana, Nebraska,
Nevada, New Mexico, North Dakota, Oregon, South Dakota,
Texas (areas of Western Texas only), Utah, Washington, and
Wyoming

Key Personnel
President. . . . . Billy Maynard
Media Contact . . . . Molly Tuttle
molly.m.tuttle@healthnet.com

100 Health Net Insurance

P.O. Box 10420
Van Nuys, CA 91410-0420
Toll-Free: 877-527-8409
www.healthnet.com
Subsidiary of: Centene Corporation
For Profit Organization: Yes

Healthplan and Services Defined
PLAN TYPE: Multiple
Model Type: Network
Plan Specialty: Behavioral Health

Type of Coverage
Commercial, Individual, Medicare, Supplemental Medicare,
Medi-Cal

Geographic Areas Served
Arizona, California, Oregon, Washington

101 Health Net, Inc.

21281 Burbank Boulevard
Woodland Hills, CA 91367
Phone: 818-676-6775
Fax: 818-676-6992
www.healthnet.com
Subsidiary of: Centene Corporation
For Profit Organization: Yes
Year Founded: 1977
Total Enrollment: 6,100,000

Healthplan and Services Defined
PLAN TYPE: HMO
Model Type: IPA, Group
Plan Specialty: Behavioral Health, PBM, Substance abuse
and employee assistance programs.
Benefits Offered: Behavioral Health, Chiropractic, Dental,
Disease Management, Prescription, Vision, Wellness,
Benefits vary according to plan
Offers Demand Management Patient Information Service:
Yes

Type of Coverage
Commercial, Individual, Medicare, Supplemental Medicare,
Health Net Medi-Cal
Catastrophic Illness Benefit: Covered

Type of Payment Plans Offered
POS, DFFS, FFS

Geographic Areas Served
Nationwide, including the District of Columbia

Peer Review Type
Utilization Review: Yes
Second Surgical Opinion: Yes
Case Management: Yes

Publishes and Distributes Report Card: Yes

Accreditation Certification
NCQA
TJC Accreditation, Medicare Approved, Utilization Review,
Pre-Admission Certification, State Licensure, Quality
Assurance Program

Key Personnel
President/CEO . . . . Jay Gellert
Chief Financial Officer . . . . Joseph C. Capezza
EVP/COO . . . . James Woys
Contact, Federal Services . . . . Molly Tuttle
molly.tuttle@healthnet.com

Specialty Managed Care Partners
Enters into Contracts with Regional Business Coalitions: Yes

102　Health Plan of San Joaquin

7751 South Manthey Road
French Camp, CA 95231-9802
Toll-Free: 888-936-7526
Phone: 209-942-6340
Fax: 209-942-6305
www.hpsj.com
Secondary Address: 1025 J. Street, Modesto, CA 95354
Non-Profit Organization: Yes
Year Founded: 1996
Number of Primary Care Physicians: 180
Number of Referral/Specialty Physicians: 1,400
Total Enrollment: 109,000
State Enrollment: 109,000

Healthplan and Services Defined
PLAN TYPE: HMO
Benefits Offered: Behavioral Health, Dental, Inpatient SNF,
Podiatry, Prescription, Vision, Wellness

Offers Demand Management Patient Information Service: Yes
DMPI Services Offered: 24 Hour Nurse Advice Hotline

Type of Coverage
Commercial, Medicaid, Medi-Cal

Geographic Areas Served
San Joaquin and Stanislaus counties

Key Personnel
CEO. . . . . Amy Shin
Medical Director . . . . Dorcas C. Yao, MD
VP, External Affairs . . . . David Hurst

103　Health Plan of San Mateo

801 Gateway Boulevard
Suite 100
South San Francisco, CA 94080
Toll-Free: 800-750-4776
Phone: 650-616-0050
Fax: 650-616-0060
info@hpsm.org
www.hpsm.org
Non-Profit Organization: Yes
Year Founded: 1987
Number of Affiliated Hospitals: 12
Number of Primary Care Physicians: 197
Total Enrollment: 87,740
State Enrollment: 87,740

Healthplan and Services Defined
PLAN TYPE: HMO
Model Type: IPA
Benefits Offered: Dental, Disease Management, Long-Term
Care, Prescription, Vision, Wellness

Type of Coverage
Medi-Cal, Healthy Families, Healthy

Type of Payment Plans Offered
Capitated, FFS

Geographic Areas Served
San Mateo county

Key Personnel
CEO. . . . . Maya Altman
CFO . . . . Ron Robinson
CIO Director . . . . Eben Yong
Chief Medical Officer . . . . Margaret Beed, MD

104　Health Services Los Angeles County

313 N Figueroa Street
Los Angeles, CA 90012
dhs.lacounty.gov/wps/portal/dhs
Subsidiary of: Los Angeles County Department of Health
Services
Non-Profit Organization: Yes
Federally Qualified: Yes
Number of Affiliated Hospitals: 4

Healthplan and Services Defined
PLAN TYPE: Other
Model Type: municipal health system

Plan Specialty: Juvenile Justice System, children in Foster Care

Benefits Offered: Disease Management, Prescription, Wellness, AIDS Drug Assistance Program; Pediatrics

Type of Coverage

Catastrophic Illness Benefit: Unlimited

Geographic Areas Served

Los Angeles County

Subscriber Information

Average Monthly Fee Per Subscriber

(Employee + Employer Contribution):

Employee Only (Self): $143.05

Employee & 1 Family Member: $286.15

Employee & 2 Family Members: $332.01

Average Subscriber Co-Payment:

Primary Care Physician: $5.00

Prescription Drugs: $4.00

Home Health Care Max. Days/Visits Covered: Unlimited

Nursing Home Max. Days/Visits Covered: 60 days

Network Qualifications

Pre-Admission Certification: Yes

Peer Review Type

Utilization Review: Yes

Second Surgical Opinion: Yes

Case Management: Yes

Accreditation Certification

TJC Accreditation, Medicare Approved, Utilization Review, State Licensure, Quality Assurance Program

Key Personnel

Director . . . . Mitchell Katz, MD

Chief Financial Officer . . . . Allan Wecker

Chief Operations Officer . . . . Christina Ghaly, MD

Chief Information Officer . . . . Kevin Lynch

Chief Medical Officer . . . . Hal F. Yee Jr., MD

---

105 Humana Health Insurance of California

1 Park Plaza

Suite 470

Irvine, CA 92614

Phone: 949-623-1447

www.humana.com

Secondary Address: 970 West 190th Street, Suite 425, Torrance, CA 90502, 424-246-4834

Subsidiary of: Humana

For Profit Organization: Yes

Healthplan and Services Defined

PLAN TYPE: HMO/PPO

Model Type: Network

Plan Specialty: Dental, Vision

Benefits Offered: Dental, Prescription, Vision, Life, LTD, STD, Benefits vary according to plan

Type of Coverage

Commercial, Medicare

Geographic Areas Served

Statewide

Accreditation Certification

URAC, NCQA, CORE

Key Personnel

Western Division Leader . . . . Mark El-Tawil

California Mrkt President. . . . . Jim Brown

---

106 Inter Valley Health Plan

300 S Park Avenue

P.O. Box 6002

Pomona, CA 91769-6002

Toll-Free: 800-251-8191

info@ivhp.com

www.ivhp.com

Non-Profit Organization: Yes

Year Founded: 1979

Owned by an Integrated Delivery Network (IDN): No

Federally Qualified: Yes

Number of Affiliated Hospitals: 24

Number of Primary Care Physicians: 1,161

Number of Referral/Specialty Physicians: 4,791

Total Enrollment: 14,600

Healthplan and Services Defined

PLAN TYPE: Medicare

Model Type: Network

Benefits Offered: Behavioral Health, Dental, Home Care, Inpatient SNF, Physical Therapy, Prescription, Psychiatric, Transplant, Wellness

Type of Coverage

Medicare

Catastrophic Illness Benefit: Unlimited

Type of Payment Plans Offered

Capitated

Geographic Areas Served

Southern California counties including Los Angeles, Riverside, San Bernardino, and Orange

Network Qualifications

Pre-Admission Certification: No

Peer Review Type

Utilization Review: Yes

Second Surgical Opinion: Yes

Case Management: Yes

Accreditation Certification

URAC, PBGH, CCHRI

TJC Accreditation, Medicare Approved, Utilization Review, State Licensure, Quality Assurance Program

Key Personnel

President and CEO . . . . Ron Bolding

VP and CFO . . . . Paul Biberkraut

VP, Health Plan Operation . . . . Susan Tenorio

Chief Medical Officer . . . . Kenneth E. Smith, MD, MBA

Average Claim Compensation

Physician's Fees Charged: 75%

Hospital's Fees Charged: 55%

Specialty Managed Care Partners

Vision Service Plan

107   Kaiser Permanente

1 Kaiser Plaza
Oakland, CA 94612
Phone: 510-271-5910
www.kaiserpermanente.org
Non-Profit Organization: Yes
Year Founded: 1945
Number of Affiliated Hospitals: 39
Number of Primary Care Physicians: 17,791
Total Enrollment: 11,800,000
State Enrollment: 8,521,345

Healthplan and Services Defined
    PLAN TYPE: HMO/PPO
    Model Type: Group
    Benefits Offered: Dental, Disease Management, Home Care,
        Inpatient SNF, Long-Term Care, Physical Therapy,
        Podiatry, Prescription, Psychiatric, Transplant, Vision,
        Wellness, Benefits vary according to plan
    Offers Demand Management Patient Information Service:
        Yes

Type of Coverage
    Commercial, Individual, Medicare, Supplemental Medicare,
        Medicaid
    Catastrophic Illness Benefit: Covered

Type of Payment Plans Offered
    POS

Geographic Areas Served
    California, Colorado, Georgia, Hawaii, Maryland, Oregon,
    Virginia, Washington and the District of Columbia

Network Qualifications
    Pre-Admission Certification: Yes

Peer Review Type
    Utilization Review: Yes
    Second Surgical Opinion: Yes
    Case Management: Yes

Publishes and Distributes Report Card: Yes

Accreditation Certification
    NCQA
    TJC Accreditation, Medicare Approved, Utilization Review,
        Pre-Admission Certification, State Licensure, Quality
        Assurance Program

Key Personnel
    Chairman/CEO . . . . Bernard Tyson
    EVP/CIO . . . . Richard Daniels
    EVP/CFO . . . . Kathy Lancaster
    EVP/CMO . . . . Patrick Courneya, MD
    Media Contact . . . . Jessie Mangaliman
        510-301-5414

Specialty Managed Care Partners
    Enters into Contracts with Regional Business Coalitions: No

108   Kaiser Permanente Northern California

1950 Franklin Street
Oakland, CA 94612
Phone: 510-987-1000
thrive.kaiserpermanente.org/care-near-northern-california

Subsidiary of: Kaiser Permanente
Non-Profit Organization: Yes
Year Founded: 1945
Number of Affiliated Hospitals: 21
Number of Primary Care Physicians: 8,500
Total Enrollment: 118,000,000
State Enrollment: 4,131,326

Healthplan and Services Defined
    PLAN TYPE: HMO/PPO
    Model Type: Group, Network
    Benefits Offered: Disease Management, Home Care, Inpatient
        SNF, Long-Term Care, Physical Therapy, Podiatry,
        Prescription, Psychiatric, Transplant, Vision, Wellness

Type of Coverage
    Commercial, Individual, Medicare, Medicaid

Type of Payment Plans Offered
    POS, Combination FFS & DFFS

Geographic Areas Served
    Alameda, Amador, Contra Costa, El Dorado, Fresno, Kings,
    Madera, Marin, Mariposa, Napa, Placer, Sacramento, San
    Francisco, San Joaquin, San Mateo, Santa Clara, Solano,
    Sonoma, Stanislaus, Sutter, Tulcare, Yolo & Yuba counties

Subscriber Information
    Average Monthly Fee Per Subscriber
        (Employee + Employer Contribution):
            Employee Only (Self): Varies by plan

Network Qualifications
    Pre-Admission Certification: Yes

Publishes and Distributes Report Card: Yes

Accreditation Certification
    TJC Accreditation, Medicare Approved, Utilization Review,
        Pre-Admission Certification, State Licensure, Quality
        Assurance Program

Key Personnel
    President, No.California . . . . Janet Liang
    Executive Medic. Director . . . . Edward M. Ellison, MD
    Media Contact . . . . Jessie Mangaliman
        510-301-5414

Specialty Managed Care Partners
    Enters into Contracts with Regional Business Coalitions: Yes

109   Kaiser Permanente Southern California

9455 Clairemont Mesa Boulevard
San Diego, CA 92123
thrive.kaiserpermanente.org/care-near-you/southern-califor
ni
Subsidiary of: Kaiser Permanente
Non-Profit Organization: Yes
Year Founded: 1945
Number of Affiliated Hospitals: 15
Number of Primary Care Physicians: 7,274
Total Enrollment: 11,800,000
State Enrollment: 4,390,019

Healthplan and Services Defined
    PLAN TYPE: Multiple

Model Type: Network
Benefits Offered: Disease Management, Home Care,
   Inpatient SNF, Long-Term Care, Physical Therapy,
   Podiatry, Prescription, Psychiatric, Transplant, Vision,
   Wellness

Type of Coverage
Commercial, Individual, Medicare, Medicaid

Geographic Areas Served
Antelope Valley, Baldwin Park, Downey, Kern County, Los
Angeles, Orange County, Panorama City, Riverside County,
San Bernadino County, San Diego, South Bay, Ventura
County, West Los Angeles, Woodland Hills

Key Personnel
President, South. Cali . . . . Julie Miller-Phipps
Media Contact . . . . Lowell Goodman
   626-405-3004

110   Kern Family Health Care

5701 Truxtun Avenue
Suite 201
Bakersfield, CA 93309
Toll-Free: 800-391-2000
Phone: 661-664-5000
louiei@khs-net.com
www.kernfamilyhealthcare.com
Subsidiary of: Kern Health Systems
Non-Profit Organization: Yes
Number of Affiliated Hospitals: 10
Number of Primary Care Physicians: 213
Number of Referral/Specialty Physicians: 400
Total Enrollment: 97,000
State Enrollment: 90,074

Healthplan and Services Defined
   PLAN TYPE: HMO
   Model Type: Network
   Benefits Offered: Dental, Disease Management, Prescription,
      Vision, Wellness
   Offers Demand Management Patient Information Service:
      Yes
   DMPI Services Offered: 24 Hour Nurse Advice Hotline

Type of Coverage
Individual, Medicaid, Medi-Cal

Key Personnel
Chief Executive Officer . . . . Douglas A. Hayward
Chief Financial Officer . . . . Robert Landis
Chief Operations Officer . . . . Alan Avery
Manager, Marketing . . . . Louis Iturriria
   661-664-5120
   louiei@khs-net.com

111   L.A. Care Health Plan

1055 W 7th Street
10th Floor
Los Angeles, CA 90017
Toll-Free: 888-839-9909
www.lacare.org
Non-Profit Organization: Yes

Year Founded: 1997
Total Enrollment: 2,000,000

Healthplan and Services Defined
   PLAN TYPE: HMO
   Benefits Offered: Behavioral Health, Dental, Home Care,
      Inpatient SNF, Physical Therapy, Prescription, Transplant,
      Vision, Wellness, Asthma Care; Cancer Clinical Trials;
      Diabetic Care; Diagnostic/Labs/Imaging Services; Durable
      Medical Equipment; Hospice

Type of Coverage
Individual, Medicare, Medicaid

Key Personnel
Chief Executive Officer . . . . John Baackes
COO . . . . Dino Kasdagly
Chief Financial Officer . . . . Marie Montgomery
Chief Medical Officer . . . . Richard Seidman
General Counsel . . . . Augustavia Haydel
Chief Compliance Officer . . . . Tom Mapp

112   L.A. Care Health Plan

1055 W 7th Street
10th Floor
Los Angeles, CA 90017
Toll-Free: 888-452-2273
www.lacare.org
Non-Profit Organization: Yes
Year Founded: 1997
Number of Affiliated Hospitals: 83
Number of Primary Care Physicians: 3,555
Number of Referral/Specialty Physicians: 6,286
Total Enrollment: 857,252
State Enrollment: 836,724

Healthplan and Services Defined
   PLAN TYPE: HMO
   Model Type: Staff
   Benefits Offered: Dental, Home Care, Podiatry, Prescription,
      Vision, Comprehensive Health Coverage, Medical

Type of Coverage
Medicaid, Medi-Cal, L.A. Care Covered, Cal Me

Geographic Areas Served
Los Angeles County

Key Personnel
CEO . . . . John Baackes
COO . . . . Dino Kasdagly
CFO . . . . Marie Montgomery
General Counsel . . . . Augustavia J. Haydel
Chief Medical Officer . . . . Richard Seidman, MD, MPH
CIO . . . . Tom Schwaninger
Media Contact . . . . Amy Gurango
   213-694-1250
   agurango@lacare.org

113 Lakeside Community Healthcare Network
191 S Buena Vista Street
Suite 200
Burbank, CA 91505-4542
Toll-Free: 818-637-2000
info@lakesidecommunityhealthcare.com
www.lakesidemed.com
For Profit Organization: Yes
Year Founded: 1997
Number of Primary Care Physicians: 300
Number of Referral/Specialty Physicians: 1,500
Total Enrollment: 250,000
State Enrollment: 250,000

Healthplan and Services Defined
PLAN TYPE: HMO
Model Type: IPA

Geographic Areas Served
San Fernando, San Gabriel, and Santa Clarita Valleys. Parts of Ventura and San Bernadino counties

Key Personnel
President/CEO .... Francesco Federico, MD
EVP, Corporate Dev............. Keith S Richman, MD
COO .... Joan Rose, MPH
CFO............................. Kermit Newman
SVP, Medical Operations .... Jeffrey Hay
Medical Director .... Ziad Dabuni, MD
Chief Medical Officer .... Bernard Siegel, MD
Media Contact....................... Pamela Pollock
pam.pollock@lakesidecommunityhealthcare.

114 Landmark Healthplan of California
P.O. Box 130028
Sacramento, CA 95853
Toll-Free: 800-298-4875
Fax: 800-547-9784
www.lhp-ca.com
For Profit Organization: Yes
Year Founded: 1985
Number of Referral/Specialty Physicians: 4,500
Total Enrollment: 150,000

Healthplan and Services Defined
PLAN TYPE: HMO/PPO
Model Type: IPA, Network
Plan Specialty: Chiropractic, Acupuncture
Benefits Offered: Chiropractic, Acupuncture

Type of Payment Plans Offered
Combination FFS & DFFS

Geographic Areas Served
Statewide

Network Qualifications
Pre-Admission Certification: Yes

Peer Review Type
Utilization Review: Yes
Case Management: Yes

Key Personnel
President/CEO .... George W. Vieth, Jr

VP/CFO......................... Thomas P. Klammer
Sales................................ Greg Clure
800-298-4875
Sales@LHP-CA.com

115 Liberty Dental Plan of California
340 Commerce
Suite 100
Irvine, CA 92602
Toll-Free: 888-703-6999
www.libertydentalplan.com
Mailing Address: P.O. Box 26110, Santa Ana, CA 92799-6110
For Profit Organization: Yes
Year Founded: 2001
Total Enrollment: 3,000,000

Healthplan and Services Defined
PLAN TYPE: Dental
Other Type: Dental HMO
Plan Specialty: Dental
Benefits Offered: Dental

Type of Coverage
Commercial, Individual, Medicare, Medicaid, Medi-Cal

Geographic Areas Served
Statewide

Accreditation Certification
NCQA

Key Personnel
Dental Director................... Richard Hague, DMD

116 Managed Health Network, Inc.
2370 Kerner Boulevard
San Rafael, CA 94901
Toll-Free: 800-327-2133
productinfo@mhn.com
www.mhn.com
Subsidiary of: Health Net, Inc.
For Profit Organization: Yes
Number of Affiliated Hospitals: 1,400
Number of Primary Care Physicians: 55,000
Total Enrollment: 7,300,000

Healthplan and Services Defined
PLAN TYPE: Other
Plan Specialty: Behavioral Health, Substance abuse and employee assistance programs (EAPs).
Benefits Offered: Behavioral Health, Disease Management, Wellness, Work/life balance, employee productivity and organizational effectiveness.

Geographic Areas Served
Nationwide

Accreditation Certification
URAC

Key Personnel
Director, Clinical Op. .... Nancy Mann
VP, Marketing & Comms................ Gina Clemente
Chief Medical Officer .... Ian Shaffer, MD
Chief Sales Officer .... Gidget L. A. Peddie

117 March Vision Care

6701 Center Drive W
Suite 790
Los Angeles, CA 90045
Toll-Free: 866-376-6780
Phone: 310-216-2300
marchinfo@marchvisioncare.com
www.marchvisioncare.com
For Profit Organization: Yes

Healthplan and Services Defined
PLAN TYPE: Vision
Plan Specialty: Vision
Benefits Offered: Vision

Type of Coverage
Commercial, Medicare, Medicaid

Geographic Areas Served
Nationwide

Key Personnel
Founder & CEO . . . . Glenville A March, Jr, MD
Founder & CEO . . . . Cabrini T March, MD

118 Medcore Medical Group

2609 E Hammer Lane
Stockton, CA 95210
Toll-Free: 877-963-2673
Phone: 209-320-2650
Fax: 209-320-2644
medcoreipa.com
Year Founded: 1985

Healthplan and Services Defined
PLAN TYPE: Other
Model Type: Network

Geographic Areas Served
San Joaquin County

Key Personnel
Chief Operating Officer . . . . Maria Martinez

119 Medica HealthCare Plans, Inc

9100 S Dadeland Boulevard
Suite 1250
Miami, FL 33156
Toll-Free: 800-407-9069
Fax: 800-517-6924
MemberServices@uhcsouthflorida.com
www.medicaplans.com
Mailing Address: P.O. Box 56-6596, Miami, FL 33156
Total Enrollment: 12,000

Healthplan and Services Defined
PLAN TYPE: Medicare
Benefits Offered: Chiropractic, Dental, Disease Management,
Inpatient SNF, Podiatry, Prescription, Psychiatric, Vision,
Wellness

Type of Coverage
Medicare, Supplemental Medicare

Geographic Areas Served
Miami-Dade & Broward counties

Key Personnel
Chief Medical Officer . . . . Orlando Lopez-Fernandez, Jr.

120 Molina Healthcare

200 Oceangate
Suite 100
Long Beach, CA 90802
Toll-Free: 888-562-5442
Phone: 562-435-3666
www.molinahealthcare.com
For Profit Organization: Yes

Healthplan and Services Defined
PLAN TYPE: Medicare
Other Type: Madicaid
Benefits Offered: Disease Management, Physical Therapy,
Wellness

Type of Coverage
Medicare, Supplemental Medicare, Medicaid

Geographic Areas Served
California, Florida, Illinois, Michigan, Ohio, Puerto Rico,
New Mexico, New York, South Carolina, Texas, Utah,
Washington and Wisconsin

Key Personnel
Chief Executive Officer . . . . Joseph White
Chief Operating Officer . . . . Terry Bayer
SVP, Relations/Marketing . . . . Juan Jos, Orellana
Chief Information Officer . . . . Rick Hopfer

121 Molina Healthcare of California

200 Oceangate
Suite 100
Long Beach, CA 90802
Toll-Free: 800-526-8196
Phone: 562-435-3666
www.molinahealthcare.com
Subsidiary of: Molina Healthcare, Inc.
For Profit Organization: Yes
Year Founded: 1980

Healthplan and Services Defined
PLAN TYPE: Medicare
Model Type: Network
Plan Specialty: Dental, PBM, Vision, Integrated
Medicare/Medicaid (Duals)
Benefits Offered: Dental, Prescription, Vision, Wellness, Life

Type of Coverage
Individual, Medicare, Supplemental Medicare, Medicaid

Geographic Areas Served
Statewide

122   Molina Medicaid Solutions

200 Oceangate
Suite 100
Long Beach, CA 90802
Toll-Free: 888-562-5442
Phone: 562-435-3666
www.molinahealthcare.com
Subsidiary of: Molina Healthcare, Inc.
For Profit Organization: Yes
Year Founded: 2010

Healthplan and Services Defined
   PLAN TYPE: Medicare

Type of Coverage
   Medicaid information management sys

Geographic Areas Served
   Idaho, Louisiana, Maine, New Jersey, West Virginia

Key Personnel
   Chief Executive Officer . . . . Joseph W. White
   Chief Operating Officer . . . . Terry Bayer
   General Counsel. . . . . Jeff D. Barlow
   SVP, Relations/Marketing . . . . Juan Jos, Orellana
   Chief Information Officer . . . . Rick Hopfer

123   On Lok Lifeways

1333 Bush Street
San Francisco, CA 94109
Phone: 415-292-8888
Fax: 415-292-8745
info@onlok.org
www.onlok.org
Non-Profit Organization: Yes
Year Founded: 1971
Number of Affiliated Hospitals: 7
Number of Primary Care Physicians: 10
Number of Referral/Specialty Physicians: 100
Total Enrollment: 1,000
State Enrollment: 942

Healthplan and Services Defined
   PLAN TYPE: HMO
   Model Type: Staff
   Benefits Offered: Dental, Home Care, Long-Term Care,
      Physical Therapy, Podiatry, Prescription, Vision, Wellness

Type of Coverage
   Medicaid
   Catastrophic Illness Benefit: Covered

Geographic Areas Served
   San Francisco, Fremont, Newark, Union City and Santa Clara
   County

Accreditation Certification
   TJC Accreditation, Medicare Approved, Utilization Review,
      Pre-Admission Certification, State Licensure, Quality
      Assurance Program

Key Personnel
   CEO . . . . Grace Li, MHA
   CFO . . . . Gary Campanella, MBA
   COO . . . . David C. Nolan

Chief, Gov. Affairs . . . . Eileen Kunz, MPH
Chief Medical Officer . . . . Jay Luxenberg, MD
CIO . . . . Neal Wright, MBA

124   Optimum HealthCare, Inc

5403 North Church Avenue
Tampa, FL 33614
Toll-Free: 866-245-5360
Fax: 813-506-6150
www.youroptimumhealthcare.com
Mailing Address: P.O. Box 151137, Tampa, FL 33684

Healthplan and Services Defined
   PLAN TYPE: HMO

Type of Coverage
   Medicare, Medicaid

Geographic Areas Served
   Brevard, Broward, Charlotte, Citrus, Clay, Collier, Dade, De
   Soto, Duval, Escambia, Hernando, Hillsborough, Indian
   River, Lake, Lee, Manatee, Marion, Martin, Orange, Osceola,
   Palm Beach, Pasco, Pinellas, Polk, Sarasota, Seminole, St.
   Lucie, Sumter and Volusia counties

Accreditation Certification
   NCQA

125   Pacific Foundation for Medical Care

3510 Unocal Place
Suite 108
Santa Rosa, CA 95403
Toll-Free: 800-548-7677
Phone: 707-525-4281
Fax: 707-525-4311
jnacol@rhs.org
pfmc.org
Non-Profit Organization: Yes
Year Founded: 1957
Number of Primary Care Physicians: 34,000

Healthplan and Services Defined
   PLAN TYPE: Multiple
   Model Type: Network
   Plan Specialty: EPO, PPO, LOCO

Geographic Areas Served
   counties: Alameda, Butte, Colusa, Contra Costa, El Dorado,
   Glenn, Imperial, Lake, Lassen, Marin, Mendocino, Modoc,
   Napa, Nevada, Placer, Plumas, Sacramento, San Diego, San
   Francisco, Shasta, Sierra, Siskiyou, Solano, Sonoma, Sutter,
   Tehama, Trinity, Yolo, Yuba

Network Qualifications
   Pre-Admission Certification: Yes

Peer Review Type
   Utilization Review: Yes
   Second Surgical Opinion: Yes
   Case Management: Yes

Publishes and Distributes Report Card: No

Key Personnel
   President. . . . . Dan Lightfoot, MD

Medical Director . . . . William Pitt, MD
Contact. . . . . Kathy Pass
   705-525-4281
   kpass@rhs.org

Specialty Managed Care Partners
Enters into Contracts with Regional Business Coalitions: No

126 Pacific Health Alliance

1525 Rollins Road
Suite B
Burlingame, CA 94010
Toll-Free: 800-533-4742
Fax: 650-375-5820
pha@pacifichealthalliance.com
www.pacifichealthalliance.com
For Profit Organization: Yes
Year Founded: 1986
Number of Affiliated Hospitals: 400
Number of Primary Care Physicians: 50,000
Number of Referral/Specialty Physicians: 1,500
Total Enrollment: 338,000
State Enrollment: 197,000

Healthplan and Services Defined
   PLAN TYPE: PPO
   Model Type: Group
   Plan Specialty: Behavioral Health, Chiropractic, EPO, Lab,
      Worker's Compensation, UR
   Benefits Offered: Behavioral Health, Chiropractic, Dental,
      Home Care, Inpatient SNF, Long-Term Care, Physical
      Therapy, Podiatry, Psychiatric, Transplant, Vision,
      Worker's Compensation

Type of Coverage
   Commercial, Individual, Indemnity

Type of Payment Plans Offered
   DFFS, FFS

Geographic Areas Served
   Nationwide

Network Qualifications
   Pre-Admission Certification: Yes

Peer Review Type
   Utilization Review: Yes
   Second Surgical Opinion: Yes
   Case Management: Yes

Publishes and Distributes Report Card: No

Accreditation Certification
   TJC Accreditation, Medicare Approved, Utilization Review,
      Pre-Admission Certification, State Licensure, Quality
      Assurance Program

Average Claim Compensation
   Physician's Fees Charged: 70%
   Hospital's Fees Charged: 75%

Specialty Managed Care Partners
   Daughters of Charity, Saint Rose Hospital, San Monterry
   Enters into Contracts with Regional Business Coalitions: No

127 Partnership HealthPlan of California

4665 Business Center Drive
Fairfield, CA 94534-1675
Toll-Free: 800-863-4155
Fax: 707-863-4177
www.partnershiphp.org
Secondary Address: 3688 Avtech Parkway, Redding, CA
   96002, 855-798-8760
Non-Profit Organization: Yes
Year Founded: 1994
Total Enrollment: 560,000

Healthplan and Services Defined
   PLAN TYPE: Other
   Other Type: Medi-Cal
   Benefits Offered: Behavioral Health, Chiropractic, Dental,
      Home Care, Inpatient SNF, Long-Term Care, Podiatry,
      Prescription, Vision, Durable Medical Equipment; Hospice;
      Prenatal Care; Substance Abuse; Transportation; Labs &
      Imaging; Pediatrics; and more

Type of Coverage
   Individual, Medicare, Medicaid

Geographic Areas Served
   counties: Del Norte, Humboldt, Lake, Lassen, Marin,
   Mendocino, Modoc, Napa, Shasta, Siskiyou, Solano, Sonoma,
   Trinity and Yolo

Accreditation Certification
   NCQA

Key Personnel
   Chief Executive Officer. . . . . Liz Gibboney
   Chief Operating Officer . . . . Sonja Bjork
   Chief Financial Officer . . . . Patti McFarland
   Administrative Officer. . . . . Sue Monez
   Chief Information Officer. . . . . Kirt Kemp
   Chief Medical Officer. . . . . Robert Moore, MD

128 Premier Access Insurance/Access Dental

P.O. Box 659010
Sacramento, CA 95865-9010
Toll-Free: 888-634-6074
Phone: 916-920-2500
Fax: 916-563-9000
info@premierlife.com
www.premierppo.com
Subsidiary of: Guardian Life Insurance Co.
For Profit Organization: Yes
Year Founded: 1989
Number of Primary Care Physicians: 1,000
Total Enrollment: 125,000

Healthplan and Services Defined
   PLAN TYPE: PPO
   Other Type: Dental
   Model Type: Network
   Plan Specialty: Dental
   Benefits Offered: Dental

Type of Payment Plans Offered
   FFS

Geographic Areas Served
California, Nevada, Utah, Arizona

Accreditation Certification
TJC Accreditation, Medicare Approved, Utilization Review, Pre-Admission Certification, State Licensure, Quality Assurance Program

Key Personnel
President & CEO . . . . Deanna M. Mulligan

129   Primecare Dental Plan

10700 Civic Center Drive
Suite 100-A
Rancho Cucamonga, CA 91730
Toll-Free: 800-937-3400
contact@primecaredental.net
www.primecaredental.net
For Profit Organization: Yes
Year Founded: 1983
Physician Owned Organization: Yes
Total Enrollment: 17,000

Healthplan and Services Defined
PLAN TYPE: Dental
Model Type: Staff
Plan Specialty: Dental
Benefits Offered: Dental
Offers Demand Management Patient Information Service: Yes

Type of Coverage
Commercial, Individual

Type of Payment Plans Offered
DFFS, Capitated

Geographic Areas Served
Alameda, Butte, Colusa, Contra Costa, El Dorado, Fresno, Glenn, Kern, Kings, Los Angeles, Madera, Mariposa, Merced Monterey, Napa, Nevada, Orange, Placer, Riverside, Sacramento, San Benito, San Bernardino, San Diego, San Francisco, San Joaquin, San Luis Opispo, San Mateo, Santa Barbara, Santa Clara, Santa Cruz, Shasta, Siskiyou, Solano, Sonoma, Stanislaus, Sutter, Tehama, Tuolumne, Tulare, Ventura, Yolo, and Yuba counties

Network Qualifications
Pre-Admission Certification: Yes

Peer Review Type
Utilization Review: Yes

Publishes and Distributes Report Card: No

Accreditation Certification
URAC, NCQA
Utilization Review

Specialty Managed Care Partners
Enters into Contracts with Regional Business Coalitions: No

130   PTPN

26635 W Agoura Road
Suite 250
Calabasas, CA 91302
Toll-Free: 800-766-7876
info@ptpn.com
www.ptpn.com
Year Founded: 1985
Number of Primary Care Physicians: 3,500

Healthplan and Services Defined
PLAN TYPE: PPO
Other Type: Rehab Network
Model Type: Network
Plan Specialty: Outpatient Rehabilitation (Physical, Occupational and Speech Therapy)
Benefits Offered: Physical Therapy, Worker's Compensation, Occupational Therapy; Speech Therapy; Physical Therapy; Hand Therapy; Speech/Language Therapy; and Pediatric Therapy

Type of Payment Plans Offered
DFFS

Geographic Areas Served
Nationwide

Network Qualifications
Minimum Years of Practice: 3

Peer Review Type
Utilization Review: Yes

Accreditation Certification
NCQA

Key Personnel
President. . . . . Michael Weinper
Vice President . . . . Nancy Rothenberg
Quality Assurance. . . . . Michel Kaye

131   San Francisco Health Plan

50 Beale Street
12th Floor
San Francisco, CA 94119
Phone: 415-547-7818
Fax: 415-547-7826
www.sfhp.org
Mailing Address: P.O. Box 194247, San Francisco, CA 94119
Year Founded: 1994
Number of Affiliated Hospitals: 6
Number of Primary Care Physicians: 2,300
Total Enrollment: 55,000
State Enrollment: 55,000

Healthplan and Services Defined
PLAN TYPE: HMO
Benefits Offered: Dental, Disease Management, Prescription, Vision, Wellness

Type of Coverage
Medicare, Medicaid, Medi-Cal, Healthy Families, Healthy

Geographic Areas Served
San Francisco

Key Personnel

Chief Executive Officer	John F Grgurina, Jr
Chief Operating Officer	Deena Louie
Compliance Officer	Nina Maruyama
Human Res Consultant	Kate Gormley
Dir, Accounting	Skip Bishop
Dir, Technology Services	Cecil Newton
Dir, Business Services	Van Wong
Dir, Qual & Performance	Tammy Fisher

132 Santa Clara Family Health Foundations Inc

210 E Hacienda Avenue
Campbell, CA 95008-6617
Toll-Free: 800-260-2055
Phone: 408-376-2000
www.scfhp.com
Non-Profit Organization: Yes
Year Founded: 1997
Number of Affiliated Hospitals: 6
Number of Primary Care Physicians: 983
Number of Referral/Specialty Physicians: 3,356
Total Enrollment: 250,000
State Enrollment: 250,000

Healthplan and Services Defined
  PLAN TYPE: HMO
  Benefits Offered: Behavioral Health, Disease Management,
    Long-Term Care, Prescription, Wellness
  Offers Demand Management Patient Information Service:
    Yes
  DMPI Services Offered: 24 hour nurse advice line

Type of Coverage
  Commercial, Medicaid, Medicare Advantage SNP, Medi-Cal,
  H

Geographic Areas Served
  Santa Clara County

Subscriber Information
  Average Monthly Fee Per Subscriber
    (Employee + Employer Contribution):
      Employee & 2 Family Members: $18 max per family

Key Personnel

CEO	Christine Tomcala
Chief Information Officer	Jonathan Tomayo
Chief Medical Officer	Jeff Robertson
Member/Medical Operations	Patricia McClelland
Pharmacy Director	Johanna Liu
Operations Director	Lori Andersen

Specialty Managed Care Partners
  Medimpact

133 Sant, Community Physicians

7370 N Palm
Suite 101
Fresno, CA 93711
Toll-Free: 800-652-2900
Phone: 559-228-5400
Fax: 559-228-2958
www.santehealth.net

Year Founded: 1980
Number of Primary Care Physicians: 1,200
Total Enrollment: 120,000

Healthplan and Services Defined
  PLAN TYPE: HMO/PPO
  Model Type: IPA
  Benefits Offered: Wellness

Type of Payment Plans Offered
  FFS

Geographic Areas Served
  Fresno, Madera and Kings counties

Network Qualifications
  Pre-Admission Certification: Yes

Peer Review Type
  Utilization Review: Yes
  Case Management: Yes

Publishes and Distributes Report Card: Yes

Accreditation Certification
  TJC Accreditation, Medicare Approved, Utilization Review,
    Pre-Admission Certification, State Licensure, Quality
    Assurance Program

Specialty Managed Care Partners
  Enters into Contracts with Regional Business Coalitions: Yes

134 SCAN Health Plan

3800 Kilroy Airport Way
Suite 100
Long Beach, CA 90806
Toll-Free: 800-559-3500
www.scanhealthplan.com
Non-Profit Organization: Yes
Year Founded: 1977
Number of Affiliated Hospitals: 151
Number of Primary Care Physicians: 6,560
Number of Referral/Specialty Physicians: 17,186
Total Enrollment: 128,272
State Enrollment: 12,283

Healthplan and Services Defined
  PLAN TYPE: HMO
  Plan Specialty: Medicare
  Benefits Offered: Vision

Type of Coverage
  Medicare

Geographic Areas Served
  California & Arizona

Subscriber Information
  Average Annual Deductible Per Subscriber:
    Medicare: $0
  Average Subscriber Co-Payment:
    Primary Care Physician: $0-$5
    Hospital ER: $75
    Home Health Care: $0
    Nursing Home: $0
    Nursing Home Max. Days/Visits Covered: 100

Key Personnel
Chief Executive Officer .... Christopher Wing
Chief Financial Officer .... Vinod Mohan
President .... Bill Roth
Chief Medical Executive................ Romilla Batra

135 Sharp Health Plan
8520 Tech Way
Suite 200
San Diego, CA 92123
Toll-Free: 800-359-2002
Phone: 858-499-8300
www.sharphealthplan.com
Subsidiary of: Sharp HealthCare
Non-Profit Organization: Yes
Year Founded: 1992
Total Enrollment: 49,000
State Enrollment: 49,000

Healthplan and Services Defined
PLAN TYPE: HMO
Model Type: Network
Benefits Offered: Prescription, Vision, Wellness

Type of Coverage
Medicare

Geographic Areas Served
San Diego and Southern Riverside counties

Key Personnel
CEO & President .... Melissa Hayden Cook
Vice President/CFO .... Rita Datko
Vice President/COO .... Leslie Pels-Beck
VP/Chief, Business Dev................. Michael Bryd
VP, Chief Medical Officer .... Cary Shames

136 Stanislaus Foundation for Medical Care
2339 St Pauls Way
Modesto, CA 95355
Phone: 209-527-1704
Fax: 209-527-5861
sms@stanislausmedicalsociety.com
www.stanislausmedicalsociety.com
Non-Profit Organization: Yes
Year Founded: 1957
Physician Owned Organization: Yes
Number of Affiliated Hospitals: 400
Number of Primary Care Physicians: 27,000
Number of Referral/Specialty Physicians: 5,000

Healthplan and Services Defined
PLAN TYPE: PPO
Model Type: Network
Benefits Offered: Dental, Prescription, Vision, Worker's
Compensation
Offers Demand Management Patient Information Service:
Yes

Geographic Areas Served
Stanislaus, Tuolumne counties

Network Qualifications
Pre-Admission Certification: Yes

Publishes and Distributes Report Card: No

Key Personnel
President of SFMC .... David Shiba, MD
President of SMS .... Ronald Arakelian, MD
Director .... Kathleen Eve, MD

Specialty Managed Care Partners
Enters into Contracts with Regional Business Coalitions: No

137 Superior Vision
11101 White Rock Road
Rancho Cordova, CA 95670
Toll-Free: 800-507-3800
contactus@supervision.com
www.superiorvision.com
Secondary Address: Corporate Headquarters, 939 Elkridge
Landing Road, Suite 200, Linthicum, MD 21090,
800-243-1401
For Profit Organization: Yes
Year Founded: 1993

Healthplan and Services Defined
PLAN TYPE: Vision
Model Type: Group
Plan Specialty: Vision
Benefits Offered: Vision

Type of Coverage
Commercial, Indemnity, Medicaid, Catastrophic

Geographic Areas Served
Nationwide

Accreditation Certification
AAPI, NCQA

Key Personnel
Chief Executive Officer .... Kirk Rothrock
Chief Information Officer................. Greg Pontius
Chief Financial Officer .... Brian Silverberg
SVP, Operations..................... Glen McDonald
VP, Provider Relations .... Zon Dunn
VP, Marketing..................... Kathleen McMinn
VP, Sales .... Thomas Luchetta

138 Taylor Benefits
4820 Harwood Road
Suite 130
San Jose, CA 95124
Toll-Free: 800-903-6066
Phone: 408-358-7502
Fax: 408-723-8201
taylorbenefitsinsurance.com
Year Founded: 1987

Healthplan and Services Defined
PLAN TYPE: Multiple
Benefits Offered: Behavioral Health, Dental, Inpatient SNF,
Long-Term Care, Prescription, Vision, Wellness, Life,
Short-and-long-term disability; Substance Abuse; Maternity
& Newborn Care; Rehabiliation; Labs; Pediatrics

Geographic Areas Served
Plans available for employers statewide

Key Personnel
Principal............................... Todd Taylor
todd@taylorbenefits.net
Administrative Assistant .... Ronda Agpaoa
ronda@taylorbenefits.net
Principal .... Jennifer Taylor
jennifer@taylorbenefits.net

139   Trinity Health of California

Saint Agnes Medical Center
1303 E Herndon Avenue
Fresno, CA 93720
Phone: 559-450-3000
www.trinity-health.org
Secondary Address: 20555 Victor Parkway, Livonia, MI
48152-7018, 734-343-1000
Subsidiary of: Trinity Health
Non-Profit Organization: Yes
Year Founded: 2013
Total Enrollment: 30,000,000

Healthplan and Services Defined
PLAN TYPE: Other
Benefits Offered: Disease Management, Home Care,
Long-Term Care, Psychiatric, Hospice programs, PACE
(Program of All Inclusive Care for the Elderly)

Geographic Areas Served
San Joaquin Valley

Key Personnel
President/CEO, SAMC .... Nancy Hollingsworth, RN
Chief Financial Officer .... Michael Prusiatis
Chief Admin Officer .... Stacy Vaillancourt
Chief Medical Officer .... W. Eugene Egerton, MD

140   United Concordia of California

21700 Oxnard Street
Suite 500
Woodland Hills, CA 91367
Phone: 818-710-9400
www.unitedconcordia.com
For Profit Organization: Yes
Year Founded: 1971
Number of Primary Care Physicians: 96,000
Total Enrollment: 7,800,000

Healthplan and Services Defined
PLAN TYPE: Dental
Model Type: Network
Plan Specialty: Dental
Benefits Offered: Dental

Type of Coverage
Commercial, Individual, Military personnel & families

Geographic Areas Served
Nationwide

Accreditation Certification
URAC

141   UnitedHealthcare of Northern California

2300 Clayton Road
Concord, CA 94520
Toll-Free: 866-574-6088
www.uhc.com/contact-us/california
Subsidiary of: UnitedHealth Group
For Profit Organization: Yes

Healthplan and Services Defined
PLAN TYPE: HMO/PPO
Model Type: Network
Plan Specialty: Behavioral Health, Dental, Disease
Management, PBM, Vision
Benefits Offered: Behavioral Health, Dental, Disease
Management, Long-Term Care, Prescription, Vision,
Wellness, Life, LTD, STD

Type of Coverage
Commercial, Individual, Medicare, Supplemental Medicare,
Medicaid, Family, Group
Catastrophic Illness Benefit: Covered

Type of Payment Plans Offered
DFFS, Capitated

Geographic Areas Served
Statewide

Subscriber Information
Average Monthly Fee Per Subscriber
(Employee + Employer Contribution):
Employee Only (Self): Varies
Employee & 1 Family Member: Varies
Employee & 2 Family Members: Varies
Medicare: Varies
Average Annual Deductible Per Subscriber:
Employee Only (Self): Varies
Employee & 1 Family Member: Varies
Employee & 2 Family Members: Varies
Medicare: Varies

Publishes and Distributes Report Card: Yes

Accreditation Certification
NCQA
TJC Accreditation, Utilization Review, State Licensure

Key Personnel
CEO, UHCC California................ Kevin Kandalaft

Specialty Managed Care Partners
Enters into Contracts with Regional Business Coalitions: Yes

142   UnitedHealthcare of Southern California

5757 Plaza Drive
Cypress, CA 90630
Toll-Free: 866-574-6088
www.uhc.com/contact-us/california
Subsidiary of: UnitedHealth Group
For Profit Organization: Yes

Healthplan and Services Defined
PLAN TYPE: HMO/PPO
Model Type: Network
Plan Specialty: Behavioral Health, Dental, Disease
Management, PBM, Vision

Benefits Offered: Behavioral Health, Dental, Disease
Management, Long-Term Care, Prescription, Vision,
Wellness, Life, LTD, STD

Type of Coverage
Commercial, Individual, Medicare, Supplemental Medicare,
Medicaid, Family, Group
Catastrophic Illness Benefit: Unlimited

Type of Payment Plans Offered
POS

Geographic Areas Served
Statewide

Network Qualifications
Pre-Admission Certification: Yes

Peer Review Type
Utilization Review: Yes
Second Surgical Opinion: Yes
Case Management: Yes

Publishes and Distributes Report Card: Yes

Accreditation Certification
NCQA
TJC Accreditation, Medicare Approved, Utilization Review,
Pre-Admission Certification, State Licensure, Quality
Assurance Program

Key Personnel
CEO, UHCC California. . . . . Kevin Kandalaft

Specialty Managed Care Partners
Enters into Contracts with Regional Business Coalitions: Yes

---

143   University HealthCare Alliance
7999 Gateway Boulevard
Suite 200
Newark, CA 95460
uha_communications@stanfordhealthcare.org
universityhealthcarealliance.org
For Profit Organization: Yes
Year Founded: 1996

Healthplan and Services Defined
PLAN TYPE: PPO
Model Type: Network

Geographic Areas Served
San Francisco Bay area

Key Personnel
Chief Medical Officer . . . . Bryan Bohman
Administrative Officer . . . . Catherine Krna
VP, Operations. . . . . Gaguik Khachatourian

---

144   Ventura County Health Care Plan
2220 E Gonzales Rd
Suite 210 B
Oxnard, CA 93036
Toll-Free: 800-600-8247
Phone: 805-981-5050
www.vchealthcareplan.org
Non-Profit Organization: Yes
Year Founded: 1993

Healthplan and Services Defined
PLAN TYPE: HMO
Benefits Offered: Behavioral Health, Disease Management,
Prescription, Wellness

Geographic Areas Served
Ventura County

Accreditation Certification
NCQA

---

145   Vision Plan of America
3255 Wilshire Boulevard
Suite 1610
Los Angeles, CA 90010
Toll-Free: 800-400-4872
Fax: 213-384-0084
info@visionplanofamerica.com
www.visionplanofamerica.com
For Profit Organization: Yes
Year Founded: 1986

Healthplan and Services Defined
PLAN TYPE: Vision
Model Type: IPA
Plan Specialty: Dental, Vision
Benefits Offered: Dental, Vision

Type of Coverage
Commercial, Individual

Type of Payment Plans Offered
POS, Capitated

Geographic Areas Served
Nationwide

Peer Review Type
Case Management: Yes

Key Personnel
President and CEO . . . . Stuart Needleman, OD
CFO . . . . Phillip Needleman
Manager . . . . Milori Lopez Duarte
Optometric Director. . . . . Adolphus Lages, OD
Provider Relations . . . . Mayra Castillo

---

146   VSP Vision Care
3333 Quality Drive
Rancho Cordova, CA 95670
Toll-Free: 800-877-7195
vsp.com
Year Founded: 1955

Healthplan and Services Defined
PLAN TYPE: Vision
Plan Specialty: Vision
Benefits Offered: Vision

Geographic Areas Served
Nationwide, Canada, Australia, and the UK

Key Personnel
Chief Executive Officer. . . . . Robert Lynch
President . . . . Kate Renwick-Espinosa

147 Western Dental Services

530 South Main Street
Orange, CA 92868
Toll-Free: 800-579-3783
corporate@westerndental.com
www.westerndental.com
Year Founded: 1903
Number of Primary Care Physicians: 1,700
Number of Referral/Specialty Physicians: 1,400
Total Enrollment: 315,440

Healthplan and Services Defined
PLAN TYPE: Dental
Other Type: Dental HMO
Model Type: Staff, IPA
Plan Specialty: Dental
Benefits Offered: Dental

Type of Coverage
Indemnity

Type of Payment Plans Offered
POS, Combination FFS & DFFS

Geographic Areas Served
California, Arizona, and Nevada

Subscriber Information
Average Monthly Fee Per Subscriber
(Employee + Employer Contribution):
Employee Only (Self): $9.25
Employee & 1 Family Member: $10.50
Employee & 2 Family Members: $12.00

Network Qualifications
Pre-Admission Certification: Yes

Peer Review Type
Utilization Review: Yes
Second Surgical Opinion: Yes
Case Management: Yes

Publishes and Distributes Report Card: No

Accreditation Certification
Utilization Review

Key Personnel
CEO . . . . Daniel D. Crowley
Senior VP/CFO . . . . Bill Dembereckyj
COO . . . . Lisa Dawe
SVP/General Counsel . . . . Jeffrey Miller
VP, Real Estate . . . . Andrew Eddy
Chief Dental Officer . . . . John Luther
Chief Marketing Officer . . . . Joshua Marder
CIO . . . . Preet M. Takkar

Average Claim Compensation
Physician's Fees Charged: 80%

Specialty Managed Care Partners
Enters into Contracts with Regional Business Coalitions: No

148 Western Health Advantage

2349 Gateway Oaks Drive
Suite 100
Sacramento, CA 95833
Toll-Free: 888-227-5942
Phone: 916-563-2250
memberservices@westernhealth.com
www.westernhealth.com
Non-Profit Organization: Yes
Year Founded: 1996
Total Enrollment: 92,000
State Enrollment: 92,000

Healthplan and Services Defined
PLAN TYPE: HMO
Model Type: Network
Benefits Offered: Disease Management, Prescription,
Wellness, 24/7 Nurse hotline, 24/7 Travel Assistance

Geographic Areas Served
Sacramento, Yolo, Solano, western El Dorado, western Placer
counties

Key Personnel
President & CEO . . . . Garry Maisel
Chief Financial Officer . . . . Rita Ruecker
Chief Legal Officer . . . . Rebecca Downing
Chief Marketing/Branding . . . . Rick Heron
Chief Medical Officer . . . . Don Hufford
Chief Client Services . . . . Glenn Hamburg
CIO . . . . Ali Darugar
Chief Sales Officer . . . . Bill Figenshu

Health Insurance Coverage Status and Type of Coverage by Age

Category	All Persons		Under 18 years		Under 65 years	
	Number	%	Number	%	Number	%
Total population	5,448	-	1,331	-	4,720	-
Covered by some type of health insurance	5,038 *(15)*	92.5 *(0.3)*	1,274 *(7)*	95.7 *(0.4)*	4,315 *(14)*	91.4 *(0.3)*
Covered by private health insurance	3,823 *(23)*	70.2 *(0.4)*	849 *(12)*	63.8 *(0.9)*	3,392 *(22)*	71.9 *(0.5)*
Employer-based	3,011 *(25)*	55.3 *(0.5)*	697 *(12)*	52.4 *(0.9)*	2,795 *(24)*	59.2 *(0.5)*
Direct purchase	775 *(17)*	14.2 *(0.3)*	120 *(6)*	9.0 *(0.5)*	551 *(14)*	11.7 *(0.3)*
TRICARE	222 *(8)*	4.1 *(0.2)*	55 *(4)*	4.1 *(0.3)*	161 *(7)*	3.4 *(0.2)*
Covered by public health insurance	1,786 *(20)*	32.8 *(0.4)*	474 *(12)*	35.6 *(0.9)*	1,089 *(20)*	23.1 *(0.4)*
Medicaid	1,056 *(20)*	19.4 *(0.4)*	469 *(13)*	35.2 *(0.9)*	977 *(20)*	20.7 *(0.4)*
Medicare	804 *(6)*	14.8 *(0.1)*	7 *(2)*	0.5 *(0.1)*	108 *(5)*	2.3 *(0.1)*
VA Care	130 *(5)*	2.4 *(0.1)*	2 *(1)*	0.1 *(0.1)*	69 *(5)*	1.5 *(0.1)*
Not covered at any time during the year	410 *(14)*	7.5 *(0.3)*	57 *(6)*	4.3 *(0.4)*	404 *(14)*	8.6 *(0.3)*

Note: Numbers in thousands; Figures cover civilian noninstitutionalized population in 2016; N/A indicates that data was not available; Z represents or rounds to zero; Margin of error appears in parenthesis and is calculated using replicate weights.
Source: U.S. Census Bureau, American Community Survey, Table HIC-4_ACS. Health Insurance Coverage Status and Type of Coverage by State—All People: 2008 to 2016, Table HIC-5_ACS. Health Insurance Coverage Status and Type of Coverage by State—Children Under 18: 2008 to 2016, Table HIC-6_ACS. Health Insurance Coverage Status and Type of Coverage by State—Persons Under 65: 2008 to 2016

Colorado

149 Aetna Health of Colorado

151 Farmington Avenue
Hartford, CT 06156
Toll-Free: 800-872-3862
Phone: 860-273-0123
www.aetna.com
Subsidiary of: Aetna Inc.
For Profit Organization: Yes
Year Founded: 1987

Healthplan and Services Defined
PLAN TYPE: HMO/PPO
Other Type: POS
Model Type: Network
Plan Specialty: Behavioral Health, Vision
Benefits Offered: Behavioral Health, Dental, Disease
    Management, Home Care, Physical Therapy, Podiatry,
    Prescription, Vision, Worker's Compensation, Life

Type of Coverage
Commercial, Student health

Type of Payment Plans Offered
POS, Capitated, FFS, Combination FFS & DFFS

Geographic Areas Served
Statewide

Peer Review Type
Case Management: Yes

Publishes and Distributes Report Card: Yes

Accreditation Certification
TJC Accreditation, Medicare Approved, Utilization Review,
    Pre-Admission Certification, State Licensure, Quality
    Assurance Program

Key Personnel
CEO.................................. Mark Bertolini

Specialty Managed Care Partners
Enters into Contracts with Regional Business Coalitions: Yes

150 American Dental Group

6755 Earl Drive
Suite 108
Colorado Springs, CO 80918
Toll-Free: 800-633-3010
Phone: 719-633-3000
info@adgincco.com
www.adgincco.com
For Profit Organization: Yes
Year Founded: 1992
Physician Owned Organization: Yes

Healthplan and Services Defined
PLAN TYPE: Dental
Other Type: Vision
Model Type: Group
Plan Specialty: Dental, Vision
Benefits Offered: Dental, Vision

Type of Coverage
Commercial, Individual

Type of Payment Plans Offered
DFFS, FFS, Combination FFS & DFFS

Geographic Areas Served
Colorado, Maryland

151 Anthem Blue Cross & Blue Shield of Colorado

700 Broadway
Suite 600
Denver, CO 80203
Phone: 303-831-2131
Fax: 303-831-3069
www.anthem.com
Subsidiary of: Anthem, Inc.
For Profit Organization: Yes
Year Founded: 1978

Healthplan and Services Defined
PLAN TYPE: HMO/PPO
Model Type: Network
Plan Specialty: Behavioral Health, Dental, Disease
    Management, Lab, PBM, Vision, Radiology
Benefits Offered: Behavioral Health, Dental, Disease
    Management, Inpatient SNF, Physical Therapy,
    Prescription, Psychiatric, Transplant, Vision, Wellness, Life,
    Benefits vary according to plan

Type of Coverage
Commercial, Individual, Medicare, Supplemental Medicare

Geographic Areas Served
Statewide

Accreditation Certification
URAC, NCQA

Key Personnel
President/GM Colorado................. Mike Ramseier

152 Behavioral Healthcare

1290 Chambers Road
Aurora, CO 80011
Toll-Free: 844-818-2485
Phone: 303-361-8100
Fax: 303-364-2240
bhicares.org
Non-Profit Organization: Yes

Healthplan and Services Defined
PLAN TYPE: Other
Plan Specialty: Behavioral Health
Benefits Offered: Behavioral Health

Type of Coverage
Medicaid

Geographic Areas Served
Adams, Arapahoe and Douglas counties, and the city of
    Aurora

Key Personnel
Chief Executive Officer.................. Pat Steadman

Chief Financial Officer . . . . Jennifer Lacov
Chief Medical Officer . . . . Ronald Morley
Quality Improvement . . . . Clara Cabanis
Clinical Services . . . . Katie Herrmann
Provider Relations . . . . Teresa Summers

153 Beta Health Association, Inc.

9725 E Hampden Avenue
Suite 400
Denver, CO 80231
Toll-Free: 800-807-0706
Phone: 303-744-3007
www.betadental.com
For Profit Organization: Yes
Year Founded: 1990
Physician Owned Organization: Yes

Healthplan and Services Defined
  PLAN TYPE: Multiple
  Plan Specialty: Dental, Vision
  Benefits Offered: Dental, Vision, Life, LTD, STD

Type of Coverage
  Commercial, Individual, Indemnity
  Catastrophic Illness Benefit: Unlimited

Geographic Areas Served
  48 states

Publishes and Distributes Report Card: Yes

Accreditation Certification
  State Dental Board

Key Personnel
  President & CEO. . . . . Rod Henningsen

Specialty Managed Care Partners
  Enters into Contracts with Regional Business Coalitions: Yes

154 Boulder Valley Individual Practice Association

6676 Gunpark Drive
Suite B
Boulder, CO 80301
Phone: 303-530-3405
Fax: 303-530-2441
www.bvipa.com
Non-Profit Organization: Yes
Year Founded: 1978
Physician Owned Organization: Yes
Number of Affiliated Hospitals: 4
Number of Primary Care Physicians: 487
Number of Referral/Specialty Physicians: 190
Total Enrollment: 60,000

Healthplan and Services Defined
  PLAN TYPE: PPO
  Model Type: IPA
  Offers Demand Management Patient Information Service:
    Yes

Type of Payment Plans Offered
  POS

Geographic Areas Served
  Boulder, Lafayette, Longmont & Louisville

Network Qualifications
  Pre-Admission Certification: Yes

Peer Review Type
  Utilization Review: Yes
  Second Surgical Opinion: Yes
  Case Management: Yes

Publishes and Distributes Report Card: No

Accreditation Certification
  TJC Accreditation, Utilization Review, State Licensure

Key Personnel
  President . . . . Susan Roach, MD
  Vice President . . . . Drigan Weider, MD
  Medical Director . . . . Laird Cagan, MD

Specialty Managed Care Partners
  Enters into Contracts with Regional Business Coalitions: No

155 Bright Health Colorado

219 N 2nd Street
Suite 310
Minneapolis, MN 55401
Phone: 844-691-6143
brighthealthplan.com
Year Founded: 2016
Number of Primary Care Physicians: 5,000

Healthplan and Services Defined
  PLAN TYPE: HMO
  Benefits Offered: Prescription, Wellness

Geographic Areas Served
  Statewide

Key Personnel
  Chief Executive Officer . . . . Bob Sheehy
  Chief Medical Officer . . . . Tom Valdivia
  President . . . . Kyle Rolfing

156 Cigna HealthCare of Colorado

Denver Centerpoint I
3900 E Mexico Avenue
Denver, CO 80210
Toll-Free: 800-997-1654
Phone: 303-782-1500
www.cigna.com
For Profit Organization: Yes
Number of Affiliated Hospitals: 80

Healthplan and Services Defined
  PLAN TYPE: HMO
  Other Type: POS
  Plan Specialty: Behavioral Health, Dental, Vision
  Benefits Offered: Behavioral Health, Dental, Disease
    Management, Prescription, Vision, Wellness, Life, LTD,
    STD
  Offers Demand Management Patient Information Service: Yes

Type of Coverage
  Commercial, Individual

Catastrophic Illness Benefit: Covered

Type of Payment Plans Offered
POS, Combination FFS & DFFS

Network Qualifications
Pre-Admission Certification: Yes

Peer Review Type
Utilization Review: Yes
Second Surgical Opinion: Yes
Case Management: Yes

Publishes and Distributes Report Card: Yes

Accreditation Certification
NCQA
TJC Accreditation, Medicare Approved, Utilization Review, Pre-Admission Certification, State Licensure, Quality Assurance Program

Key Personnel
Chairman & CEO . . . . David M. Cordani

Specialty Managed Care Partners
Enters into Contracts with Regional Business Coalitions: Yes

157 Colorado Access
11100 E Bethany Drive
Aurora, CO 80014
Toll-Free: 800-511-5010
customer.service@coaccess.com
www.coaccess.com
Non-Profit Organization: Yes
Year Founded: 1994

Healthplan and Services Defined
PLAN TYPE: HMO
Benefits Offered: Behavioral Health, Dental, Disease Management, Psychiatric, Wellness

Type of Coverage
Medicaid

Geographic Areas Served
Statewide

Key Personnel
President/CEO. . . . . Marshall Thomas, MD
CFO . . . . Philip J Reed
COO. . . . . April Abrahamson
VP of Legal Services . . . . Ann Edelman
Chief Medical Officer/SVP. . . . . Alexis Giese, MD
CIO . . . . Don Couch

158 Colorado Choice Health Plans
700 Main Street
Suite 100
Alamosa, CO 81101
Toll-Free: 800-475-8466
Phone: 719-589-3696
Fax: 719-589-4901
coloradochoicehp.com
Non-Profit Organization: Yes
Year Founded: 1972
Total Enrollment: 5,000

Healthplan and Services Defined
PLAN TYPE: HMO
Benefits Offered: Dental, Disease Management, Home Care, Inpatient SNF, Podiatry, Prescription, Vision, Wellness, Life

Type of Coverage
Commercial, Individual, Medicare

Geographic Areas Served
Southern Colorado, San Luis Valley, Arkansas Valley, Durango, Pueblo, Colorado Springs, Denver

Key Personnel
CEO . . . . Cynthia Palmer
CFO. . . . . Mary Catron
VP of Operations. . . . . Jennifer Mueller
Medical Director . . . . Maria Soto, MD
VP of Tech/Infrastructure . . . . Craig Stevens
VP of Sales/Marketing . . . . Paul Roberts

159 Colorado Health Partnerships
9925 Federal Drive
Suite 100
Colorado Springs, CO 80921
Toll-Free: 800-804-5008
www.coloradohealthpartnerships.com
Non-Profit Organization: Yes
Year Founded: 1995
Number of Affiliated Hospitals: 8
Total Enrollment: 326,000

Healthplan and Services Defined
PLAN TYPE: HMO
Plan Specialty: Behavioral Health
Benefits Offered: Behavioral Health

Type of Coverage
Medicaid

Geographic Areas Served
Alamosa, Archuleta, Baca, Bent, Chaffee, Conejos, Costilla, Crowley, Custer, Delta, Dolores, Eagle, El Paso, Fremont, Garfield, Grand, Gunnison, Hinsdale, Huerfano, Jackson, Kiowa, Lake, La Plata, Las Animas, Mesa, Mineral, Moffat, Montezuma, Montrose, Otero, Ouray, Park, Pitkin, Pueblo, Prowers, Rio Blanco, Rio Grande, Routt, Saguache, San Juan, San Miguel, Summit and Teller counties

Accreditation Certification
URAC

Key Personnel
Executive Director. . . . . Arnold Salazar
719-587-0899
Quality Assurance . . . . Erica Arnold-Miller
719-538-1430
Medical Director . . . . Peter Brodrick
719-538-1430
Provider Relations . . . . Alma Mejorado
719-538-1430

160　Coventry Health Care of Colorado

6720-B Rockledge Drive
Suite 700
Bethesda, MD 20817
Phone: 301-581-0600
www.coventryhealthcare.com
Subsidiary of: Aetna Inc.
For Profit Organization: Yes

Healthplan and Services Defined
PLAN TYPE: HMO/PPO
Model Type: Network
Plan Specialty: Behavioral Health, Dental, Worker's
Compensation
Benefits Offered: Behavioral Health, Dental, Prescription,
Wellness, Worker's Compensation

Type of Coverage
Commercial, Medicare, Medicaid

Geographic Areas Served
Statewide

Key Personnel
Chief Executive Officer . . . . Mark T. Bertolini
President . . . . Karen S. Lynch
Chief Financial Officer . . . . Shawn M. Guertin
Operations & Technology . . . . Meg McCarthy
Chief Medical Officer . . . . Harold L. Paz
General Counsel . . . . Thomas Sabatino Jr.
Government Services . . . . Fran S. Soistman

161　Delta Dental of Colorado

4582 S Ulster Street
Suite 800
Denver, CO 80237
Toll-Free: 800-233-0860
customer_service@ddpco.com
www.deltadentalco.com
Non-Profit Organization: Yes
Year Founded: 1958
Number of Primary Care Physicians: 3,200
State Enrollment: 1,000,000

Healthplan and Services Defined
PLAN TYPE: Dental
Model Type: Network
Plan Specialty: Dental
Benefits Offered: Dental

Type of Coverage
Commercial, Individual

Type of Payment Plans Offered
DFFS

Geographic Areas Served
Statewide

Publishes and Distributes Report Card: Yes

Key Personnel
President & CEO . . . . Helen Drexler
Chief Financial Officer . . . . Greg Vochis
Network/Clinical Mgmt. . . . . Cheryl Lerner, MD
General Counsel . . . . Dave Gerbus

VP, Sales & Marketing . . . . Jean Lawhead

162　Denver Health Medical Plan

777 Bannock Street
Denver, CO 80204-4507
Phone: 303-602-2100
www.denverhealthmedicalplan.com
Non-Profit Organization: Yes
Year Founded: 1997
Total Enrollment: 15,000

Healthplan and Services Defined
PLAN TYPE: HMO
Benefits Offered: Chiropractic, Home Care, Inpatient SNF,
Physical Therapy, Podiatry, Psychiatric, Transplant, Vision,
Wellness

Type of Coverage
Commercial, Medicare, Medicare Advantage, CHP+

Key Personnel
Chief Executive Officer . . . . Robin D. Wittenstein
Marketing/PR Officer . . . . Rob Borland
Chief Nursing Officer . . . . Kathy Boyle
Chief Financial Officer . . . . Peg Burnett
Director of Public Health . . . . Bill Burman
Chief Operating Officer . . . . Timothy J. Harlin

163　Humana Health Insurance of Colorado

8033 N Academy Boulevard
Colorado Springs, CO 80920
Toll-Free: 800-871-6270
Phone: 719-532-7700
Fax: 719-531-7089
www.humana.com
Secondary Address: 6300 S Syracuse Way, Suite 555,
Centennial, CO 80111, 866-355-6152
For Profit Organization: Yes
Year Founded: 1987

Healthplan and Services Defined
PLAN TYPE: HMO/PPO
Plan Specialty: Dental, Vision
Benefits Offered: Dental, Disease Management, Transplant,
Vision

Type of Coverage
Commercial, Individual, Group, Medicare

Geographic Areas Served
Statewide

Accreditation Certification
URAC, NCQA

Key Personnel
President & CEO . . . . Bruce D. Broussard
Chief Medical Officer . . . . Roy A. Beveridge
Chief Consumer Officer . . . . Jody L. Bilney
Human Resources . . . . Tim Huval
Chief Financial Officer . . . . Brian Kane
Chief Information Officer . . . . Brian LeClaire
General Counsel . . . . Christopher M. Todoroff

164 Kaiser Permanente Northern Colorado

10350 E Dakota Avenue
Denver, CO 80247-1314
Toll-Free: 800-476-2167
thrive.kaiserpermanente.org/care-near-northern-colorado
Subsidiary of: Kaiser Permanente
Non-Profit Organization: Yes
Year Founded: 1969
Number of Primary Care Physicians: 1,121
Total Enrollment: 11,800,000
State Enrollment: 675,279

Healthplan and Services Defined
PLAN TYPE: HMO
Model Type: Network
Benefits Offered: Disease Management, Home Care,
    Inpatient SNF, Long-Term Care, Physical Therapy,
    Podiatry, Prescription, Psychiatric, Transplant, Vision,
    Wellness, Benefits vary according to plan

Type of Coverage
Commercial, Individual, Medicare, Supplemental Medicare,
    Medicaid

Geographic Areas Served
Denver, Boulder, Fort Collins, Loveland, Greeley and
    surrounding areas

Accreditation Certification
NCQA

Key Personnel
Executive Med. Director . . . . Margaret Ferguson, MD
President, Colorado Area . . . . Roland Lyon
Media Contact . . . . Amy Whited
    303-344-7518

165 Kaiser Permanente Southern Colorado

10350 E Dakota Avenue
Denver, CO 80247
Toll-Free: 800-476-2167
thrive.kaiserpermanente.org/care-near-southern-colorado
Subsidiary of: Kaiser Permanente
Non-Profit Organization: Yes
Year Founded: 1969
Number of Primary Care Physicians: 1,121
Total Enrollment: 11,800,000
State Enrollment: 675,279

Healthplan and Services Defined
PLAN TYPE: HMO/PPO
Model Type: Network
Benefits Offered: Disease Management, Home Care,
    Inpatient SNF, Long-Term Care, Physical Therapy,
    Podiatry, Prescription, Psychiatric, Transplant, Vision,
    Wellness, Benefits vary according to plan

Type of Coverage
Commercial, Individual, Medicare, Supplemental Medicare,
    Medicaid

Geographic Areas Served
Colorado Springs, Pueblo

Accreditation Certification
NCQA

Key Personnel
President, Colorado Area . . . . Roland Lyon
Executive Med. Director . . . . Margaret Ferguson, MD
Media Contact . . . . Amy Whited
    303-344-7518

166 Pueblo Health Care

400 W 16th Street
Pueblo, CO 81003
Phone: 719-584-4000
www.pueblohealthcare.com
Number of Primary Care Physicians: 270

Healthplan and Services Defined
PLAN TYPE: PPO
Model Type: Network

Geographic Areas Served
Pueblo Market Area

Key Personnel
Executive Director . . . . Ann Bellah
    719-584-4371
    ann_bellah@parkviewmc.com
Provider Relations . . . . Sandra Proud
    719-584-4642
    sandra_proud@parkviewmc.com
President . . . . Bruce Johnson, MD
    719-566-3535

167 Rocky Mountain Health Plans

2775 Crossroads Boulevard
Grand Junction, CO 81506-8712
Toll-Free: 800-346-4643
Phone: 970-243-7050
www.rmhp.org
Mailing Address: P.O. Box 10600, Grand Junction, CO
    81502-5600
Subsidiary of: Rocky Mountain Health Maintenance
    Organization
Non-Profit Organization: Yes
Year Founded: 1974
Owned by an Integrated Delivery Network (IDN): Yes
Number of Affiliated Hospitals: 107
Number of Primary Care Physicians: 2,643
Number of Referral/Specialty Physicians: 6,866
Total Enrollment: 236,962
State Enrollment: 236,962

Healthplan and Services Defined
PLAN TYPE: HMO/PPO
Other Type: HSA
Model Type: Mixed
Benefits Offered: Disease Management, Home Care,
    Prescription, Wellness

Type of Coverage
Commercial, Individual, Medicare, Supplemental Medicare
Catastrophic Illness Benefit: Unlimited

Type of Payment Plans Offered
FFS

Geographic Areas Served
Statewide

Network Qualifications
Minimum Years of Practice: 3
Pre-Admission Certification: Yes

Peer Review Type
Utilization Review: Yes
Second Surgical Opinion: Yes
Case Management: Yes

Publishes and Distributes Report Card: Yes

Accreditation Certification
NCQA
Medicare Approved, Utilization Review, Pre-Admission
Certification, State Licensure, Quality Assurance Program

Key Personnel
President/CEO . . . . Steven ErkenBrack
COO. . . . . Laurel Walters
CFO. . . . . Pat Duncan
VP, Human Resources . . . . Jan Rohr
VP, Legal & Govt Affairs. . . . . Mike Huotari
Chief Marketing Officer. . . . . Neil Waldron
Chief Medical Officer. . . . . Kevin R Fitzgerald, MD

Specialty Managed Care Partners
Delta Dental, Landmark Chiropractic, Vision Service Plan,
Life Strategies

---

168   United Concordia of Colorado
P.O. Box 69420
Harrisburg, PA 17106-9420
Toll-Free: 800-332-0366
www.unitedconcordia.com
For Profit Organization: Yes
Year Founded: 1971
Number of Primary Care Physicians: 96,000

Healthplan and Services Defined
PLAN TYPE: Dental
Model Type: Network
Plan Specialty: Dental
Benefits Offered: Dental

Type of Coverage
Commercial, Individual, Military personnel & families

Geographic Areas Served
Nationwide

Accreditation Certification
URAC

---

169   UnitedHealthcare of Colorado
6465 S Greenwood Plaza Boulevard
Suite 300
Centennial, CO 80111
Toll-Free: 800-516-3344
www.uhc.com/contact-us/colorado
Subsidiary of: UnitedHealth Group

Healthplan and Services Defined
PLAN TYPE: HMO/PPO
Model Type: Network
Plan Specialty: Behavioral Health, Dental, Disease
Management, MSO, PBM, Vision
Benefits Offered: Behavioral Health, Chiropractic,
Complementary
Medicine, Dental, Disease Management, Home Care,
Inpatient SNF, Long-Term Care, Physical Therapy,
Podiatry, Prescription, Psychiatric, Transplant,
Vision, Wellness, AD&D, Life, Benefits vary
according to plan

Type of Coverage
Commercial, Individual, Medicare, Medicaid, Family,
Military, Veterans, Group,

Type of Payment Plans Offered
DFFS, FFS, Combination FFS & DFFS

Geographic Areas Served
HMO: Front Range Colorado; PPO/POS: Statewide

Subscriber Information
Average Monthly Fee Per Subscriber
(Employee + Employer Contribution):
Employee Only (Self): Varies

Network Qualifications
Pre-Admission Certification: Yes

Peer Review Type
Case Management: Yes

Publishes and Distributes Report Card: Yes

Accreditation Certification
URAC, NCQA
State Licensure, Quality Assurance Program

Average Claim Compensation
Physician's Fees Charged: 70%
Hospital's Fees Charged: 55%

Specialty Managed Care Partners
United Behavioral Health
Enters into Contracts with Regional Business Coalitions: No

Health Insurance Coverage Status and Type of Coverage by Age

Category	All Persons		Under 18 years		Under 65 years	
	Number	%	Number	%	Number	%
Total population	3,525	-	804	-	2,969	-
Covered by some type of health insurance	3,353 *(11)*	95.1 *(0.3)*	781 *(5)*	97.2 *(0.5)*	2,799 *(11)*	94.3 *(0.4)*
Covered by private health insurance	2,536 *(19)*	71.9 *(0.5)*	530 *(10)*	66.0 *(1.2)*	2,187 *(18)*	73.7 *(0.6)*
Employer-based	2,129 *(21)*	60.4 *(0.6)*	478 *(10)*	59.5 *(1.3)*	1,920 *(20)*	64.7 *(0.7)*
Direct purchase	464 *(11)*	13.2 *(0.3)*	52 *(4)*	6.4 *(0.5)*	290 *(9)*	9.8 *(0.3)*
TRICARE	46 *(4)*	1.3 *(0.1)*	10 *(2)*	1.2 *(0.3)*	31 *(4)*	1.0 *(0.1)*
Covered by public health insurance	1,234 *(18)*	35.0 *(0.5)*	282 *(10)*	35.1 *(1.3)*	702 *(18)*	23.7 *(0.6)*
Medicaid	724 *(18)*	20.5 *(0.5)*	281 *(10)*	35.0 *(1.3)*	649 *(18)*	21.8 *(0.6)*
Medicare	605 *(5)*	17.2 *(0.1)*	2 *(1)*	0.2 *(0.1)*	74 *(5)*	2.5 *(0.2)*
VA Care	54 *(3)*	1.5 *(0.1)*	Z *(Z)*	Z *(Z)*	21 *(2)*	0.7 *(0.1)*
Not covered at any time during the year	172 *(11)*	4.9 *(0.3)*	23 *(4)*	2.8 *(0.5)*	170 *(11)*	5.7 *(0.4)*

Note: Numbers in thousands; Figures cover civilian noninstitutionalized population in 2016; N/A indicates that data was not available; Z represents or rounds to zero; Margin of error appears in parenthesis and is calculated using replicate weights.
Source: U.S. Census Bureau, American Community Survey, Table HIC-4_ACS. Health Insurance Coverage Status and Type of Coverage by State—All People: 2008 to 2016, Table HIC-5_ACS. Health Insurance Coverage Status and Type of Coverage by State—Children Under 18: 2008 to 2016, Table HIC-6_ACS. Health Insurance Coverage Status and Type of Coverage by State—Persons Under 65: 2008 to 2016

Connecticut

170 Aetna Health of Connecticut

151 Farmington Avenue
Hartford, CT 06156-3475
Toll-Free: 800-872-3862
Phone: 860-273-0123
www.aetna.com
Subsidiary of: Aetna Inc.
For Profit Organization: Yes
Year Founded: 1853

Healthplan and Services Defined
PLAN TYPE: HMO/PPO
Other Type: POS
Model Type: Network
Plan Specialty: Behavioral Health, Dental, EPO, Lab, PBM, Vision, Radiology
Benefits Offered: Behavioral Health, Dental, Disease Management, Long-Term Care, Physical Therapy, Podiatry, Prescription, Psychiatric, Vision, Wellness, Life, LTD, STD

Type of Coverage
Commercial, Medicare, Medicaid, Student health

Geographic Areas Served
Statewide

Key Personnel
Chief Executive Officer . . . . Mark Bertolini
President . . . . Karen S. Lynch
EVP/CFO . . . . Shawn M. Guertin
EVP/General Counsel . . . . Thomas J. Sabatino, Jr.
EVP/Chief Medical Officer . . . . Harold L. Paz, MD

171 Aetna Inc.

151 Farmington Avenue
Hartford, CT 06156
Toll-Free: 800-872-3862
Phone: 860-273-0123
www.aetna.com
For Profit Organization: Yes
Year Founded: 1853
Number of Affiliated Hospitals: 5,667
Number of Primary Care Physicians: 664,301
Total Enrollment: 46,700,000

Healthplan and Services Defined
PLAN TYPE: Multiple
Other Type: POS
Model Type: Network
Plan Specialty: Behavioral Health, Dental, Lab, PBM, Vision, Radiology
Benefits Offered: Behavioral Health, Dental, Disease Management, Long-Term Care, Physical Therapy, Podiatry, Prescription, Psychiatric, Vision, Wellness, Life, LTD, STD

Type of Coverage
Commercial, Medicare, Medicaid, Public sector, Retirees, Part-time,

Type of Payment Plans Offered
FFS

Geographic Areas Served
Nationwide

Key Personnel
CEO . . . . Mark Bertolini
President . . . . Karen Lynch
EVP/CFO . . . . Shawn Guertin
EVP/General Counsel . . . . Thomas Sabatino, Jr
EVP/Chief Medical Officer . . . . Harold Paz, MD

172 Aetna Medicare

c/o Aetna Inc.
151 Farmington Avenue
Hartford, CT 06156
Toll-Free: 855-335-1407
www.aetnamedicare.com
Secondary Address: Aetna Inc., P.O. Box 14088, Lexington, KY 40512, 800-633-4227
Subsidiary of: Aetna Inc.
For Profit Organization: Yes

Healthplan and Services Defined
PLAN TYPE: Medicare
Model Type: Network
Benefits Offered: Chiropractic, Dental, Disease Management, Home Care, Inpatient SNF, Physical Therapy, Prescription, Psychiatric, Vision, Wellness

Type of Coverage
Individual, Medicare, Supplemental Medicare

Geographic Areas Served
Available in multiple states

Subscriber Information
Average Monthly Fee Per Subscriber
    (Employee + Employer Contribution):
        Employee Only (Self): Varies
        Medicare: Varies
Average Annual Deductible Per Subscriber:
        Employee Only (Self): Varies
        Medicare: Varies
Average Subscriber Co-Payment:
        Primary Care Physician: Varies
        Non-Network Physician: Varies
        Prescription Drugs: Varies
        Hospital ER: Varies
        Home Health Care: Varies
        Home Health Care Max. Days/Visits Covered: Varies

Key Personnel
CEO . . . . Mark Bertolini

173 Aetna Student Health

151 Farmington Avenue
Hartford, CT 06156
Toll-Free: 877-437-6535
www.aetnastudenthealth.com
Subsidiary of: Aetna Inc.
For Profit Organization: Yes

Healthplan and Services Defined
PLAN TYPE: HMO/PPO
Other Type: POS
Model Type: Network
Plan Specialty: Disease Management, Vision
Benefits Offered: Dental, Prescription, Vision, Wellness, Life

Type of Coverage
Individual

Geographic Areas Served
Nationwide

Key Personnel
Chief Executive Officer . . . . Mark T. Bertolini
President . . . . Karen S. Lynch
Chief Financial Officer . . . . Shawn M. Guertin
Operations & Technology . . . . Meg McCarthy
Chief Medical Officer . . . . Harold L. Paz
General Counsel . . . . Thomas Sabatino Jr.
Government Services . . . . Fran S. Soistman

174   Anthem Blue Cross & Blue Shield of Connecticut
108 Leigus Road
Wallingford, CT 06492
Toll-Free: 800-922-4670
www.anthem.com
Subsidiary of: Anthem, Inc.
For Profit Organization: Yes

Healthplan and Services Defined
PLAN TYPE: HMO/PPO
Model Type: Network
Plan Specialty: Behavioral Health, Dental, Disease Management, Lab, PBM, Vision, Radiology
Benefits Offered: Behavioral Health, Dental, Disease Management, Inpatient SNF, Physical Therapy, Prescription, Psychiatric, Transplant, Vision, Wellness, Life

Type of Coverage
Commercial, Individual, Medicare, Supplemental Medicare, Catastrophic

Geographic Areas Served
Statewide

Accreditation Certification
URAC, NCQA

Key Personnel
President/CEO . . . . Joseph Swedish

175   CareCentrix
20 Church Street
12th Floor
Hartford, CT 06103
Toll-Free: 800-808-1902
carecentrix.com
Secondary Address: 100 First Stamford Place, 2nd Floor W, Stamford, CT 06902
Year Founded: 1996
Number of Primary Care Physicians: 8,000

Healthplan and Services Defined
PLAN TYPE: HMO
Benefits Offered: Home Care, Physical Therapy, Durable Medical Equipment; Occupational & Respiratory Therapy; Orthotics; Prosthetics

Geographic Areas Served
Arizona, Connecticut, Florida, Georgia, Kansas, and New York

Key Personnel
Chief Executive Officer . . . . John Driscoll
Chief Data Officer . . . . Tej Anand
Chief Medical Officer . . . . Michael Cantor
Chief Operating Officer . . . . Mary Daschner
Chief Customer Officer . . . . Tom Gaffney

176   Cigna Corporation
900 Cottage Grove Road
Bloomfield, CT 06002
Toll-Free: 800-997-1654
www.cigna.com
For Profit Organization: Yes
Year Founded: 1982

Healthplan and Services Defined
PLAN TYPE: Multiple
Benefits Offered: Behavioral Health, Dental, Disease Management, Prescription, Vision, Wellness, AD&D, Life, LTD, STD

Type of Coverage
Commercial, Individual, Medicare, Supplemental Medicare, Medicaid, Part-time and hourly workers; Union

Geographic Areas Served
Nationwide

Accreditation Certification
URAC, NCQA

Key Personnel
Chairman & CEO . . . . David M. Cordani

177   Cigna-HealthSpring Medicare
900 Cottage Grove Road
Bloomfield, CT 06002
Toll-Free: 800-668-3813
cigna.com/medicare
For Profit Organization: Yes

Healthplan and Services Defined
PLAN TYPE: Medicare
Benefits Offered: Prescription

Type of Coverage
Medicare, Supplemental Medicare

Geographic Areas Served
Nationwide

Key Personnel
Chairman & CEO . . . . David M. Cordani

178 ConnectiCare

175 Scott Swamp Road
P.O. Box 4050
Farmington, CT 06034-4050
Toll-Free: 800-251-7722
Phone: 860-674-5757
info@connecticare.com
www.connecticare.com
For Profit Organization: Yes
Year Founded: 1981
Owned by an Integrated Delivery Network (IDN): Yes

Healthplan and Services Defined
PLAN TYPE: HMO/PPO
Other Type: POS
Model Type: IPA, HMO, POS
Plan Specialty: Disease Management, Vision, UR
Benefits Offered: Behavioral Health, Chiropractic,
Complementary Medicine, Dental, Disease Management,
Home Care, Inpatient SNF, Physical Therapy, Podiatry,
Prescription, Psychiatric, Transplant, Vision, Wellness

Type of Coverage
Commercial, Individual, Medicare, Medicare Advantage
Catastrophic Illness Benefit: Unlimited

Type of Payment Plans Offered
Capitated, FFS

Geographic Areas Served
Statewide

Peer Review Type
Utilization Review: Yes
Second Surgical Opinion: Yes
Case Management: Yes

Publishes and Distributes Report Card: Yes

Accreditation Certification
TJC, NCQA
Utilization Review, Pre-Admission Certification, State
Licensure, Quality Assurance Program

Key Personnel
President & CoO . . . . Eric Galvin
SVP, Sales & Marketing . . . . Bert Wachtelhaussen
SVP, Human Resources . . . . Cheryl Hutchinson
Chief Medical Officer . . . . Wayne Rawlins

Average Claim Compensation
Physician's Fees Charged: 100%
Hospital's Fees Charged: 100%

Specialty Managed Care Partners
United Behavioral Health, Express Scripts
Enters into Contracts with Regional Business Coalitions: No

Employer References
Federal Government, Hartford Insurance Company, United
Technologies, State of Connecticut

179 Coventry Health Care of Connecticut

6730-B Rockledge Drive
Suite 700
Bethesda, MD 20817
www.coventryhealthcare.com
Subsidiary of: Aetna Inc.
For Profit Organization: Yes

Healthplan and Services Defined
PLAN TYPE: HMO/PPO
Model Type: Network
Plan Specialty: Behavioral Health, Dental, Worker's
Compensation
Benefits Offered: Behavioral Health, Dental, Prescription,
Vision, Wellness, Worker's Compensation

Type of Coverage
Commercial, Medicare, Medicaid

Geographic Areas Served
Statewide

180 Harvard Pilgrim Health Care Connecticut

City Place II
185 Asylum Street, 2nd Floor
Hartford, CT 06103
Toll-Free: 888-888-4742
www.harvardpilgrim.org
Non-Profit Organization: Yes
Year Founded: 1973
Number of Affiliated Hospitals: 179
Number of Referral/Specialty Physicians: 53,000

Healthplan and Services Defined
PLAN TYPE: HMO
Benefits Offered: Prescription

Geographic Areas Served
Statewide

Peer Review Type
Utilization Review: Yes
Second Surgical Opinion: No
Case Management: Yes

Publishes and Distributes Report Card: No

Accreditation Certification
TJC Accreditation, Medicare Approved, Utilization Review,
Pre-Admission Certification, State Licensure, Quality
Assurance Program

Key Personnel
President & CEO . . . . Eric H. Schultz
Chief Financial Officer . . . . Charles Goheen
Chief Legal Officer . . . . Tisa Hughes
Chief Information Officer . . . . Deborah A. Norton
VP, Marketing . . . . Richard O'Connor
Human Resources . . . . Cynthia Ring
SVP, Sales & Marketing . . . . Beth Roberts
Chief Medical Officer . . . . Michael Sherman, MD

Specialty Managed Care Partners
Enters into Contracts with Regional Business Coalitions: No

181   Humana Health Insurance of Connecticut

1 International Boulevard
Suite 904
Mahwah, NJ 07495
Toll-Free: 800-967-2370
Fax: 201-934-1369
www.humana.com
Subsidiary of: Humana
For Profit Organization: Yes

Healthplan and Services Defined
   PLAN TYPE: HMO/PPO
   Model Type: Network
   Plan Specialty: Dental, Vision
   Benefits Offered: Dental, Vision, Life, LTD, STD

Type of Coverage
   Commercial

Geographic Areas Served
   Connecticut is covered by the New Jersey branch

Accreditation Certification
   URAC, NCQA, CORE

Key Personnel
   President . . . . Bruce Broussard
   Chief Medical Officer. . . . . Roy A. Beveridge
   Chief Consumer Officer. . . . . Jody L. Bilney
   Human Resources. . . . . Tim Huval
   Chief Financial Officer . . . . Brian Kane
   Chief Information Officer . . . . Brian LeClaire
   General Counsel. . . . . Christopher M. Todoroff

182   Oxford Health Plans

48 Monroe Turnpike
Trumbull, CT 06611
Toll-Free: 800-444-6222
Phone: 203-459-9100
www.oxhp.com
For Profit Organization: Yes
Year Founded: 1984
Owned by an Integrated Delivery Network (IDN): Yes

Healthplan and Services Defined
   PLAN TYPE: HMO/PPO
   Model Type: IPA, Network, POS
   Benefits Offered: Behavioral Health, Chiropractic,
      Complementary Medicine, Dental, Disease Management,
      Home Care, Inpatient SNF, Podiatry, Prescription,
      Psychiatric, Transplant, Vision, Wellness
   Offers Demand Management Patient Information Service:
      Yes

Type of Coverage
   Commercial, Individual, Indemnity, Medicare, Catastrophic
   Catastrophic Illness Benefit: Varies per case

Type of Payment Plans Offered
   FFS

Geographic Areas Served
   Connecticut: Fairfield, New Haven, Litchfield, Hartford,
   Middlesex, New London, Tolland & Windham counties; New
   Jersey: Essex, Hudson, Middlesex, Monmouth, Morris,

Ocean, Passaic & Somerset counties; New York: Bronx,
Dutchess, Kings, Nassau, New York, Putnam, Queens,
Richmond, Rockland, Suffolk, & Westchester counties

Peer Review Type
   Utilization Review: Yes
   Second Surgical Opinion: Yes
   Case Management: Yes

Publishes and Distributes Report Card: Yes

Accreditation Certification
   NCQA
   TJC Accreditation, Medicare Approved, Utilization Review,
      Pre-Admission Certification, State Licensure, Quality
      Assurance Program

Key Personnel
   Chief Executive Officer. . . . . David S. Wichmann
   Chief Operating Officer . . . . Dan Schumacher
   Chief Strategy Officer . . . . John Cosgriff
   Communications Officer . . . . Kirsten Gorsuch
   Chief Medical Officer. . . . . Sam Ho
   Chief Legal Officer . . . . Thad Johnson
   Chief Information Officer . . . . Phil McKoy
   Chief Financial Officer. . . . . Jeff Putnam

Specialty Managed Care Partners
   Enters into Contracts with Regional Business Coalitions: Yes

183   Trinity Health of Connecticut

1000 Asylum Avenue
5th Floor
Hartford, CT 06105
Phone: 860-714-1900
www.trinity-health.org
Subsidiary of: Trinity Health
Non-Profit Organization: Yes
Year Founded: 2013
Number of Affiliated Hospitals: 3
Number of Primary Care Physicians: 900
Total Enrollment: 30,000,000

Healthplan and Services Defined
   PLAN TYPE: Other
   Benefits Offered: Disease Management, Home Care,
      Long-Term Care, Psychiatric, Hospice programs, PACE
      (Program of All Inclusive Care for the Elderly)

Key Personnel
   President/CEO . . . . Christopher Dadlez

184   UnitedHealthcare of Connecticut

185 Asylum Street
Hartford, CT 06103
Phone: 860-702-5000
www.uhc.com/contact-us/connecticut
Subsidiary of: UnitedHealth Group
For Profit Organization: Yes
Year Founded: 1991

Healthplan and Services Defined
   PLAN TYPE: HMO/PPO
   Model Type: Network

Plan Specialty: Behavioral Health, Dental, Disease
   Management, PBM, Vision
Benefits Offered: Behavioral Health, Dental, Disease
   Management, Long-Term Care, Prescription, Vision,
   Wellness, Life, LTD, STD

Type of Coverage
   Individual, Medicare, Supplemental Medicare, Medicaid,
   Catastrophic, Family, Military, Veterans, Group,

Geographic Areas Served
   Statewide

Key Personnel
   President & CEO . . . . David Wichmann
   Chief Operating Officer . . . . Dan Schumacher
   Chief Strategy Officer . . . . John Cosgriff
   Communications Officer . . . . Kirsten Gorsuch
   Chief Medical Officer. . . . . Sam Ho
   Chief Legal Officer . . . . Thad Johnson
   Chief Information Officer . . . . Phil McKoy
   Chief Financial Officer. Jeff Putnam

Health Insurance Coverage Status and Type of Coverage by Age

Category	All Persons		Under 18 years		Under 65 years	
	Number	%	Number	%	Number	%
Total population	938	-	217	-	775	-
Covered by some type of health insurance	885 *(5)*	94.3 *(0.5)*	211 *(2)*	96.9 *(0.8)*	724 *(5)*	93.4 *(0.6)*
Covered by private health insurance	670 *(9)*	71.4 *(1.0)*	140 *(5)*	64.5 *(2.0)*	559 *(8)*	72.1 *(1.1)*
Employer-based	566 *(11)*	60.3 *(1.2)*	124 *(5)*	56.9 *(2.3)*	491 *(11)*	63.4 *(1.4)*
Direct purchase	120 *(7)*	12.8 *(0.7)*	14 *(3)*	6.6 *(1.4)*	72 *(6)*	9.2 *(0.8)*
TRICARE	29 *(4)*	3.1 *(0.4)*	5 *(2)*	2.5 *(0.9)*	18 *(4)*	2.3 *(0.5)*
Covered by public health insurance	348 *(9)*	37.1 *(1.0)*	80 *(5)*	36.7 *(2.2)*	191 *(9)*	24.6 *(1.2)*
Medicaid	190 *(9)*	20.3 *(1.0)*	79 *(5)*	36.4 *(2.2)*	171 *(9)*	22.1 *(1.1)*
Medicare	181 *(3)*	19.3 *(0.4)*	2 *(1)*	0.7 *(0.4)*	23 *(3)*	3.0 *(0.3)*
VA Care	17 *(2)*	1.8 *(0.2)*	Z *(Z)*	Z *(Z)*	7 *(1)*	0.9 *(0.2)*
Not covered at any time during the year	53 *(5)*	5.7 *(0.5)*	7 *(2)*	3.1 *(0.8)*	52 *(4)*	6.6 *(0.6)*

Note: Numbers in thousands; Figures cover civilian noninstitutionalized population in 2016; N/A indicates that data was not available; Z represents or rounds to zero; Margin of error appears in parenthesis and is calculated using replicate weights.
Source: U.S. Census Bureau, American Community Survey, Table HIC-4_ACS. Health Insurance Coverage Status and Type of Coverage by State—All People: 2008 to 2016, Table HIC-5_ACS. Health Insurance Coverage Status and Type of Coverage by State—Children Under 18: 2008 to 2016, Table HIC-6_ACS. Health Insurance Coverage Status and Type of Coverage by State—Persons Under 65: 2008 to 2016

Delaware

185　Aetna Health of Delaware
151 Farmington Avenue
Hartford, CT 06156
Toll-Free: 800-872-3862
Phone: 860-273-0123
www.aetna.com
Subsidiary of: Aetna Inc.
For Profit Organization: Yes
State Enrollment: 27,179

Healthplan and Services Defined
PLAN TYPE: HMO/PPO
Other Type: POS
Model Type: Network
Plan Specialty: Behavioral Health, Dental, EPO, Lab, PBM, Vision, Radiology
Benefits Offered: Behavioral Health, Dental, Disease Management, Long-Term Care, Physical Therapy, Podiatry, Prescription, Psychiatric, Wellness, Life, LTD, STD, As of 2018 Aetna will no longer be offering plans in the state of Delaware

Type of Coverage
Commercial, Individual, Supplemental Medicare, Student health

Type of Payment Plans Offered
POS, FFS

Geographic Areas Served
Statewide

Key Personnel
CEO . . . . Mark Bertolini

186　Delta Dental of Delaware
One Delta Drive
Mechanicsburg, PA 17055-6999
Toll-Free: 800-932-0783
www.deltadentalins.com
Non-Profit Organization: Yes

Healthplan and Services Defined
PLAN TYPE: Dental
Other Type: Dental PPO
Plan Specialty: Dental
Benefits Offered: Dental

Type of Coverage
Commercial, Individual

Geographic Areas Served
Statewide

Key Personnel
President & CEO . . . . Tony Barth
Chief Financial Officer . . . . Michael Castro
Chief Legal Officer . . . . Michael Hankinson
EVP, Sales & Marketing . . . . Belinda Martinez
Chief Operating Officer . . . . Nilesh Patel

187　Highmark BCBS Delaware
Fifth Avenue Place
120 Fifth Avenue
Pittsburgh, PA 15222-3099
Phone: 412-544-7000
www.highmarkbcbsde.com
Non-Profit Organization: Yes
Year Founded: 1935

Healthplan and Services Defined
PLAN TYPE: HMO/PPO
Model Type: IPA, Network
Benefits Offered: Dental, Disease Management, Prescription, Vision, Wellness

Type of Coverage
Commercial, Individual, Medicare, Supplemental Medicare

Type of Payment Plans Offered
Combination FFS & DFFS

Geographic Areas Served
Statewide

Key Personnel
President . . . . Deborah L. Rice-Johnson
Chief Medical Officer . . . . Charles Deshazer, MD

188　Humana Health Insurance of Delaware
5000 Ritter Road
Suite 101
Mechanicsburg, PA 17055
Toll-Free: 866-355-5861
Phone: 717-766-6040
Fax: 717-795-1951
www.humana.com
Subsidiary of: Humana
For Profit Organization: Yes

Healthplan and Services Defined
PLAN TYPE: HMO/PPO
Model Type: Network
Plan Specialty: Dental, Vision
Benefits Offered: Dental, Vision, Life, LTD, STD

Type of Coverage
Commercial

Geographic Areas Served
Statewide. Delaware is covered by the Pennsylvannia branch

Accreditation Certification
URAC, NCQA, CORE

Key Personnel
President & CEO . . . . Bruce Broussard
Chief Medical Officer . . . . Roy A. Beveridge
Chief Consumer Officer . . . . Jody L. Bilney
Human Resources . . . . Tim Huval
Chief Financial Officer . . . . Brian Kane
Chief Information Officer . . . . Brian LeClaire
General Counsel . . . . Christopher M. Todoroff
Chief Accounting Officer . . . . Cynthia H. Zipperie

189 Mid-Atlantic Behavioral Health

910 S Chapel Street
Suite 102
Newark, DE 19713
Phone: 302-224-1400
www.midatlanticbh.com
Secondary Address: 3521 Silverside Road, Suite 2F1,
    Wilmington, DE 19810, 302-224-1400

Healthplan and Services Defined
PLAN TYPE: Multiple
Plan Specialty: Behavioral Health
Benefits Offered: Behavioral Health, Psychiatric

Type of Payment Plans Offered
FFS

Geographic Areas Served
Maryland, Virginia, West Virginia, North Carolina,
Pennsylvania, Delaware & Washington DC

Network Qualifications
Minimum Years of Practice: 2
Pre-Admission Certification: Yes

Peer Review Type
Utilization Review: No
Second Surgical Opinion: No
Case Management: No

Publishes and Distributes Report Card: No

Accreditation Certification
TJC Accreditation, Medicare Approved, Utilization Review,
    Pre-Admission Certification, State Licensure, Quality
    Assurance Program

Key Personnel
Practive Director . . . . Traci Bolander, Psy. D

Specialty Managed Care Partners
Enters into Contracts with Regional Business Coalitions: No

190 Trinity Health of Delaware

St. Francis Healthcare
701 North Clayton Street
Wilmington, DE 19805
Phone: 302-421-4100
www.trinity-health.org
Subsidiary of: Trinity Health
Non-Profit Organization: Yes
Year Founded: 2013
Total Enrollment: 30,000,000

Healthplan and Services Defined
PLAN TYPE: Other
Benefits Offered: Disease Management, Home Care,
    Long-Term Care, Psychiatric, Hospice programs, PACE
    (Program of All Inclusive Care for the Elderly)

Key Personnel
Chief Executive Officer . . . . Richard J. Gilfillian
Chief Financial Officer . . . . Benjamin R. Carter
Human Resources . . . . Edmund F. Hodge
General Counsel . . . . Paul G. Neumann
Chief Clinical Officer . . . . Daniel J. Roth

Chief Operating Officer . . . . Michael A. Slubowski

191 UnitedHealthcare Community Plan Delaware

UnitedHealthcare Customer Service
P.O. Box 29675
Hot Springs, AR 71903-9802
Toll-Free: 877-877-8159
www.uhccommunityplan.com/de.html
Subsidiary of: UnitedHealth Group

Healthplan and Services Defined
PLAN TYPE: HMO
Benefits Offered: Dental, Home Care, Long-Term Care,
    Physical Therapy, Prescription, Vision, Wellness, Hearing,
    Labs & X-rays, Diabetic Support

Type of Coverage
Medicaid

Geographic Areas Served
Statewide

Key Personnel
Chief Executive Officer . . . . Steve Nelson
Chief Operating Officer . . . . Dan Schumacher
Chief Strategy Officer . . . . John Cosgriff
Communications Officer . . . . Kirsten Gorsuch
Chief Medical Officer . . . . Sam Ho
Chief Legal Officer . . . . Thad Johnson
Chief Information Officer . . . . Phil McKoy

Health Insurance Coverage Status and Type of Coverage by Age

Category	All Persons		Under 18 years		Under 65 years	
	Number	%	Number	%	Number	%
Total population	671	-	131	-	594	-
Covered by some type of health insurance	645 *(4)*	96.1 *(0.6)*	127 *(3)*	96.9 *(1.3)*	568 *(4)*	95.7 *(0.7)*
Covered by private health insurance	459 *(8)*	68.4 *(1.3)*	69 *(4)*	52.9 *(3.1)*	409 *(8)*	68.9 *(1.4)*
Employer-based	384 *(9)*	57.3 *(1.4)*	59 *(5)*	44.7 *(3.4)*	347 *(9)*	58.4 *(1.5)*
Direct purchase	85 *(5)*	12.6 *(0.7)*	9 *(2)*	7.0 *(1.5)*	67 *(5)*	11.3 *(0.8)*
TRICARE	14 *(2)*	2.0 *(0.3)*	3 *(1)*	2.2 *(0.7)*	10 *(2)*	1.7 *(0.3)*
Covered by public health insurance	249 *(8)*	37.1 *(1.2)*	63 *(4)*	48.2 *(3.4)*	178 *(8)*	30.0 *(1.4)*
Medicaid	190 *(9)*	28.3 *(1.3)*	63 *(4)*	47.9 *(3.4)*	169 *(8)*	28.5 *(1.4)*
Medicare	86 *(2)*	12.8 *(0.3)*	1 *(Z)*	0.5 *(0.4)*	15 *(2)*	2.6 *(0.3)*
VA Care	11 *(2)*	1.7 *(0.3)*	Z *(Z)*	0.2 *(0.2)*	6 *(1)*	1.0 *(0.2)*
Not covered at any time during the year	26 *(4)*	3.9 *(0.6)*	4 *(2)*	3.1 *(1.3)*	26 *(4)*	4.3 *(0.7)*

Note: Numbers in thousands; Figures cover civilian noninstitutionalized population in 2016; N/A indicates that data was not available; Z represents or rounds to zero; Margin of error appears in parenthesis and is calculated using replicate weights.
Source: U.S. Census Bureau, American Community Survey, Table HIC-4_ACS. Health Insurance Coverage Status and Type of Coverage by State—All People: 2008 to 2016, Table HIC-5_ACS. Health Insurance Coverage Status and Type of Coverage by State—Children Under 18: 2008 to 2016, Table HIC-6_ACS. Health Insurance Coverage Status and Type of Coverage by State—Persons Under 65: 2008 to 2016

District of Columbia

192   Aetna Health of District of Columbia
151 Farmington Avenue
Hartford, CT 06156
Toll-Free: 800-872-3862
Phone: 860-273-0123
www.aetna.com
Subsidiary of: Aetna Inc.
For Profit Organization: Yes

Healthplan and Services Defined
PLAN TYPE: HMO/PPO
Other Type: POS
Model Type: Network
Plan Specialty: Behavioral Health, EPO, Lab, PBM,
    Radiology
Benefits Offered: Behavioral Health, Dental, Disease
    Management, Long-Term Care, Physical Therapy,
    Podiatry, Prescription, Psychiatric, Vision, Wellness, Life,
    LTD, STD

Type of Coverage
Commercial, Student health

Geographic Areas Served
Statewide

Key Personnel
CEO................................. Mark Bertolini

193   AmeriHealth Caritas District of Columbia
1120 Vermont Avenue NW
Suite 200
Washington, DC 20005
Toll-Free: 800-408-7511
Phone: 202-408-4720
www.amerihealthcaritasdc.com
For Profit Organization: Yes
Year Founded: 1987

Healthplan and Services Defined
PLAN TYPE: Other
Plan Specialty: Behavioral Health, Dental
Benefits Offered: Prescription

Type of Coverage
Medicaid

Geographic Areas Served
District of Columbia

Publishes and Distributes Report Card: Yes

Accreditation Certification
NCQA

Key Personnel
Market President .... Karen M. Dale
Finance Director .... Terrence J. Cunningham
Compliance Director .... Brian Geesaman
Local Operations Director .... James R. Christian
Dental Director...................... Nathan Fletcher
Chief Medical Officer .... Lavdena Adams, MD

Specialty Managed Care Partners
Enters into Contracts with Regional Business Coalitions: Yes

194   Delta Dental of the District of Columbia
One Delta Drive
Mechanicsburg, PA 17055-6999
Toll-Free: 800-932-0783
www.deltadentalins.com
Non-Profit Organization: Yes

Healthplan and Services Defined
PLAN TYPE: Dental
Other Type: Dental PPO
Plan Specialty: Dental
Benefits Offered: Dental

Type of Coverage
Commercial, Individual

Geographic Areas Served
District of Columbia

Key Personnel
President & CEO......................... Tony Barth
Chief Financial Officer .... Michael Castro
Chief Legal Officer .... Michael Hankinson
EVP, Sales & Marketing .... Belinda Martinez
Chief Operating Officer .... Nilesh Patel

195   Quality Plan Administrators
7824 Eastern Avenue NW
Suite 100
Washington, DC 20012
Toll-Free: 800-900-4112
Phone: 202-722-2744
Fax: 202-291-5703
quality@qpatpa.com
qualityplanadmin.com
For Profit Organization: Yes
Year Founded: 1986
Number of Primary Care Physicians: 175
Total Enrollment: 90,000

Healthplan and Services Defined
PLAN TYPE: HMO/PPO
Plan Specialty: Dental, Vision
Benefits Offered: Dental, Vision

Type of Coverage
Commercial, Government, municipalities, correct

Key Personnel
President/CEO................... Milton Bernard, DDS

196   UnitedHealthcare Community Plan Capital Area
P.O. Box 29675
Hot Springs, AR 71903-9802
Toll-Free: 866-790-9424
www.uhccommunityplan.com/dc.html
Subsidiary of: UnitedHealth Group

Healthplan and Services Defined
PLAN TYPE: PPO
Model Type: Network
Benefits Offered: Dental, Podiatry, Prescription, Vision, 24hr Nurse Line

Type of Coverage
Medicare, Supplemental Medicare, Medicaid

Geographic Areas Served
District of Columbia

---

197   UnitedHealthcare of the District of Columbia
800 King Farm Boulevard
Suite 600
Rockville, MD 20850
Toll-Free: 877-842-3210
Fax: 410-540-8381
md_dc_de_provider_relations@uhc.com
www.uhc.com/contact-us/district-of-columbia
Subsidiary of: UnitedHealth Group
Non-Profit Organization: Yes
Year Founded: 1976

Healthplan and Services Defined
PLAN TYPE: HMO/PPO
Model Type: Network
Benefits Offered: Disease Management, Prescription, Wellness

Geographic Areas Served
Statewide. The District of Columbia is covered by the Maryland branch

Subscriber Information
Average Monthly Fee Per Subscriber
(Employee + Employer Contribution):
Employee Only (Self): $104.00-135.00
Employee & 1 Family Member: $143.00-184.00
Employee & 2 Family Members: $331.00-440.00
Medicare: $112.00-156.00
Average Annual Deductible Per Subscriber:
Employee Only (Self): $100.00-250.00
Employee & 1 Family Member: $500.00-1500.00
Employee & 2 Family Members: $200.00-500.00
Medicare: $0
Average Subscriber Co-Payment:
Primary Care Physician: $5.00/10.00
Non-Network Physician: Deductible
Prescription Drugs: $5.00/10.00
Hospital ER: $25.00/50.00
Home Health Care: $5.00/10.00

Network Qualifications
Pre-Admission Certification: Yes

Peer Review Type
Utilization Review: Yes
Second Surgical Opinion: Yes
Case Management: Yes

Publishes and Distributes Report Card: Yes

Accreditation Certification
TJC Accreditation, Medicare Approved, Utilization Review, Pre-Admission Certification, State Licensure, Quality Assurance Program

Key Personnel
President . . . . David Wichmann
Chief Operating Officer. . . . . Dan Schummacher
Chief Strategy Officer . . . . John Cosgriff
Communications Officer . . . . Kirsten Gorsuch
Chief Medical Officer. . . . . Sam Ho
Chief Legal Officer . . . . Thad Johnson
Chief Information Officer . . . . Phil McKoy
Chief Financial Officer. . . . . Jeff Putnam

Specialty Managed Care Partners
Enters into Contracts with Regional Business Coalitions: Yes

HMO/PPO DIRECTORY

Health Insurance Coverage Status and Type of Coverage by Age

Category	All Persons		Under 18 years		Under 65 years	
	Number	%	Number	%	Number	%
Total population	20,294	-	4,386	-	16,274	-
Covered by some type of health insurance	17,750 *(47)*	87.5 *(0.2)*	4,098 *(17)*	93.4 *(0.4)*	13,783 *(47)*	84.7 *(0.3)*
Covered by private health insurance	12,663 *(61)*	62.4 *(0.3)*	2,340 *(26)*	53.3 *(0.6)*	10,578 *(60)*	65.0 *(0.4)*
Employer-based	9,107 *(55)*	44.9 *(0.3)*	1,839 *(23)*	41.9 *(0.5)*	8,086 *(53)*	49.7 *(0.3)*
Direct purchase	3,567 *(40)*	17.6 *(0.2)*	439 *(15)*	10.0 *(0.3)*	2,420 *(39)*	14.9 *(0.2)*
TRICARE	716 *(17)*	3.5 *(0.1)*	130 *(8)*	3.0 *(0.2)*	438 *(14)*	2.7 *(0.1)*
Covered by public health insurance	7,629 *(48)*	37.6 *(0.2)*	1,908 *(26)*	43.5 *(0.6)*	3,777 *(47)*	23.2 *(0.3)*
Medicaid	3,858 *(48)*	19.0 *(0.2)*	1,888 *(26)*	43.0 *(0.6)*	3,284 *(44)*	20.2 *(0.3)*
Medicare	4,380 *(16)*	21.6 *(0.1)*	27 *(3)*	0.6 *(0.1)*	533 *(13)*	3.3 *(0.1)*
VA Care	610 *(14)*	3.0 *(0.1)*	8 *(2)*	0.2 *(Z)*	255 *(10)*	1.6 *(0.1)*
Not covered at any time during the year	2,544 *(47)*	12.5 *(0.2)*	288 *(16)*	6.6 *(0.4)*	2,491 *(47)*	15.3 *(0.3)*

Note: Numbers in thousands; Figures cover civilian noninstitutionalized population in 2016; N/A indicates that data was not available; Z represents or rounds to zero; Margin of error appears in parenthesis and is calculated using replicate weights.
Source: U.S. Census Bureau, American Community Survey, Table HIC-4_ACS. Health Insurance Coverage Status and Type of Coverage by State—All People: 2008 to 2016, Table HIC-5_ACS. Health Insurance Coverage Status and Type of Coverage by State—Children Under 18: 2008 to 2016, Table HIC-6_ACS. Health Insurance Coverage Status and Type of Coverage by State—Persons Under 65: 2008 to 2016

Florida

198　Aetna Health of Florida

151 Farmington Avenue
Hartford, CT 06156
Toll-Free: 800-872-3862
Phone: 860-273-0123
www.aetna.com
Subsidiary of: Aetna Inc.
For Profit Organization: Yes

Healthplan and Services Defined
　PLAN TYPE: HMO/PPO
　Other Type: POS
　Model Type: Network
　Plan Specialty: Behavioral Health, Dental, EPO, Lab, PBM,
　　Vision, Radiology
　Benefits Offered: Behavioral Health, Dental, Disease
　　Management, Long-Term Care, Physical Therapy,
　　Podiatry, Prescription, Psychiatric, Wellness, Life, LTD,
　　STD

Type of Coverage
　Commercial, Medicare, Medicaid, Catastrophic, Student
　health

Geographic Areas Served
　Statewide

Key Personnel
　CEO . . . . Mark Bertolini

199　Amerigroup Florida

4200 W Cypress Street
Suite 900
Tampa, FL 33607
Toll-Free: 800-600-4441
Phone: 813-830-6900
www.myamerigroup.com/fl
Subsidiary of: Anthem, Inc.
For Profit Organization: Yes

Healthplan and Services Defined
　PLAN TYPE: Other
　Model Type: Network
　Plan Specialty: Behavioral Health, Dental, Disease
　　Management, Lab, Vision, Managed health care for people
　　in public programs. Mental health and substance abuse
　　services.
　Benefits Offered: Behavioral Health, Dental, Disease
　　Management, Long-Term Care, Podiatry, Prescription,
　　Vision, Wellness, Transportation; Art Therapy; Hearing
　　Aids Batteires

Type of Coverage
　Medicaid

Key Personnel
　EVP/Pres., Gov. Business . . . . Peter D. Haytaian
　Chief Financial Officer . . . . Scott Anglin
　VP, Human Resources . . . . Jenn Crenshaw
　Information Technology . . . . Jeff Schrecengost

200　AvMed

9400 S Dadeland Boulevard
Miami, FL 33156
Toll-Free: 800-477-8768
Phone: 305-671-5437
www.avmed.org
Subsidiary of: SantaFe HealthCare, Inc.
Non-Profit Organization: Yes
Year Founded: 1969
Total Enrollment: 340,000
State Enrollment: 340,000

Healthplan and Services Defined
　PLAN TYPE: Medicare
　Plan Specialty: Dental, Nurse On Call Program
　Benefits Offered: Behavioral Health, Dental, Prescription,
　　Wellness

Type of Coverage
　Medicare

Type of Payment Plans Offered
　POS

Geographic Areas Served
　Miami-Dade counties

Subscriber Information
　Average Annual Deductible Per Subscriber:
　　Employee Only (Self): $0
　　Employee & 1 Family Member: $0
　　Employee & 2 Family Members: $0
　　Medicare: $0

Accreditation Certification
　NCQA

Key Personnel
　President & CEO . . . . Michael P. Gallagher
　President & COO . . . . James M. Repp
　SVP, Human Resources . . . . Kay Ayers
　Chief Information Officer . . . . Jim Simpson
　SVP, Financial Officer . . . . Randall L. Stuart
　SVP, Medical Officer . . . . Ann O. Wehr
　SVP, General Counsel. . . . . Steven M. Ziegler

Specialty Managed Care Partners
　Enters into Contracts with Regional Business Coalitions: No

201　AvMed Ft. Lauderdale

13450 W Sunrise Boulevard
Suite 370
Ft. Lauderdale, FL 33323
Toll-Free: 800-477-8768
Phone: 954-462-2520
www.avmed.org
Non-Profit Organization: Yes
Year Founded: 1973
Federally Qualified: Yes
Total Enrollment: 340,000
State Enrollment: 340,000

Healthplan and Services Defined
　PLAN TYPE: Medicare
　Model Type: IPA

Plan Specialty: Nurse On Call Program
Benefits Offered: Behavioral Health, Dental, Disease
    Management, Prescription, Wellness

Type of Coverage
Medicare

Geographic Areas Served
Broward County

Accreditation Certification
TJC, NCQA

Key Personnel
President & CEO . . . . Michael P. Gallagher
Chief Operating Officer . . . . James M. Repp
SVP, Human Resources . . . . Kay Ayers
SVP, Information Officer . . . . Jim Simpson
SVP, Financial Officer . . . . Randall L. Stuart
SVP, Medical Officer . . . . Ann O. Wehr
SVP, General Counsel. . . . . Steven M. Ziegler

202 AvMed Gainesville

4300 NW 89th Boulevard
Gainesville, FL 32606
Toll-Free: 800-477-8768
Phone: 352-372-8400
www.avmed.org
Non-Profit Organization: Yes
Year Founded: 1986
Total Enrollment: 340,000
State Enrollment: 340,000

Healthplan and Services Defined
  PLAN TYPE: HMO
Model Type: IPA
Plan Specialty: Nurse On Call Program
Benefits Offered: Behavioral Health, Dental, Disease
    Management, Prescription, Wellness

Type of Coverage
Commercial, Individual
Catastrophic Illness Benefit: Unlimited

Type of Payment Plans Offered
POS, DFFS, Combination FFS & DFFS

Geographic Areas Served
Alachua, Bradford, Citrus, Columbia, Dixie, Gilchrist,
Hamilton, Levy, Marion, Suwannee and Union counties

Accreditation Certification
NCQA

Key Personnel
President & CEO . . . . Michael P. Gallagher
Chief Operating Officer . . . . James M. Repp
SVP, Human Resources . . . . Kay Ayers
Chief Information Officer. . . . . Jim Simpson
SVP, Financial Officer . . . . Randall L. Stuart

Average Claim Compensation
Physician's Fees Charged: 85%
Hospital's Fees Charged: 70%

Specialty Managed Care Partners
Enters into Contracts with Regional Business Coalitions: No

203 AvMed Jacksonville

1300 Riverplace Boulevard
Suite 640
Jacksonville, FL 32207
Toll-Free: 800-477-8768
Phone: 904-858-1300
www.avmed.org
Non-Profit Organization: Yes
Year Founded: 1969
Federally Qualified: Yes
Total Enrollment: 340,000
State Enrollment: 340,000

Healthplan and Services Defined
  PLAN TYPE: HMO
Plan Specialty: Nurse On Call Program
Benefits Offered: Behavioral Health, Dental, Disease
    Management, Prescription, Wellness

Type of Coverage
Commercial, Individual

Geographic Areas Served
Baker, Clay, Duval, Nassau and St. Johns counties

Peer Review Type
Second Surgical Opinion: Yes
Case Management: Yes

Publishes and Distributes Report Card: Yes

Accreditation Certification
NCQA

Key Personnel
President & CEO . . . . Michael P. Gallagher
Chief Operating Officer . . . . James M. Repp
SVP, Human Resources . . . . Kay Ayers
Chief Information Officer. . . . . Jim Simpson
SVP, Financial Officer . . . . Randall L. Stuart
SVP, Medical Officer . . . . Ann O. Wehr
SVP, General Counsel. . . . . Steven M. Ziegler

204 AvMed Orlando

1800 Pembrook Drive
Suite 190
Orlando, FL 32810
Toll-Free: 800-477-8767
Phone: 407-539-0007
www.avmed.org
Non-Profit Organization: Yes
Year Founded: 1988
Total Enrollment: 340,000
State Enrollment: 340,000

Healthplan and Services Defined
  PLAN TYPE: HMO
Benefits Offered: Behavioral Health, Dental, Disease
    Management, Prescription, Wellness

Type of Coverage
Commercial, Individual

Type of Payment Plans Offered
FFS, Combination FFS & DFFS

Geographic Areas Served

Orange, Osceola and Seminole counties

Accreditation Certification

NCQA

Key Personnel

President & CEO . . . . Michael P. Gallagher
Chief Operating Officer . . . . James M. Repp
SVP, Human Resources . . . . Kay Ayers
Chief Information Officer . . . . Jim Simpson
SVP, Financial Officer . . . . Randall L. Stuart
SVP, Medical Officer . . . . Ann O. Wehr
SVP, General Counsel . . . . Steven M. Ziegler

Specialty Managed Care Partners

Enters into Contracts with Regional Business Coalitions: Yes

205 AvMed Pembroke Pines

340 S Flamingo Road
Pembroke Pines, FL 33027
Toll-Free: 800-477-8767
Phone: 954-986-1700
www.avmed.org
Non-Profit Organization: Yes
Year Founded: 1969
Federally Qualified: Yes
Total Enrollment: 340,000
State Enrollment: 340,000

Healthplan and Services Defined
  PLAN TYPE: Medicare
  Plan Specialty: Nurse On Call Program
  Benefits Offered: Behavioral Health, Dental, Disease
    Management, Prescription, Wellness

Type of Coverage

Medicare

Key Personnel

President & CEO . . . . Michael P. Gallagher
SVP, Member Services . . . . Kay Ayers
SVP, Underwriting . . . . Brad Bentley
SVP, Sales & Marketing . . . . James M. Repp
SVP/CFO . . . . Randall L. Stuart
SVP/Chief Medical Officer . . . . . . Ann O. Wehr, MD, FACP
SVP/General Counsel . . . . Steven M. Ziegler
SVP/Chief Info Officer . . . . Tony Tardugno

206 AvMed Tampa Bay

1511 North Westshore Boulevard
Suite 450
Tampa, FL 33607
Toll-Free: 800-477-8768
Phone: 813-281-5650
www.avmed.org
Non-Profit Organization: Yes
Year Founded: 1969
Federally Qualified: Yes
Total Enrollment: 340,000
State Enrollment: 340,000

Healthplan and Services Defined
  PLAN TYPE: HMO
  Plan Specialty: Nurse On Call Program
  Benefits Offered: Behavioral Health, Dental, Disease
    Management, Prescription, Wellness

Geographic Areas Served

Hernando, Hillsborough, Lee, Pasco, Pinellas, Polk and
Sarasota counties

Network Qualifications

Pre-Admission Certification: Yes

Accreditation Certification

NCQA

Key Personnel

President & CEO . . . . Michael P. Gallagher
Chief Operating Officer . . . . James M. Repp
SVP, Human Resources . . . . Kay Ayers
Chief Information Officer . . . . Jim Simpson
SVP, Financial Officer . . . . Randall L. Stuart
SVP, Medical Officer . . . . Ann O. Wehr
SVP, General Counsel . . . . Steven M. Ziegler

Specialty Managed Care Partners

Enters into Contracts with Regional Business Coalitions: Yes

207 Capital Health Plan

2140 Centerville Place
Tallahassee, FL 32308
Phone: 850-383-3311
memberservices@chp.org
www.capitalhealth.com
Subsidiary of: Blue Cross Blue Shield of Florida
Non-Profit Organization: Yes
Year Founded: 1982
Owned by an Integrated Delivery Network (IDN): Yes
Number of Primary Care Physicians: 150
Number of Referral/Specialty Physicians: 400
Total Enrollment: 125,000
State Enrollment: 125,000

Healthplan and Services Defined
  PLAN TYPE: HMO
  Model Type: Staff, Mixed Model
  Plan Specialty: Chiropractic, Lab, Vision, Radiology, UR
  Benefits Offered: Behavioral Health, Chiropractic, Disease
    Management, Home Care, Inpatient SNF, Physical Therapy,
    Podiatry, Prescription, Psychiatric, Transplant, Vision,
    Wellness

Type of Coverage

Commercial, Medicare, Supplemental Medicare, Catastrophic
Catastrophic Illness Benefit: Unlimited

Geographic Areas Served

Calhoun, Franklin, Gadsden, Jefferson, Leon, Liberty and
Wakulla counties

Peer Review Type

Second Surgical Opinion: Yes

Publishes and Distributes Report Card: Yes

Accreditation Certification

NCQA

Key Personnel

President & CEO . . . . John Hogan

Specialty Managed Care Partners

Enters into Contracts with Regional Business Coalitions: Yes

208 CareCentrix: Florida

9119 Corporate Lake Drive
Suite 300
Tampa, FL 33634
Toll-Free: 800-808-1902
carecentrix.com
Year Founded: 1996
Number of Primary Care Physicians: 8,000

Healthplan and Services Defined

PLAN TYPE: HMO
Benefits Offered: Home Care, Physical Therapy, Durable
Medical Equipment; Occupational & Respiratory Therapy;
Orthotics; Prosthetics

Key Personnel

Chief Executive Officer . . . . John Driscoll
Chief Data Officer. . . . . Tej Anand
Chief Medical Officer. . . . . Michael Cantor
Chief Operating Officer . . . . Mary Daschner
Chief Customer Officer . . . . Tom Gaffney

209 CarePlus Health Plans

11430 NW 20th Street
Suite 300
Miami, FL 33172
Toll-Free: 800-794-5907
cphp_memberservices@careplus-hp.com
www.careplushealthplans.com
Subsidiary of: Humana
Year Founded: 2003
Total Enrollment: 111,000
State Enrollment: 111,000

Healthplan and Services Defined

PLAN TYPE: Medicare
Benefits Offered: Prescription

Type of Coverage

Medicare

Geographic Areas Served

Miami-Dade, Broward, Palm Beach, Hillsborough, Pinellas,
Pasco, Polk, Lake, Marion, Sumter, Orange, Osceola,
Seminole, Brevard, Indian River, Martin, Okeechobee, St.
Lucie and Duval counties

Accreditation Certification

AAAHC

Key Personnel

Regional President . . . . David Jarboe

210 Cigna HealthCare of Florida

900 Cottage Grove Road
Bloomfield, CT 06002
Toll-Free: 800-997-1654
www.cigna.com
For Profit Organization: Yes

Healthplan and Services Defined

PLAN TYPE: HMO
Other Type: POS
Model Type: Network
Benefits Offered: Dental, Disease Management, Prescription,
Transplant, Vision, Wellness, Life, LTD, STD

Type of Coverage

Commercial, Individual

Type of Payment Plans Offered

POS, DFFS, FFS, Combination FFS & DFFS

Network Qualifications

Minimum Years of Practice: 3

Peer Review Type

Second Surgical Opinion: Yes
Case Management: Yes

Publishes and Distributes Report Card: Yes

Accreditation Certification

NCQA
TJC Accreditation, Medicare Approved, Utilization Review,
Pre-Admission Certification, State Licensure, Quality
Assurance Program

Key Personnel

President & CEO . . . . David M. Cordani

211 Coventry Health Care of Florida

1340 Concord Terrace
Sunrise, FL 33323
Toll-Free: 866-847-8235
chcflorida.coventryhealthcare.com
Subsidiary of: Aetna Inc.
For Profit Organization: Yes
Total Enrollment: 5,000,000
State Enrollment: 375,000

Healthplan and Services Defined

PLAN TYPE: HMO/PPO
Model Type: Network
Plan Specialty: Behavioral Health, Dental, Worker's
Compensation
Benefits Offered: Behavioral Health, Dental, Prescription,
Wellness, Worker's Compensation

Type of Coverage

Individual, Medicare, Medicaid

Type of Payment Plans Offered

POS

Geographic Areas Served

Greater Miami area, Greater Fort Lauderdale area, Boca
Raton, Boynton Beach, Clearwater, Gainesville, Ocala,
Pensacola, Port Saint Lucie, St. Petersburg, Tallahassee,
Tampa, Wellington, West Palm Beach

Accreditation Certification
URAC

Key Personnel
Chairman & CEO . . . . Mark T. Bertolini
President . . . . Karen S. Lynch
Chief Financial Officer . . . . Shawn M. Guertin
Operations & Technology . . . . Meg McCarthy
Chief Medical Officer . . . . Harold L. Paz
General Counsel . . . . Thomas Sabatino Jr.
Government Services . . . . Fran S. Soistman

212 Dimension Health

5881 NW 151st Street
Suite 201
Hialeah, FL 33014
Toll-Free: 800-483-4992
Phone: 305-823-7664
info@dimensionhealth.com
www.dimensionhealth.com
Year Founded: 1985
Number of Affiliated Hospitals: 51

Healthplan and Services Defined
PLAN TYPE: PPO
Model Type: Network
Benefits Offered: Disease Management, Wellness, Worker's
Compensation

Type of Coverage
Commercial

Type of Payment Plans Offered
POS, DFFS, Capitated, FFS, Combination FFS & DFFS

Network Qualifications
Pre-Admission Certification: Yes

Peer Review Type
Utilization Review: Yes
Second Surgical Opinion: Yes
Case Management: Yes

Publishes and Distributes Report Card: No

Key Personnel
President & CEO . . . . Charles A. Lindgren
VP, Network Development . . . . Creta Diehs
Office Manager . . . . Rosemary Osorio
rosorio@dimensionhealth.com

Average Claim Compensation
Physician's Fees Charged: 110%

Specialty Managed Care Partners
Enters into Contracts with Regional Business Coalitions: No

213 Florida Blue

PO Box 1798
Jacksonville, FL 32231-0014
Toll-Free: 877-352-5830
www.floridablue.com
Subsidiary of: Blue Cross and Blue Shield of Florida, Inc.
Non-Profit Organization: Yes
Year Founded: 1985

Owned by an Integrated Delivery Network (IDN): Yes

Healthplan and Services Defined
PLAN TYPE: HMO
Plan Specialty: Dental
Benefits Offered: Behavioral Health, Chiropractic,
Complementary Medicine, Dental, Disease Management,
Home Care, Inpatient SNF, Physical Therapy, Podiatry,
Prescription, Psychiatric, Transplant, Wellness, AD&D,
Life, Critical illness
Offers Demand Management Patient Information Service: Yes
DMPI Services Offered: Nurse Line 24x7x365, Health
Coaching, Support for Chronic Conditions, Health Risk
Assessments, Web Tools & Resources

Type of Coverage
Commercial, Individual, Indemnity, Medicare

Type of Payment Plans Offered
FFS

Geographic Areas Served
Statewide

Subscriber Information
Average Subscriber Co-Payment:
Primary Care Physician: Varies
Non-Network Physician: Varies
Prescription Drugs: Varies
Hospital ER: Varies
Home Health Care: Varies
Nursing Home: Varies

Network Qualifications
Pre-Admission Certification: Yes

Peer Review Type
Utilization Review: Yes

Publishes and Distributes Report Card: No

Accreditation Certification
Utilization Review

Key Personnel
CEO . . . . Patrick Geraghty
Chairman . . . . Steven T. Halverson
Chief Operating Officer . . . . Catherine P. Bessant

Specialty Managed Care Partners
Prime Therapeutics, LLC-PBM and Mental Health Network
(MHnet), Health Dialog, Accordant and Quest Diagnostics
Enters into Contracts with Regional Business Coalitions: Yes

Employer References
State of Florida, Gevity HR (formerly Staff Leasing), Publix,
Lincare, Miami Dade County

214 Florida Health Care Plans

1340 Ridgewood Avenue
Holly Hill, FL 32117
Toll-Free: 800-352-9824
Fax: 386-676-7119
www.fhcp.com
Subsidiary of: Blue Cross Blue Shield of Florida
Non-Profit Organization: Yes
Year Founded: 1974

Owned by an Integrated Delivery Network (IDN): Yes
Federally Qualified: Yes

Healthplan and Services Defined
  PLAN TYPE: HMO
  Benefits Offered: Behavioral Health, Chiropractic, Dental, Disease Management, Home Care, Inpatient SNF, Podiatry, Prescription, Psychiatric, Transplant, Vision, Wellness

Type of Coverage
  Commercial, Individual, Medicare, Supplemental Medicare
  Catastrophic Illness Benefit: Varies per case

Geographic Areas Served
  Volusia, Flagler, Brevard and Seminole counties

Publishes and Distributes Report Card: Yes

Accreditation Certification
  TJC, NCQA

Key Personnel
  President & CEO . . . . Wendy Myers, MD
  Chief Financial Officer. . . . . David Schandel
  Chief Medical Officer . . . . Joseph Zuckerman, MD
  Chief Information Officer . . . . Tim Moylan
  Compliance Officer . . . . Robert Gilliland
  Quality Management . . . . Joann Adams
  Legal Counsel . . . . Pamerla Thomas

Specialty Managed Care Partners
  Enters into Contracts with Regional Business Coalitions: Yes

215 Freedom Health

5403 N Church Avenue
Tampa, FL 33614
Toll-Free: 800-401-2740
Fax: 813-506-6150
www.freedomhealth.com
Mailing Address: P.O. Box 151137, Tampa, FL 33684
Physician Owned Organization: Yes

Healthplan and Services Defined
  PLAN TYPE: Medicare
  Benefits Offered: Prescription, Wellness

Type of Coverage
  Supplemental Medicare, Medicaid

Geographic Areas Served
  Brevard, Broward, Charlotte, Citrus, Collier, Hernando, Hillsborough, Indian River, Lake, Lee, Manatee, Marion, Martin, Miami-Dade, Orange, Osceola, Palm Beach, Pasco, Pinellas, Polk, Sarasota, Seminole, St. Lucie, Sumter and Volusia counties

Accreditation Certification
  NCQA

Key Personnel
  CEO . . . . Rupesh Shah

216 Health First Health Plans

6450 US Highway 1
Rockledge, FL 32955
Toll-Free: 800-716-7737
www.healthfirsthealthplans.org

Non-Profit Organization: Yes
Year Founded: 1995
Number of Affiliated Hospitals: 8
Number of Referral/Specialty Physicians: 3,000

Healthplan and Services Defined
  PLAN TYPE: Medicare
  Benefits Offered: Behavioral Health, Chiropractic, Disease Management, Home Care, Inpatient SNF, Long-Term Care, Physical Therapy, Podiatry, Prescription, Psychiatric, Transplant, Vision, Wellness

Type of Coverage
  Commercial, Medicare
  Catastrophic Illness Benefit: Covered

Type of Payment Plans Offered
  FFS

Geographic Areas Served
  Brevard and Indian River counties

Peer Review Type
  Utilization Review: Yes
  Second Surgical Opinion: Yes
  Case Management: Yes

Accreditation Certification
  NCQA

Key Personnel
  President & CEO. . . . . Steven P. Johnson
  Chief Strategy Officer . . . . Drew Rector
  Chief Physician Officer . . . . Jeffrey Stalnaker
  Chief Financial Officer . . . . Joe Felkner
  Chief Information Officer . . . . Alex Popowycz

Average Claim Compensation
  Physician's Fees Charged: 110%

Specialty Managed Care Partners
  SXC, Ameripharm

Employer References
  Boeing/McDonnell Douglas Corp., ITT, Computer Science Raytheon, Intersil Corp.

217 Health First Medicare Plans

6450 US Highway 1
Rockledge, FL 32955
Toll-Free: 800-716-7737
www.health-first.org/health_plans/medicare
Subsidiary of: Health First
Year Founded: 1997
Number of Referral/Specialty Physicians: 1,100

Healthplan and Services Defined
  PLAN TYPE: Medicare
  Other Type: HMO-POS

Type of Coverage
  Medicare

Geographic Areas Served
  Brevard and Indian River counties

Key Personnel
  President & CEO. . . . . Steven P. Johnson

Chief Strategy Officer . . . . Drew Rector
Chief Financial Officer . . . . Joe Felkner
Chief Physician Officer . . . . Jeffrey Stalnaker
Chief Information Officer . . . . Alex Popowycz

218 Healthchoice

55 W Gore Street
Orlando, FL 32801
Toll-Free: 800-635-4345
Phone: 407-481-7100
Fax: 407-481-7190
hcweb@orlandohealth.com
www.healthchoiceorlando.org
Subsidiary of: Orlando Health
For Profit Organization: Yes
Year Founded: 1984
Number of Affiliated Hospitals: 9

Healthplan and Services Defined
 PLAN TYPE: PPO
 Plan Specialty: Behavioral Health, Worker's Compensation,
  UR, Pediatrics
 Benefits Offered: Behavioral Health, Disease Management

Type of Coverage
 Commercial
 Catastrophic Illness Benefit: Varies per case

Type of Payment Plans Offered
 FFS

Geographic Areas Served
 Central Florida

Peer Review Type
 Utilization Review: Yes
 Second Surgical Opinion: Yes
 Case Management: Yes

Publishes and Distributes Report Card: Yes

Accreditation Certification
 AAAHC
 TJC Accreditation, Medicare Approved, Utilization Review,
  Pre-Admission Certification, State Licensure, Quality
  Assurance Program

Specialty Managed Care Partners
 Enters into Contracts with Regional Business Coalitions: Yes

219 HealthSun

3250 Mary Street
Suite 400
Coconut Grove, FL 33133
Phone: 305-234-9292
www.healthsun.com
Subsidiary of: Anthem, Inc.
Year Founded: 2005
Number of Affiliated Hospitals: 19

Healthplan and Services Defined
 PLAN TYPE: Medicare
 Benefits Offered: Prescription, Transportation Services

Type of Coverage
 Medicare

Geographic Areas Served
 Miami-Dade and Broward counties

Key Personnel
 Chief Executive Officer . . . . Ron Schutzen

220 HealthSun Health Plans

3250 Mary Street
Suite 400
Coconut Grove, FL 33133
Phone: 305-234-9292
Fax: 305-234-9275
www.health-sun.com
Year Founded: 2004

Healthplan and Services Defined
 PLAN TYPE: Medicare
 Other Type: HMO

Type of Coverage
 Medicare

Geographic Areas Served
 Miami-Dade and Broward counties

221 Humana Health Insurance Company of Florida, Inc.

Doral Concourse Building
8400 NW 36th Street, Suite 350
Doral, FL 33166
Toll-Free: 800-462-7587
Phone: 305-698-3100
Fax: 305-698-3169
www.humana.com
Secondary Address: Carollwood Center, 10037 N Dale Mabry
 Highway, Tampa, FL 33618, 813-463-4220
Subsidiary of: Humana
For Profit Organization: Yes
Year Founded: 1962

Healthplan and Services Defined
 PLAN TYPE: HMO/PPO
 Model Type: IPA
 Plan Specialty: Dental, Vision
 Benefits Offered: Dental, Disease Management, Prescription,
  Vision, Wellness, Life, LTD, STD

Type of Coverage
 Commercial, Individual

Type of Payment Plans Offered
 POS

Geographic Areas Served
 Statewide

Subscriber Information
 Average Annual Deductible Per Subscriber:
  Employee Only (Self): $0
  Medicare: $0
 Average Subscriber Co-Payment:
  Primary Care Physician: $10.00

Prescription Drugs: $7.00
Hospital ER: $25.00

Network Qualifications
Pre-Admission Certification: Yes

Peer Review Type
Utilization Review: Yes
Second Surgical Opinion: Yes
Case Management: Yes

Publishes and Distributes Report Card: Yes

Accreditation Certification
URAC, NCQA, CORE
TJC Accreditation, Medicare Approved, Utilization Review,
Pre-Admission Certification, State Licensure, Quality
Assurance Program

Key Personnel
President & CEO. . . . . Bruce Broussard
Chief Medical Officer. . . . . Roy A. Beveridge
Chief Consumer Officer. . . . . Jody L. Bilney
Human Resources. . . . . Tim Huval
Chief Financial Officer . . . . Brian Kane
Chief Information Officer . . . . Brian LeClaire
General Counsel. . . . . Christopher M. Todoroff
Chief Accounting Officer . . . . Cynthia H. Zipperie

Specialty Managed Care Partners
Enters into Contracts with Regional Business Coalitions: Yes

---

222 Leon Medical Centers Health Plan

8600 NW 41st Street
Suite 201
Doral, FL 33166
Toll-Free: 866-393-5366
Phone: 305-229-7461
membersupport@lmchealthplans.com
www.lmchealthplans.com
Subsidiary of: HealthSpring, Inc.
For Profit Organization: Yes
Year Founded: 1996
Number of Affiliated Hospitals: 5
Number of Primary Care Physicians: 1,200
Total Enrollment: 27,000

Healthplan and Services Defined
PLAN TYPE: HMO
Benefits Offered: Chiropractic, Dental, Inpatient SNF,
Podiatry, Prescription, Psychiatric, Vision, Wellness

Type of Coverage
Supplemental Medicare, Medicare Advantage

Geographic Areas Served
Miami-Dade County

Key Personnel
President/CEO. . . . . Henry Hernandez
henry.hernandez@lmchealthplans.com
Vice President, IT . . . . Jennifer Velasquez
jennifer.velasquez@lmchealthplans.com
COO . . . . Guillermo Gurdian
guillermo.gurdian@lmchealthplans.com

VP, Claims . . . . Luis Fernandez
luis.fernandez@lmchealthplans.com
Director of Finance . . . . Mercy Kirkpatrick
mercy.kirpatrick@lmchealthplans.com
Medical Director . . . . Alina Campos, MD
alina.campos@lmchealthplans.com

---

223 Liberty Dental Plan of Florida

PO Box 15149
Tampa, FL 33684-5149
Toll-Free: 888-352-7924
Fax: 888-334-6034
www.libertydentalplan.com
For Profit Organization: Yes
Total Enrollment: 2,000,000

Healthplan and Services Defined
PLAN TYPE: Dental
Other Type: Dental HMO
Plan Specialty: Dental
Benefits Offered: Dental

Type of Coverage
Commercial, Medicare, Medicaid, Unions

Geographic Areas Served
Statewide

Accreditation Certification
NCQA

Key Personnel
President & CEO. . . . . Amir Neshat
Executive Vice President . . . . John Carvelli
Chief Financial Officer . . . . Maja Kapic
General Counsel . . . . Lisa Wright
Chief Dental Officer. . . . . Richard Goren
Chief Operating Officer . . . . Nico Alvarez
Dental Director . . . . Richard Hague

---

224 Magellan Complete Care of Florida

4800 North Scottdale Road
Suite 4400
Scottsdale, AZ 85251
Toll-Free: 800-327-8613
www.magellancompletecareoffl.com
For Profit Organization: Yes

Healthplan and Services Defined
PLAN TYPE: Other
Benefits Offered: Psychiatric

Type of Coverage
Medicaid, Specialty plan for individuals with

Geographic Areas Served
Statewide

Key Personnel
Chairman & CEO. . . . . Barry M. Smith
Chief Financial Officer . . . . Jonathan N. Rubin
General Counsel . . . . Daniel N. Gregoire
Human Resources. . . . . Caskie Lewis-Clapper
Chief Medical Officer . . . . Karen Amstutz
Chief Information Officer . . . . Srini Koushik

225   Molina Healthcare of Florida

8300 NW 33rd Street
Suite 400
Miami, FL 33122
Toll-Free: 866-422-2541
www.molinahealthcare.com
Subsidiary of: Molina Healthcare, Inc.
For Profit Organization: Yes

Healthplan and Services Defined
    PLAN TYPE: Medicare
    Model Type: Network
    Plan Specialty: Dental, PBM, Vision, Integrated
        Medicare/Medicaid (Duals)
    Benefits Offered: Dental, Prescription, Vision, Wellness, Life

Type of Coverage
    Individual, Medicare, Supplemental Medicare, Medicaid

Geographic Areas Served
    Statewide

Key Personnel
    Chief Executive Officer . . . . Joseph W. White
    Chief Operating Officer . . . . Terry Bayer
    General Counsel. . . . . Jeff D. Barlow
    SVP, Relations/Marketing . . . . Juan Jos, Orellana
    Chief Information Officer . . . . Rick Hopfer

226   Neighborhood Health Partnership

7600 Corporate Center Drive
Miami, FL 33126
Toll-Free: 877-972-8845
www.neighborhood-health.com
Subsidiary of: UnitedHealthcare
For Profit Organization: Yes
Year Founded: 1993
Number of Primary Care Physicians: 1,282
Total Enrollment: 108,000
State Enrollment: 141,178

Healthplan and Services Defined
    PLAN TYPE: HMO
    Other Type: POS
    Plan Specialty: Behavioral Health, Chiropractic
    Benefits Offered: Disease Management, Home Care,
        Transplant, Durable Medical Equipment

Type of Coverage
    Commercial, Medicare

Type of Payment Plans Offered
    Capitated

Geographic Areas Served
    Orange, Seminole, Osceola, Flagler, Lake, Volusia,
    Hillsborough, Pasco, Pinellas, Sarasota, Polk, Hernando, and
    Lee counties

Peer Review Type
    Utilization Review: Yes

Publishes and Distributes Report Card: Yes

Accreditation Certification
    NCQA

Key Personnel
    President & CEO . . . . David Wichmann
    Chief Operating Officer . . . . Dan Schumacher
    Chief Strategy Officer . . . . John Cosgriff
    Communications Officer . . . . Kirsten Gorsuch
    Chief Medical Officer. . . . . Sam Ho
    Chief Legal Officer . . . . Thad Johnson
    Chief Information Officer . . . . Phil McKoy

227   One Call Care Management

841 Prudential Drive
Suite 900
Jacksonville, FL 32207
Toll-Free: 800-848-1989
www.onecallcm.com
Secondary Address: 8501 Fallbrook Avenue, West Hills, CA
91304
For Profit Organization: Yes
Year Founded: 1993

Healthplan and Services Defined
    PLAN TYPE: Other
    Plan Specialty: Worker's Compensation
    Benefits Offered: Worker's Compensation

Type of Payment Plans Offered
    POS, DFFS, FFS, Combination FFS & DFFS

Geographic Areas Served
    Nationwide

Network Qualifications
    Pre-Admission Certification: Yes

Publishes and Distributes Report Card: No

Accreditation Certification
    Utilization Review, Quality Assurance Program

Key Personnel
    President & CEO. . . . . Dale Wolf
    Chief Financial Officer . . . . Rick McCook
    Chief Operating Officer . . . . Chris Watson
    Sales & Marketing Officer. . . . . Robert Zeccardi
    Chief Product Officer. Will Smith
    Chief Strategy Officer. . . . . Pat Rowland

Specialty Managed Care Partners
    Enters into Contracts with Regional Business Coalitions: No

228   Preferred Care Partners

9100 South Dadeland Boulevard
Suite 1250
Miami, FL 33156
Toll-Free: 866-231-7201
Fax: 888-659-0618
MemberServices@uhcsouthflorida.com
www.mypreferredcare.com
Mailing Address: P.O. Box 56-5748, Miami, FL 33256
Number of Affiliated Hospitals: 27
Number of Primary Care Physicians: 1,500
Total Enrollment: 45,000

Healthplan and Services Defined
    PLAN TYPE: Multiple

Benefits Offered: Dental, Prescription, Vision, Hearing,
Transportation, Fitness Programs

Type of Coverage
Supplemental Medicare

Geographic Areas Served
Miami-Dade, Broward, and Palm Beach counties

Accreditation Certification
URAC

Key Personnel
President. . . . . Justo Luis Pozo
CEO . . . . Joseph L Caruncho
COO. . . . . Annette Onorati

---

229   Trinity Health of Florida

BayCare Health System
2985 Drew Street
Clearwater, FL 33759
Toll-Free: 800-229-2273
www.trinity-health.org
Secondary Address: Holy Cross Hospital, 4725 N Federal
Highway, Fort Lauderdale, FL 33308
Subsidiary of: Trinity Health
Non-Profit Organization: Yes
Year Founded: 2013
Total Enrollment: 30,000,000

Healthplan and Services Defined
PLAN TYPE: Other
Benefits Offered: Disease Management, Home Care,
Long-Term Care, Psychiatric, Hospice programs, PACE
(Program of All Inclusive Care for the Elderly)

Geographic Areas Served
South Florida

Key Personnel
Chief Executive Officer . . . . Richard J. Gilfillan
Chief Financial Officer. . . . . Benjamin R. Carter
Human Resources. . . . . Edmund F. Hodge
General Counsel . . . . Paul G. Neumann
Chief Clinical Officer. . . . . Daniel J. Roth
Chief Operating Officer . . . . Michael A. Slubowski

---

230   United Concordia of Florida

3501 E Frontage Road
Tampa, FL 33607
Phone: 813-313-4464
www.unitedconcordia.com
For Profit Organization: Yes
Year Founded: 1971
Total Enrollment: 7,800,000

Healthplan and Services Defined
PLAN TYPE: Dental
Plan Specialty: Dental
Benefits Offered: Dental

Type of Coverage
Commercial, Individual, Military personnel & families

Geographic Areas Served
Nationwide

Accreditation Certification
URAC

Key Personnel
President & COO . . . . Timothy J. Constantine
Contact. . . . . Beth Rutherford
717-260-7659
beth.rutherford@ucci.com

---

231   UnitedHealthcare of Florida

10151 Deerwood Park
Building 100, Suite 420
Jacksonville, FL 32256
Toll-Free: 800-250-6178
www.uhc.com/contact-us/florida
Secondary Address: 495 North Keller Road, Maitland, FL
32751, 800-899-6500
Subsidiary of: UnitedHealth Group
For Profit Organization: Yes
Owned by an Integrated Delivery Network (IDN): Yes

Healthplan and Services Defined
PLAN TYPE: HMO/PPO
Model Type: Network
Plan Specialty: Behavioral Health, Dental, Disease
Management, PBM, Vision
Benefits Offered: Behavioral Health, Chiropractic, Dental,
Disease Management, Home Care, Inpatient SNF, Physical
Therapy, Podiatry, Prescription, Psychiatric, Transplant,
Vision, Wellness, AD&D, Life, LTD, STD

Type of Coverage
Commercial, Individual, Medicare, Supplemental Medicare,
Medicaid, Catastrophic, Family, Military, Veterans, Group,

Geographic Areas Served
Statewide

Subscriber Information
Average Monthly Fee Per Subscriber
(Employee + Employer Contribution):
Employee Only (Self): Varies

Peer Review Type
Case Management: Yes

Accreditation Certification
TJC, NCQA

Key Personnel
President . . . . David Wichmann
Chief Operating Officer . . . . Dan Schumacher
Chief Strategy Officer . . . . John Cosgriff
Communications Officer . . . . Kirsten Gorsuch
Chief Medical Officer. . . . . Sam Ho
Chief Legal Officer . . . . Thad Johnson
Chief Information Officer . . . . Phil McKoy
Chief Financial Officer. . . . . Jeff Putnam

Specialty Managed Care Partners
Own Network
Enters into Contracts with Regional Business Coalitions: Yes

232 UnitedHealthcare of South Florida

3100 SW 145th Avenue
Miramar, FL 33027
Toll-Free: 800-310-7622
www.uhc.com/contact-us/florida
Subsidiary of: UnitedHealth Group
For Profit Organization: Yes
Year Founded: 1970

Healthplan and Services Defined
  PLAN TYPE: HMO/PPO
  Model Type: Network
  Plan Specialty: ASO, Behavioral Health, Chiropractic,
    Dental, Disease Management, PBM, Vision
  Benefits Offered: Behavioral Health, Chiropractic,
    Complementary Medicine, Dental, Disease Management,
    Long-Term Care, Physical Therapy, Podiatry, Prescription,
    Psychiatric, Vision, Wellness, AD&D, Life, LTD, STD

Type of Coverage
  Commercial, Individual, Medicare, Supplemental Medicare,
    Medicaid, Catastrophic, Family, Military, Veterans, Group,
  Catastrophic Illness Benefit: Varies per case

Type of Payment Plans Offered
  POS, DFFS, Capitated, FFS, Combination FFS & DFFS

Geographic Areas Served
  Palm Beach, Broward & Dade counties

Subscriber Information
  Average Subscriber Co-Payment:
      Primary Care Physician: $5.00-15.00
      Non-Network Physician: Varies
      Prescription Drugs: $5.00-10.00
      Hospital ER: $100.00

Network Qualifications
  Pre-Admission Certification: Yes

Peer Review Type
  Utilization Review: Yes
  Second Surgical Opinion: Yes
  Case Management: Yes

Publishes and Distributes Report Card: Yes

Accreditation Certification
  AAAHC, URAC, NCQA
  TJC Accreditation, Medicare Approved, Utilization Review,
    Pre-Admission Certification, State Licensure, Quality
    Assurance Program

Key Personnel
  President . . . . David Wichmann
  Chief Operating Officer . . . . Dan Schumacher
  Chief Strategy Officer . . . . John Cosgriff
  Communications Officer . . . . Kirsten Gorsuch
  Chief Medical Officer. . . . . Sam Ho
  Chief Legal Officer . . . . Thad Johnson
  Chief Information Officer . . . . Phil McKoy
  Chief Financial Officer. . . . . Jeff Putnam

Specialty Managed Care Partners
  Enters into Contracts with Regional Business Coalitions: No

233 WellCare Health Plans

8735 Henderson Road
Tampa, FL 33634
Toll-Free: 866-334-7927
www.wellcare.com
For Profit Organization: Yes
Total Enrollment: 3,700,000

Healthplan and Services Defined
  PLAN TYPE: Medicare
  Model Type: Network
  Plan Specialty: Dental, PBM, Vision, Integrated
    Medicare/Medicaid (Duals)
  Benefits Offered: Dental, Prescription, Vision, Wellness, Life

Type of Coverage
  Individual, Medicare, Supplemental Medicare, Medicaid

Geographic Areas Served
  Nationwide

Accreditation Certification
  URAC

Key Personnel
  Chief Executive Officer . . . . Ken Burdick
  Chief Financial Officer. Drew Asher
  Chief Information Officer. . . . . Darren Ghanayem
  General Counsel. . . . . Anat Hakim
  Chief Medical Officer . . . . Mark Lennay

Health Insurance Coverage Status and Type of Coverage by Age

Category	All Persons		Under 18 years		Under 65 years	
	Number	%	Number	%	Number	%
Total population	10,121	-	2,661	-	8,790	-
Covered by some type of health insurance	8,811 *(30)*	87.1 *(0.3)*	2,482 *(14)*	93.3 *(0.5)*	7,494 *(29)*	85.2 *(0.3)*
Covered by private health insurance	6,710 *(40)*	66.3 *(0.4)*	1,488 *(21)*	55.9 *(0.8)*	5,920 *(35)*	67.3 *(0.4)*
Employer-based	5,338 *(42)*	52.7 *(0.4)*	1,240 *(22)*	46.6 *(0.8)*	4,900 *(39)*	55.7 *(0.4)*
Direct purchase	1,369 *(28)*	13.5 *(0.3)*	196 *(12)*	7.3 *(0.4)*	978 *(25)*	11.1 *(0.3)*
TRICARE	410 *(15)*	4.0 *(0.1)*	104 *(7)*	3.9 *(0.3)*	305 *(15)*	3.5 *(0.2)*
Covered by public health insurance	3,170 *(31)*	31.3 *(0.3)*	1,086 *(22)*	40.8 *(0.8)*	1,896 *(30)*	21.6 *(0.3)*
Medicaid	1,818 *(31)*	18.0 *(0.3)*	1,061 *(22)*	39.9 *(0.8)*	1,621 *(30)*	18.4 *(0.3)*
Medicare	1,557 *(11)*	15.4 *(0.1)*	29 *(5)*	1.1 *(0.2)*	285 *(10)*	3.2 *(0.1)*
VA Care	256 *(8)*	2.5 *(0.1)*	7 *(2)*	0.3 *(0.1)*	145 *(7)*	1.7 *(0.1)*
Not covered at any time during the year	1,310 *(30)*	12.9 *(0.3)*	179 *(13)*	6.7 *(0.5)*	1,297 *(30)*	14.8 *(0.3)*

Note: Numbers in thousands; Figures cover civilian noninstitutionalized population in 2016; N/A indicates that data was not available; Z represents or rounds to zero; Margin of error appears in parenthesis and is calculated using replicate weights.
Source: U.S. Census Bureau, American Community Survey, Table HIC-4_ACS. Health Insurance Coverage Status and Type of Coverage by State—All People: 2008 to 2016, Table HIC-5_ACS. Health Insurance Coverage Status and Type of Coverage by State—Children Under 18: 2008 to 2016, Table HIC-6_ACS. Health Insurance Coverage Status and Type of Coverage by State—Persons Under 65: 2008 to 2016

Georgia

234 Aetna Health of Georgia
151 Farmington Avenue
Hartford, CT 06156
Toll-Free: 800-872-3862
Phone: 860-273-0123
www.aetna.com
Subsidiary of: Aetna Inc.
For Profit Organization: Yes

Healthplan and Services Defined
PLAN TYPE: HMO/PPO
Other Type: POS
Model Type: Network
Plan Specialty: Behavioral Health, Dental, EPO, Lab, PBM, Vision, Radiology
Benefits Offered: Behavioral Health, Dental, Disease Management, Long-Term Care, Physical Therapy, Podiatry, Prescription, Psychiatric, Vision, Wellness, Life, LTD, STD

Type of Coverage
Commercial, Medicare, Supplemental Medicare, Medicaid, Catastrophic, Student health

Geographic Areas Served
Statewide

Key Personnel
CEO . . . . Mark Bertolini

235 Alliant Health Plans
1503 N Tibbs Road
Dalton, GA 30720
Toll-Free: 800-811-4793
Phone: 706-629-3744
Fax: 706-671-2873
information@alliantplans.com
www.alliantplans.com
Non-Profit Organization: Yes
Year Founded: 1998
Physician Owned Organization: Yes
Number of Affiliated Hospitals: 9,999
Number of Primary Care Physicians: 500,000
Total Enrollment: 15,000
State Enrollment: 15,000

Healthplan and Services Defined
PLAN TYPE: HMO/PPO
Model Type: PSHCC

Type of Coverage
Commercial, Individual

Geographic Areas Served
Statewide

Key Personnel
Chief Executive Officer . . . . Mark Mixer
Chief Operating Officer . . . . Amanda Reed
Chief Financial Officer . . . . Joe Caldwell

236 Amerigroup Georgia
303 Perimeter Center North
Suite 400
Atlanta, GA 30346
Toll-Free: 800-600-4441
GAmembers@amerigroup.com
www.myamerigroup.com/ga
Subsidiary of: Anthem, Inc.
For Profit Organization: Yes
Year Founded: 2006

Healthplan and Services Defined
PLAN TYPE: HMO
Benefits Offered: Prescription

Type of Coverage
Medicaid, PeachCare for Kids, Planning for He

Accreditation Certification
NCQA

237 Anthem Blue Cross & Blue Shield of Georgia
3350 Peachtree Road
Atlanta, GA 30326
Toll-Free: 866-755-2680
Phone: 404-842-8000
www.anthem.com
For Profit Organization: Yes

Healthplan and Services Defined
PLAN TYPE: HMO/PPO
Model Type: Network
Plan Specialty: ASO, Behavioral Health, Chiropractic, Dental, Disease Management, Lab, PBM, Vision, Radiology, Worker's Compensation, UR
Benefits Offered: Behavioral Health, Chiropractic, Dental, Disease Management, Home Care, Inpatient SNF, Physical Therapy, Podiatry, Prescription, Psychiatric, Transplant, Vision, Wellness, Worker's Compensation, Life

Type of Coverage
Commercial, Individual, Medicare, Supplemental Medicare, Medicaid, Catastrophic

Geographic Areas Served
Statewide

Accreditation Certification
URAC, NCQA

Key Personnel
President & CEO . . . . Scott P. Serota
Chief Financial Officer . . . . Robert Kolodgy
Human Resources . . . . Maureen A. Cahill
Chief Medical Officer. . . . . Trent Haywood
General Counsel. . . . . Scott Nehs

238 Blue Cross Blue Shield of Georgia
3350 Peachtree Road
Atlanta, GA 30326
Phone: 404-842-8000
www.anthem.com
Secondary Address: 6087 Technology Parkway, Suite 2000, Columbus, GA 31907, 706-286-8470

Subsidiary of: Anthem, Inc.

Healthplan and Services Defined
PLAN TYPE: HMO/PPO
Model Type: Network
Plan Specialty: Behavioral Health, Dental, Disease
   Management, Lab, PBM, Vision, Radiology
Benefits Offered: Behavioral Health, Dental, Disease
   Management, Inpatient SNF, Physical Therapy,
   Prescription, Psychiatric, Transplant, Vision, Wellness, Life

Type of Coverage
Commercial, Individual, Medicare, Supplemental Medicare,
   Catastrophic

Geographic Areas Served
Statewide

Accreditation Certification
URAC

Key Personnel
President & CEO . . . . Scott P. Serota
Chief Financial Officer . . . . Robert Kolodgy
Human Resources . . . . Maureen A. Cahill
Chief Medical Officer. . . . . Trent Haywood
General Counsel. . . . . Scott Nehs

239   CompBenefits Corporation
100 Mansell Court East
Suite 400
Roswell, GA 30076
Toll-Free: 800-295-6279
Phone: 404-365-0074
Fax: 404-233-2366
www.compbenefits.com
Subsidiary of: Humana
Year Founded: 1978
Owned by an Integrated Delivery Network (IDN): Yes

Healthplan and Services Defined
PLAN TYPE: HMO/PPO
Model Type: Network, HMO, PPO, POS, TPA
Plan Specialty: ASO, Dental, Vision
Benefits Offered: Dental, Vision

Type of Coverage
Commercial, Individual

Type of Payment Plans Offered
DFFS, Capitated, FFS

Publishes and Distributes Report Card: Yes

Key Personnel
President & CEO . . . . Bruce D. Broussard
Chief Medical Officer. . . . . Roy A. Beveridge
Chief Consumer Officer. . . . . Jody L. Bilney
Human Resources. . . . . Tim Huval
Chief Financial Officer . . . . Brian Kane
Chief Information Officer . . . . Brian LeClaire
General Counsel . . . . Christopher M. Todoroff

Specialty Managed Care Partners
Enters into Contracts with Regional Business Coalitions: Yes

Employer References
Royal Caribbean Cruise Line, Tupperware

240   Coventry Health Care of Georgia
1100 Circle 75 Parkway
Suite 1400
Atlanta, GA 30339
Phone: 678-202-2100
chcgeorgia.coventryhealthcare.com
Subsidiary of: Aetna Inc.
For Profit Organization: Yes
Year Founded: 1994
Number of Affiliated Hospitals: 111
Number of Primary Care Physicians: 31,000
Total Enrollment: 5,000,000
State Enrollment: 200,000

Healthplan and Services Defined
PLAN TYPE: HMO/PPO
Other Type: POS
Model Type: Network
Plan Specialty: Behavioral Health, Dental, Worker's
   Compensation
Benefits Offered: Behavioral Health, Dental, Prescription,
   Wellness, Worker's Compensation

Type of Coverage
Commercial, Individual, Medicare, Supplemental Medicare,
   Medicaid

Type of Payment Plans Offered
POS

Geographic Areas Served
Serves more than 100 counties in Georgia including Greater
   Atlanta, Augusta, Brunswick, Columbia, Columbus, Macon,
   Savannah and Valdosta

Publishes and Distributes Report Card: Yes

Accreditation Certification
AAAHC, URAC

Key Personnel
Chairman & CEO . . . . Mark T. Bertolini
President. . . . . Karen S. Lynch
Chief Financial Officer . . . . Shawn M. Guertin
Operations & Technology . . . . Meg McCarthy
Chief Medical Officer . . . . Harold L. Paz
General Counsel. Thomas Sabatino
Government Services . . . . Fran S. Soistman

Specialty Managed Care Partners
Enters into Contracts with Regional Business Coalitions: Yes

241   Delta Dental Insurance Company
1130 Sanctuary Parkway
Suite 600
Alpharetta, GA 30009
Toll-Free: 800-521-2651
www.deltadentalins.com
Non-Profit Organization: Yes

Healthplan and Services Defined
PLAN TYPE: Dental

Plan Specialty: Dental
Benefits Offered: Dental

Type of Coverage
Commercial, Individual

Type of Payment Plans Offered
POS, DFFS, FFS

Geographic Areas Served
Alabama, Florida, Georgia, Louisiana, Mississippi, Montana, Nevada, Texas and Utah

Key Personnel
President & CEO . . . . Tony Barth
Chief Financial Officer . . . . Michael Castro
Chief Operating Officer . . . . Nilesh Patel
Chief Legal Officer . . . . Michael Hankinson
Sales & Marketing Officer. . . . . Belinda Martinez
EVP & Chief Sales & Mktg. . . . . Belinda Martinez

242　Humana Employers Health Plan of Georgia, Inc.

1200 Ashwood Parkway
Suite 180
Atlanta, GA 30338
Toll-Free: 800-986-9527
Phone: 770-508-2388
Fax: 770-391-1423
www.humana.com
Subsidiary of: Humana
For Profit Organization: Yes
Year Founded: 1961

Healthplan and Services Defined
PLAN TYPE: HMO/PPO
Model Type: Network
Plan Specialty: Dental, Vision
Benefits Offered: Behavioral Health, Chiropractic, Dental, Disease Management, Prescription, Psychiatric, Transplant, Vision, Wellness, Worker's Compensation, Life, LTD, STD

Type of Coverage
Commercial, Individual, Medicare, Supplemental Medicare

Geographic Areas Served
Statewide

Accreditation Certification
URAC, NCQA, CORE

Key Personnel
President & CEO. . . . . Bruce Broussard
Chief Medical Officer. . . . . Roy A. Beveridge
Chief Consumer Officer. . . . . Jody L. Bilney
Human Resources. . . . . Tim Huval
Chief Financial Officer . . . . Brian Kane
Chief Information Officer . . . . Brian LeClaire
General Counsel . . . . Christopher M. Todoroff
Chief Accounting Officer . . . . Cynthia H. Zipperie

243　Kaiser Permanente Georgia

2525 Cumberland Parkway SE
Atlanta, GA 30305
Toll-Free: 800-611-1811
Phone: 404-365-0966
thrive.kaiserpermanente.org/care-near-georgia
Subsidiary of: Kaiser Permanente
Non-Profit Organization: Yes
Year Founded: 1985
Number of Primary Care Physicians: 450
State Enrollment: 269,962

Healthplan and Services Defined
PLAN TYPE: HMO
Model Type: Network
Benefits Offered: Disease Management, Prescription, Vision, Wellness

Type of Coverage
Commercial, Individual, Medicare, Supplemental Medicare, Medicaid

Geographic Areas Served
Atlanta, Athens

Key Personnel
Chief Medical Director . . . . Edward M. Ellison
Executive Director/CEO . . . . Richard S. Isaacs
Chief Operating Officer . . . . Chris Grant

244　Northeast Georgia Health Partners

465 EE Butler Parkway
Gainesville, GA 30501
Phone: 770-219-6600
Fax: 770-219-6609
www.healthpartnersnetwork.com
Non-Profit Organization: Yes
Number of Affiliated Hospitals: 6
Number of Primary Care Physicians: 750
Number of Referral/Specialty Physicians: 75

Healthplan and Services Defined
PLAN TYPE: PPO
Benefits Offered: Behavioral Health, Home Care, Physical Therapy, Podiatry, Prescription, Psychiatric, Wellness, Labs; Occupational & Speech Therapy; Durable Medical Equipment; Hearing Center

Type of Coverage
Commercial

Geographic Areas Served
Banks, Barrow, Dawson, Forsyth, Gwinnett (City of Buford only), Habersham, Hall, Jackson, Lumpkin, Rabun, Stephens, Towns, Union and White counties

Accreditation Certification
NCQA

Key Personnel
Vice President. . . . . Steven McNeilly
Executive Director . . . . Wanda Katich
Operations Manager . . . . Kathryn Riner
Project Manager . . . . Jennifer Nicholson

245 Secure Health PPO Newtork

577 Mulberry Street
Suite 1000
Macon, GA 31201
Toll-Free: 800-648-7563
Phone: 478-314-2400
www.shpg.com
Mailing Address: P.O. Box 4088, Macon, GA 31028
For Profit Organization: Yes
Year Founded: 1992
Physician Owned Organization: Yes
Number of Affiliated Hospitals: 16
Number of Primary Care Physicians: 950
Total Enrollment: 68,000
State Enrollment: 68,000

Healthplan and Services Defined
PLAN TYPE: PPO
Other Type: TPA
Benefits Offered: Disease Management, Prescription,
Wellness, EAP

Type of Coverage
Commercial

Geographic Areas Served
Statewide

Peer Review Type
Utilization Review: Yes
Case Management: Yes

Accreditation Certification
URAC

Key Personnel
President/CEO . . . . Albert Ertel
VP Business Development . . . . Steven M. Clement

246 Trinity Health of Georgia

Saint Mary's Health Care System
1230 Baxter Street
Athens, GA 30606
Phone: 706-389-3000
www.trinity-health.org
Subsidiary of: Trinity Health
Non-Profit Organization: Yes
Year Founded: 2013
Total Enrollment: 30,000,000

Healthplan and Services Defined
PLAN TYPE: Other
Benefits Offered: Disease Management, Home Care,
Long-Term Care, Psychiatric, Hospice programs, PACE
(Program of All Inclusive Care for the Elderly)

Geographic Areas Served
Atlanta and Southeast Georgia

Key Personnel
Chief Executive Officer . . . . Richard J. Gilfillan
Chief Financial Officer. . . . . Benjamin R. Carter
Human Resources. . . . . Edmund F. Hodge
General Counsel . . . . Paul G. Neumann
Chief Clinical Officer. . . . . Daniel J. Roth

Chief Operating Officer . . . . Michael A. Slubowski

247 United Concordia of Georgia

9635 Ventana Way
Suite 100
Alpharetta, GA 30022
Phone: 678-893-8650
www.unitedconcordia.com
For Profit Organization: Yes
Year Founded: 1971
Total Enrollment: 7,800,000

Healthplan and Services Defined
PLAN TYPE: Dental
Plan Specialty: Dental
Benefits Offered: Dental

Type of Coverage
Commercial, Individual, Military personnel & families

Geographic Areas Served
Nationwide

Accreditation Certification
URAC

Key Personnel
President & COO . . . . Timothy J. Constantine
Contact. . . . . Beth Rutherford
717-260-7659
beth.rutherford@ucci.com

248 UnitedHealthcare of Georgia

3720 Davinci Court
Suite 300
Norcross, GA 30092
Phone: 770-300-3501
www.uhc.com/contact-us/georgia
Subsidiary of: UnitedHealth Group
For Profit Organization: Yes
Year Founded: 1980

Healthplan and Services Defined
PLAN TYPE: HMO/PPO
Model Type: Network
Plan Specialty: Behavioral Health, Dental, Disease
Management, PBM, Vision
Benefits Offered: Behavioral Health, Dental, Disease
Management, Long-Term Care, Physical Therapy,
Prescription, Vision, Wellness, Life, LTD, STD

Type of Coverage
Individual, Medicare, Supplemental Medicare, Medicaid,
Catastrophic, Family, Military, Veterans, Group,
Catastrophic Illness Benefit: Unlimited

Type of Payment Plans Offered
POS, FFS

Geographic Areas Served
Statewide

Network Qualifications
Pre-Admission Certification: Yes

Peer Review Type
Utilization Review: Yes
Case Management: Yes

Publishes and Distributes Report Card: Yes

Accreditation Certification
NCQA
TJC Accreditation, Medicare Approved, Utilization Review,
Pre-Admission Certification, State Licensure, Quality
Assurance Program

Key Personnel
President . . . . David Wichmann
Chief Operating Officer . . . . Dan Schumacher
Chief Strategy Officer . . . . John Cosgriff
Communications Officer . . . . Kirsten Gorsuch
Chief Medical Officer. . . . . Sam Ho
Chief Legal Officer . . . . Thad Johnson
Chief Information Officer . . . . Phil McKoy
Chief Financial Officer. . . . . Jeff Putnam

Specialty Managed Care Partners
Enters into Contracts with Regional Business Coalitions: Yes

HMO/PPO DIRECTORY
HAWAII

Health Insurance Coverage Status and Type of Coverage by Age

Category	All Persons		Under 18 years		Under 65 years	
	Number	%	Number	%	Number	%
Total population	1,379	-	323	-	1,140	-
Covered by some type of health insurance	1,330 *(6)*	96.5 *(0.4)*	315 *(3)*	97.5 *(0.7)*	1,092 *(6)*	95.8 *(0.5)*
Covered by private health insurance	1,065 *(10)*	77.2 *(0.7)*	229 *(5)*	70.9 *(1.6)*	898 *(10)*	78.8 *(0.9)*
Employer-based	879 *(12)*	63.8 *(0.9)*	179 *(6)*	55.6 *(1.9)*	755 *(12)*	66.2 *(1.0)*
Direct purchase	169 *(8)*	12.2 *(0.6)*	25 *(3)*	7.7 *(0.8)*	111 *(7)*	9.7 *(0.6)*
TRICARE	125 *(7)*	9.1 *(0.5)*	45 *(4)*	13.9 *(1.2)*	105 *(7)*	9.2 *(0.6)*
Covered by public health insurance	469 *(10)*	34.1 *(0.7)*	101 *(5)*	31.4 *(1.6)*	244 *(9)*	21.4 *(0.8)*
Medicaid	244 *(10)*	17.7 *(0.7)*	100 *(5)*	31.1 *(1.6)*	215 *(9)*	18.8 *(0.8)*
Medicare	247 *(3)*	17.9 *(0.3)*	1 *(Z)*	0.2 *(0.1)*	22 *(2)*	1.9 *(0.2)*
VA Care	34 *(3)*	2.5 *(0.2)*	1 *(1)*	0.2 *(0.2)*	18 *(2)*	1.6 *(0.2)*
Not covered at any time during the year	49 *(5)*	3.5 *(0.4)*	8 *(2)*	2.5 *(0.7)*	48 *(5)*	4.2 *(0.5)*

Note: Numbers in thousands; Figures cover civilian noninstitutionalized population in 2016; N/A indicates that data was not available; Z represents or rounds to zero; Margin of error appears in parenthesis and is calculated using replicate weights.
Source: U.S. Census Bureau, American Community Survey, Table HIC-4_ACS. Health Insurance Coverage Status and Type of Coverage by State—All People: 2008 to 2016, Table HIC-5_ACS. Health Insurance Coverage Status and Type of Coverage by State—Children Under 18: 2008 to 2016, Table HIC-6_ACS. Health Insurance Coverage Status and Type of Coverage by State—Persons Under 65: 2008 to 2016

Hawaii

249 Aetna Health of Hawaii
151 Farmington Avenue
Hartford, CT 06156
Toll-Free: 800-872-3862
Phone: 860-273-0123
www.aetna.com
Subsidiary of: Aetna Inc.
For Profit Organization: Yes

Healthplan and Services Defined
PLAN TYPE: PPO
Other Type: POS
Model Type: Network
Plan Specialty: Behavioral Health, EPO, Lab, PBM,
   Radiology
Benefits Offered: Behavioral Health, Dental, Disease
   Management, Long-Term Care, Physical Therapy,
   Podiatry, Prescription, Psychiatric, Vision, Wellness, Life,
   LTD, STD

Type of Coverage
Commercial, Catastrophic, Student health

Geographic Areas Served
Statewide

Key Personnel
CEO . . . . Mark Bertolini

250 AlohaCare
1357 Kapiolani Boulevard
Suite 1250
Honolulu, HI 96814
Toll-Free: 866-973-7418
Phone: 808-973-1657
Fax: 877-316-6376
www.alohacare.org
Secondary Address: 210 Imi Kala Street, Suite 206, Wailuku,
   HI 96793
Non-Profit Organization: Yes
Year Founded: 1994
Number of Primary Care Physicians: 2,200
Total Enrollment: 70,000

Healthplan and Services Defined
PLAN TYPE: HMO
Benefits Offered: Dental, Prescription, Vision, Wellness,
   Hearing; X-rays & Labs; Acupuncture; 24-hour Nurse
   Advice Line

Type of Coverage
Medicare, Supplemental Medicare

Geographic Areas Served
Oahu, Kauai, Molokai, Lanai, Maui, Hawaii

Peer Review Type
Case Management: Yes

Publishes and Distributes Report Card: Yes

Key Personnel
Chairman . . . . Richard Bettini

Vice Chair . . . . Emmanuel Kintu
Treasurer . . . . Richard Taaffe
Secretary . . . . David Derauf

251 AlohaCare Advantage Plus
1357 Kapiolani Boulevard
Suite 1250
Honolulu, HI 96814
Toll-Free: 866-973-6395
Phone: 808-973-1657
www.alohacare.org
Non-Profit Organization: Yes
Year Founded: 1994

Healthplan and Services Defined
PLAN TYPE: Medicare
Other Type: HMO SNP
Benefits Offered: Prescription

Type of Coverage
Medicare, Part A, B, and D

Geographic Areas Served
Oahu, Kauai, Molokai, Lanai, Maui, Hawaii

Key Personnel
Chairman . . . . Richard Bettini
Vice Chair . . . . Emmanuel Kintu
Treasure . . . . Richard Taafee
Secretary . . . . David Derauf

252 Coventry Health Care of Hawaii
6720-B Rockledge Drive
Suite 700
Bethesda, MD 20817
Phone: 301-581-0600
www.coventryhealthcare.com
Subsidiary of: Aetna Inc.
For Profit Organization: Yes

Healthplan and Services Defined
PLAN TYPE: HMO/PPO
Model Type: Network
Plan Specialty: Behavioral Health, Dental, Worker's
   Compensation
Benefits Offered: Behavioral Health, Dental, Prescription,
   Wellness, Worker's Compensation

Type of Coverage
Commercial, Medicare, Medicaid

Geographic Areas Served
Statewide

Key Personnel
Chief Executive Officer . . . . Mark T. Bertolini
President . . . . Karen S. Lynch
Chief Financial Officer . . . . Shawn M. Guertin
Operations & Technology . . . . Meg McCarthy
Chief Medical Officer . . . . Harold L. Paz
General Counsel . . . . Thomas Sabatino Jr.
Government Services . . . . Fran S. Soistman

253   Hawaii Medical Assurance Association

737 Bishop Street
Suite 1200
Honolulu, HI 96813
Toll-Free: 800-621-6998
Phone: 808-591-0088
Fax: 808-591-0463
www.hmaa.com
Secondary Address: Customer Service Center , 888-941-4622
For Profit Organization: Yes
Year Founded: 1989

Healthplan and Services Defined
PLAN TYPE: PPO
Benefits Offered: Chiropractic, Dental, Prescription, Vision, Wellness, AD&D, Life, Acupuncture

Type of Coverage
Commercial

Accreditation Certification
URAC

Key Personnel
Chairman, COO, CFO . . . . John Henry Felix
Director. . . . . Gail Mukaihata Hannemann
Director . . . . Dennis Y.C. Kwan
Director . . . . Warren Price III
President & CEO . . . . William C. McCorriston

254   Hawaii Medical Service Association

HMSA Building
818 Keeaumoku Street
Honolulu, HI 96814
hmsa.com
Secondary Address: HMSA, P.O. Box 860, Honolulu, HI 96808
State Enrollment: 700,000

Healthplan and Services Defined
PLAN TYPE: HMO/PPO
Benefits Offered: Dental, Prescription, Vision, Wellness

Type of Coverage
Commercial, Individual, Medicare, Medicaid

Key Personnel
President & CEO . . . . Michael A. Gold
Chief Operating Officer . . . . Michael B. Stollar
Chief Health Officer. . . . . Mark M. Mugiishi
Chief Information Officer . . . . Dick Escue
Chief Financial Officer . . . . Gina L. Marting
General Counsel . . . . Jennifer A. Walker

255   Humana Health Insurance of Hawaii

733 Bishop Street
Suite 2100
Honolulu, HI 96813
Phone: 808-540-2570
Fax: 808-548-7618
www.humana.com
Subsidiary of: Humana
For Profit Organization: Yes

Healthplan and Services Defined
PLAN TYPE: HMO/PPO
Model Type: Network
Plan Specialty: Dental, Vision
Benefits Offered: Dental, Vision, Life, LTD, STD

Type of Coverage
Commercial

Geographic Areas Served
Statewide

Accreditation Certification
URAC, NCQA, CORE

Key Personnel
President & CEO. Bruce Broussard
Chief Medical Officer. . . . . Roy A. Beveridge
Chief Consumer Officer. . . . . Jody L. Bilney
Human Resources. . . . . Tim Huval
Chief Financial Officer . . . . Brian Kane
Chief Information Officer . . . . Brian LeClaire
General Counsel . . . . Christopher M. Todoroff
Chief Accounting Officer . . . . Cynthia H. Zipperie

256   Kaiser Permanente Hawaii

1010 Pensacola Street
Honolulu, HI 96814
Toll-Free: 800-432-2000
www.kpinhawaii.org
Subsidiary of: Kaiser Permanente
Non-Profit Organization: Yes
Year Founded: 1958
Number of Primary Care Physicians: 500
State Enrollment: 242,978

Healthplan and Services Defined
PLAN TYPE: HMO
Model Type: Group
Plan Specialty: Obstetrics/gynecology, orthopedics, cardiothoracic and vascular surgery, neurosurgery, oncology, gastroenterology
Benefits Offered: Chiropractic, Complementary Medicine, Disease Management, Prescription, Vision, Wellness, Worker's Compensation
Offers Demand Management Patient Information Service: Yes

Type of Coverage
Commercial, Individual, Medicare, Medicaid
Catastrophic Illness Benefit: Unlimited

Type of Payment Plans Offered
POS, Capitated, FFS

Geographic Areas Served
Big Island, Maui, Molokai & Lanai, Oahu, Kauai

Subscriber Information
Average Subscriber Co-Payment:
Home Health Care Max. Days/Visits Covered: Unlimited
Nursing Home: Skilled nursing fac.
Nursing Home Max. Days/Visits Covered: Skilled nursing fac.

Network Qualifications
Pre-Admission Certification: No

Peer Review Type
Utilization Review: Yes
Case Management: Yes

Publishes and Distributes Report Card: Yes

Accreditation Certification
NCQA, UNICEF/WHO Baby Friendly
TJC Accreditation, Medicare Approved, Utilization Review,
　State Licensure, Quality Assurance Program

Key Personnel
Chief Medical Director . . . . Edward M. Ellison
Executive Director/CEO . . . . Richard S. Isaacs
Chief Operating Officer . . . . Chris Grant

Specialty Managed Care Partners
Enters into Contracts with Regional Business Coalitions: Yes

257　UnitedHealthcare of Hawaii
5901 Lincoln Drive, MN012-N123
Edina, MN 55436
Toll-Free: 866-432-5992
www.uhc.com/contact-us/hawaii
Subsidiary of: UnitedHealth Group
For Profit Organization: Yes
Year Founded: 1986

Healthplan and Services Defined
PLAN TYPE: HMO/PPO
Model Type: Network
Plan Specialty: Behavioral Health, Dental, Disease
　Management, PBM, Vision
Benefits Offered: Behavioral Health, Dental, Disease
　Management, Long-Term Care, Prescription, Vision,
　Wellness, Life, LTD, STD

Type of Coverage
Medicare, Supplemental Medicare, Medicaid, Catastrophic,
　Family, Military, Veterans, Group,
Catastrophic Illness Benefit: Covered

Type of Payment Plans Offered
DFFS, Capitated

Geographic Areas Served
Statewide. Hawaii is covered by the Minnesota branch

Subscriber Information
Average Monthly Fee Per Subscriber
　(Employee + Employer Contribution):
　　Employee Only (Self): $120.00
　　Employee & 1 Family Member: $240.00
　　Employee & 2 Family Members: $375.00
Average Annual Deductible Per Subscriber:
　　Employee & 2 Family Members: Varies
Average Subscriber Co-Payment:
　　Primary Care Physician: $5.00-10.00
　　Prescription Drugs: $5.00/10.00/25.00
　　Hospital ER: $50.00
　　Nursing Home Max. Days/Visits Covered: 120 per year

Publishes and Distributes Report Card: Yes

Accreditation Certification
NCQA
TJC Accreditation, Utilization Review, State Licensure

Key Personnel
President . . . . David Wichmann
Chief Operating Officer . . . . Dan Schumacher
Chief Strategy . . . . John Cosgriff
Communications Officer . . . . Kirsten Gorsuch
Chief Medical Officer. . . . . Sam Ho
Chief Legal Officer . . . . Thad Johnson
Chief Information Officer . . . . Phil McKoy
Chief Financial Officer. . . . . Jeff Putnam

Specialty Managed Care Partners
Enters into Contracts with Regional Business Coalitions: Yes

HMO/PPO DIRECTORY

Health Insurance Coverage Status and Type of Coverage by Age

Category	All Persons		Under 18 years		Under 65 years	
	Number	%	Number	%	Number	%
Total population	1,663	-	460	-	1,410	-
Covered by some type of health insurance	1,495 *(9)*	89.9 *(0.5)*	438 *(5)*	95.1 *(0.8)*	1,244 *(8)*	88.2 *(0.6)*
Covered by private health insurance	1,166 *(15)*	70.1 *(0.9)*	284 *(8)*	61.7 *(1.7)*	1,008 *(14)*	71.5 *(1.0)*
Employer-based	859 *(17)*	51.7 *(1.0)*	232 *(9)*	50.3 *(1.9)*	801 *(17)*	56.8 *(1.2)*
Direct purchase	319 *(10)*	19.2 *(0.6)*	50 *(6)*	10.9 *(1.2)*	216 *(10)*	15.3 *(0.7)*
TRICARE	53 *(5)*	3.2 *(0.3)*	12 *(2)*	2.6 *(0.5)*	33 *(4)*	2.3 *(0.3)*
Covered by public health insurance	543 *(13)*	32.6 *(0.8)*	175 *(9)*	38.0 *(2.1)*	298 *(12)*	21.1 *(0.9)*
Medicaid	293 *(14)*	17.6 *(0.8)*	174 *(9)*	37.8 *(2.0)*	261 *(13)*	18.5 *(0.9)*
Medicare	283 *(4)*	17.0 *(0.2)*	2 *(1)*	0.5 *(0.2)*	39 *(4)*	2.8 *(0.3)*
VA Care	52 *(4)*	3.1 *(0.2)*	Z *(Z)*	0.1 *(0.1)*	22 *(3)*	1.6 *(0.2)*
Not covered at any time during the year	168 *(8)*	10.1 *(0.5)*	22 *(4)*	4.9 *(0.8)*	166 *(8)*	11.8 *(0.6)*

Note: Numbers in thousands; Figures cover civilian noninstitutionalized population in 2016; N/A indicates that data was not available; Z represents or rounds to zero; Margin of error appears in parenthesis and is calculated using replicate weights.
Source: U.S. Census Bureau, American Community Survey, Table HIC-4_ACS. Health Insurance Coverage Status and Type of Coverage by State—All People: 2008 to 2016, Table HIC-5_ACS. Health Insurance Coverage Status and Type of Coverage by State—Children Under 18: 2008 to 2016, Table HIC-6_ACS. Health Insurance Coverage Status and Type of Coverage by State—Persons Under 65: 2008 to 2016

Idaho

258 Aetna Health of Idaho

151 Farmington Avenue
Hartford, CT 06156
Toll-Free: 800-872-3862
Phone: 860-273-0123
www.aetna.com
Secondary Address: 6730-B Rockledge Drive, Suite 700,
Bethesda, MD 20817, 301-581-0600
Subsidiary of: Aetna Inc.
For Profit Organization: Yes

Healthplan and Services Defined
PLAN TYPE: PPO
Other Type: POS
Model Type: Network
Plan Specialty: Behavioral Health, EPO, Lab, PBM,
Radiology
Benefits Offered: Behavioral Health, Dental, Disease
Management, Long-Term Care, Physical Therapy,
Podiatry, Prescription, Psychiatric, Vision, Wellness, Life,
LTD, STD

Type of Coverage
Commercial, Student health

Type of Payment Plans Offered
POS, FFS

Geographic Areas Served
Statewide

Key Personnel
CEO . . . . Mark Bertolini

259 Blue Cross of Idaho Health Service, Inc.

3000 East Pine Avenue
Meridian, ID 83642
Toll-Free: 800-274-4018
Phone: 208-345-4550
Fax: 208-331-7582
www.bcidaho.com
Mailing Address: PO Box 7408, Boise, ID 83707
Subsidiary of: Blue Cross and Blue Shield Association
Non-Profit Organization: Yes
Year Founded: 1945
Number of Affiliated Hospitals: 44
Number of Primary Care Physicians: 1,631
Total Enrollment: 563,000
State Enrollment: 563,000

Healthplan and Services Defined
PLAN TYPE: HMO/PPO
Model Type: IPA, Group, Network
Plan Specialty: ASO, Chiropractic, Dental, Disease
Management
Benefits Offered: Chiropractic, Dental, Disease Management,
Prescription, Vision, Wellness

Type of Coverage
Commercial, Individual, Indemnity, Medicare, Supplemental
Medicare

Type of Payment Plans Offered
POS, DFFS, FFS

Geographic Areas Served
Statewide

Subscriber Information
Average Subscriber Co-Payment:
Prescription Drugs: Varies
Hospital ER: Varies
Home Health Care: Varies
Nursing Home: Varies

Network Qualifications
Pre-Admission Certification: Yes

Peer Review Type
Utilization Review: Yes
Case Management: Yes

Publishes and Distributes Report Card: Yes

Accreditation Certification
TJC Accreditation, Pre-Admission Certification, State
Licensure

Key Personnel
President & CEO . . . . Charlene Maher
Chief Financial Officer . . . . Ralph Woodard
VP actuarial Services . . . . David J. Hutchins
General Counsel . . . . Steven Tobiason
EVP, Marketing & Sales . . . . David Jeppesen
Chief Medical Officer . . . . Rhonda Robinson-Beale, MD
VP, Sales . . . . Rex Warwick

Specialty Managed Care Partners
Wellpoint Pharmacy Management, Dental through Blue Cross
of Idaho, Vision through VSP, Life Insurance, EAP through
Business Psychology Associates
Enters into Contracts with Regional Business Coalitions: No

260 Delta Dental of Idaho

555 East Parkcenter Boulevard
Boise, ID 83706
Toll-Free: 800-356-7586
Phone: 208-489-3580
customerservice@deltadentalid.com
www.deltadentalid.com
Non-Profit Organization: Yes
Year Founded: 1971

Healthplan and Services Defined
PLAN TYPE: Dental
Other Type: Dental PPO
Model Type: Network
Plan Specialty: Dental
Benefits Offered: Dental

Type of Coverage
Commercial, Individual, Medicare

Type of Payment Plans Offered
DFFS

Geographic Areas Served
Statewide

Network Qualifications
Pre-Admission Certification: Yes

Publishes and Distributes Report Card: Yes

Key Personnel
President & CEO . . . . Jean De Luca
Director of Sales . . . . Don Murray
dmurray@deltadentalid.com

261 Humana Health Insurance of Idaho
1505 South Eagle Road
Suite 120
Meridian, ID 83642
Phone: 208-319-3400
Fax: 208-888-7298
www.humana.com
Subsidiary of: Humana
For Profit Organization: Yes

Healthplan and Services Defined
PLAN TYPE: HMO/PPO
Model Type: Network
Plan Specialty: Dental, Vision
Benefits Offered: Dental, Vision, Life, LTD, STD

Type of Coverage
Commercial

Geographic Areas Served
Statewide

Accreditation Certification
URAC, NCQA, CORE

Key Personnel
President & CEO. Bruce Broussard
Chief Medical Officer. . . . . Roy A. Beveridge
Chief Consumer Officer. . . . . Jody L. Bilney
Human Resources. . . . . Tim Huval
Chief Financial Officer . . . . Brian Kane
Chief Information Officer . . . . Brian LeClaire
General Counsel. . . . . Christopher M. Todoroff

262 Molina Medicaid Solutions
9415 W Golden Trout
Boise, ID 83704
Phone: 208-373-1300
www.molinahealthcare.com
Subsidiary of: Molina Healthcare, Inc.
For Profit Organization: Yes

Healthplan and Services Defined
PLAN TYPE: Medicare

Type of Coverage
Medicaid information management sys

Geographic Areas Served
Statewide

Key Personnel
Chief Executive Officer . . . . Joseph W. White
Chief Operating Officer . . . . Terry Bayer
General Counsel. . . . . Jeff D. Barlow
SVP, Relations/Marketing . . . . Juan Jos, Orellana

Chief Information Officer . . . . Rick Hopfer

263 Primary Health Medical Group
10482 W Carlton Bay Drive
Garden City, ID 83714
Toll-Free: 800-481-9777
Phone: 208-955-6500
Fax: 208-955-6502
information@primaryhealth.com
www.primaryhealth.com
Year Founded: 1996
Physician Owned Organization: Yes

Healthplan and Services Defined
PLAN TYPE: Multiple
Model Type: IPA
Plan Specialty: ASO
Benefits Offered: Behavioral Health, Chiropractic, Dental,
Disease Management, Home Care, Inpatient SNF, Physical
Therapy, Podiatry, Prescription, Psychiatric, Transplant,
Vision, Wellness, AD&D, Life

Type of Coverage
Commercial, Individual, Indemnity

Type of Payment Plans Offered
POS, DFFS

Geographic Areas Served
Southwest Idaho

Accreditation Certification
NCQA

Key Personnel
Chief Operating Officer . . . . Steve Judy
Director of Information . . . . Paul Castronova

264 Regence BlueShield of Idaho
PO Box 1106
Lewiston, ID 83501
Toll-Free: 888-232-5763
Phone: 208-746-2671
Fax: 208-798-2097
www.regence.com
Subsidiary of: Regence
Non-Profit Organization: Yes
Total Enrollment: 2,400,000
State Enrollment: 160,000

Healthplan and Services Defined
PLAN TYPE: Multiple
Model Type: Network
Benefits Offered: Dental, Prescription, Vision, Wellness, Life,
Preventive Care

Type of Coverage
Commercial, Individual, Supplemental Medicare

Accreditation Certification
URAC

Key Personnel
President . . . . Scott Kreiling
Chief Marketing Officer. . . . . Carol Kruse

Chief Medical Officer . . . . Richard Popiel

265 Trinity Health of Idaho

Saint Adolphus Health System
1055 N Curtis Road
Boise, ID 83706
Toll-Free: 855-220-0432
Phone: 208-367-2121
www.trinity-health.org
Secondary Address: Oakland Mercy Hospital, 601 East 2nd
   Street, Oakland, NE 68045, 402-685-5601
Subsidiary of: Trinity Health
Non-Profit Organization: Yes
Year Founded: 2013
Number of Affiliated Hospitals: 4
Number of Primary Care Physicians: 1,400
Total Enrollment: 30,000,000
State Enrollment: 700,000

Healthplan and Services Defined
PLAN TYPE: Other
   Benefits Offered: Disease Management, Home Care,
      Long-Term Care, Psychiatric, Hospice programs, PACE
      (Program of All Inclusive Care for the Elderly)

Geographic Areas Served
   Boise and Nampa, Idaho and Ontario and Baker City,
   Oregon, and Nebraska

Key Personnel
   Chief Executive Officer . . . . Richard J. Gilfillan
   Chief Financial Officer. . . . . Benjamin R. Carter
   Human Resources. . . . . Edmund F. Hodge
   General Counsel . . . . Paul G. Neumann
   Chief Clinical Officer. . . . . Daniel J. Roth
   Chief Operating Officer . . . . Michael A. Slubowski

266 UnitedHealthcare of Idaho

205 East Watertower Lane
Meridian, ID 83642
Toll-Free: 866-432-5992
www.uhc.com/contact-us/idaho
Subsidiary of: UnitedHealth Group
For Profit Organization: Yes
Year Founded: 1986

Healthplan and Services Defined
PLAN TYPE: HMO/PPO
   Model Type: Network
   Plan Specialty: Behavioral Health, Dental, Disease
      Management, PBM, Vision
   Benefits Offered: Behavioral Health, Dental, Disease
      Management, Long-Term Care, Prescription, Vision,
      Wellness, Life, LTD, STD

Type of Coverage
   Individual, Medicare, Supplemental Medicare, Medicaid,
      Catastrophic, Family, Military, Veterans, Group,
   Catastrophic Illness Benefit: Covered

Type of Payment Plans Offered
   DFFS, Capitated

Geographic Areas Served
   Statewide

Subscriber Information
   Average Monthly Fee Per Subscriber
      (Employee + Employer Contribution):
         Employee Only (Self): $120.00
         Employee & 1 Family Member: $240.00
         Employee & 2 Family Members: $375.00
   Average Annual Deductible Per Subscriber:
      Employee & 2 Family Members: Varies
   Average Subscriber Co-Payment:
      Primary Care Physician: $5.00-10.00
      Prescription Drugs: $5.00/10.00/25.00
      Hospital ER: $50.00
      Nursing Home Max. Days/Visits Covered: 120 per year

Publishes and Distributes Report Card: Yes

Accreditation Certification
   NCQA
   TJC Accreditation, Utilization Review, State Licensure

Key Personnel
   President . . . . David Wichmann
   Chief Operating Officer . . . . Dan Schumacher
   Chief Strategy Officer . . . . John Cosgriff
   Communications Officer . . . . Kirsten Gorsuch
   Chief Medical Officer. . . . . Sam Ho
   Chief Legal Officer . . . . Thad Johnson
   Chief Information Officer . . . . Phil McKoy
   Chief Financial Officer. . . . . Jeff Putnam

Specialty Managed Care Partners
   Enters into Contracts with Regional Business Coalitions: Yes

Health Insurance Coverage Status and Type of Coverage by Age

Category	All Persons		Under 18 years		Under 65 years	
	Number	%	Number	%	Number	%
Total population	12,620	-	3,095	-	10,812	-
Covered by some type of health insurance	11,804 *(20)*	93.5 *(0.2)*	3,013 *(8)*	97.4 *(0.2)*	10,011 *(19)*	92.6 *(0.2)*
Covered by private health insurance	8,884 *(40)*	70.4 *(0.3)*	1,931 *(21)*	62.4 *(0.7)*	7,757 *(37)*	71.7 *(0.3)*
Employer-based	7,382 *(39)*	58.5 *(0.3)*	1,728 *(19)*	55.8 *(0.6)*	6,778 *(35)*	62.7 *(0.3)*
Direct purchase	1,751 *(24)*	13.9 *(0.2)*	211 *(10)*	6.8 *(0.3)*	1,118 *(20)*	10.3 *(0.2)*
TRICARE	139 *(7)*	1.1 *(0.1)*	29 *(4)*	0.9 *(0.1)*	91 *(7)*	0.8 *(0.1)*
Covered by public health insurance	4,292 *(35)*	34.0 *(0.3)*	1,183 *(21)*	38.2 *(0.7)*	2,562 *(34)*	23.7 *(0.3)*
Medicaid	2,550 *(34)*	20.2 *(0.3)*	1,173 *(21)*	37.9 *(0.7)*	2,349 *(32)*	21.7 *(0.3)*
Medicare	1,994 *(12)*	15.8 *(0.1)*	15 *(3)*	0.5 *(0.1)*	265 *(11)*	2.5 *(0.1)*
VA Care	211 *(7)*	1.7 *(0.1)*	3 *(1)*	0.1 *(Z)*	85 *(4)*	0.8 *(Z)*
Not covered at any time during the year	817 *(20)*	6.5 *(0.2)*	82 *(7)*	2.6 *(0.2)*	801 *(19)*	7.4 *(0.2)*

Note: Numbers in thousands; Figures cover civilian noninstitutionalized population in 2016; N/A indicates that data was not available; Z represents or rounds to zero; Margin of error appears in parenthesis and is calculated using replicate weights.

Source: U.S. Census Bureau, American Community Survey, Table HIC-4_ACS. Health Insurance Coverage Status and Type of Coverage by State—All People: 2008 to 2016, Table HIC-5_ACS. Health Insurance Coverage Status and Type of Coverage by State—Children Under 18: 2008 to 2016, Table HIC-6_ACS. Health Insurance Coverage Status and Type of Coverage by State—Persons Under 65: 2008 to 2016

Illinois

267 Aetna Health of Illinois

151 Farmington Avenue
Hartford, CT 06156
Toll-Free: 800-872-3862
Phone: 860-273-0123
www.aetna.com
Subsidiary of: Aetna Inc.
For Profit Organization: Yes

Healthplan and Services Defined
PLAN TYPE: HMO/PPO
Other Type: POS
Model Type: Network
Plan Specialty: Behavioral Health, Dental, EPO, Lab, PBM,
Vision, Radiology
Benefits Offered: Behavioral Health, Dental, Disease
Management, Long-Term Care, Physical Therapy,
Podiatry, Prescription, Psychiatric, Vision, Wellness, Life,
LTD, STD

Type of Coverage
Commercial, Student health

Geographic Areas Served
Statewide

Key Personnel
CEO . . . . Mark Bertolini

268 Blue Cross & Blue Shield of Illinois

300 East Randolph Street
Chicago, IL 60601-5099
Toll-Free: 866-977-7378
www.bcbsil.com
Subsidiary of: Health Care Service Corporation
Year Founded: 1936
Total Enrollment: 8,100,000
State Enrollment: 8,100,000

Healthplan and Services Defined
PLAN TYPE: HMO/PPO
Benefits Offered: Disease Management, Physical Therapy,
Prescription, Wellness

Type of Coverage
Commercial, Individual, Supplemental Medicare, Medicaid,
Healthy Kids, Healthy Families

Type of Payment Plans Offered
POS, FFS

Geographic Areas Served
Statewide

Key Personnel
President BCBS Illinois . . . . Maurice Smith

Specialty Managed Care Partners
Prime Therapeutics

269 BlueCross BlueShield Association

225 North Michigan Avenue
Chicago, IL 60601
Toll-Free: 888-630-2583
www.bcbs.com
Total Enrollment: 105,000,000

Healthplan and Services Defined
PLAN TYPE: Medicare
Benefits Offered: Chiropractic, Disease Management, Home
Care, Inpatient SNF, Physical Therapy, Podiatry,
Prescription, Psychiatric, Wellness

Type of Coverage
Individual, Medicare

Geographic Areas Served
Nationwide, including the District of Columbia and Puerto
Rico

Subscriber Information
Average Monthly Fee Per Subscriber
(Employee + Employer Contribution):
Employee Only (Self): Varies
Medicare: Varies
Average Annual Deductible Per Subscriber:
Employee Only (Self): Varies
Medicare: Varies
Average Subscriber Co-Payment:
Primary Care Physician: Varies
Non-Network Physician: Varies
Prescription Drugs: Varies
Hospital ER: Varies
Home Health Care: Varies
Home Health Care Max. Days/Visits Covered: Varies
Nursing Home: Varies
Nursing Home Max. Days/Visits Covered: Varies

Key Personnel
President & CEO . . . . Scott P. Serota
Chief Financial Officer . . . . Robert Kolodgy
Human Resources . . . . Maureen A. Cahill
Chief Medical Officer. . . . . Trent Haywood
General Counsel. . . . . Scott Nehs

270 Cigna HealthSpring CarePlan of Illinois

175 W Jackson Boulevard
Suite 1750
Chicago, IL 60604
Toll-Free: 866-487-4331
wecanhelp@healthspring.com
www.careplanil.com
Year Founded: 2004
Physician Owned Organization: Yes
Total Enrollment: 13,000
State Enrollment: 13,000

Healthplan and Services Defined
PLAN TYPE: Medicare

Type of Coverage
Medicare, Supplemental Medicare

Geographic Areas Served
Greater Chicago

Key Personnel
President & CEO . . . . David M. Cordani

---

271 CNA
CNA Center
333 S Wabash Avenue
Chicago, IL 60604
Toll-Free: 877-262-2727
Phone: 312-822-5000
www.cna.com
Year Founded: 1987
Owned by an Integrated Delivery Network (IDN): Yes

Healthplan and Services Defined
PLAN TYPE: Other
Model Type: Network
Plan Specialty: Dental, Disease Management, Lab, MSO, Vision, Radiology, Worker's Compensation, UR
Benefits Offered: Behavioral Health, Chiropractic, Dental, Disease Management, Home Care, Inpatient SNF, Long-Term Care, Physical Therapy, Podiatry, Prescription, Psychiatric, Transplant, Vision, Wellness, Worker's Compensation, AD&D, Life, LTD, STD

Type of Coverage
Commercial, Individual, Indemnity, Medicaid, Catastrophic

Type of Payment Plans Offered
POS

Network Qualifications
Pre-Admission Certification: Yes

Peer Review Type
Utilization Review: Yes
Case Management: Yes

Publishes and Distributes Report Card: Yes

Accreditation Certification
URAC
TJC Accreditation, Pre-Admission Certification

Key Personnel
Chairman & CEO . . . . Thomas F. Motamed

Specialty Managed Care Partners
Enters into Contracts with Regional Business Coalitions: Yes

---

272 CoreSource
400 Field Drive
Lake Forest, IL 60045
Toll-Free: 800-832-3332
Phone: 847-604-9200
www.coresource.com
Subsidiary of: Trustmark
Year Founded: 1980
Total Enrollment: 1,100,000

Healthplan and Services Defined
PLAN TYPE: PPO
Other Type: TPA
Model Type: Network

Plan Specialty: Benefits Administration
Benefits Offered: Behavioral Health, Dental, Home Care, Prescription, Transplant, Vision, Wellness

Type of Coverage
Commercial

Geographic Areas Served
Nationwide

Accreditation Certification
URAC
Utilization Review, Pre-Admission Certification

Key Personnel
President . . . . Nancy Eckrich
Chief Clinical Leader. . . . . Meera Atkins
Chief Operating Officer. . . . . Lloyd Sarrel
Chief Financial Officer. . . . . Clare Smith
Chief Information Officer . . . . Brooke Terry
VP, Marketing. . . . . Steve Horvath
Human Resources . . . . Dave Kenney

---

273 Coventry Health Care of Illinois
2110 Fox Drive
Suite A
Champaign, IL 61820
Toll-Free: 800-431-1211
Phone: 217-366-5551
Fax: 217-366-5410
infochcil@cvty.com
chcillinois.coventryhealthcare.com
Secondary Address: 4507 Sterling Avenue, Suite 205, Peoria, IL 61615, 866-895-7412
Subsidiary of: Aetna Inc.
For Profit Organization: Yes
Year Founded: 1984

Healthplan and Services Defined
PLAN TYPE: HMO
Model Type: Network
Plan Specialty: Behavioral Health, Dental, Worker's Compensation
Benefits Offered: Behavioral Health, Dental, Wellness, Worker's Compensation

Type of Coverage
Commercial, Individual, Medicare, Supplemental Medicare, Medicaid

Type of Payment Plans Offered
POS, DFFS, Capitated, FFS, Combination FFS & DFFS

Geographic Areas Served
Bond, Boone, Calhoun, Champaign, Christian, Clark, Clinton, Coles, Crawford, Cumberland, DeWitt, Douglas, Edgar, Effingham, Fayette, Ford, Greene, Iroquois, Jasper, Jersey, Kankakee, LaSalle, Lee, Logan, Macon, Macoupin, Madison, Marshall, McLean, Menard, Monroe, Montgomery, Morgan, Moultrie, Ogle, Peoria, Piatt, Sangaman, Saint Clair, Shelby, Stark, Stephenson, Tazewell, Vermilion, Washington, Whiteside, Will, Winnebago, Woodford counties

Network Qualifications
Pre-Admission Certification: Yes

Peer Review Type
Utilization Review: Yes
Second Surgical Opinion: Yes
Case Management: Yes

Accreditation Certification
NCQA
TJC Accreditation, Medicare Approved, Utilization Review,
Pre-Admission Certification, State Licensure, Quality
Assurance Program

Key Personnel
Chairman & CEO . . . . Mark T. Bertolini
President . . . . Karen S. Lynch
Chief Financial Officer . . . . Shawn M. Guertin
Operations & Technology . . . . Meg McCarthy
Chief Medical Officer . . . . Harold L. Paz
General Counsel . . . . Thomas Sabatino Jr.
Government Services . . . . Fran S. Soistman

Employer References
Horace Mann, Verizon, Pepsi, Sarah Bush Lincoln Health,
Walgreen's

274   Delta Dental of Illinois
111 Shuman Boulevard
Naperville, IL 60563
Toll-Free: 800-323-1743
Phone: 630-718-4700
askdelta@deltadentalil.com
www.deltadentalil.com
Non-Profit Organization: Yes
Year Founded: 1967
State Enrollment: 2,000,000

Healthplan and Services Defined
PLAN TYPE: Dental
Other Type: Dental PPO
Model Type: Network
Plan Specialty: Dental
Benefits Offered: Dental

Type of Coverage
Commercial, Individual

Geographic Areas Served
Statewide

Peer Review Type
Utilization Review: Yes

Key Personnel
President & CEO . . . . Bernard Glossy

275   Dental Network of America
701 E. 22nd Street
Suite 300
Lombard, IL 60148
Toll-Free: 800-972-7565
Phone: 630-691-1133
general_inquiry@dnoa.com
www.dnoa.com
Subsidiary of: Health Care Service Corporation
For Profit Organization: Yes

Year Founded: 1985
Federally Qualified: Yes
Number of Primary Care Physicians: 80,000
Total Enrollment: 6,200,000

Healthplan and Services Defined
PLAN TYPE: Dental
Other Type: TPA, Dental PPO
Plan Specialty: ASO, Dental, Dental, Fully Insured
Benefits Offered: Dental

Type of Coverage
Commercial, Individual, Indemnity, Group

Type of Payment Plans Offered
Capitated

Geographic Areas Served
Nationwide

Network Qualifications
Pre-Admission Certification: Yes

Peer Review Type
Utilization Review: Yes

Key Personnel
CEO/President, HCSO . . . . Paula Steiner

276   HCSC Insurance Services Company
300 E Randolph Street
Chicago, IL 60601
Toll-Free: 800-654-7385
Phone: 312-653-6000
hcsc.com
Subsidiary of: Blue Cross Blue Shield Association
Non-Profit Organization: Yes
Year Founded: 1936
Number of Primary Care Physicians: 233,000

Healthplan and Services Defined
PLAN TYPE: HMO
Benefits Offered: Behavioral Health, Dental, Disease
Management, Psychiatric, Wellness

Geographic Areas Served
Illinois, Montana, New Mexico, Oklahoma, and Texas

Key Personnel
President & CEO . . . . Paula Steiner
EVP, Plan Operations. . . . . Colleen Reitan
SVP, Clinical Officer. . . . . Opella Ernest, MD
SVP, Financial Officer. . . . . Eric Feldstein
SVP, Human Resources. . . . . Nazneen Razi
SVP, Chief Legal Officer. . . . . Blair Todt
SVP, Compliance Officer. . . . . Thomas Lubben
Media Contact . . . . Kristen Cunningham
312-653-1686
kristen_cunningham@hcsc.net
Media Contact . . . . Greg Thompson
312-653-7581
greg_thompson@hcsc.net

277　Health Alliance

301 S Vine Street
Urbana, IL 61801
Toll-Free: 877-686-1168
www.healthalliance.org
For Profit Organization: Yes
Year Founded: 1980
Physician Owned Organization: Yes
Federally Qualified: Yes

Healthplan and Services Defined
PLAN TYPE: HMO/PPO
Plan Specialty: Dental, Vision
Benefits Offered: Dental, Disease Management, Vision,
　Wellness

Type of Coverage
Commercial, Individual, Medicare, Medicaid

Geographic Areas Served
Illinois and Central Iowa

Publishes and Distributes Report Card: Yes

Accreditation Certification
NCQA

278　Health Alliance Medicare

301 S Vine Street
Urbana, IL 61801
Toll-Free: 888-382-9771
memberservices@healthalliance.org
www.healthalliance.org
Year Founded: 1997
Number of Primary Care Physicians: 3,000
Total Enrollment: 255,494

Healthplan and Services Defined
PLAN TYPE: Medicare
Other Type: HMO/PPO
Benefits Offered: Prescription

Type of Coverage
Medicare, Supplemental Medicare

Accreditation Certification
NCQA

279　Health Care Service Corporation

300 E Randolph Street
Chicago, IL 60601
Toll-Free: 800-654-7385
www.hcsc.com
For Profit Organization: Yes
Year Founded: 1975
Total Enrollment: 15,000,000
State Enrollment: 15,000,000

Healthplan and Services Defined
PLAN TYPE: HMO/PPO
Model Type: Network
Plan Specialty: Chiropractic, Dental, Disease Management,
　Lab, Vision, Radiology, UR

Benefits Offered: Chiropractic, Dental, Disease Management,
　Home Care, Inpatient SNF, Physical Therapy, Podiatry,
　Prescription, Psychiatric, Transplant, Vision, Wellness,
　AD&D, Life, LTD, STD

Type of Coverage
Commercial, Individual, Indemnity, Supplemental Medicare,
　Catastrophic

Geographic Areas Served
Illinois, Montana, New Mexico, Oklahoma, Texas

Peer Review Type
Second Surgical Opinion: Yes

Accreditation Certification
NCQA

Key Personnel
President & CEO . . . . Paula Steiner
Senior VP & CFO . . . . Eric Feldstein
EVP, Plan Operations. . . . . Colleen Reitan

280　Humana Health Insurance of Illinois

2301 22nd Street
Suite 301
Oak Brook, IL 60523
Toll-Free: 800-569-2492
Phone: 630-794-5950
Fax: 630-794-0107
www.humana.com
For Profit Organization: Yes
Year Founded: 1972

Healthplan and Services Defined
PLAN TYPE: HMO/PPO
Model Type: Network
Plan Specialty: Behavioral Health, Chiropractic, Dental,
　Disease Management, Lab, PBM, Vision, Worker's
　Compensation, UR
Benefits Offered: Behavioral Health, Chiropractic,
　Complementary Medicine, Dental, Disease Management,
　Home Care, Inpatient SNF, Long-Term Care, Physical
　Therapy, Prescription, Psychiatric, Transplant, Vision,
　Wellness, Worker's Compensation, AD&D, Life, LTD, STD

Type of Coverage
Commercial, Individual, Indemnity, Medicare, Supplemental
　Medicare, Medicaid, Catastrophic

Type of Payment Plans Offered
POS, DFFS, Capitated, FFS

Network Qualifications
Pre-Admission Certification: Yes

Peer Review Type
Utilization Review: Yes
Second Surgical Opinion: Yes
Case Management: Yes

Publishes and Distributes Report Card: Yes

Accreditation Certification
URAC, NCQA, CORE

TJC Accreditation, Medicare Approved, Utilization Review,
Pre-Admission Certification, State Licensure, Quality
Assurance Program

Key Personnel
President & CEO . . . . Bruce D. Broussard
Chief Medical Officer. . . . . Roy A. Beveridge
Chief Consumer Officer. . . . . Jody L. Bilney
Human Resources. . . . . Tim Huval
Chief Financial Officer . . . . Brian Kane
Chief Information Officer . . . . Brian LeClaire
General Counsel. . . . . Christopher M. Todoroff

Specialty Managed Care Partners
Behavioral Health, Disease Management, PBM, Worker's
Compensation
Enters into Contracts with Regional Business Coalitions: Yes
Midwest Business Group on Health, Mercer Coalition

281 Liberty Dental Plan of Illinois
PO Box 401086
Las Vegas, NV 89140
Toll-Free: 888-352-7924
www.libertydentalplan.com
For Profit Organization: Yes
Total Enrollment: 2,000,000

Healthplan and Services Defined
PLAN TYPE: Dental
Other Type: Dental HMO
Plan Specialty: Dental
Benefits Offered: Dental

Type of Coverage
Commercial, Medicare, Medicaid, Unions

Geographic Areas Served
Statewide

Accreditation Certification
NCQA

Key Personnel
President & CEO. . . . . Amir Neshat
Executive Vice President . . . . John Carvelli
Chief Financial Officer . . . . Maja Kapic
General Counsel . . . . Lisa Wright
Chief Operating Officer . . . . Nico Alvarez
Chief Dental Officer. . . . . Richard Goren
Dental Director . . . . Richard Hague

282 Meridian Health Plan of Illinois
333 S Wabash Avenue
Suite 2900
Chicago, IL 60604
Toll-Free: 866-606-3700
memberservices.il@mhplan.com
www.mhplan.com
Total Enrollment: 750,000
State Enrollment: 240,000

Healthplan and Services Defined
PLAN TYPE: Medicare

Type of Coverage
Medicare, Medicaid

Geographic Areas Served
Statewide

Accreditation Certification
URAC, NCQA

Key Personnel
President . . . . Karen Brach

283 Molina Healthcare of Illinois
1520 Kensington Road
Suite 212
Oak Brook, IL 60523
Toll-Free: 888-858-2156
www.molinahealthcare.com
Secondary Address: 1 West Old State Capital Plaza, Suite 300,
Springfield, IL 62701
Subsidiary of: Molina Healthcare, Inc.
For Profit Organization: Yes

Healthplan and Services Defined
PLAN TYPE: Medicare
Model Type: Network
Plan Specialty: Dental, PBM, Vision, Integrated
Medicare/Medicaid (Duals)
Benefits Offered: Dental, Prescription, Vision, Wellness, Life

Type of Coverage
Individual, Medicare, Supplemental Medicare, Medicaid

Geographic Areas Served
Statewide

Key Personnel
Chief Executive Officer . . . . Joseph W. White
Chief Operating Officer . . . . Terry Bayer
General Counsel. Jeff D. Barlow
SVP, Relations/Marketing . . . . Juan Jos, Orellana
Chief Information Officer . . . . Rick Hopfer

284 OptumRx
1600 McConnor Parkway
Schaumburg, IL 60173-6801
Toll-Free: 800-788-4863
Phone: 224-231-1000
www.catamaranrx.com
Secondary Address: 2300 Main Street, Irvine, CA 92614

Healthplan and Services Defined
PLAN TYPE: Other
Other Type: PBM
Benefits Offered: Prescription

Key Personnel
CEO, OptumRx. . . . . John Prince

285 OSF Healthcare
800 NE Glen Oak Avenue
Peoria, IL 61603-3200
Phone: 309-655-2321
www.osfhealthcare.org

Subsidiary of: Sisters of the Third Order of St Francis
Non-Profit Organization: Yes
Number of Affiliated Hospitals: 11
Number of Primary Care Physicians: 700
Number of Referral/Specialty Physicians: 50
Total Enrollment: 1,500,000

Healthplan and Services Defined
  PLAN TYPE: HMO
  Model Type: Network
  Plan Specialty: Integrated Healthcare Network of Facilities
  Benefits Offered: Disease Management, Wellness

Geographic Areas Served
  Illinois and Michigan

Key Personnel
  CEO. . . . . Kevin Schoeplein
  COO . . . . Bob Sehring

---

286   Preferred Network Access

1510 W 75th Street
Suite 250
Darien, IL 60561
Phone: 630-493-0905
www.pna-usa.com
For Profit Organization: Yes
Year Founded: 1995
Number of Affiliated Hospitals: 113
Number of Primary Care Physicians: 34,000
Number of Referral/Specialty Physicians: 250
Total Enrollment: 316,000
State Enrollment: 316,000

Healthplan and Services Defined
  PLAN TYPE: PPO
  Plan Specialty: Group, Health
  Benefits Offered: Home Care, Physical Therapy, Wellness,
    Worker's Compensation, Occupational Health

Type of Coverage
  Commercial

Geographic Areas Served
  Illinois, Indiana, Wisconsin

Key Personnel
  President. . . . . Joseph M Zerega

---

287   Trinity Health of Illinois

Mercy Health System
2525 S Michigan Avenue
Chicago, IL 60616
Phone: 312-567-2000
www.trinity-health.org
Secondary Address: Layola University Medical Center, 2160
  S First Avenue, Maywood, IL 60153, 888-584-7888
Subsidiary of: Trinity Health
Non-Profit Organization: Yes
Year Founded: 2013
Total Enrollment: 30,000,000

Healthplan and Services Defined
  PLAN TYPE: Other

Benefits Offered: Disease Management, Home Care,
  Long-Term Care, Psychiatric, Hospice programs, PACE
  (Program of All Inclusive Care for the Elderly)

Geographic Areas Served
  Greater Chicago

Key Personnel
  Chief Executive Officer . . . . Richard J. Gilfillan
  Chief Financial Officer. . . . . Benjamin R. Carter
  Human Resources. . . . . Edmund F. Hodge
  General Counsel . . . . Paul G. Neumann
  Chief Clinical Officer. . . . . Daniel J. Roth
  Chief Operating Officer . . . . Michael A. Slubowski

---

288   Trustmark Companies

400 Field Drive
Lake Forest, IL 60045
Phone: 847-615-1500
Fax: 847-615-3910
www.trustmarkcompanies.com
For Profit Organization: Yes
Year Founded: 1913
Federally Qualified: Yes
Total Enrollment: 475,000

Healthplan and Services Defined
  PLAN TYPE: PPO
  Other Type: Self-funded
  Model Type: Network
  Plan Specialty: Behavioral Health, Dental, Lab
  Benefits Offered: Behavioral Health, Dental, Disease
    Management, Prescription, Vision, Wellness, AD&D, Life,
    LTD, STD, Major Medical, Nurse Line, Health Advocacy
    Service

Type of Coverage
  Commercial, Indemnity

Type of Payment Plans Offered
  FFS

Geographic Areas Served
  Nationwide

Network Qualifications
  Pre-Admission Certification: Yes

Peer Review Type
  Utilization Review: Yes
  Second Surgical Opinion: Yes

Accreditation Certification
  TJC Accreditation, Utilization Review, State Licensure

Key Personnel
  SVP, CIO . . . . Dan Simpson
  President, CEO. . . . . Joe Pray
  SVP, CFO. . . . . Phil Goss
  SVP, General Counsel . . . . Steve Auburn
  SVP, Marketing Officer . . . . Jim Coleman
  SVP, Chief Human Resource. . . . . Kristin Zelkowitz

289 UniCare Illinois

233 S Wacker Drive
Chicago, IL 60606
Phone: 312-234-8000
www.unicare.com
Subsidiary of: Anthem, Inc.
For Profit Organization: Yes
Year Founded: 1995

Healthplan and Services Defined
  PLAN TYPE: HMO/PPO
  Model Type: Network
  Benefits Offered: Behavioral Health, Chiropractic,
    Complementary
Medicine, Dental, Disease Management, Home Care,
Inpatient SNF, Long-Term Care, Physical Therapy,
Podiatry, Prescription, Psychiatric, Transplant,
Vision, Wellness, Worker's Compensation, AD&D,
Life, LTD, STD

Type of Coverage
  Commercial, Individual, Medicare, Supplemental Medicare

Type of Payment Plans Offered
  POS

Geographic Areas Served
  Statewide

Network Qualifications
  Pre-Admission Certification: Yes

Peer Review Type
  Utilization Review: Yes
  Second Surgical Opinion: Yes

Accreditation Certification
  URAC, NCQA
  TJC Accreditation, State Licensure

Specialty Managed Care Partners
  Enters into Contracts with Regional Business Coalitions: Yes

Geographic Areas Served
  Statewide

Key Personnel
  President . . . . David Wichmann
  Chief Operating Officer . . . . Dan Schumacher
  Chief Strategy Officer . . . . John Cosgriff
  Communications Officer . . . . Kirsten Gorsuch
  Chief Medical Officer. . . . . Sam Ho
  Chief Legal Officer . . . . Thad Johnson
  Chief Information Officer . . . . Phil McKoy
  Chief Financial Officer. Jeff Putnam

290 UnitedHealthcare of Illinois

200 E Randolph Street
Suite 5300
Chicago, IL 60601-6602
Toll-Free: 877-842-3210
Phone: 312-803-5900
www.uhc.com/contact-us/illinois
Subsidiary of: UnitedHealth Group
For Profit Organization: Yes

Healthplan and Services Defined
  PLAN TYPE: HMO/PPO
  Model Type: Network
  Plan Specialty: Behavioral Health, Dental, Disease
    Management, PBM, Vision
  Benefits Offered: Behavioral Health, Chiropractic, Dental,
    Disease Management, Home Care, Inpatient SNF,
    Long-Term Care, Podiatry, Prescription, Psychiatric,
    Transplant, Vision, Wellness, Life, LTD, STD

Type of Coverage
  Individual, Medicare, Supplemental Medicare, Medicaid,
    Catastrophic, Family, Military, Veterans, Group,

Health Insurance Coverage Status and Type of Coverage by Age

Category	All Persons		Under 18 years		Under 65 years	
	Number	%	Number	%	Number	%
Total population	6,535	-	1,671	-	5,578	-
Covered by some type of health insurance	6,005 *(17)*	91.9 *(0.3)*	1,573 *(10)*	94.1 *(0.5)*	5,053 *(17)*	90.6 *(0.3)*
Covered by private health insurance	4,624 *(28)*	70.8 *(0.4)*	1,048 *(15)*	62.7 *(0.9)*	4,005 *(27)*	71.8 *(0.5)*
Employer-based	3,832 *(30)*	58.6 *(0.5)*	953 *(16)*	57.0 *(0.9)*	3,536 *(29)*	63.4 *(0.5)*
Direct purchase	916 *(17)*	14.0 *(0.3)*	104 *(6)*	6.2 *(0.4)*	534 *(15)*	9.6 *(0.3)*
TRICARE	98 *(7)*	1.5 *(0.1)*	18 *(3)*	1.1 *(0.2)*	62 *(6)*	1.1 *(0.1)*
Covered by public health insurance	2,177 *(22)*	33.3 *(0.3)*	591 *(14)*	35.3 *(0.8)*	1,249 *(22)*	22.4 *(0.4)*
Medicaid	1,183 *(21)*	18.1 *(0.3)*	585 *(14)*	35.0 *(0.8)*	1,091 *(22)*	19.6 *(0.4)*
Medicare	1,123 *(9)*	17.2 *(0.1)*	10 *(2)*	0.6 *(0.1)*	196 *(7)*	3.5 *(0.1)*
VA Care	151 *(6)*	2.3 *(0.1)*	1 *(Z)*	0.1 *(Z)*	62 *(4)*	1.1 *(0.1)*
Not covered at any time during the year	530 *(17)*	8.1 *(0.3)*	99 *(8)*	5.9 *(0.5)*	524 *(17)*	9.4 *(0.3)*

Note: Numbers in thousands; Figures cover civilian noninstitutionalized population in 2016; N/A indicates that data was not available; Z represents or rounds to zero; Margin of error appears in parenthesis and is calculated using replicate weights.
Source: U.S. Census Bureau, American Community Survey, Table HIC-4_ACS. Health Insurance Coverage Status and Type of Coverage by State—All People: 2008 to 2016, Table HIC-5_ACS. Health Insurance Coverage Status and Type of Coverage by State—Children Under 18: 2008 to 2016, Table HIC-6_ACS. Health Insurance Coverage Status and Type of Coverage by State—Persons Under 65: 2008 to 2016

Indiana

291   Aetna Health of Indiana

151 Farmington Avenue
Hartford, CT 06156
Toll-Free: 800-872-3862
Phone: 860-273-0123
www.aetna.com
Subsidiary of: Aetna Inc.
For Profit Organization: Yes
Year Founded: 1995

Healthplan and Services Defined
PLAN TYPE: HMO/PPO
Other Type: POS
Model Type: Network
Plan Specialty: Dental, Vision
Benefits Offered: Chiropractic, Complementary Medicine,
   Dental, Home Care, Inpatient SNF, Long-Term Care,
   Podiatry, Prescription, Psychiatric, Transplant, Vision,
   Wellness

Type of Coverage
Commercial, Student health

Geographic Areas Served
Statewide

Key Personnel
CEO . . . . Mark Bertolini

292   American Health Network

10689 N Pennsylvania Street
Suite 200
Indianapolis, IN 46280
Toll-Free: 888-255-2246
Phone: 317-580-6309
www.ahni.com
Secondary Address: 2500 Corporate Exchange, Suite 100,
   Columbus, OH 43229, 800-880-5896
Year Founded: 1994
Number of Primary Care Physicians: 200

Healthplan and Services Defined
PLAN TYPE: PPO
Plan Specialty: Lab, Vision, Family medicine, general
   surgery, pain management, pediatrics
Benefits Offered: Physical Therapy

Type of Payment Plans Offered
Capitated

Geographic Areas Served
Indiana and Ohio

Accreditation Certification
TJC Accreditation, State Licensure

Key Personnel
President . . . . Ben Park, MD

293   Anthem Blue Cross & Blue Shield of Indiana

4681 Masons Ridge Road
Lafayette, IN 47909
Phone: 317-315-5448
www.anthem.com
Subsidiary of: Anthem, Inc.
For Profit Organization: Yes
Year Founded: 1990
Number of Affiliated Hospitals: 105
Number of Primary Care Physicians: 3,532
Number of Referral/Specialty Physicians: 8,475
Total Enrollment: 900,000

Healthplan and Services Defined
PLAN TYPE: HMO/PPO
Model Type: Network
Benefits Offered: Behavioral Health, Chiropractic,
   Complementary Medicine, Dental, Disease Management,
   Home Care, Inpatient SNF, Physical Therapy, Podiatry,
   Prescription, Psychiatric, Transplant, Vision, Wellness

Type of Coverage
Medicare, Supplemental Medicare

Type of Payment Plans Offered
DFFS, FFS, Combination FFS & DFFS

Geographic Areas Served
Statewide

Subscriber Information
Average Annual Deductible Per Subscriber:
     Employee Only (Self): Varies $250-$5000
     Employee & 2 Family Members: Varies $2500-$10000
Average Subscriber Co-Payment:
     Primary Care Physician: Varies $25/20%
     Non-Network Physician: 20%
     Prescription Drugs: Varies $15/$30/$0
     Hospital ER: 20%
     Home Health Care: 20%
     Home Health Care Max. Days/Visits Covered: 100 days
     Nursing Home Max. Days/Visits Covered: 60 days

Network Qualifications
Pre-Admission Certification: Yes

Peer Review Type
Utilization Review: Yes
Second Surgical Opinion: No
Case Management: Yes

Publishes and Distributes Report Card: Yes

Accreditation Certification
URAC, NCQA
TJC Accreditation, Medicare Approved, Utilization Review,
   Pre-Admission Certification, State Licensure, Quality
   Assurance Program

Key Personnel
President & CEO . . . . Scott P. Serota
Chief Financial Officer . . . . Robert Kolodgy
Human Resources . . . . Maureen A. Cahill
Chief Medical Officer . . . . Trent Haywood
General Counsel . . . . Scott Nehs

294   Anthem, Inc.

120 Monument Circle
Indianapolis, IN 46204
Toll-Free: 800-331-1476
www.antheminc.com
For Profit Organization: Yes
Year Founded: 2004

Healthplan and Services Defined
PLAN TYPE: HMO/PPO
Model Type: Network
Plan Specialty: Behavioral Health, Dental, Vision
Benefits Offered: Behavioral Health, Dental, Vision, Life,
LTD, STD

Type of Coverage
Commercial, Individual, Medicare, Supplemental Medicare,
Medicaid, Federal employee program

Key Personnel
President & CEO . . . . Joseph Swedish
EVP & CFO. . . . . John Gallina
EVP & CAO. . . . . Gloria McCarthy
EVP & Clinical Officer . . . . Craig Samitt
General Counsel . . . . Thomas Zielinski

295   Ascension At Home

St Vincent Home Health & Hospice
2015 Jackson Street
Anderson, IN 46016
Phone: 765-646-8179
Fax: 765-648-3805
ascensionathome.com
Subsidiary of: Ascension
Non-Profit Organization: Yes

Healthplan and Services Defined
PLAN TYPE: Other
Plan Specialty: Disease Management
Benefits Offered: Dental, Disease Management, Home Care,
Wellness, Abulance & Transportation; Nursing Service;
Short-and-long-term care management planning; Hospice

Geographic Areas Served
Texas, Alabama, Indiana, Kansas, Michigan, Mississipi,
Oklahoma, Wisconsin

Key Personnel
President. . . . . Kirk Allen
Dir., Home Health Service . . . . Darcy Burthay

296   CareSource Indiana

135 N Pennsylvania Street
Suite 1300
Indianapolis, IN 46204
Toll-Free: 877-438-4479
Phone: 317-982-6400
www.caresource.com
Non-Profit Organization: Yes
Total Enrollment: 1,000,000

Healthplan and Services Defined
PLAN TYPE: Medicare

Benefits Offered: Dental, Disease Management, Prescription,
Vision, 24-hour Nurse Advice Line; Durable Medical
Equipment

Type of Coverage
Medicare, Medicaid

Geographic Areas Served
Statewide

Key Personnel
President & CEO . . . . Pamela Morris
General Counsel . . . . Mark Chilson
Administrative Officer . . . . Dan McCabe
Chief Information Officer . . . . Paul Stoddard
EVP, COO, CFO . . . . L. Tarlton Thomas III

297   Coventry Health Care of Indiana

6720-B Rockledge Drive
Suite 700
Bethesda, MD 20817
Phone: 301-581-0600
www.coventryhealthcare.com
Subsidiary of: Aetna Inc.
For Profit Organization: Yes

Healthplan and Services Defined
PLAN TYPE: HMO/PPO
Model Type: Network
Plan Specialty: Behavioral Health, Dental, Worker's
Compensation
Benefits Offered: Behavioral Health, Dental, Prescription,
Wellness, Worker's Compensation

Type of Coverage
Commercial, Medicare, Medicaid

Geographic Areas Served
Statewide

Key Personnel
Chief Executive Officer. . . . . Mark T. Bertolini
President. . . . . Karen S. Lynch
Chief Financial Officer . . . . Shawn M. Guertin
Operations & Technology . . . . Meg McCarthy
Chief Medical Officer . . . . Harold L. Paz
General Counsel . . . . Thomas Sabatino Jr.
Government Services . . . . Fran S. Soistman

298   Deaconess Health Plans

600 Mary St Evanville
Evansville, IN 47747
Phone: 812-450-5000
www.deaconess.com
Year Founded: 1892
Physician Owned Organization: Yes
Number of Affiliated Hospitals: 6

Healthplan and Services Defined
PLAN TYPE: PPO
Model Type: Network
Plan Specialty: Behavioral Health, Chiropractic
Benefits Offered: Disease Management, Wellness

Type of Coverage
Individual

Geographic Areas Served
Illinois, Indiana, Kentucky

Peer Review Type
Utilization Review: Yes
Second Surgical Opinion: No
Case Management: Yes

Accreditation Certification
TJC Accreditation, Medicare Approved, Utilization Review, Pre-Admission Certification, State Licensure, Quality Assurance Program

Key Personnel
President.............................. James R. Porter
Chief Executive Officer................. Shawn McCoy
Chief Financial Officer .... Cheryl Wathen
Chief Operating Officer .... Lynn Lingafelter

Average Claim Compensation
Physician's Fees Charged: 1%
Hospital's Fees Charged: 1%

299 Encore Health Network

8520 Allison Pointe Boulevard
Suite 200
Indianapolis, IN 46250-4299
Toll-Free: 888-574-8180
Phone: 317-621-4250
Fax: 317-621-2388
encoreconnect.com
Subsidiary of: The HealthCare Group, LLC
Year Founded: 1986

Healthplan and Services Defined
PLAN TYPE: PPO
Benefits Offered: Worker's Compensation

Type of Coverage
Commercial, Individual

Geographic Areas Served
Select Indiana markets

Key Personnel
President .... Bruce Smiley

300 Golden Rule Insurance

7440 Woodland Drive
Indianapolis, IN 46278
Toll-Free: 888-545-5205
uhc.com
Subsidiary of: UnitedHealthcare

Healthplan and Services Defined
PLAN TYPE: HMO/PPO

Geographic Areas Served
Available in 40 states and the District of Columbia

Key Personnel
Chief Executive Officer .... Steve Nelson

301 Healthy Indiana Plan

Toll-Free: 877-438-4479
www.in.gov/fssa/hip
Year Founded: 2007

Healthplan and Services Defined
PLAN TYPE: HMO
Benefits Offered: Behavioral Health, Disease Management, Home Care, Inpatient SNF, Prescription, Wellness

Type of Coverage
Individual

Geographic Areas Served
Statewide

302 Humana Health Insurance of Indiana

7035 E 96th Street
Suite F
Indianapolis, IN 46250
Toll-Free: 866-355-6170
Phone: 317-558-5670
Fax: 502-508-8169
www.humana.com
Secondary Address: 7525 E Virginia Street, Suite 430, Evansville, IN 47715, 888-652-9151
For Profit Organization: Yes
Year Founded: 1986

Healthplan and Services Defined
PLAN TYPE: HMO/PPO
Model Type: IPA
Benefits Offered: Disease Management, Wellness

Type of Coverage
Commercial, Individual, Medicare, Medicaid

Geographic Areas Served
(Southern Indiana) Boone, Clark, Crawford, Delaware, Dubois, Floyd, Gibson, Hamilton, Hancock, Harrison, Hendricks, Howard, Jackson, Jefferson, Jennings, Johnson, Knox, Lake, LaPorte, Madison, Marrion, Morgan, Orange, Pike, Porter, Posey, Scott, Shelby, Spencer, Tipton, Vanderburgh, Warrick, Washington

Accreditation Certification
URAC, NCQA, CORE

Key Personnel
President & CEO .... Bruce D. Broussard
Chief Medical Officer................. Roy A. Beveridge
Chief Consumer Officer................. Jody L. Bilney
Human Resources....................... Tim Huval
Chief Financial Officer .... Brian Kane
Chief Information Officer .... Brian LeClaire
General Counsel............... Christopher M. Todoroff

303 Mid America Health

1499 Windhorst Way
Suite 100
Greenwood, IN 46143
Toll-Free: 888-309-8239
Fax: 317-972-7969
mahweb.com

For Profit Organization: Yes
Year Founded: 1986

Healthplan and Services Defined
PLAN TYPE: Multiple
Plan Specialty: Behavioral Health, Dental, Vision

Geographic Areas Served
Correctional facilities, county jails, military installations and long-term care facilities nationwide

Key Personnel
President........................... Patrick Murphy
patrick@mahweb.com
VP of Operations .... Jose Lopez
jlopez@mahweb.com
Marketing/Sales Director............. Elizabeth McClure
emcclure@mahweb.com

304   Parkview Total Health

Toll-Free: 800-666-4449
Phone: 260-266-5510
www.parkviewtotalhealth.com
Non-Profit Organization: Yes
Year Founded: 1992

Healthplan and Services Defined
PLAN TYPE: PPO
Benefits Offered: Disease Management, Wellness

Type of Coverage
Commercial

Geographic Areas Served
Indiana & Northwestern Ohio

Network Qualifications
Pre-Admission Certification: Yes

Peer Review Type
Utilization Review: Yes
Second Surgical Opinion: No
Case Management: Yes

Accreditation Certification
TJC Accreditation, Medicare Approved, Utilization Review, Pre-Admission Certification, State Licensure, Quality Assurance Program

Key Personnel
Wellness Coordinator .... Courntey Drummond

Employer References
Parkview Hospitals, East Allen County Schools, Guardian Industries, Chore Timer Brook, Tomkins

305   Physicians Health Plan of Northern Indiana

8101 W Jefferson Boulevard
Fort Wayne, IN 46804
Toll-Free: 800-982-6257
Phone: 260-432-6690
Fax: 260-432-0493
custsvc@phpni.com
www.phpni.com
Non-Profit Organization: Yes
Year Founded: 1983

Physician Owned Organization: Yes
Federally Qualified: Yes

Healthplan and Services Defined
PLAN TYPE: HMO
Model Type: IPA, POS
Benefits Offered: Behavioral Health, Dental, Disease Management, Home Care, Physical Therapy, Podiatry, Prescription, Psychiatric, Transplant, Vision, Wellness, AD&D, Life, LTD, STD
Offers Demand Management Patient Information Service: Yes

Type of Coverage
Commercial, Individual
Catastrophic Illness Benefit: Unlimited

Type of Payment Plans Offered
POS, DFFS, FFS, Combination FFS & DFFS

Geographic Areas Served
40 Northern Indiana counties

Peer Review Type
Utilization Review: Yes
Case Management: Yes

Publishes and Distributes Report Card: Yes

Accreditation Certification
Utilization Review, Pre-Admission Certification, State Licensure, Quality Assurance Program

Key Personnel
Chairman .... James C. Stevens
Vice-Chairwoman .... Theresa A. Gutierrez
Secretary........................... Karl R. LePan
Treasurer .... Michael R. DeWald

Specialty Managed Care Partners
Enters into Contracts with Regional Business Coalitions: Yes

306   Renaissance Dental

P.O. Box 1596
Indianapolis, IN 46206-4596
Toll-Free: 800-963-4596
Fax: 800-963-4597
renaissancedental.com

Healthplan and Services Defined
PLAN TYPE: Dental
Plan Specialty: Dental
Benefits Offered: Dental

Type of Coverage
Supplemental Medicare

Geographic Areas Served
Georgia, Indiana, Kentucky, Michigan, New Mexico, New York, North Carolina, Ohio, and Tennessee

Key Personnel
President & CEO................... Robert P. Mulligan

307　Sagamore Health Network

11595 N Meridian Street
Suite 600
Carmel, IN 46032
Toll-Free: 800-364-3469
Phone: 317-573-2900
www.sagamorehn.com
Subsidiary of: Cigna
Year Founded: 1985

Healthplan and Services Defined
　PLAN TYPE: PPO
　Model Type: IPA

Geographic Areas Served
　Entire state of Indiana, Kentucky, Illinois, Michigan and
　Ohio

Accreditation Certification
　URAC
　TJC Accreditation, Medicare Approved, Utilization Review,
　　Pre-Admission Certification, State Licensure, Quality
　　Assurance Program

308　SIHO Insurance Services

417 Washington Street
Columbus, IN 47201
Toll-Free: 800-443-2980
Phone: 812-378-7070
memberservices@siho.org
www.siho.org
Mailing Address: P.O. Box 1787, Columbus, IN 47202-1787
Non-Profit Organization: Yes
Year Founded: 1987
Physician Owned Organization: Yes

Healthplan and Services Defined
　PLAN TYPE: HMO
　Model Type: IPA, Network, POS
　Plan Specialty: ASO, Dental, Disease Management, Vision
　Benefits Offered: Behavioral Health, Chiropractic, Dental,
　　Disease Management, Home Care, Inpatient SNF,
　　Long-Term Care, Physical Therapy, Prescription,
　　Transplant, Vision, Wellness, AD&D, Life, STD

Type of Coverage
　Individual, Indemnity, Medicaid
　Catastrophic Illness Benefit: Unlimited

Type of Payment Plans Offered
　POS, DFFS, FFS

Geographic Areas Served
　Bloomington, Columbus, Evansville, Indianapolis and
　Seymour

Network Qualifications
　Pre-Admission Certification: Yes

Peer Review Type
　Utilization Review: Yes
　Case Management: Yes

Publishes and Distributes Report Card: Yes

Accreditation Certification
　TJC Accreditation, Utilization Review, Pre-Admission
　　Certification, State Licensure

Key Personnel
　Chief Executive Officer. . . . . Dave Barker
　VP of Medical Management . . . . Hoskins Mary

Specialty Managed Care Partners
　Caremark Rx
　Enters into Contracts with Regional Business Coalitions: Yes

Employer References
　Columbus Regional Hospital, Enkei America, Seymour
　　Memorial Hospital, Seymour Tubing

309　Trinity Health of Indiana

Saint Joseph Health System
5215 Holy Cross Parkway
Mishawaka, IN 46545
Toll-Free: 855-887-5633
Phone: 574-335-5000
www.trinity-health.org
Subsidiary of: Trinity Health
Non-Profit Organization: Yes
Year Founded: 2013
Total Enrollment: 30,000,000

Healthplan and Services Defined
　PLAN TYPE: Other
　Benefits Offered: Disease Management, Home Care,
　　Long-Term Care, Psychiatric, Hospice programs, PACE
　　(Program of All Inclusive Care for the Elderly)

Geographic Areas Served
　North Central Indiana

Key Personnel
　Chief Executive Officer . . . . Richard J. Gilfillan
　Chief Financial Officer. . . . . Benjamin R. Carter
　Human Resources. . . . . Edmund F. Hodge
　General Counsel . . . . Paul G. Neumann
　Chief Clinical Officer. . . . . Daniel J. Roth
　Chief Operating Officer . . . . Michael A. Slubowski

310　UnitedHealthcare of Indiana

7440 Woodland Drive
Dept 100
Indianapolis, IN 46278
Toll-Free: 800-382-5445
www.uhc.com/contact-us/indiana
Subsidiary of: UnitedHealth Group
For Profit Organization: Yes
Year Founded: 1986

Healthplan and Services Defined
　PLAN TYPE: HMO/PPO
　Model Type: Network
　Plan Specialty: Behavioral Health, Dental, Disease
　　Management, PBM, Vision
　Benefits Offered: Behavioral Health, Chiropractic, Dental,
　　Disease Management, Home Care, Inpatient SNF,

Long-Term Care, Podiatry, Prescription, Psychiatric,
Transplant, Vision, Wellness, Life, LTD, STD

Type of Coverage

Commercial, Individual, Medicare, Supplemental Medicare,
Medicaid, Catastrophic, Family, Military, Veterans, Group,

Type of Payment Plans Offered

POS

Geographic Areas Served

Statewide

Subscriber Information

Average Monthly Fee Per Subscriber
(Employee + Employer Contribution):
Employee Only (Self): Varies per plan
Employee & 2 Family Members: Variers per plan
Average Annual Deductible Per Subscriber:
Employee Only (Self): Varies per plan
Employee & 2 Family Members: Varies per plan
Average Subscriber Co-Payment:
Primary Care Physician: Varies per plan

Accreditation Certification

TJC

Key Personnel

President . . . . David Wichmann
Chief Operating Officer . . . . Dan Schumacher
Chief Strategy Officer . . . . John Cosgriff
Communications Officer . . . . Kirsten Gorsuch
Chief Medical Officer. . . . . Sam Ho
Chief Legal Officer . . . . Thad Johnson
Chief Information Officer . . . . Phil McKoy
Chief Financial Officer. . . . . Jeff Putnam

Health Insurance Coverage Status and Type of Coverage by Age

Category	All Persons		Under 18 years		Under 65 years	
	Number	%	Number	%	Number	%
Total population	3,091	-	773	-	2,600	-
Covered by some type of health insurance	2,960 *(8)*	95.7 *(0.2)*	753 *(5)*	97.4 *(0.4)*	2,469 *(8)*	95.0 *(0.3)*
Covered by private health insurance	2,327 *(17)*	75.3 *(0.6)*	526 *(9)*	68.0 *(1.2)*	1,999 *(17)*	76.9 *(0.6)*
Employer-based	1,859 *(18)*	60.1 *(0.6)*	472 *(10)*	61.1 *(1.3)*	1,743 *(18)*	67.0 *(0.7)*
Direct purchase	530 *(12)*	17.1 *(0.4)*	57 *(4)*	7.4 *(0.5)*	296 *(11)*	11.4 *(0.4)*
TRICARE	52 *(5)*	1.7 *(0.2)*	10 *(2)*	1.3 *(0.3)*	34 *(4)*	1.3 *(0.2)*
Covered by public health insurance	1,069 *(16)*	34.6 *(0.5)*	275 *(10)*	35.5 *(1.3)*	589 *(16)*	22.7 *(0.6)*
Medicaid	591 *(15)*	19.1 *(0.5)*	272 *(10)*	35.2 *(1.3)*	539 *(15)*	20.7 *(0.6)*
Medicare	545 *(5)*	17.6 *(0.2)*	3 *(1)*	0.4 *(0.1)*	66 *(4)*	2.5 *(0.2)*
VA Care	79 *(3)*	2.5 *(0.1)*	2 *(1)*	0.2 *(0.1)*	29 *(2)*	1.1 *(0.1)*
Not covered at any time during the year	132 *(8)*	4.3 *(0.2)*	20 *(3)*	2.6 *(0.4)*	131 *(8)*	5.0 *(0.3)*

Note: Numbers in thousands; Figures cover civilian noninstitutionalized population in 2016; N/A indicates that data was not available; Z represents or rounds to zero; Margin of error appears in parenthesis and is calculated using replicate weights.
Source: U.S. Census Bureau, American Community Survey, Table HIC-4_ACS. Health Insurance Coverage Status and Type of Coverage by State—All People: 2008 to 2016, Table HIC-5_ACS. Health Insurance Coverage Status and Type of Coverage by State—Children Under 18: 2008 to 2016, Table HIC-6_ACS. Health Insurance Coverage Status and Type of Coverage by State—Persons Under 65: 2008 to 2016

Iowa

311 Aetna Health of Iowa

151 Farmington Avenue
Hartford, CT 06156
Toll-Free: 800-872-3862
Phone: 860-273-0123
www.aetna.com
Secondary Address: 6730-B Rockledge Drive, Suite 700, Bethesda, MD 20817, 301-581-0600
Subsidiary of: Aetna Inc.
For Profit Organization: Yes

Healthplan and Services Defined
PLAN TYPE: PPO
Other Type: POS
Model Type: Network
Plan Specialty: Behavioral Health, Dental, EPO, Lab, PBM, Vision, Radiology
Benefits Offered: Behavioral Health, Dental, Disease Management, Long-Term Care, Physical Therapy, Podiatry, Prescription, Psychiatric, Vision, Wellness, Life, LTD, STD

Type of Coverage
Commercial, Student health

Type of Payment Plans Offered
POS, FFS

Geographic Areas Served
Statewide

Key Personnel
CEO . . . . Mark Bertolini

312 Amerigroup Iowa

PO Box 71099
Clive, IA 50325
Toll-Free: 800-338-8366
www.myamerigroup.com/ia
Subsidiary of: Anthem, Inc.
For Profit Organization: Yes

Healthplan and Services Defined
PLAN TYPE: HMO
Model Type: Network
Plan Specialty: Behavioral Health, Disease Management, Lab, Vision, Managed health care for people in public programs. Mental health and substance abuse services.
Benefits Offered: Behavioral Health, Disease Management, Physical Therapy, Podiatry, Prescription, Vision, Wellness

Type of Coverage
Medicaid

Key Personnel
Executive Vice President . . . . Peter D. Haytaian

313 Coventry Health Care of Iowa

4320 114th Street
Urbandale, IA 50322-5408
Toll-Free: 800-470-6352
Phone: 515-225-1234
chciowa.coventryhealthcare.com
Subsidiary of: Aetna Inc.
For Profit Organization: Yes

Healthplan and Services Defined
PLAN TYPE: HMO/PPO
Model Type: Network
Plan Specialty: Behavioral Health, Dental, Worker's Compensation
Benefits Offered: Behavioral Health, Dental, Prescription, Wellness, Worker's Compensation

Type of Coverage
Commercial, Individual, Medicare, Medicaid

Geographic Areas Served
Central Iowa & South Dakota

Key Personnel
Chief Executive Officer . . . . Mark T. Bertolini
President . . . . Karen S. Lynch
Chief Financial Officer . . . . Shawn M. Guertin
Operations & Technology . . . . Meg McCarthy
Chief Medical Officer . . . . Harold L. Paz
General Counsel . . . . Thomas Sabatino Jr.
Government Servives . . . . Fran S. Soistman

314 Delta Dental of Iowa

P.O. Box 9010
Johnston, IA 50131-9010
Phone: 800-544-0718
Fax: 888-264-1440
www.deltadentalia.com
Non-Profit Organization: Yes
Year Founded: 1970

Healthplan and Services Defined
PLAN TYPE: Dental
Other Type: Dental PPO
Model Type: Network
Plan Specialty: Dental
Benefits Offered: Dental

Type of Coverage
Commercial

Type of Payment Plans Offered
DFFS

Geographic Areas Served
Statewide

Publishes and Distributes Report Card: Yes

Key Personnel
President & CEO . . . . Jeff Russell
VP, Operations . . . . Liz Myers
VP & Dental Director . . . . Jeffrey Chaffin
VP, Finance & Controller . . . . Sherry Perkins
VP, Marketing . . . . April Schmaltz
VP, Technology . . . . Todd Herren

315   hawk-i Healthy and Well Kids in Iowa

Toll-Free: 800-257-8563
Fax: 515-457-7701
hawk-i@dhs.state.ia.us
www.hawk-i.org

Healthplan and Services Defined
PLAN TYPE: HMO
Plan Specialty: Chiropractic, Dental, Vision
Benefits Offered: Behavioral Health, Chiropractic, Dental,
Home Care, Prescription, Vision, Wellness

Geographic Areas Served
Statewide

316   Humana Health Insurance of Iowa

1415 Kimberly Road
Bettendorf, IA 52722
Toll-Free: 866-653-7275
Phone: 563-344-1242
Fax: 563-355-0730
www.humana.com
For Profit Organization: Yes
Year Founded: 1961
Federally Qualified: Yes

Healthplan and Services Defined
PLAN TYPE: HMO/PPO
Model Type: Staff
Plan Specialty: Dental
Benefits Offered: Behavioral Health, Chiropractic, Dental,
Disease Management, Prescription, Psychiatric, Wellness,
Worker's Compensation, Life, LTD, STD

Type of Coverage
Commercial, Individual, Supplemental Medicare

Accreditation Certification
URAC, NCQA, CORE

Key Personnel
President & CEO . . . . Bruce D. Broussard
Chief Medical Officer. . . . . Roy A. Beveridge
Chief Consumer Officer. . . . . Jody L. Bilney
Human Resources. . . . . Tim Huval
Chief Financial Officer . . . . Brian Kane
Chief Information Officer . . . . Brian LeClaire
General Counsel. . . . . Christopher M. Todoroff

317   Medical Associates

1500 Associates Drive
Dubuque, IA 52002
Toll-Free: 800-648-6868
Phone: 563-584-3000
www.mahealthcare.com
Non-Profit Organization: Yes
Year Founded: 1982
Physician Owned Organization: Yes
Number of Primary Care Physicians: 170
Number of Referral/Specialty Physicians: 1,000
Total Enrollment: 45,000

Healthplan and Services Defined
PLAN TYPE: HMO
Model Type: Group
Plan Specialty: EPO
Benefits Offered: Behavioral Health, Chiropractic,
Complementary Medicine, Home Care, Inpatient SNF,
Physical Therapy, Podiatry, Prescription, Psychiatric,
Transplant, Vision, Wellness

Type of Coverage
Commercial, Indemnity, Medicare, Supplemental Medicare

Type of Payment Plans Offered
POS

Geographic Areas Served
Iowa-Wisconsin-Illinois tri-state area

Accreditation Certification
NCQA

Key Personnel
CEO . . . . John Tallent
Director of Finance . . . . Jill Mitchell
Chief Operating Officer . . . . Zach Keeling

318   Mercy Health Network

1755 59th Place
West Des Moines, IA 50266
Phone: 515-358-8027
Fax: 515-358-8931
mhninfo@mercydesmoines.org
www.mercyhealthnetwork.com
Year Founded: 1998
Number of Affiliated Hospitals: 15

Healthplan and Services Defined
PLAN TYPE: HMO
Plan Specialty: Lab, Cardiac Care
Benefits Offered: Disease Management, Home Care, Physical
Therapy, Prescription, Wellness

Type of Coverage
Individual

Geographic Areas Served
Clinton, Des Moines, Dubuque, North Iowa, Sioux City

Key Personnel
Chief Executive Officer. . . . . Bob Ritz
SVP, Human Resources . . . . Barbara Gessel
bgessel@mercydesmoines.org
VP of Marketing . . . . Janell Pittman
jpittman@mercydesmoines.org
VP, General Counsel . . . . Marcia Smith

319   Sanford Health Plan

300 Cherapa Place
Suite 201
Sioux Falls, SD 57103
Toll-Free: 877-305-5463
Phone: 605-328-6868
memberservices@sanfordhealth.org
www.sanfordhealthplan.org
Mailing Address: P.O. Box 91110, Sioux Falls, SD 57109-1110

Non-Profit Organization: Yes
Year Founded: 1996
Total Enrollment: 50,000

Healthplan and Services Defined
  PLAN TYPE: HMO
  Model Type: IPA
  Plan Specialty: Commercial Group
  Benefits Offered: Disease Management, Home Care,
    Long-Term Care, Prescription, Wellness

Type of Coverage
  Commercial, Individual, Medicare, Supplemental Medicare,
    Sec 125, TPA, Individual, Lg Group

Geographic Areas Served
  Northwest Iowa, Southwest Minnesota, South Dakota

Accreditation Certification
  NCQA

---

320   Trinity Health of Iowa
Mercy Medical Center
1410 N Fourth Street
Clinton, IA 52732
Phone: 563-244-5555
www.trinity-health.org
Subsidiary of: Trinity Health
Non-Profit Organization: Yes
Year Founded: 2013

Healthplan and Services Defined
  PLAN TYPE: Other
  Benefits Offered: Disease Management, Home Care,
    Long-Term Care, Psychiatric, Hospice programs, PACE
    (Program of All Inclusive Care for the Elderly)

Geographic Areas Served
  Statewide

Key Personnel
  Chief Executive Officer . . . . Richard J. Gilfillan
  Chief Financial Officer. . . . . Benjamin R. Carter
  Human Resources. . . . . Edmund F. Hodge
  General Counsel . . . . Paul G. Neumann
  Chief Clinical Officer. . . . . Daniel J. Roth
  Chief Operating Officer . . . . Michael A. Slubowski

---

321   UnitedHealthcare of Iowa
1089 Jordan Creek Parkway
Suite 320
West Des Moines, IA 50266
Toll-Free: 800-669-1830
www.uhc.com/contact-us/iowa
Subsidiary of: UnitedHealth Group
For Profit Organization: Yes
Year Founded: 1984

Healthplan and Services Defined
  PLAN TYPE: HMO/PPO
  Model Type: Network
  Plan Specialty: Behavioral Health, Dental, Disease
    Management, PBM, Vision

Benefits Offered: Behavioral Health, Dental, Disease
  Management, Long-Term Care, Prescription, Vision,
  Wellness, Life, LTD, STD

Type of Coverage
  Commercial, Individual, Indemnity, Medicare, Supplemental
    Medicare, Medicaid, Catastrophic, Family, Military,
    Veterans, Group,

Type of Payment Plans Offered
  POS, DFFS, FFS

Geographic Areas Served
  Statewide

Network Qualifications
  Pre-Admission Certification: Yes

Peer Review Type
  Utilization Review: Yes
  Second Surgical Opinion: Yes
  Case Management: Yes

Publishes and Distributes Report Card: Yes

Accreditation Certification
  TJC Accreditation, Medicare Approved, Utilization Review,
    Pre-Admission Certification, State Licensure, Quality
    Assurance Program

Key Personnel
  President . . . . David Wichmann
  Chief Operating Officer . . . . Dan Schumacher
  Chief Strategy Officer . . . . John Cosgriff
  Communications Officer . . . . Kirsten Gorsuch
  Chief Medical Officer. . . . . Sam Ho
  Chieg Legal Officer. . . . . Thad Johnson
  Chief Information Officer . . . . Phil McKoy
  Chief Financial Officer. . . . . Jeff Putnam

---

322   Wellmark Blue Cross Blue Shield
1331 Grand Avenue
Des Moines, IA 50309
Toll-Free: 800-524-9242
Phone: 515-376-4500
www.wellmark.com
Year Founded: 1939

Healthplan and Services Defined
  PLAN TYPE: HMO
  Model Type: IPA
  Plan Specialty: ASO, Chiropractic, Disease Management,
    Lab, Vision, Radiology, UR
  Benefits Offered: Chiropractic, Disease Management, Home
    Care, Inpatient SNF, Physical Therapy, Podiatry,
    Prescription, Psychiatric, Transplant, Vision, Wellness
  Offers Demand Management Patient Information Service: Yes

Type of Coverage
  Commercial, Individual, Indemnity, Medicare, Supplemental
    Medicare, Medicaid

Type of Payment Plans Offered
  POS, Capitated

Geographic Areas Served

Statewide except Alamakee, Winneshiek, Fayette, Des Moines and Dubuque counties

Network Qualifications

Pre-Admission Certification: Yes

Peer Review Type

Utilization Review: Yes

Publishes and Distributes Report Card: Yes

Accreditation Certification

URAC, NCQA

TJC Accreditation, Medicare Approved, Utilization Review, Pre-Admission Certification, State Licensure, Quality Assurance Program

Key Personnel

Chairman & CEO . . . . John D. Forsyth
Chief Financial Officer . . . . David Brown
Chief Information Officer . . . . Paul Eddy
Admin. & Legal Officer . . . . Cory R. Harris
Chief Operating Officer . . . . Vicki Signor

Health Insurance Coverage Status and Type of Coverage by Age

Category	All Persons		Under 18 years		Under 65 years	
	Number	%	Number	%	Number	%
Total population	2,851	-	758	-	2,431	-
Covered by some type of health insurance	2,602 *(9)*	91.3 *(0.3)*	724 *(5)*	95.5 *(0.4)*	2,185 *(9)*	89.9 *(0.4)*
Covered by private health insurance	2,142 *(16)*	75.1 *(0.6)*	521 *(9)*	68.7 *(1.1)*	1,860 *(16)*	76.5 *(0.7)*
Employer-based	1,652 *(19)*	58.0 *(0.7)*	433 *(10)*	57.2 *(1.3)*	1,546 *(18)*	63.6 *(0.8)*
Direct purchase	499 *(14)*	17.5 *(0.5)*	73 *(7)*	9.7 *(0.9)*	306 *(14)*	12.6 *(0.6)*
TRICARE	116 *(6)*	4.1 *(0.2)*	33 *(3)*	4.4 *(0.4)*	87 *(6)*	3.6 *(0.2)*
Covered by public health insurance	831 *(13)*	29.2 *(0.5)*	239 *(9)*	31.5 *(1.2)*	423 *(13)*	17.4 *(0.5)*
Medicaid	401 *(13)*	14.1 *(0.4)*	236 *(9)*	31.1 *(1.2)*	359 *(12)*	14.8 *(0.5)*
Medicare	476 *(4)*	16.7 *(0.2)*	3 *(1)*	0.4 *(0.2)*	68 *(4)*	2.8 *(0.2)*
VA Care	72 *(4)*	2.5 *(0.1)*	1 *(Z)*	0.1 *(0.1)*	32 *(3)*	1.3 *(0.1)*
Not covered at any time during the year	249 *(9)*	8.7 *(0.3)*	34 *(3)*	4.5 *(0.4)*	247 *(9)*	10.1 *(0.4)*

Note: Numbers in thousands; Figures cover civilian noninstitutionalized population in 2016; N/A indicates that data was not available; Z represents or rounds to zero; Margin of error appears in parenthesis and is calculated using replicate weights.
Source: U.S. Census Bureau, American Community Survey, Table HIC-4_ACS. Health Insurance Coverage Status and Type of Coverage by State—All People: 2008 to 2016, Table HIC-5_ACS. Health Insurance Coverage Status and Type of Coverage by State—Children Under 18: 2008 to 2016, Table HIC-6_ACS. Health Insurance Coverage Status and Type of Coverage by State—Persons Under 65: 2008 to 2016

Kansas

323 Advance Insurance Company of Kansas

1133 SW Topeka Boulevard
Topeka, KS 66629
Toll-Free: 800-530-5989
Phone: 785-273-9804
Fax: 785-290-0727
claims@advanceinsurance.com
www.advanceinsurance.com
Subsidiary of: Blue Cross & Blue Shield of Kansas
For Profit Organization: Yes
Total Enrollment: 134,000

Healthplan and Services Defined
  PLAN TYPE: Multiple
  Benefits Offered: AD&D, Life, LTD, STD

Key Personnel
  President & CEO . . . . Andrew C. Corbin

324 Aetna Health of Kansas

151 Farmington Avenue
Hartford, CT 06156
Toll-Free: 800-872-3862
Phone: 860-273-0123
www.aetna.com
Secondary Address: 6730-B Rockledge Drive, Suite 700,
  Bethesda, MD 20817, 301-581-0600
Subsidiary of: Aetna Inc.
For Profit Organization: Yes

Healthplan and Services Defined
  PLAN TYPE: HMO/PPO
  Other Type: POS
  Model Type: Network
  Plan Specialty: Behavioral Health, Dental, EPO, Lab, PBM,
    Vision, Radiology
  Benefits Offered: Behavioral Health, Dental, Disease
    Management, Long-Term Care, Physical Therapy,
    Podiatry, Prescription, Psychiatric, Vision, Wellness, Life,
    LTD, STD

Type of Coverage
  Commercial, Medicare, Medicaid, Student health

Geographic Areas Served
  Statewide

Key Personnel
  CEO . . . . Mark Bertolini

325 Aetna Health of Kansas

151 Farmington Avenue
Hartford, CT 06156
Toll-Free: 800-872-3862
Phone: 860-273-0123
www.aetna.com
Secondary Address: 6730-B Rockledge Drive, Suite 700,
  Bethesda, MD 20817, 301-581-0600
Subsidiary of: Aetna Inc.
For Profit Organization: Yes

Healthplan and Services Defined
  PLAN TYPE: HMO/PPO
  Other Type: POS
  Model Type: Network
  Plan Specialty: Behavioral Health, Dental, EPO, Lab, PBM,
    Vision, Radiology
  Benefits Offered: Behavioral Health, Dental, Disease
    Management, Long-Term Care, Physical Therapy, Podiatry,
    Prescription, Psychiatric, Vision, Wellness, Life, LTD, STD

Type of Coverage
  Commercial, Student health

Type of Payment Plans Offered
  POS, FFS

Geographic Areas Served
  Statewide

Key Personnel
  CEO . . . . Mark Bertolini

326 Ascension At Home

Via Christi Home Health
555 S Washington, Suite 103
Wichita, KS 67211
Phone: 316-268-8588
Fax: 316-264-1265
ascensionathome.com
Non-Profit Organization: Yes

Healthplan and Services Defined
  PLAN TYPE: Other
  Plan Specialty: Disease Management
  Benefits Offered: Dental, Disease Management, Home Care,
    Wellness, Ambulance & Transportation; Nursing Service;
    Short-and-long-term care management planning; Hospice

Geographic Areas Served
  Texas, Alabama, Indiana, Kansas, Michigan, Mississippi,
  Oklahoma, Wisconsin

Key Personnel
  President . . . . Kirk Allen
  Dir., Home Health Service . . . . Darcy Burthay

327 Blue Cross and Blue Shield of Kansas

1133 SW Topeka Boulevard
Topeka, KS 66629
Toll-Free: 800-432-3990
Phone: 785-291-4180
Fax: 785-290-0754
www.bcbsks.com
For Profit Organization: Yes
Year Founded: 1942
State Enrollment: 880,000

Healthplan and Services Defined
  PLAN TYPE: HMO
  Model Type: Staff
  Benefits Offered: Chiropractic, Disease Management,
    Inpatient SNF, Podiatry, Psychiatric, Wellness

Type of Coverage
  Commercial, Individual

Geographic Areas Served
All counties in Kansas except Johnson and Wyandotte

Subscriber Information
Average Annual Deductible Per Subscriber:
Employee Only (Self): $1,000
Employee & 2 Family Members: $2,000
Average Subscriber Co-Payment:
Primary Care Physician: $15.00
Prescription Drugs: $5.00
Hospital ER: $50.00

Accreditation Certification
TJC, URAC

Key Personnel
President & CEO . . . . Andrew Corbin

328 CareCentrix: Kansas
6130 Sprint Parkway
Suite 200
Overland Park, KS 66211
Toll-Free: 800-808-1902
carecentrix.com
Year Founded: 1996
Number of Primary Care Physicians: 8,000

Healthplan and Services Defined
PLAN TYPE: HMO
Benefits Offered: Home Care, Physical Therapy, Durable
Medical Equipment; Occupational & Respiratory Therapy;
Orthotics; Prosthetics

Key Personnel
Chief Executive Officer . . . . John Driscoll
Chief Data Officer. . . . . Tej Anand
Chief Medical Officer. . . . . Michael Cantor
Chief Operating Officer . . . . Mary Daschner
Chief Customer Officer . . . . Tom Gaffney

329 Coventry Health Care of Kansas
8535 East 21st Street N
Wichita, KS 67206
Toll-Free: 800-289-0345
chckansas.coventryhealthcare.com
Secondary Address: 9401 Indian Creek Parkway, Suite 1300,
Overland Park, KS 66210, 800-969-3343
Subsidiary of: Aetna Inc.
For Profit Organization: Yes
Year Founded: 1976

Healthplan and Services Defined
PLAN TYPE: HMO/PPO
Other Type: POS
Plan Specialty: Behavioral Health, Dental, Worker's
Compensation
Benefits Offered: Behavioral Health, Dental, Prescription,
Wellness, Worker's Compensation, Alternative and
complementary care services include discounts on massage
therapy, acupuncture and chiropractic services.

Type of Coverage
Commercial, Individual, Medicare, Supplemental Medicare,
Medicaid
Catastrophic Illness Benefit: Covered

Type of Payment Plans Offered
DFFS

Geographic Areas Served
Kansas, Missouri, Oklahoma

Subscriber Information
Average Monthly Fee Per Subscriber
(Employee + Employer Contribution):
Employee Only (Self): Varies
Average Annual Deductible Per Subscriber:
Employee & 2 Family Members: None
Average Subscriber Co-Payment:
Primary Care Physician: $10.00
Prescription Drugs: $5.00/15.00
Hospital ER: $50
Home Health Care: None
Nursing Home: None

Peer Review Type
Second Surgical Opinion: Yes
Case Management: Yes

Publishes and Distributes Report Card: Yes

Accreditation Certification
URAC, NCQA
Medicare Approved, Utilization Review, Pre-Admission
Certification, State Licensure, Quality Assurance Program

Key Personnel
Chairman & CEO . . . . Mark T. Bertolini
President. . . . . Karen S. Lynch
Chief Financial Officer . . . . Shawn M. Guertin
Operations & Technology . . . . Meg McCarthy
Chief Medical Officer . . . . Harold L. Paz
General Counsel . . . . Thomas Sabatino Jr.
Government Services . . . . Fran S. Soistman

Specialty Managed Care Partners
Enters into Contracts with Regional Business Coalitions: Yes

330 Delta Dental of Kansas
1619 N Waterfront Parkway
P.O. Box 789769
Wichita, KS 67278-9769
Toll-Free: 800-234-3375
Phone: 316-264-4511
Fax: 316-462-3392
moreinfo@deltadentalks.com
www.deltadentalks.com
Secondary Address: 11300 Tomahawk Creek Parkway,
Pinnacle Corporate Centre, Suite 350, Leawood, KS 66211,
913-381-4928
Non-Profit Organization: Yes
Year Founded: 1972

Healthplan and Services Defined
PLAN TYPE: Dental
Other Type: Dental PPO

Model Type: Network
Plan Specialty: Dental
Benefits Offered: Dental

Type of Coverage
Commercial, Individual

Type of Payment Plans Offered
DFFS

Geographic Areas Served
Statewide

Network Qualifications
Pre-Admission Certification: Yes

Publishes and Distributes Report Card: Yes

Key Personnel
President & CEO.....................Michael Herbert
EVP & Managing Director ....Dean Newton
Chief Financial Officer...................Michael Ellis
Chief Operating Officer..................Patrick Tuttle
In-House Counsel.....................Jennifer Bauer
VP, Information......................Bob Ebenkamp

331 Health Partners of Kansas

550 N Lorraine Street
Wichita, KS 67214
Phone: 316-652-1327
www.hpkansas.com
Subsidiary of: Wesley Medical Center
For Profit Organization: Yes
Year Founded: 1987
Number of Affiliated Hospitals: 149
Number of Primary Care Physicians: 1,000
Number of Referral/Specialty Physicians: 6,000
Total Enrollment: 95,000
State Enrollment: 95,000

Healthplan and Services Defined
PLAN TYPE: PPO
Model Type: IPA, Network
Benefits Offered: Worker's Compensation, Network Rental, Provider Servicing, Provider Credentialing

Type of Coverage
Catastrophic Illness Benefit: Maximum $1M

Type of Payment Plans Offered
POS, DFFS, Capitated, FFS, Combination FFS & DFFS

Geographic Areas Served
Statewide

Network Qualifications
Pre-Admission Certification: Yes

Peer Review Type
Utilization Review: Yes
Second Surgical Opinion: Yes
Case Management: Yes

Key Personnel
President ....Gaylee Dolloff
Vice President.....................Teresa Montenegro
Provider Services ....Angie Newton

Specialty Managed Care Partners
Enters into Contracts with Regional Business Coalitions: No

332 Humana Health Insurance of Kansas

7311 W 132nd Street
Suite 200
Overland Park, KS 66213
Toll-Free: 800-842-6188
Phone: 913-217-3300
Fax: 913-217-3245
www.humana.com
For Profit Organization: Yes
Year Founded: 1985

Healthplan and Services Defined
PLAN TYPE: HMO/PPO
Model Type: IPA
Plan Specialty: Dental, Vision
Benefits Offered: Dental, Disease Management, Prescription, Vision, Wellness, Life, LTD, STD

Type of Coverage
Commercial, Individual

Geographic Areas Served
Kansas City metro area

Subscriber Information
Average Monthly Fee Per Subscriber
(Employee + Employer Contribution):
Employee Only (Self): $150.44
Employee & 1 Family Member: $354.06
Employee & 2 Family Members: $354.06
Medicare: $196.48
Average Subscriber Co-Payment:
Primary Care Physician: $5.00
Non-Network Physician: Not covered
Prescription Drugs: $5.00
Hospital ER: $25.00
Home Health Care: $0
Nursing Home: $0
Nursing Home Max. Days/Visits Covered: 60 days

Accreditation Certification
URAC, NCQA, CORE

Key Personnel
President & CEO.....................Bruce Broussard
Chief Medical Officer.................Roy A. Beveridge
Chief Consumer Officer.................Jody L. Bilney
Human Resources........................Tim Huval
Chief Financial Officer ....Brian Kane
Chief Information Officer................Brian Leclaire
General Counsel ....Christopher M. Todoroff

Average Claim Compensation
Physician's Fees Charged: 70%
Hospital's Fees Charged: 60%

Specialty Managed Care Partners
Enters into Contracts with Regional Business Coalitions: Yes

333 Mercy Clinic Kansas

220 N Pennsylviania
Columbus, KS 66725
Phone: 620-429-2545
mercy.net
Subsidiary of: IBM Watson Health
Non-Profit Organization: Yes
Number of Affiliated Hospitals: 44
Number of Primary Care Physicians: 700
Number of Referral/Specialty Physicians: 2,000

Healthplan and Services Defined
PLAN TYPE: HMO
Benefits Offered: Behavioral Health, Disease Management,
Home Care, Physical Therapy, Podiatry, Vision, Wellness,
Non-Surgical Weight Loss; Urgent Care; Dermatology;
Rehabilitation; Breast Cancer; Orthopedics; Ostoclerosis;
Pediatrics

Geographic Areas Served
Arkansas, Kansas, Missouri, and Oklahoma

Key Personnel
General Manager . . . . Deborah DiSanzo

334 PCC Preferred Chiropractic Care

555 North McLean Boulevard
Suite 200
Wichita, KS 67203
Toll-Free: 800-611-3048
Phone: 316-263-7800
Fax: 316-263-7814
providerrelations@pccnetwork.com
www.pccnetwork.com
For Profit Organization: Yes
Year Founded: 1984
Physician Owned Organization: No
Federally Qualified: No
Number of Primary Care Physicians: 3,500
Total Enrollment: 5,000,000

Healthplan and Services Defined
PLAN TYPE: PPO
Model Type: Network
Plan Specialty: Chiropractic
Benefits Offered: Chiropractic, Disease Management,
Wellness, Worker's Compensation
Offers Demand Management Patient Information Service:
Yes
DMPI Services Offered: Chiropractic, Physical Therapy

Type of Coverage
Medicaid

Type of Payment Plans Offered
POS, DFFS, Capitated, FFS, Combination FFS & DFFS

Geographic Areas Served
Nationwide

Network Qualifications
Pre-Admission Certification: No

Peer Review Type
Utilization Review: Yes

Second Surgical Opinion: Yes
Case Management: No

Publishes and Distributes Report Card: No

Accreditation Certification
URAC, NCQA

Key Personnel
President and CEO . . . . Brad Dopps, DC

Average Claim Compensation
Physician's Fees Charged: 80%

Specialty Managed Care Partners
Enters into Contracts with Regional Business Coalitions: Yes

Employer References
Preferred Health Systems, fiserv, Health Partners of Kansas

335 Preferred Mental Health Management

7309 E 21st N Street
Suite 110
Wichita, KS 67206
Toll-Free: 800-819-9571
Phone: 316-262-0444
providerrelations@pmhm.com
www.pmhm.com
Subsidiary of: Family Health America
Year Founded: 1987
Number of Affiliated Hospitals: 1,900
Number of Primary Care Physicians: 10,500
Number of Referral/Specialty Physicians: 4,000
Total Enrollment: 400,000

Healthplan and Services Defined
PLAN TYPE: Multiple
Model Type: Network
Plan Specialty: Mental Health
Benefits Offered: Behavioral Health, Prescription, Psychiatric,
Substance Abuse
Offers Demand Management Patient Information Service: Yes

Type of Coverage
Work

Geographic Areas Served
Nationwide including Puerto Rico

Network Qualifications
Minimum Years of Practice: 6
Pre-Admission Certification: Yes

Peer Review Type
Utilization Review: Yes

Publishes and Distributes Report Card: Yes

Accreditation Certification
URAC, NCQA
TJC Accreditation, Utilization Review, Pre-Admission
Certification, State Licensure, Quality Assurance Program

Key Personnel
President and CEO . . . . Les Ruthven, PhD
316-262-0444

Specialty Managed Care Partners
Enters into Contracts with Regional Business Coalitions: No

336 Preferred Vision Care

P.O. Box 26025
Overland Park, KS 66225-6025
Phone: 913-451-1672
Fax: 913-451-1704
customerservice@preferredvisioncare.com
preferredvisioncare.com
For Profit Organization: Yes
Owned by an Integrated Delivery Network (IDN): Yes

Healthplan and Services Defined
PLAN TYPE: Vision
Other Type: PPO
Model Type: Network
Plan Specialty: Vision
Benefits Offered: Vision

Type of Coverage
Commercial
Catastrophic Illness Benefit: Unlimited

Type of Payment Plans Offered
POS, DFFS

Network Qualifications
Pre-Admission Certification: No

Peer Review Type
Utilization Review: Yes
Second Surgical Opinion: Yes
Case Management: Yes

Publishes and Distributes Report Card: Yes

Accreditation Certification
URAC
Quality Assurance Program

Key Personnel
CEO . . . . Michele G. Disser, RN

Specialty Managed Care Partners
Enters into Contracts with Regional Business Coalitions: Yes

337 ProviDRs Care Network

1102 S Hillside
Wichita, KS 67211
Toll-Free: 800-801-9772
Phone: 316-683-4111
customerservice@providrscare.net
www.providrscare.net
Subsidiary of: Medical Society Medical Review Foundation
For Profit Organization: Yes
Year Founded: 1985
Physician Owned Organization: Yes
Number of Affiliated Hospitals: 157
Number of Primary Care Physicians: 11,000
Number of Referral/Specialty Physicians: 700
Total Enrollment: 152,000

Healthplan and Services Defined
PLAN TYPE: PPO
Model Type: Group
Benefits Offered: Behavioral Health, Chiropractic, Home
Care, Physical Therapy, Podiatry, Psychiatric, Transplant,
Worker's Compensation

Type of Coverage
Commercial, Individual

Type of Payment Plans Offered
POS

Geographic Areas Served
Kansas, Southwest Missouri; parts of Oklahoma and
Nebraska; 1 county in Colorado

Subscriber Information
Average Monthly Fee Per Subscriber
(Employee + Employer Contribution):
Employee Only (Self): $3.00
Employee & 1 Family Member: $3.00
Employee & 2 Family Members: $3.00
Average Annual Deductible Per Subscriber:
Employee Only (Self): Varies
Employee & 1 Family Member: Varies
Average Subscriber Co-Payment:
Primary Care Physician: Varies
Non-Network Physician: Varies
Prescription Drugs: Varies
Hospital ER: Varies

Network Qualifications
Pre-Admission Certification: Yes

Peer Review Type
Utilization Review: Yes
Second Surgical Opinion: Yes
Case Management: No

Publishes and Distributes Report Card: No

Accreditation Certification
URAC
TJC Accreditation, Medicare Approved, Utilization Review,
Pre-Admission Certification, State Licensure, Quality
Assurance Program

Key Personnel
Chief Executive Officer . . . . Karen Cox
316-683-0665
karencox@providrscare.net
Operations Coordinataor. . . . . Kirsten Haas
316-683-0679
kirstenhaas@providrscare.net
Support Specialist . . . . Jeanne Hingst
jeannehingst@providrscare.net
Director of Operations . . . . Nikki Sade
316-683-0805
nikkisade@providrscare.net

Specialty Managed Care Partners
Enters into Contracts with Regional Business Coalitions: No

Employer References
Western Resources, Kansas Health Insurance Association,
Medicalodges, County of Reno Kansas, National
Cooperative of Refineries Association

338 UniCare Kansas

825 Kansas Avenue
Suite 101
Topeka, KS 66608-1210
Toll-Free: 877-864-2273
www.unicare.com
Secondary Address: 327 North Hillside Road, Wichita, KS
67214
Subsidiary of: Anthem, Inc.
For Profit Organization: Yes
Year Founded: 1995

Healthplan and Services Defined
PLAN TYPE: HMO/PPO
Model Type: Network
Benefits Offered: Behavioral Health, Chiropractic,
Complementary Medicine, Dental, Disease Management,
Home Care, Inpatient SNF, Long-Term Care, Physical
Therapy, Podiatry, Prescription, Psychiatric, Transplant,
Vision, Wellness, Life, LTD, STD

Type of Coverage
Commercial, Individual, Medicare, Supplemental Medicare,
Medicaid

Type of Payment Plans Offered
POS

Geographic Areas Served
Illinois: Cook, DuPage, Kane, Kankakee, Kendall, Lake,
McHenry, Will counties. Indiana: Lake, Porter counties

Network Qualifications
Pre-Admission Certification: Yes

Peer Review Type
Utilization Review: Yes
Second Surgical Opinion: Yes
Case Management: Yes

Publishes and Distributes Report Card: Yes

Accreditation Certification
URAC, NCQA
TJC Accreditation, Utilization Review, Pre-Admission
Certification, State Licensure, Quality Assurance Program

Specialty Managed Care Partners
WellPoint Pharmacy Management, WellPoint Dental
Services, WellPoint Behavioral Health
Enters into Contracts with Regional Business Coalitions: Yes

339 UnitedHealthcare of Kansas

10895 Grandview Drive
Suite 200
Overland Park, KS 66210
Toll-Free: 888-340-9716
www.uhc.com/contact-us/kansas
Subsidiary of: UnitedHealth Group
For Profit Organization: Yes

Healthplan and Services Defined
PLAN TYPE: HMO/PPO
Model Type: Network
Plan Specialty: Behavioral Health, Dental, Disease
Management, PBM, Vision

Benefits Offered: Behavioral Health, Dental, Disease
Management, Long-Term Care, Prescription, Vision,
Wellness, Life, LTD, STD

Type of Coverage
Individual, Medicare, Supplemental Medicare, Medicaid,
Catastrophic, Family, Military, Veterans, Group,

Geographic Areas Served
Statewide

Key Personnel
President . . . . David Wichmann
Chief Operating Officer. . . . . Dan Schummacher
Chief Strategy Officer . . . . John Cosgriff
Communications Officer . . . . Kirsten Gorsuch
Chief Medical Officer. . . . . Sam Ho
Chief Legal Officer . . . . Thad Johnson
Chief Information Officer . . . . Phil McKoy
Chief Financial Officer. Jeff Putnam

Health Insurance Coverage Status and Type of Coverage by Age

Category	All Persons		Under 18 years		Under 65 years	
	Number	%	Number	%	Number	%
Total population	4,354	-	1,080	-	3,689	-
Covered by some type of health insurance	4,131 *(10)*	94.9 *(0.2)*	1,045 *(6)*	96.7 *(0.4)*	3,468 *(10)*	94.0 *(0.3)*
Covered by private health insurance	2,842 *(26)*	65.3 *(0.6)*	619 *(13)*	57.3 *(1.2)*	2,424 *(24)*	65.7 *(0.7)*
Employer-based	2,324 *(25)*	53.4 *(0.6)*	534 *(12)*	49.5 *(1.1)*	2,095 *(23)*	56.8 *(0.6)*
Direct purchase	542 *(12)*	12.4 *(0.3)*	68 *(5)*	6.3 *(0.5)*	318 *(10)*	8.6 *(0.3)*
TRICARE	132 *(9)*	3.0 *(0.2)*	29 *(4)*	2.7 *(0.3)*	89 *(8)*	2.4 *(0.2)*
Covered by public health insurance	1,873 *(24)*	43.0 *(0.5)*	473 *(13)*	43.8 *(1.2)*	1,224 *(24)*	33.2 *(0.7)*
Medicaid	1,165 *(23)*	26.7 *(0.5)*	467 *(13)*	43.2 *(1.2)*	1,080 *(22)*	29.3 *(0.6)*
Medicare	834 *(7)*	19.2 *(0.2)*	11 *(2)*	1.0 *(0.2)*	186 *(7)*	5.0 *(0.2)*
VA Care	124 *(5)*	2.8 *(0.1)*	2 *(1)*	0.2 *(0.1)*	56 *(4)*	1.5 *(0.1)*
Not covered at any time during the year	223 *(10)*	5.1 *(0.2)*	35 *(4)*	3.3 *(0.4)*	221 *(10)*	6.0 *(0.3)*

Note: Numbers in thousands; Figures cover civilian noninstitutionalized population in 2016; N/A indicates that data was not available; Z represents or rounds to zero; Margin of error appears in parenthesis and is calculated using replicate weights.
Source: U.S. Census Bureau, American Community Survey, Table HIC-4_ACS. Health Insurance Coverage Status and Type of Coverage by State—All People: 2008 to 2016, Table HIC-5_ACS. Health Insurance Coverage Status and Type of Coverage by State—Children Under 18: 2008 to 2016, Table HIC-6_ACS. Health Insurance Coverage Status and Type of Coverage by State—Persons Under 65: 2008 to 2016

Kentucky

340 Aetna Health of Kentucky

151 Farmington Avenue
Hartford, CT 06156
Toll-Free: 800-872-3862
Phone: 860-273-0123
www.aetna.com
Subsidiary of: Aetna Inc.
For Profit Organization: Yes

Healthplan and Services Defined
PLAN TYPE: HMO/PPO
Other Type: POS
Model Type: Network
Plan Specialty: Behavioral Health, EPO, Lab, PBM,
Radiology
Benefits Offered: Behavioral Health, Dental, Disease
Management, Long-Term Care, Physical Therapy,
Podiatry, Prescription, Psychiatric, Vision, Wellness, Life,
LTD, STD

Type of Coverage
Commercial, Medicaid, Student health

Type of Payment Plans Offered
POS, FFS

Geographic Areas Served
Statewide

Key Personnel
CEO . . . . Mark Bertolini

341 Anthem Blue Cross & Blue Shield of Kentucky

1792 Alysheba Way
Suite 200
Lexington, KY 40509
Phone: 866-755-2680
www.anthem.com
Subsidiary of: Anthem, Inc.
For Profit Organization: Yes

Healthplan and Services Defined
PLAN TYPE: HMO/PPO
Model Type: Network
Plan Specialty: Behavioral Health, Dental, Disease
Management, Lab, PBM, Vision, Radiology
Benefits Offered: Behavioral Health, Dental, Disease
Management, Inpatient SNF, Physical Therapy,
Prescription, Psychiatric, Transplant, Vision, Wellness, Life

Type of Coverage
Commercial, Individual, Medicare, Supplemental Medicare,
Catastrophic

Geographic Areas Served
Statewide

Accreditation Certification
URAC, NCQA

Key Personnel
President & CEO . . . . Scott P. Serota

Chief Financial Officer . . . . Robert Kolodgy
Human Resources . . . . Maureen A. Cahill
Chief Medical Officer . . . . Trent Haywood
General Counsel . . . . Scott Nehs

342 Baptist Health Plan

651 Perimeter Drive
Suite 300
Lexington, KY 40517
Toll-Free: 800-787-2680
cservice@baptisthealthplan.com
www.baptisthealthplan.com
Subsidiary of: Baptist Health Care Systems
Non-Profit Organization: Yes
Year Founded: 1993
Number of Affiliated Hospitals: 40
Number of Primary Care Physicians: 764
Number of Referral/Specialty Physicians: 1,000
Total Enrollment: 136,472
State Enrollment: 65,428

Healthplan and Services Defined
PLAN TYPE: HMO/PPO
Other Type: POS
Model Type: Network
Plan Specialty: ASO, Behavioral Health, Dental, EPO, MSO,
PBM, Vision
Benefits Offered: Chiropractic, Disease Management, Home
Care, Inpatient SNF, Physical Therapy, Podiatry,
Prescription, Transplant, Vision, Wellness, Occupational &
Speech Therapy; Hospice; Durable Medical Equipment

Type of Coverage
Commercial, Medicare

Type of Payment Plans Offered
POS, Combination FFS & DFFS

Geographic Areas Served
Bullitt, Estill, Fayette, Garrard, Henry, Hopkins, Jefferson,
Jessamine, Madison, Mercer, Oldham, Rockcastle, Shelby,
Spencer, Trimble, Webster, Whitley, Woodford counties

Peer Review Type
Second Surgical Opinion: Yes
Case Management: Yes

Publishes and Distributes Report Card: Yes

Accreditation Certification
TJC Accreditation, Medicare Approved, Utilization Review,
Pre-Admission Certification, State Licensure, Quality
Assurance Program

Key Personnel
President . . . . James S Fritz

343 CareSource Kentucky

10200 Forest Green Boulevard
Suite 400
Louisville, KY 40223
Phone: 502-213-4700
www.caresource.com
Non-Profit Organization: Yes

Total Enrollment: 1,000,000

Healthplan and Services Defined
PLAN TYPE: Medicare
Benefits Offered: Chiropractic, Dental, Podiatry, Prescription, Psychiatric, Vision

Type of Coverage
Medicare, Medicaid

Geographic Areas Served
Statewide

Key Personnel
President & CEO . . . . Pamela Morris
Kentucky Director. . . . . Michael Taylor
Administrative Officer . . . . Dan McCabe
Chief Information Officer . . . . Paul Stoddard
EVP, COO, CFO . . . . L. Tarlton Thomas III

---

344   CoventryCares of Kentucky
9900 Corporate Campus Drive
Suite 1000
Louisville, KY 40223
Phone: 502-622-7577
Subsidiary of: Coventry Health & Life Insurance Co.
Non-Profit Organization: Yes

Healthplan and Services Defined
PLAN TYPE: HMO/PPO
Other Type: MCO, POS
Benefits Offered: Behavioral Health, Dental, Disease Management, Physical Therapy, Prescription, Wellness, Worker's Compensation

Type of Coverage
Medicaid

Type of Payment Plans Offered
FFS

Geographic Areas Served
Statewide

Subscriber Information
Average Subscriber Co-Payment:
Primary Care Physician: Varies
Hospital ER: Varies
Home Health Care: Varies
Home Health Care Max. Days/Visits Covered: Varies
Nursing Home: Varies
Nursing Home Max. Days/Visits Covered: Varies

Key Personnel
Chairman & CEO . . . . Mark T. Bertolini
President. . . . . Karen S. Lynch
Chief Financial Officer . . . . Shawn M. Guertin
Operations & Technology . . . . Meg McCarthy
Chief Medical Officer . . . . Harold L. Paz
General Counsel . . . . Thomas Sabatino Jr.
Government Services . . . . Fran S. Soistman

---

345   Delta Dental of Kentucky
10100 Linn Station Road
Louisville, KY 40223
Toll-Free: 800-955-2030
Fax: 877-224-0052
www.deltadentalky.com
Non-Profit Organization: Yes
Year Founded: 1966

Healthplan and Services Defined
PLAN TYPE: Dental
Other Type: Dental PPO
Model Type: IPA
Plan Specialty: Dental
Benefits Offered: Dental

Type of Coverage
Commercial, Individual

Type of Payment Plans Offered
DFFS

Geographic Areas Served
Statewide

Peer Review Type
Utilization Review: Yes
Second Surgical Opinion: Yes
Case Management: Yes

Publishes and Distributes Report Card: Yes

Key Personnel
Intereim CEO . . . . Jude Thompson
VP, Chief Finance Officer . . . . Russell Skaggs
Chief Operating Officer . . . . Tammy York-Day
VP & General Counsel . . . . John Weeks
VP, Sales & Marketing . . . . Brian Hart

Specialty Managed Care Partners
Enters into Contracts with Regional Business Coalitions: Yes

---

346   Humana Inc.
1918 Hikes Lane
Suite 101
Louisville, KY 40218
Phone: 502-479-6580
www.humana.com
Secondary Address: 2530 Sir Barton Way, Suite 100, Lexington, KY 40509, 800-941-6172
For Profit Organization: Yes

Healthplan and Services Defined
PLAN TYPE: HMO/PPO
Model Type: Network
Plan Specialty: Dental, Vision
Benefits Offered: Dental, Prescription, Vision, Life, LTD, STD

Type of Coverage
Commercial, Individual, Medicare, Supplemental Medicare

Geographic Areas Served
Statewide

Accreditation Certification
URAC, NCQA

Key Personnel

President & CEO . . . . Bruce D. Broussard
Executive VP & COO. . . . . James E. Murray
Senior VP & CFO . . . . Brian Kane

347 Humana Medicare

Humana Correspondence Office
P.O. Box 14601
Lexington, KY 40512-4601
Toll-Free: 888-371-9538
www.humana.com/medicare
Subsidiary of: Humana
For Profit Organization: Yes

Healthplan and Services Defined
  PLAN TYPE: Medicare
  Benefits Offered: Chiropractic, Dental, Home Care, Inpatient
    SNF, Physical Therapy, Podiatry, Prescription, Psychiatric,
    Vision, Wellness

Type of Coverage
  Individual, Medicare, Supplemental Medicare

Geographic Areas Served
  Available in multiple states

Subscriber Information
  Average Monthly Fee Per Subscriber
    (Employee + Employer Contribution):
      Employee Only (Self): Varies
      Medicare: Varies
  Average Annual Deductible Per Subscriber:
      Employee Only (Self): Varies
      Medicare: Varies
  Average Subscriber Co-Payment:
      Primary Care Physician: Varies
      Non-Network Physician: Varies
      Prescription Drugs: Varies
      Hospital ER: Varies
      Home Health Care: Varies
      Home Health Care Max. Days/Visits Covered: Varies
      Nursing Home: Varies
      Nursing Home Max. Days/Visits Covered: Varies

Accreditation Certification
  URAC, NCQA, CORE

Key Personnel

President & CEO. Bruce Broussard
Chief Medical Officer. . . . . Roy A. Beveridge
Chief Consumer Officer. . . . . Judy L. Bilney
Human Resources. . . . . Tim Huval
Chief Financial Officer . . . . Brian Kane
Chief Information Officer . . . . Brian LeClaire
General Counsel . . . . Christopher M. Todoroff

348 Passport Health Plan

5100 Commerce Crossings Drive
Louisville, KY 40229
Toll-Free: 800-578-0603
Phone: 502-585-7900
www.passporthealthplan.com
Subsidiary of: AmeriHealth Mercy Health Plan

Non-Profit Organization: Yes
Year Founded: 1997
Total Enrollment: 170,000
State Enrollment: 170,000

Healthplan and Services Defined
  PLAN TYPE: HMO

Geographic Areas Served
  Jefferson, Oldham, Trimble, Carroll, Henry, Shelby, Spencer,
  Bullitt, Nelson, Washington, Marion, Larue, Hardin, Grayson,
  Meade, Breckinridge counties

Accreditation Certification
  NCQA

Key Personnel

Chief Executive Officer. . . . . Mark B. Carter
Chief Financial Officer . . . . David A. Stanley
VP/Chief Medical Officer . . . . . . Stephen J. Houghland, MD
VP/Chief Communications . . . . Jill Joseph Bell
VP, Human Resources . . . . Gary Bensing
Chief Operations Officer . . . . Carl Felix

349 Preferred Health Plan, Inc.

9520 Ormsby Station Road
Suite 300
Louisville, KY 40223
Toll-Free: 800-832-8212
Phone: 502-339-7500
Fax: 502-339-8716
www.phpinc.com
For Profit Organization: Yes
Year Founded: 1983
Total Enrollment: 110,000
State Enrollment: 110,000

Healthplan and Services Defined
  PLAN TYPE: PPO
  Other Type: TPA
  Model Type: Network
  Plan Specialty: ASO, Dental, PBM, Vision, UR
  Benefits Offered: TPA Services

Type of Coverage
  Commercial

Type of Payment Plans Offered
  DFFS

Geographic Areas Served
  Nationwide

Network Qualifications
  Pre-Admission Certification: Yes

Publishes and Distributes Report Card: No

Accreditation Certification
  Medicare Approved, Utilization Review, Pre-Admission
    Certification, State Licensure, Quality Assurance Program

Specialty Managed Care Partners
  Enters into Contracts with Regional Business Coalitions: No

350 Rural Carrier Benefit Plan

P.O. Box 7404
London, KY 40742
Toll-Free: 800-638-8432
www.rcbphealth.com
Subsidiary of: Aetna

Healthplan and Services Defined
PLAN TYPE: PPO
Benefits Offered: Disease Management, Prescription, Vision, Wellness, Cancer Treatment; Kidney Dialysis; 24-hour Nurse Line; Travel Assistance Program; Healthy Maternity; Quest Lab Program

Type of Coverage
Commercial, Individual

Type of Payment Plans Offered
Capitated, FFS

Subscriber Information
Average Monthly Fee Per Subscriber
(Employee + Employer Contribution):
Employee Only (Self): $73.11
Employee & 2 Family Members: $119.87
Average Annual Deductible Per Subscriber:
Employee & 2 Family Members: $350.00
Average Subscriber Co-Payment:
Primary Care Physician: 10%
Prescription Drugs: $20 - $30
Hospital ER: $0

Key Personnel
Chief Executive Officer . . . . Mark T. Bertolini
President . . . . Karen S. Lynch
Chief Financial Officer . . . . Shawn M. Guertin
Operations & Technology . . . . Meg McCarthy
Chief Medical Officer . . . . Harold L. Paz
EVP, General Counsel . . . . Thomas J. Sabatino Jr.
Government Services . . . . Fran S. Soistman

351 UnitedHealthcare of Kentucky

230 Lexington Green Circle
Suite 400
Lexington, KY 40503
Toll-Free: 800-357-0978
Phone: 859-825-6132
Fax: 859-825-6174
www.uhc.com/contact-us/kentucky
Subsidiary of: UnitedHealth Group
For Profit Organization: Yes
Year Founded: 1986

Healthplan and Services Defined
PLAN TYPE: HMO/PPO
Model Type: Network
Plan Specialty: Behavioral Health, Dental, Disease Management, PBM, Vision
Benefits Offered: Behavioral Health, Chiropractic, Dental, Disease Management, Long-Term Care, Prescription, Vision, Wellness, Life, LTD, STD

Type of Coverage
Individual, Medicare, Supplemental Medicare, Medicaid, Catastrophic, Family, Military, Veterans, Group, Catastrophic Illness Benefit: Maximum $1M

Type of Payment Plans Offered
POS

Geographic Areas Served
Central Kentucky: 99 counties

Subscriber Information
Average Monthly Fee Per Subscriber
(Employee + Employer Contribution):
Employee Only (Self): $139.00
Employee & 1 Family Member: $282.00
Employee & 2 Family Members: $445.00
Medicare: $0
Average Annual Deductible Per Subscriber:
Employee Only (Self): $0
Employee & 1 Family Member: $0
Employee & 2 Family Members: $0
Average Subscriber Co-Payment:
Primary Care Physician: $10.00
Non-Network Physician: Not covered
Prescription Drugs: $7.00
Hospital ER: $50.00
Home Health Care: 20%
Nursing Home: Not covered

Network Qualifications
Pre-Admission Certification: Yes

Peer Review Type
Utilization Review: Yes
Second Surgical Opinion: No
Case Management: Yes

Publishes and Distributes Report Card: Yes

Accreditation Certification
TJC Accreditation, Utilization Review, Pre-Admission Certification, State Licensure, Quality Assurance Program

Key Personnel
President . . . . David Wichmann
Chief Operating Officer . . . . Dan Schummacher
Chief Strategy Officer . . . . John Cosgriff
Communications Officer . . . . Kirsten Gorsuch
Chief Medical Officer . . . . Sam Ho
Chief Legal Officer . . . . Thad Johnson
Chief Information Officer . . . . Phil McKoy
Chief Financial Officer . . . . Jeff Putnam

Average Claim Compensation
Physician's Fees Charged: 1%
Hospital's Fees Charged: 1%

Specialty Managed Care Partners
Enters into Contracts with Regional Business Coalitions: Yes

Health Insurance Coverage Status and Type of Coverage by Age

Category	All Persons		Under 18 years		Under 65 years	
	Number	%	Number	%	Number	%
Total population	4,577	-	1,184	-	3,923	-
Covered by some type of health insurance	4,107 *(17)*	89.7 *(0.4)*	1,145 *(7)*	96.7 *(0.4)*	3,456 *(17)*	88.1 *(0.4)*
Covered by private health insurance	2,811 *(28)*	61.4 *(0.6)*	585 *(16)*	49.4 *(1.3)*	2,441 *(28)*	62.2 *(0.7)*
Employer-based	2,233 *(32)*	48.8 *(0.7)*	491 *(16)*	41.5 *(1.4)*	2,025 *(32)*	51.6 *(0.8)*
Direct purchase	606 *(16)*	13.2 *(0.4)*	81 *(7)*	6.8 *(0.6)*	421 *(15)*	10.7 *(0.4)*
TRICARE	117 *(7)*	2.6 *(0.1)*	28 *(3)*	2.3 *(0.3)*	80 *(6)*	2.0 *(0.1)*
Covered by public health insurance	1,811 *(24)*	39.6 *(0.5)*	611 *(16)*	51.6 *(1.3)*	1,182 *(23)*	30.1 *(0.6)*
Medicaid	1,166 *(23)*	25.5 *(0.5)*	605 *(16)*	51.1 *(1.3)*	1,062 *(21)*	27.1 *(0.5)*
Medicare	793 *(8)*	17.3 *(0.2)*	9 *(2)*	0.8 *(0.2)*	166 *(7)*	4.2 *(0.2)*
VA Care	97 *(5)*	2.1 *(0.1)*	2 *(1)*	0.1 *(0.1)*	46 *(4)*	1.2 *(0.1)*
Not covered at any time during the year	470 *(17)*	10.3 *(0.4)*	39 *(5)*	3.3 *(0.4)*	467 *(17)*	11.9 *(0.4)*

Note: Numbers in thousands; Figures cover civilian noninstitutionalized population in 2016; N/A indicates that data was not available; Z represents or rounds to zero; Margin of error appears in parenthesis and is calculated using replicate weights.
Source: U.S. Census Bureau, American Community Survey, Table HIC-4_ACS. Health Insurance Coverage Status and Type of Coverage by State—All People: 2008 to 2016, Table HIC-5_ACS. Health Insurance Coverage Status and Type of Coverage by State—Children Under 18: 2008 to 2016, Table HIC-6_ACS. Health Insurance Coverage Status and Type of Coverage by State—Persons Under 65: 2008 to 2016

Louisiana

352 Aetna Health of Louisiana

151 Farmington Avenue
Hartford, CT 06156
Toll-Free: 800-872-3862
Phone: 860-273-0123
www.aetna.com
Secondary Address: 6730-B Rockledge Drive, Suite 700,
   Bethesda, MD 20817, 301-581-0600
Subsidiary of: Aetna Inc.
For Profit Organization: Yes

Healthplan and Services Defined
PLAN TYPE: PPO
Other Type: POS
Model Type: Network
Plan Specialty: Behavioral Health, Dental, EPO, Lab, PBM,
   Vision, Radiology
Benefits Offered: Behavioral Health, Dental, Disease
   Management, Long-Term Care, Physical Therapy,
   Podiatry, Prescription, Psychiatric, Vision, Wellness, Life,
   LTD, STD

Type of Coverage
Commercial, Medicaid, Student health

Type of Payment Plans Offered
POS, FFS

Geographic Areas Served
Statewide with some exceptions

Key Personnel
CEO . . . . Mark Bertolini

353 Blue Cross and Blue Shield of Louisiana

5525 Reitz Avenue
Baton Rouge, LA 70809
Toll-Free: 800-495-2583
Phone: 225-295-2556
www.bcbsla.com
Secondary Address: 4508 Coliseum Boulvecard, Suite A,
   Alexandria, LA 71303
For Profit Organization: Yes
Year Founded: 1934
Number of Affiliated Hospitals: 39
Number of Primary Care Physicians: 962
Number of Referral/Specialty Physicians: 2,219
Total Enrollment: 1,300,000
State Enrollment: 1,300,000

Healthplan and Services Defined
PLAN TYPE: HMO/PPO
Model Type: Network
Benefits Offered: Behavioral Health, Disease Management,
   Prescription, Wellness

Type of Coverage
Commercial, Individual, Medicare, Supplemental Medicare
Catastrophic Illness Benefit: Maximum $2M

Type of Payment Plans Offered
POS

Subscriber Information
Average Subscriber Co-Payment:
   Primary Care Physician: 10%/20%
   Home Health Care: Varies

Network Qualifications
Pre-Admission Certification: Yes

Peer Review Type
Utilization Review: Yes

Publishes and Distributes Report Card: No

Accreditation Certification
URAC, NCQA
TJC Accreditation, Medicare Approved, Utilization Review,
   Pre-Admission Certification, State Licensure, Quality
   Assurance Program

Key Personnel
President & CEO . . . . I. Steven Udvarhelyi
Chairman . . . . Dan Borne
Director. . . . . C. Richard Atkins
Human Resources . . . . John E. Brown Jr.
General Counsel . . . . Michele Calandro
Chief Financial Officer. . . . . Bryan Camerlinck

Specialty Managed Care Partners
Enters into Contracts with Regional Business Coalitions: Yes

354 Coventry Health Care of Louisiana

4000 S Sherwood Forest Road
Suite 101
Baton Rouge, LA 70816
Toll-Free: 866-757-7930
Phone: 225-296-8912
chclouisiana.coventryhealthcare.com
Secondary Address: 920 Pierremont Road, Suite 308,
   Shreveport, LA 71106, 866-896-3568
Subsidiary of: Aetna Inc.
For Profit Organization: Yes

Healthplan and Services Defined
PLAN TYPE: HMO
Benefits Offered: Behavioral Health, Dental, Disease
   Management, Physical Therapy, Prescription, Wellness

Geographic Areas Served
New Orleans metropolitan area, Baton Rouge, Metairie,
   Shreveport, Slidell, Bayou Region

Accreditation Certification
URAC

Key Personnel
Chairman & CEO . . . . Mark T. Bertolini
President. . . . . Karen S. Lynch
Chief Financial Officer . . . . Shawn M. Guertin
Operations & Technology . . . . Meg McCarthy
Chief Medical Officer . . . . Harold L. Paz
General Counsel . . . . Thomas Sabatino Jr.
Government Services . . . . Fran S. Soistman

355 DINA Dental Plan

11969 Bricksome Avenue
Suite A
Baton Rouge, LA 70816
Toll-Free: 800-376-3462
Phone: 225-291-3172
Fax: 225-292-3075
info@dinadental.com
www.dinadental.com
For Profit Organization: Yes
Year Founded: 1978

Healthplan and Services Defined
 PLAN TYPE: Dental
 Model Type: Group
 Plan Specialty: Dental
 Benefits Offered: Dental

Type of Coverage
 Commercial, Individual

Geographic Areas Served
 Statewide

Peer Review Type
 Second Surgical Opinion: Yes

Publishes and Distributes Report Card: No

Specialty Managed Care Partners
 Enters into Contracts with Regional Business Coalitions: No

356 Humana Health Insurance of Louisiana

10330 Airline Highway
Baton Rouge, LA 70816
Phone: 225-442-6100
www.humana.com
Secondary Address: 910 Pierremont Road, Suite 410,
 Shreveport, LA 71106, 318-861-8609
Subsidiary of: Humana
For Profit Organization: Yes
Year Founded: 1985
Physician Owned Organization: Yes
Federally Qualified: Yes

Healthplan and Services Defined
 PLAN TYPE: HMO/PPO
 Model Type: Network
 Plan Specialty: Dental, Vision
 Benefits Offered: Behavioral Health, Chiropractic, Dental,
 Disease Management, Home Care, Inpatient SNF, Physical
 Therapy, Podiatry, Prescription, Psychiatric, Transplant,
 Vision, Wellness, Life, LTD, STD

Type of Coverage
 Commercial, Individual, Indemnity, Medicare
 Catastrophic Illness Benefit: Unlimited

Type of Payment Plans Offered
 POS, Combination FFS & DFFS

Geographic Areas Served
 Statewide, excluding Monroe

Subscriber Information
 Average Monthly Fee Per Subscriber
  (Employee + Employer Contribution):
   Employee Only (Self): $189.31
   Employee & 1 Family Member: $378.62
   Employee & 2 Family Members: $530.07
 Average Subscriber Co-Payment:
   Primary Care Physician: $15.00
   Prescription Drugs: $10/$25/$40
   Home Health Care Max. Days/Visits Covered: 60 days

Network Qualifications
 Pre-Admission Certification: Yes

Peer Review Type
 Utilization Review: Yes
 Second Surgical Opinion: Yes
 Case Management: Yes

Publishes and Distributes Report Card: Yes

Accreditation Certification
 URAC, NCQA, CORE
 Medicare Approved, Utilization Review, Pre-Admission
  Certification, State Licensure, Quality Assurance Program

Key Personnel
 President & CEO. Bruce Broussard
 Chief Medical Officer. . . . . Roy A. Beveridge
 Chief Consumer Officer. . . . . Jody L. Bilney
 Human Resources. . . . . Tim Huval
 Chief Financial Officer . . . . Brian Kane
 Chief Information Officer . . . . Brian LeClaire
 General Counsel . . . . Christopher M. Todoroff

Specialty Managed Care Partners
 CMS Healthcare, Medimpact
 Enters into Contracts with Regional Business Coalitions: Yes
 Chamber of Commerce

Employer References
 State of Louisiana, Exxon-Mobil, Shell, Chevron, Sears

357 Molina Medicaid Solutions

8495 United Plaza Boulevard
Suite 110, 280
Baton Rouge, LA 70809
Phone: 225-216-6000
www.molinahealthcare.com
Subsidiary of: Molina Healthcare, Inc.
For Profit Organization: Yes

Healthplan and Services Defined
 PLAN TYPE: Medicare

Type of Coverage
 Medicaid information management sys

Geographic Areas Served
 Statewide

Key Personnel
 Chief Executive Officer . . . . Joseph W. White
 Chief Operating Officer . . . . Terry Bayer
 General Counsel. . . . . Jeff D. Barlow
 SVP, Relations/Marketing . . . . Juan Jos, Orellana
 Chief Information Officer . . . . Rick Hopfer

358 Peoples Health

7434 Perkins Road
Suite 200
Baton Rouge, LA 70808
Toll-Free: 800-222-8600
Phone: 225-346-5704
www.peopleshealth.com
Secondary Address: Three Lakeway Center, 3838 N
Causeway Boulevard, Suite 2200, Metairie, LA 70002,
504-849-4685
For Profit Organization: Yes
Year Founded: 1994
Total Enrollment: 50,000
State Enrollment: 4,707

Healthplan and Services Defined
PLAN TYPE: HMO
Plan Specialty: Lab, Radiology
Benefits Offered: Dental, Disease Management, Home Care,
Prescription, Wellness

Type of Coverage
Commercial, Medicare

Geographic Areas Served
Statewide

Accreditation Certification
NCQA

Key Personnel
Chief Executive Officer . . . . Warren Murrell
Chief Financial Officer . . . . Kim Eller
Chief Information Officer. . . . . Colin Hulin
Marketing/Communications . . . . Nick Karl
General Counsel . . . . Donna Klein
VP, Health Services. . . . . Barbara Guerard
Chief Medical Officer . . . . Frank N. Deus
SVP, Network Development . . . . Janice Ortego

359 Starmount

8485 Goodwood Boulevard
Baton Rouge, LA 70806
Toll-Free: 888-400-9304
starmountlife.com
Mailing Address: P.O. Box 98100, Baton Rouge, LA
70898-9100

Healthplan and Services Defined
PLAN TYPE: Dental
Benefits Offered: Dental, Prescription, Vision, Life, Hearing
aids

Geographic Areas Served
Available in 41 states

Key Personnel
Chief Executive Officer . . . . Erich Sternberg
President . . . . Deborah Sternberg

360 UnitedHealthcare of Louisiana

3838 N Causeway Boulevard
Suite 2600
Metairie, LA 70002
Toll-Free: 800-826-1981
www.uhc.com/contact-us/louisiana
Subsidiary of: UnitedHealth Group
For Profit Organization: Yes
Year Founded: 1986

Healthplan and Services Defined
PLAN TYPE: HMO/PPO
Model Type: Network
Plan Specialty: Behavioral Health, Dental, Disease
Management, PBM, Vision
Benefits Offered: Behavioral Health, Dental, Disease
Management, Long-Term Care, Prescription, Vision,
Wellness, Life, LTD, STD

Type of Coverage
Individual, Medicare, Supplemental Medicare, Medicaid,
Catastrophic, Family, Military, Veterans, Group,

Geographic Areas Served
Ascension, Assumption, East Baton Rouge, East Feliciana,
Iberville, Jefferson, LaFourche, Livingston, Orleans,
Plaquemines, Point Coupee, St. Bernard, St. Charles, St.
Helena, St. James, St. Tammany, Tangipahoa, Terrabona, West
Baton Rouge, West Feliciana

Subscriber Information
Average Monthly Fee Per Subscriber
(Employee + Employer Contribution):
Employee Only (Self): $129.45
Employee & 1 Family Member: $261.04
Employee & 2 Family Members: $422.40
Average Annual Deductible Per Subscriber:
Employee Only (Self): $5.00
Average Subscriber Co-Payment:
Primary Care Physician: $10.00
Prescription Drugs: $10.00
Hospital ER: $50.00

Network Qualifications
Pre-Admission Certification: Yes

Peer Review Type
Utilization Review: Yes

Publishes and Distributes Report Card: No

Accreditation Certification
TJC Accreditation, Medicare Approved, Utilization Review,
Pre-Admission Certification, State Licensure, Quality
Assurance Program

Key Personnel
President . . . . David Wichmann
Chief Operating Officer. . . . . Dan Schummacher
Chief Strategy Officer . . . . John Cosgriff
Communication Officer. . . . . Kirsten Gorsuch
Chief Medical Officer. . . . . Sam Ho
Chief Legal Officer . . . . Thad Johnson
Chief Information Officer . . . . Phil McKoy
Chief Financial Officer. . . . . Jeff Putnam

Specialty Managed Care Partners
Enters into Contracts with Regional Business Coalitions: No

---

361 Vantage Health Plan

130 DeSiard Street
Suite 300
Monroe, LA 71201
Toll-Free: 888-823-1910
Phone: 318-361-0900
www.vantagehealthplan.com
For Profit Organization: Yes
Year Founded: 1994
Number of Referral/Specialty Physicians: 7,000
Total Enrollment: 50,000
State Enrollment: 50,000

Healthplan and Services Defined
PLAN TYPE: HMO
Plan Specialty: Lab, Radiology
Benefits Offered: Behavioral Health, Chiropractic, Disease
   Management, Home Care, Inpatient SNF, Physical
   Therapy, Prescription, Wellness, Durable Medical
   Equipment

Type of Coverage
Medicare, Supplemental Medicare

Geographic Areas Served
Statewide

Network Qualifications
Pre-Admission Certification: Yes

Key Personnel
Executive Vice President. . . . . Mike Breard
Chief Financial Officer . . . . Rhonda Haygood
Chief Information Officer . . . . Landon Wright

Specialty Managed Care Partners
Caremark Rx

---

362 Vantage Medicare Advantage

130 DeSiard Street
Suite 300
Monroe, LA 71201
Toll-Free: 866-704-0109
Phone: 318-361-0900
www.vantagehealthplan.com
Secondary Address: Customer Service & Marketing, 122 St
   John Street, Monroe, LA 71201, 318-361-0900
Year Founded: 1994
Total Enrollment: 14,000

Healthplan and Services Defined
PLAN TYPE: Medicare
Other Type: Medicare PPO
Plan Specialty: Dental, Vision
Benefits Offered: Home Care, Inpatient SNF, Prescription,
   Vision

Type of Coverage
Medicare, Supplemental Medicare

Geographic Areas Served
Bossier, Caddo, Caldwell, Jackson, Lincoln, Morehouse,
Rapides, Ouachita, richland, and Union Parishes

Key Personnel
Executive Vice President. . . . . Mike Breard
Chief Financial Officer . . . . Rhonda Haygood
Chief Information Officer . . . . Landon Wright

Health Insurance Coverage Status and Type of Coverage by Age

Category	All Persons		Under 18 years		Under 65 years	
	Number	%	Number	%	Number	%
Total population	1,317	-	274	-	1,068	-
Covered by some type of health insurance	1,211 (7)	92.0 (0.5)	261 (3)	95.2 (0.9)	962 (7)	90.1 (0.6)
Covered by private health insurance	926 (12)	70.3 (0.9)	180 (6)	65.7 (2.0)	765 (11)	71.6 (1.0)
Employer-based	720 (12)	54.7 (0.9)	159 (6)	58.0 (2.2)	645 (11)	60.4 (1.1)
Direct purchase	215 (7)	16.3 (0.6)	20 (3)	7.3 (0.9)	123 (7)	11.5 (0.6)
TRICARE	45 (5)	3.4 (0.3)	7 (2)	2.4 (0.6)	22 (4)	2.1 (0.4)
Covered by public health insurance	480 (10)	36.4 (0.7)	93 (5)	33.8 (1.9)	239 (10)	22.4 (0.9)
Medicaid	253 (10)	19.2 (0.7)	92 (5)	33.5 (1.9)	210 (9)	19.7 (0.9)
Medicare	291 (5)	22.1 (0.4)	2 (1)	0.7 (0.3)	50 (5)	4.7 (0.4)
VA Care	41 (3)	3.1 (0.2)	Z (Z)	0.1 (0.1)	16 (2)	1.5 (0.2)
Not covered at any time during the year	106 (7)	8.0 (0.5)	13 (3)	4.8 (0.9)	106 (7)	9.9 (0.6)

Note: Numbers in thousands; Figures cover civilian noninstitutionalized population in 2016; N/A indicates that data was not available; Z represents or rounds to zero; Margin of error appears in parenthesis and is calculated using replicate weights.
Source: U.S. Census Bureau, American Community Survey, Table HIC-4_ACS. Health Insurance Coverage Status and Type of Coverage by State—All People: 2008 to 2016, Table HIC-5_ACS. Health Insurance Coverage Status and Type of Coverage by State—Children Under 18: 2008 to 2016, Table HIC-6_ACS. Health Insurance Coverage Status and Type of Coverage by State—Persons Under 65: 2008 to 2016

Maine

363   Aetna Health of Maine

151 Farmington Avenue
Hartford, CT 06156
Toll-Free: 800-872-3862
Phone: 860-273-0123
www.aetna.com
Subsidiary of: Aetna Inc.
For Profit Organization: Yes

Healthplan and Services Defined
PLAN TYPE: HMO/PPO
Other Type: POS
Model Type: Network
Plan Specialty: Behavioral Health, Dental, EPO, Lab, PBM, Vision, Radiology
Benefits Offered: Behavioral Health, Dental, Disease Management, Long-Term Care, Physical Therapy, Podiatry, Prescription, Psychiatric, Vision, Wellness, Life, LTD, STD

Type of Coverage
Commercial, Medicare, Medicaid, Student health

Geographic Areas Served
Statewide

Key Personnel
CEO . . . . Mark Bertolini

364   Anthem Blue Cross & Blue Shield of Maine

2 Gannett Drive
South Portland, ME 04106
Phone: 207-536-9026
www.anthem.com
Subsidiary of: Anthem, Inc.
For Profit Organization: Yes

Healthplan and Services Defined
PLAN TYPE: HMO/PPO
Model Type: Network
Plan Specialty: Behavioral Health, Dental, Disease Management, Lab, PBM, Vision, Radiology
Benefits Offered: Behavioral Health, Dental, Disease Management, Inpatient SNF, Physical Therapy, Prescription, Psychiatric, Transplant, Vision, Wellness, Life

Type of Coverage
Commercial, Individual, Medicare, Supplemental Medicare, Catastrophic

Geographic Areas Served
Statewide

Accreditation Certification
URAC, NCQA

Key Personnel
President & CEO . . . . Scott P. Serota
Chief Financial Officer . . . . Robert Kolodgy
Human Resources . . . . Maureen A. Cahill
Chief Medical Officer. . . . . Trent Haywood
General Counsel. . . . . Scott Nehs

365   Community Health Options

150 Mill Street
Lewiston, ME 04240
Toll-Free: 855-624-6463
healthoptions.org
Secondary Address: Mail Stop 200, P.O. Box 1121, Lewiston, ME 04243
Non-Profit Organization: Yes

Healthplan and Services Defined
PLAN TYPE: HMO/PPO

Geographic Areas Served
Maine and New Hampshire

Key Personnel
President & CEO . . . . Kevin Lewis
SVP, Operations Officer . . . . Robert Hillman
SVP, Financial Officer . . . . Ed Vozzo
SVP, Medical Officer. . . . . John Yindra, MD
SVP, Information Officer . . . . Will Kilbreth
SVP, Human Resources . . . . Joyce McPhetres

366   Coventry Health Care of Maine

6720-B Rockledge Drive
Suite 700
Bethesda, MD 20817
Phone: 301-581-0600
www.coventryhealthcare.com
Subsidiary of: Aetna Inc.
For Profit Organization: Yes

Healthplan and Services Defined
PLAN TYPE: HMO/PPO
Model Type: Network
Plan Specialty: Behavioral Health, Dental, Worker's Compensation
Benefits Offered: Behavioral Health, Dental, Prescription, Wellness, Worker's Compensation

Type of Coverage
Commercial, Medicare, Medicaid

Geographic Areas Served
Statewide

Key Personnel
Chief Executive Officer. . . . . Mark T. Bertolini
President. . . . . Karen S. Lynch
Chief Financial Officer . . . . Shawn M. Guertin
Operations & Technology . . . . Meg McCarthy
Chief Medical Officer . . . . Harold L. Paz
General Counsel . . . . Thomas Sabatino Jr.
Government Services . . . . Fran S. Soistman

367   Harvard Pilgrim Health Care Maine

1 Market Street
3rd Floor
Portland, ME 04101
Toll-Free: 888-888-4742
Phone: 617-509-1000
www.harvardpilgrim.org
Non-Profit Organization: Yes

Year Founded: 1977
Number of Affiliated Hospitals: 179
Number of Referral/Specialty Physicians: 53,000

Healthplan and Services Defined
PLAN TYPE: Multiple
Model Type: Network
Plan Specialty: ASO, Behavioral Health, Chiropractic,
Dental, Disease Management, EPO, Lab, MSO, PBM,
Vision, Radiology, Worker's Compensation, UR
Benefits Offered: Behavioral Health, Chiropractic, Disease
Management, Home Care, Inpatient SNF, Long-Term Care,
Physical Therapy, Podiatry, Prescription, Psychiatric,
Transplant, Vision, Wellness

Type of Coverage
Commercial, Individual, Indemnity, Medicare, Supplemental
Medicare, Medicaid

Geographic Areas Served
Statewide

Peer Review Type
Utilization Review: Yes
Second Surgical Opinion: Yes
Case Management: Yes

Publishes and Distributes Report Card: Yes

Accreditation Certification
NCQA
TJC Accreditation, Medicare Approved, Utilization Review,
Pre-Admission Certification, State Licensure, Quality
Assurance Program

Key Personnel
President & CEO...................... Eric H. Schultz
CFO .... Charles Goheen
Chief Legal Officer .... Tisa Hughes
Chief Information Officer............ Deborah A. Norton
VP, Marketing .... Richard O'Connor
Human Resources...................... Cynthia Ring
Chief Medical Officer .... Michael Sherman
Enterprise Marketing .... Beth Roberts

Average Claim Compensation
Physician's Fees Charged: 51%
Hospital's Fees Charged: 40%

Specialty Managed Care Partners
Enters into Contracts with Regional Business Coalitions: No

368　Martin's Point HealthCare
331 Veranda Street
Portland, ME 04103
Toll-Free: 800-322-0280
Phone: 207-828-2402
www.martinspoint.org
Non-Profit Organization: Yes
Year Founded: 1981
Total Enrollment: 70,000

Healthplan and Services Defined
PLAN TYPE: Multiple
Benefits Offered: Disease Management, Prescription,
Wellness, No co-pay for: routine physical exams/hearing

tests/eye exams/mammograms/prostrate & pap exams/bone
mass/flu vaccines.

Type of Coverage
Commercial, Medicare, Military

Geographic Areas Served
Maine, New Hampshire, Vermont, Northeastern New York

Subscriber Information
Average Monthly Fee Per Subscriber
(Employee + Employer Contribution):
Employee Only (Self): Varies
Medicare: Varies
Average Annual Deductible Per Subscriber:
Employee Only (Self): Varies
Medicare: Varies
Average Subscriber Co-Payment:
Primary Care Physician: Varies
Prescription Drugs: Varies
Hospital ER: Varies

Key Personnel
President/CEO.................... David Howes, MD
Chief Financial Officer................ Dan Chojnowski
COO, Delivery System............... Sandra Monfiletto
Chief Human Resources .... Teresa Schulz
Chief Medical Officer............. Jonathan Harvey, MD

369　Molina Medicaid Solutions
189 Water Street
Augusta, ME 04330
Toll-Free: 888-321-5557
www.molinahealthcare.com
Secondary Address: 45 Commerce Drive, Augusta, ME 04330,
800-321-5557
Subsidiary of: Molina Healthcare, Inc.
For Profit Organization: Yes

Healthplan and Services Defined
PLAN TYPE: Medicare

Type of Coverage
Medicaid information management sys

Geographic Areas Served
Statewide

Key Personnel
Chief Executive Officer .... Joseph W. White
Chief Operating Officer .... Terry Bayer
General Counsel....................... Jeff D. Barlow
SVP, Relations/Marketing .... Juan Jos, Orellana
Chief Information Officer .... Rick Hopfer

370　UnitedHealthcare of Maine
475 Kilvert Street
Warwick, RI 02886
Toll-Free: 888-735-5842
www.uhc.com/contact-us/maine
Subsidiary of: UnitedHealth Group
Year Founded: 1977

Healthplan and Services Defined
PLAN TYPE: HMO/PPO

Model Type: Network

Plan Specialty: Behavioral Health, Dental, Disease
Management, Lab, PBM, Vision, Radiology

Benefits Offered: Behavioral Health, Chiropractic, Dental,
Disease Management, Long-Term Care, Physical Therapy,
Prescription, Vision, Wellness, AD&D, Life, LTD, STD

Type of Coverage

Commercial, Individual, Indemnity, Medicare, Supplemental
Medicare, Medicaid, Catastrophic, Family, Military,
Veterans, Group,

Geographic Areas Served

Statewide. Maine is covered by the Rhode Island branch

Network Qualifications

Pre-Admission Certification: Yes

Peer Review Type

Utilization Review: Yes

Second Surgical Opinion: Yes

Case Management: Yes

Publishes and Distributes Report Card: Yes

Accreditation Certification

TJC, NCQA

Key Personnel

President	David Wichmann
Chief Operating Officer	Dan Schumacher
Chief Strategy Officer	John Cosgriff
Communications Officer	Kirsten Gorsuch
Chief Medical Officer	Sam Ho
Chief Legal Officer	Thad Johnson
Chief Information Officer	Phil McKoy
Chief Financial Officer	Jeff Putnam

Specialty Managed Care Partners

Enters into Contracts with Regional Business Coalitions: Yes

Health Insurance Coverage Status and Type of Coverage by Age

Category	All Persons		Under 18 years		Under 65 years	
	Number	%	Number	%	Number	%
Total population	5,919	-	1,422	-	5,066	-
Covered by some type of health insurance	5,555 (16)	93.9 (0.3)	1,373 (8)	96.6 (0.4)	4,711 (16)	93.0 (0.3)
Covered by private health insurance	4,407 (29)	74.5 (0.5)	949 (16)	66.7 (1.1)	3,804 (27)	75.1 (0.5)
Employer-based	3,716 (28)	62.8 (0.5)	831 (15)	58.5 (1.1)	3,293 (27)	65.0 (0.5)
Direct purchase	761 (18)	12.9 (0.3)	102 (7)	7.2 (0.5)	518 (16)	10.2 (0.3)
TRICARE	213 (13)	3.6 (0.2)	48 (6)	3.4 (0.4)	155 (11)	3.1 (0.2)
Covered by public health insurance	1,889 (26)	31.9 (0.4)	474 (14)	33.3 (1.0)	1,087 (26)	21.4 (0.5)
Medicaid	1,067 (26)	18.0 (0.4)	465 (15)	32.7 (1.0)	966 (26)	19.1 (0.5)
Medicare	934 (9)	15.8 (0.1)	12 (3)	0.8 (0.2)	134 (7)	2.6 (0.1)
VA Care	115 (5)	1.9 (0.1)	1 (1)	0.1 (Z)	58 (4)	1.1 (0.1)
Not covered at any time during the year	363 (16)	6.1 (0.3)	49 (6)	3.4 (0.4)	355 (15)	7.0 (0.3)

Note: Numbers in thousands; Figures cover civilian noninstitutionalized population in 2016; N/A indicates that data was not available; Z represents or rounds to zero; Margin of error appears in parenthesis and is calculated using replicate weights.
Source: U.S. Census Bureau, American Community Survey, Table HIC-4_ACS. Health Insurance Coverage Status and Type of Coverage by State—All People: 2008 to 2016, Table HIC-5_ACS. Health Insurance Coverage Status and Type of Coverage by State—Children Under 18: 2008 to 2016, Table HIC-6_ACS. Health Insurance Coverage Status and Type of Coverage by State—Persons Under 65: 2008 to 2016

Maryland

371 Aetna Health of Maryland

151 Farmington Avenue
Hartford, CT 06156
Toll-Free: 800-872-3862
Phone: 860-273-0123
www.aetna.com
Subsidiary of: Aetna Inc.
For Profit Organization: Yes

Healthplan and Services Defined
PLAN TYPE: HMO/PPO
Other Type: POS
Model Type: Network
Plan Specialty: Behavioral Health, EPO, Lab, PBM,
  Radiology
Benefits Offered: Behavioral Health, Disease Management,
  Long-Term Care, Physical Therapy, Podiatry, Prescription,
  Psychiatric, Vision, Wellness, Life, LTD, STD

Type of Coverage
Commercial, Student health

Type of Payment Plans Offered
DFFS, Capitated, FFS

Geographic Areas Served
Statewide

Key Personnel
CEO . . . . Mark Bertolini

372 American Postal Workers Union (APWU) Health Plan

799 Cromwell Park Drive
Suite K-Z
Glen Burnie, MD 21061
Toll-Free: 800-222-2798
Fax: 410-424-1588
www.apwuhp.com
Year Founded: 1960
Number of Affiliated Hospitals: 6,000
Number of Primary Care Physicians: 600,000
Total Enrollment: 205,000
State Enrollment: 205,000

Healthplan and Services Defined
PLAN TYPE: PPO
Plan Specialty: Behavioral Health, Dental, Disease
  Management
Benefits Offered: Behavioral Health, Dental, Disease
  Management, Prescription, Wellness
Offers Demand Management Patient Information Service:
  Yes
DMPI Services Offered: 24 Hour Nurse Advisory Line

Type of Payment Plans Offered
FFS

Geographic Areas Served
Nationwide - APWU/The American Postal Workers Union
  Health Plan is health insurance for federal employees and
  retirees

Subscriber Information
Average Monthly Fee Per Subscriber
  (Employee + Employer Contribution):
    Employee Only (Self): $36.80-177.20 varies
    Employee & 2 Family Members: $82.80-398.66 varies
Average Annual Deductible Per Subscriber:
  Employee Only (Self): $250
Average Subscriber Co-Payment:
  Primary Care Physician: 15%
  Prescription Drugs: 25%
  Hospital ER: 15% - 30%
  Home Health Care Max. Days/Visits Covered: 10 - 30%

Key Personnel
President . . . . Mark Dimondstein
Director . . . . John L. Marcotte

373 Amerigroup Maryland

7550 Teague Road
Suite 500
Hanover, MD 21076
Toll-Free: 800-600-4441
Phone: 410-859-5800
www.myamerigroup.com/md
Subsidiary of: Anthem, Inc.
For Profit Organization: Yes
Year Founded: 1999

Healthplan and Services Defined
PLAN TYPE: HMO
Plan Specialty: Dental, Disease Management, Vision, Taking
  Care of Baby and Me program
Benefits Offered: Disease Management

Type of Coverage
Medicare, Medicaid

Accreditation Certification
NCQA

Key Personnel
President & CEO . . . . Peter D. Haytaian

374 Avesis: Maryland

10324 S Dolfield Road
Owings Mills, MD 21117
Toll-Free: 800-643-1132
www.avesis.com
Subsidiary of: Guardian Life Insurance Company
Year Founded: 1978
Number of Primary Care Physicians: 25,000
Total Enrollment: 3,500,000

Healthplan and Services Defined
PLAN TYPE: PPO
Other Type: Vision, Dental
Model Type: Network
Plan Specialty: Dental, Vision, Hearing
Benefits Offered: Dental, Vision

Type of Coverage
Commercial

Type of Payment Plans Offered
POS, Capitated, Combination FFS & DFFS

Geographic Areas Served
Nationwide and Puerto Rico

Publishes and Distributes Report Card: Yes

Accreditation Certification
AAAHC
TJC Accreditation

Key Personnel
Chief Executive Officer . . . . Chris Swanker
Business Development . . . . Alan Cohn

---

375 CareFirst BlueCross BlueShield

Canton Tower
1501 S Clinton Street
Baltimore, MD 21224
Toll-Free: 800-544-8703
Phone: 410-581-3000
individual.carefirst.com
Secondary Address: Union Center Plaza, 840 First Street NE,
Washington, DC 20065, 202-479-8000
Non-Profit Organization: Yes
Year Founded: 1984
Number of Primary Care Physicians: 5,000
Total Enrollment: 3,200,000

Healthplan and Services Defined
PLAN TYPE: HMO/PPO
Model Type: Network
Benefits Offered: Dental, Prescription, Vision

Type of Coverage
Commercial, Individual, Medicare
Catastrophic Illness Benefit: Unlimited

Geographic Areas Served
Maryland, the District of Columbia and parts of Northern
Virginia

Accreditation Certification
NCQA
TJC Accreditation, Medicare Approved, Utilization Review,
Pre-Admission Certification, State Licensure, Quality
Assurance Program

Key Personnel
Preisdent & CEO . . . . Chet Burrell
Chair . . . . Stephen L. Waechter
Chair . . . . Ann B. Mech
Chair . . . . Wendell L. Johns

Specialty Managed Care Partners
Enters into Contracts with Regional Business Coalitions: Yes

---

376 Coventry Health Care, Inc.

6730-B Rockledge Drive
Suite 700
Bethesda, MD 20817
Phone: 301-581-0600
coventryhealthcare.com
Subsidiary of: Aetna Inc.

For Profit Organization: Yes

Healthplan and Services Defined
PLAN TYPE: HMO/PPO
Model Type: Network
Plan Specialty: Behavioral Health, Dental, Worker's
Compensation
Benefits Offered: Behavioral Health, Dental, Prescription,
Wellness, Worker's Compensation

Type of Coverage
Commercial, Individual, Medicare, Medicaid

Geographic Areas Served
Nationwide, including the District of Columbia and Puerto
Rico

Key Personnel
Chairman & CEO . . . . Mark T. Bertolini
President . . . . Karen S. Lynch
Chief Financial Officer . . . . Shawn M. Guertin
Operations & Technology . . . . Meg McCarthy
Chief Medical Officer . . . . Harold L. Paz
General Counsel . . . . Thomas Sabatino Jr.
Government Services . . . . Fran S. Soistman

---

377 Denta-Chek of Maryland

10400 Little Patuxet Parkway
Suite 260
Columbia, MD 21044
Toll-Free: 888-478-8833
Phone: 410-997-3300
Fax: 410-997-3796
info@dentachek.com
www.dentachek.com
Non-Profit Organization: Yes
Year Founded: 1981
Number of Primary Care Physicians: 300
Number of Referral/Specialty Physicians: 200
Total Enrollment: 10,000

Healthplan and Services Defined
PLAN TYPE: Dental
Model Type: IPA
Plan Specialty: Dental
Benefits Offered: Dental

Type of Coverage
Catastrophic Illness Benefit: None

Type of Payment Plans Offered
POS, Combination FFS & DFFS

Geographic Areas Served
Statewide

Subscriber Information
Average Monthly Fee Per Subscriber
(Employee + Employer Contribution):
Employee Only (Self): $16.00
Employee & 1 Family Member: $22.00
Employee & 2 Family Members: $28.00
Medicare: $0
Average Annual Deductible Per Subscriber:
Employee Only (Self): $0

Employee & 1 Family Member: $0
Employee & 2 Family Members: $0
Medicare: $0
Average Subscriber Co-Payment:
Non-Network Physician: $0
Prescription Drugs: $0
Hospital ER: $0
Home Health Care: $0
Nursing Home: $0

Network Qualifications
Pre-Admission Certification: Yes

Peer Review Type
Utilization Review: Yes
Second Surgical Opinion: Yes
Case Management: Yes

Publishes and Distributes Report Card: No

Accreditation Certification
State Licensure, Quality Assurance Program

Specialty Managed Care Partners
Enters into Contracts with Regional Business Coalitions: No

378 Dental Benefit Providers
6220 Old Dobbin Lane
Columbia, MD 21045
Toll-Free: 800-307-7820
www.dbp.com
Secondary Address: 425 Market Street, 14th Floor, San
Francisco, CA 94105, 415-778-3800
Subsidiary of: UnitedHealth Group
For Profit Organization: Yes
Year Founded: 1984
Number of Primary Care Physicians: 125,000
Total Enrollment: 6,600,000

Healthplan and Services Defined
PLAN TYPE: Dental
Model Type: IPA
Plan Specialty: ASO, Dental, EPO, DHMO, PPO, CSO,
Preventive, Claims Repricing and Network Access
Benefits Offered: Dental

Type of Coverage
Indemnity, Medicare, Medicaid

Type of Payment Plans Offered
POS, DFFS, Capitated, FFS

Geographic Areas Served
48 states including District of Columbia, Puerto Rico and
Virgin Islands

Accreditation Certification
NCQA

Key Personnel
President, UH Dental . . . . Paul Hebert

379 First Health Part D
6730-B Rockledge Drive
Suite 700
Bethasda, MD 20817
Phone: 301-581-0600
coventry-medicare.com
Subsidiary of: Coventry Health Care
For Profit Organization: Yes

Healthplan and Services Defined
PLAN TYPE: Medicare
Benefits Offered: Prescription

Type of Coverage
Medicare, Medicare Part D

Geographic Areas Served
Nationwide

380 Kaiser Permanente Mid-Atlantic
2101 E Jefferson Street
Suite 100
Rockville, MD 20852
Phone: 301-816-2424
thrive.kaiserpermanente.org/care-near-mid-atlantic
Subsidiary of: Kaiser Permanente
Non-Profit Organization: Yes
Year Founded: 1945
Number of Primary Care Physicians: 1,100
Total Enrollment: 614,350

Healthplan and Services Defined
PLAN TYPE: Multiple
Model Type: Network
Benefits Offered: Disease Management, Prescription, Vision,
Wellness

Type of Coverage
Commercial, Individual, Medicare, Supplemental Medicare,
Medicaid

Geographic Areas Served
Virginia, Maryland and the District of Columbia

Key Personnel
President, Mid-Atlantic . . . . Kim Horn
Chief Executive Officer . . . . Richard Isaacs
Executive Vice President. . . . . Gregory A. Adams

381 Priority Partners Health Plans
6704 Curtis Court
Glen Burnie, MD 21060-9949
Toll-Free: 800-654-9728
ppcustomerservice@jhhc.com
www.ppmco.org
Subsidiary of: John Hopkins HealthCare LLC/Maryland
Community Health System
Non-Profit Organization: Yes
Year Founded: 1996
Total Enrollment: 185,000
State Enrollment: 185,000

Healthplan and Services Defined
PLAN TYPE: HMO

Benefits Offered: Behavioral Health, Dental, Prescription, Vision

Type of Coverage
Medicaid

Type of Payment Plans Offered
Capitated, FFS

Geographic Areas Served
Maryland

Peer Review Type
Second Surgical Opinion: Yes

Publishes and Distributes Report Card: Yes

Accreditation Certification
TJC, NCQA, JACHO, HMO

382 Spectera Eyecare Networks

6220 Old Dobbin Lane
Liberty 6, Suite 200
Columbia, MD 21045
Toll-Free: 800-638-3120
www.spectera.com
Mailing Address: P.O. Box 30978, Salt Lake City, UT 84130
Subsidiary of: UnitedHealth Group
For Profit Organization: Yes
Year Founded: 1964
Number of Primary Care Physicians: 24,000
Total Enrollment: 17,000,000

Healthplan and Services Defined
PLAN TYPE: Multiple
Model Type: Network
Plan Specialty: Vision
Benefits Offered: Disease Management, Vision

Type of Coverage
Commercial, Individual

Type of Payment Plans Offered
POS, DFFS, Capitated

Subscriber Information
Average Monthly Fee Per Subscriber
(Employee + Employer Contribution):
Employee Only (Self): Varies
Average Annual Deductible Per Subscriber:
Employee & 2 Family Members: Varies
Average Subscriber Co-Payment:
Primary Care Physician: Varies

Network Qualifications
Pre-Admission Certification: Yes

Publishes and Distributes Report Card: Yes

Key Personnel
CEO . . . . Paul Gaulstrand
CFO . . . . Kyle Stern
General Counsel . . . . Jennifer Lewis
Chief Sales Officer . . . . Laurida Mackenzie

Specialty Managed Care Partners
United Heath Group
Enters into Contracts with Regional Business Coalitions: No

383 Trinity Health of Maryland

Holy Cross Health
1500 Forest Glen Road
Silver Spring, MD 20910
Phone: 301-754-7000
www.trinity-health.org
Subsidiary of: Trinity Health
Non-Profit Organization: Yes
Year Founded: 2013
Total Enrollment: 30,000,000

Healthplan and Services Defined
PLAN TYPE: Other
Benefits Offered: Disease Management, Home Care,
Long-Term Care, Psychiatric, Hospice programs, PACE
(Program of All Inclusive Care for the Elderly)

Geographic Areas Served
Montgomery, Prince Georges and Howard counties

Key Personnel
Chief Executive Officer . . . . Richard J. Gilfillan
Chief Financial Officer . . . . Benjamin R. Carter
Human Resources . . . . Edmund F. Hodge
General Counsel . . . . Paul G. Neumann
Chief Clinical Officer . . . . Daniel J. Roth
Chief Operating Officer . . . . Michael A. Slubowski

384 United Concordia of Maryland

11311 McCormick Ep 4 Road
Suite 170
Hunt Valley, MD 21031
Phone: 443-866-9500
www.unitedconcordia.com
For Profit Organization: Yes
Year Founded: 1971
Total Enrollment: 7,800,000

Healthplan and Services Defined
PLAN TYPE: Dental
Plan Specialty: Dental
Benefits Offered: Dental

Type of Coverage
Commercial, Individual, Military personnel & families

Geographic Areas Served
Nationwide

Accreditation Certification
URAC

Key Personnel
President & COO . . . . Timothy J. Constantine
Contact . . . . Beth Rutherford
717-260-7659
beth.rutherford@ucci.com

385 UnitedHealthcare of Maryland

6220 Old Dobbin Lane
Columbia, MD 21045
Toll-Free: 800-307-7820
www.uhc.com/contact-us/maryland
Subsidiary of: UnitedHealth Group

Non-Profit Organization: Yes
Year Founded: 1976

Healthplan and Services Defined
PLAN TYPE: HMO/PPO
Model Type: Network
Plan Specialty: Behavioral Health, Dental, Disease
Management, PBM, Vision
Benefits Offered: Behavioral Health, Dental, Disease
Management, Long-Term Care, Prescription, Vision,
Wellness, Life, LTD, STD

Type of Coverage
Individual, Medicare, Supplemental Medicare, Medicaid,
Catastrophic, Family, Military, Veterans, Group,

Geographic Areas Served
Maryland, Virginia, and the District of Columbia

Subscriber Information
Average Monthly Fee Per Subscriber
(Employee + Employer Contribution):
Employee Only (Self): $104.00-135.00
Employee & 1 Family Member: $143.00-184.00
Employee & 2 Family Members: $331.00-440.00
Medicare: $112.00-156.00
Average Annual Deductible Per Subscriber:
Employee Only (Self): $100.00-250.00
Employee & 1 Family Member: $500.00-1500.00
Employee & 2 Family Members: $200.00-500.00
Medicare: $0
Average Subscriber Co-Payment:
Primary Care Physician: $5.00/10.00
Non-Network Physician: Deductible
Prescription Drugs: $5.00/10.00
Hospital ER: $25.00/50.00
Home Health Care: $5.00/10.00

Network Qualifications
Pre-Admission Certification: Yes

Peer Review Type
Utilization Review: Yes
Second Surgical Opinion: Yes
Case Management: Yes

Publishes and Distributes Report Card: Yes

Accreditation Certification
TJC Accreditation, Medicare Approved, Utilization Review,
Pre-Admission Certification, State Licensure, Quality
Assurance Program

Key Personnel
President . . . . David Wichmann
Chief Operating Officer. . . . . Dan Schummacher
Chief Strategy Officer . . . . John Cosgriff
Communications Officer . . . . Kirsten Gorsuch
Chief Medical Officer. . . . . Sam Ho
Chief Legal Officer . . . . Thad Johnson
Chief Information Officer . . . . Phil McKoy
Chief Financial Officer. Jeff Putnam

Specialty Managed Care Partners
Enters into Contracts with Regional Business Coalitions: Yes

Health Insurance Coverage Status and Type of Coverage by Age

Category	All Persons		Under 18 years		Under 65 years	
	Number	%	Number	%	Number	%
Total population	6,736	-	1,482	-	5,700	-
Covered by some type of health insurance	6,565 *(11)*	97.5 *(0.2)*	1,467 *(5)*	99.0 *(0.2)*	5,532 *(11)*	97.1 *(0.2)*
Covered by private health insurance	4,975 *(32)*	73.9 *(0.5)*	1,035 *(12)*	69.8 *(0.8)*	4,288 *(30)*	75.2 *(0.5)*
Employer-based	4,245 *(35)*	63.0 *(0.5)*	940 *(13)*	63.4 *(0.9)*	3,818 *(32)*	67.0 *(0.6)*
Direct purchase	912 *(18)*	13.5 *(0.3)*	110 *(5)*	7.4 *(0.4)*	573 *(16)*	10.1 *(0.3)*
TRICARE	79 *(6)*	1.2 *(0.1)*	13 *(2)*	0.9 *(0.2)*	46 *(6)*	0.8 *(0.1)*
Covered by public health insurance	2,459 *(27)*	36.5 *(0.4)*	509 *(13)*	34.3 *(0.9)*	1,476 *(27)*	25.9 *(0.5)*
Medicaid	1,583 *(27)*	23.5 *(0.4)*	506 *(13)*	34.2 *(0.8)*	1,401 *(26)*	24.6 *(0.5)*
Medicare	1,123 *(7)*	16.7 *(0.1)*	4 *(1)*	0.3 *(0.1)*	141 *(7)*	2.5 *(0.1)*
VA Care	101 *(4)*	1.5 *(0.1)*	1 *(1)*	0.1 *(Z)*	37 *(3)*	0.6 *(0.1)*
Not covered at any time during the year	171 *(10)*	2.5 *(0.2)*	15 *(3)*	1.0 *(0.2)*	168 *(11)*	2.9 *(0.2)*

Note: Numbers in thousands; Figures cover civilian noninstitutionalized population in 2016; N/A indicates that data was not available; Z represents or rounds to zero; Margin of error appears in parenthesis and is calculated using replicate weights.
Source: U.S. Census Bureau, American Community Survey, Table HIC-4_ACS. Health Insurance Coverage Status and Type of Coverage by State—All People: 2008 to 2016, Table HIC-5_ACS. Health Insurance Coverage Status and Type of Coverage by State—Children Under 18: 2008 to 2016, Table HIC-6_ACS. Health Insurance Coverage Status and Type of Coverage by State—Persons Under 65: 2008 to 2016

Massachusetts

386 Aetna Health of Massachusetts

151 Farmington Avenue
Hartford, CT 06156
Toll-Free: 800-872-3862
Phone: 860-273-0123
www.aetna.com
Subsidiary of: Aetna Inc.
For Profit Organization: Yes
Year Founded: 1987

Healthplan and Services Defined
PLAN TYPE: HMO/PPO
Other Type: POS
Model Type: IPA, Network
Plan Specialty: Behavioral Health, EPO, Lab, PBM,
    Radiology
Benefits Offered: Behavioral Health, Dental, Disease
    Management, Long-Term Care, Physical Therapy,
    Podiatry, Prescription, Psychiatric, Vision, Life, LTD, STD

Type of Coverage
Commercial, Student health
Catastrophic Illness Benefit: Covered

Geographic Areas Served
Statewide

Peer Review Type
Second Surgical Opinion: Yes
Case Management: Yes

Publishes and Distributes Report Card: Yes

Accreditation Certification
NCQA

Key Personnel
CEO . . . . Mark Bertolini

387 Araz Group

7201 West 78th Street
Bloomington, MN 55439
Toll-Free: 800-444-3005
Phone: 952-896-1200
info@araz.com
www.araz.com
For Profit Organization: Yes
Year Founded: 1982
Number of Primary Care Physicians: 71,000
Total Enrollment: 250,000
State Enrollment: 160,000

Healthplan and Services Defined
PLAN TYPE: PPO
Plan Specialty: UR
Benefits Offered: Behavioral Health, Disease Management,
    Prescription, Worker's Compensation, AD&D, LTD, STD

Type of Coverage
Commercial, Medicare

Geographic Areas Served
Minnesota, Western Wisconsin, Northern Iowa, North and
South Dakota

Accreditation Certification
Pre-Admission Certification

Key Personnel
Founder & CEO . . . . Nazie Eftekhari
President . . . . Amir Eftekhari

Specialty Managed Care Partners
Intracorp

388 Avesis: Massachusetts

790 Turnpike Street
Suite 202
North Andover, MA 01845
Toll-Free: 855-214-6777
Phone: 888-363-4824
www.avesis.com
Subsidiary of: Guardian Life Insurance Co.
Year Founded: 1978
Number of Primary Care Physicians: 25,000
Total Enrollment: 3,500,000

Healthplan and Services Defined
PLAN TYPE: PPO
Other Type: Vision, Dental
Model Type: Network
Plan Specialty: Dental, Vision
Benefits Offered: Dental, Vision

Type of Coverage
Commercial

Type of Payment Plans Offered
POS, Capitated, Combination FFS & DFFS

Geographic Areas Served
Nationwide and Puerto Rico

Publishes and Distributes Report Card: Yes

Accreditation Certification
AAAHC
TJC Accreditation

Key Personnel
Chief Executive Officer . . . . Chris Swanker
Business Development . . . . Alan Cohn

389 Blue Cross & Blue Shield of Massachusetts

101 Huntington Avenue
Suite 1300
Boston, MA 02199-7611
Toll-Free: 800-262-2583
www.bcbsma.com
Non-Profit Organization: Yes
Year Founded: 1937
Number of Affiliated Hospitals: 77
Number of Primary Care Physicians: 20,266
Total Enrollment: 3,000,000
State Enrollment: 3,000,000

Healthplan and Services Defined
PLAN TYPE: HMO
Model Type: Network
Plan Specialty: Dental, Group Medical
Benefits Offered: Behavioral Health, Chiropractic,
  Complementary Medicine, Dental, Disease Management,
  Home Care, Inpatient SNF, Long-Term Care, Physical
  Therapy, Podiatry, Prescription, Psychiatric, Transplant,
  Vision, Wellness, AD&D, Life, LTD, STD
Offers Demand Management Patient Information Service:
  Yes
DMPI Services Offered: 24-Hour Nurse Care Line

Type of Coverage
Medicare, Group Insurance

Type of Payment Plans Offered
FFS

Geographic Areas Served
Massachusetts & Southern New Hampshire

Subscriber Information
Average Monthly Fee Per Subscriber
  (Employee + Employer Contribution):
    Employee Only (Self): Varies by plan

Network Qualifications
Pre-Admission Certification: Yes

Peer Review Type
Utilization Review: Yes

Accreditation Certification
NCQA
TJC Accreditation, Medicare Approved, Utilization Review,
  Pre-Admission Certification, State Licensure

Key Personnel
President/CEO . . . . Andrew Dreyfus
COO . . . . Deborah Devaux
EVP/CFO. . . . . Andreana Santangelo
SVP/General Counsel. . . . . Stephanie Lovell
SVP, Corp Communications . . . . Jay McQuaide
Chief Physician Executive . . . . Bruce Nash
Chief Strategy Officer. . . . . Jason Robart
EVP, Sales/Marketing. . . . . Patrick Gilligan

Specialty Managed Care Partners
Express Scripts

---

390   Dentaquest
465 Medford Street
Boston, MA 02129-1454
Toll-Free: 800-417-7140
www.dentaquest.com
Subsidiary of: DentaQuest Ventures
Year Founded: 1980
Number of Primary Care Physicians: 750
Total Enrollment: 14,000,000

Healthplan and Services Defined
PLAN TYPE: Dental
Plan Specialty: Dental
Benefits Offered: Dental

Type of Coverage
Individual, Medicare, Medicaid

Geographic Areas Served
Arizona, California, Colorado, Florida, Georgia, Idaho,
  Illinois, Indiana, Kentucky, Louisiana, Maryland,
  Massachusetts, Michicgan, Minnesota, Mississippi, Missouri,
  New Hampshire, New Jersey, New Mexico, New York, Ohio,
  Rhode Island, Pennsylvania, North Carolina, South Carolina,
  Tennessee, Texas, Utah, Virginia, Washington, Wisconsin

Key Personnel
President/CEO . . . . Steve Pollock
CFO/COO . . . . James Collins
Chief Dental Officer . . . . Olivia Croom
Chief Legal Officer . . . . David Abelman
Vice President, Sales. . . . . Judd Wagner
  262-834-3757
  Judd.Wagner@improvingoralhealth.com
Director, Public Affairs . . . . Kristin LaRoche
  617-886-1458
  Kristin.LaRoche@improvingoralhealth.com

---

391   Fallon Health
10 Chestnut Street
Worcester, MA 01608
Toll-Free: 800-333-2535
Phone: 508-799-2100
contactcustomerservice@fallonhealth.org
www.fchp.org
Non-Profit Organization: Yes
Year Founded: 1977

Healthplan and Services Defined
PLAN TYPE: Multiple
Benefits Offered: Behavioral Health, Chiropractic, Dental,
  Disease Management, Home Care, Inpatient SNF, Physical
  Therapy, Podiatry, Prescription, Psychiatric, Vision,
  Wellness

Type of Coverage
Individual, Medicare, Medicaid

Geographic Areas Served
Statewide

Key Personnel
President & CEO . . . . Richard P. Burke
Senior VP & CCO. . . . . James Gentile
Senior VP & COO. . . . . Emily West
Chief Legal Counsel . . . . Mark Mosby
Chief Medical Officer . . . . Thomas H. Ebert, MD
SVP & Chief Sales Officer . . . . David Przesiek
Director, Community Rel. . . . . Kimberly Salmon
  508-368-9439
  kimberly.salmon@fallonhealth.org

---

392   Harvard Pilgrim Health Care Massachusetts
93 Worcester Street
Wellesley, MA 02481
Toll-Free: 888-888-4742
Phone: 617-509-1000
www.harvardpilgrim.org

Non-Profit Organization: Yes
Year Founded: 1977
Number of Affiliated Hospitals: 179
Number of Referral/Specialty Physicians: 53,000

Healthplan and Services Defined
  PLAN TYPE: Multiple
  Model Type: Network
  Plan Specialty: ASO, Behavioral Health, Chiropractic,
    Dental, Disease Management, EPO, Lab, MSO, PBM,
    Vision, Radiology, Worker's Compensation, UR
  Benefits Offered: Behavioral Health, Chiropractic, Disease
    Management, Home Care, Inpatient SNF, Long-Term Care,
    Physical Therapy, Podiatry, Prescription, Psychiatric,
    Transplant, Vision, Wellness

Type of Coverage
  Commercial, Individual, Indemnity, Medicare, Supplemental
    Medicare, Medicaid

Geographic Areas Served
  Statewide

Peer Review Type
  Utilization Review: Yes
  Second Surgical Opinion: Yes
  Case Management: Yes

Publishes and Distributes Report Card: Yes

Accreditation Certification
  NCQA
  TJC Accreditation, Medicare Approved, Utilization Review,
    Pre-Admission Certification, State Licensure, Quality
    Assurance Program

Key Personnel
  President & CEO...................... Eric H. Schultz
  Chief Financial Officer .... Charles Goheen
  President, Health Plans .... Deborah Hodges
  Chief Legal Officer .... Tisa Hughes
  Chief Information Officer............. Deborah A. Norton
  VP, Marketing .... Richard O'Connor
  Human Resources...................... Cynthia Ring
  SVP, Sales & Marketing .... Beth Roberts
  SVP, Medical Officer .... Michael Sherman, MD

Average Claim Compensation
  Physician's Fees Charged: 51%
  Hospital's Fees Charged: 40%

Specialty Managed Care Partners
  Enters into Contracts with Regional Business Coalitions: No

---

393   **Health New England**
One Monarch Place
Suite 1500
Springfield, MA 01144-1500
Toll-Free: 800-310-2835
Phone: 413-787-4004
healthnewengland.org
Non-Profit Organization: Yes
Year Founded: 1985
Number of Affiliated Hospitals: 22
Number of Primary Care Physicians: 4,300

Total Enrollment: 200,000
State Enrollment: 200,000

Healthplan and Services Defined
  PLAN TYPE: HMO/PPO
  Model Type: IPA
  Plan Specialty: ASO, Disease Management
  Benefits Offered: Behavioral Health, Chiropractic,
    Complementary Medicine, Dental, Disease Management,
    Home Care, Inpatient SNF, Physical Therapy, Podiatry,
    Prescription, Psychiatric, Transplant, Vision, Wellness

Type of Coverage
  Commercial, Medicare, Medicaid, Catastrophic
  Catastrophic Illness Benefit: Maximum $1M

Type of Payment Plans Offered
  POS

Geographic Areas Served
  Berkshire, Franklin, Hampden, Hampshire and Worcester
  counties in Massachusetts, and Hartford and Tolland counties
  in Connecticut

Peer Review Type
  Utilization Review: Yes
  Second Surgical Opinion: Yes
  Case Management: Yes

Publishes and Distributes Report Card: Yes

Accreditation Certification
  NCQA
  TJC Accreditation, Medicare Approved, Utilization Review,
    Pre-Admission Certification, State Licensure, Quality
    Assurance Program

Key Personnel
  President & CEO .... Maura C. McCaffrey
  VP, Sales & Marketing .... Ashley Allen
  Information Technology .... Ken Bernard
  VP, Medical Officer .... Laurie Gianturco, MD
  VP, Operations........................... Jody Gross

Average Claim Compensation
  Physician's Fees Charged: 59%
  Hospital's Fees Charged: 49%

Specialty Managed Care Partners
  Enters into Contracts with Regional Business Coalitions: No

---

394   **Health Plans, Inc.**
1500 West Park Drive
Suite 330
Westborough, MA 01581
Toll-Free: 800-532-7575
Phone: 508-752-2480
Fax: 508-754-9664
www.healthplansinc.com
Subsidiary of: Harvard Pilgrim
Year Founded: 1981

Healthplan and Services Defined
  PLAN TYPE: PPO
  Other Type: TPA
  Model Type: Network

Plan Specialty: ASO, Behavioral Health, Chiropractic, Dental, Disease Management, EPO, Lab, PBM, Vision, Radiology, UR
Benefits Offered: Home Care, Inpatient SNF, Long-Term Care, Physical Therapy, Podiatry, Prescription, Psychiatric, Transplant, Vision, Wellness, Worker's Compensation, AD&D, Life, LTD, STD

Geographic Areas Served
New England and South Carolina

Accreditation Certification
TJC Accreditation, Pre-Admission Certification

Key Personnel
President & CEO . . . . Deborah Hodges
Senior Vice President. . . . . Todd Bailey
Chief Information Officer . . . . Chuck Moulter
VP, Operations. . . . . Chris Parr
VP, Financial Operations . . . . Joan Recore

395 Humana Health Insurance of Massachusetts
1 International Boulevard
Suite 904
Mahwah, NJ 07495
Toll-Free: 800-967-2370
Fax: 201-934-1369
www.humana.com
Subsidiary of: Humana
For Profit Organization: Yes

Healthplan and Services Defined
PLAN TYPE: HMO/PPO
Model Type: Network
Plan Specialty: Dental, Vision
Benefits Offered: Dental, Vision, Life, LTD, STD

Type of Coverage
Commercial

Geographic Areas Served
Massachusetts is covered by the New Jersey branch

Accreditation Certification
URAC, NCQA, CORE

Key Personnel
President & CEO. Bruce Broussard
Chief Medical Officer. . . . . Roy A. Beveridge
Chief Consumer Officer. . . . . Jody L. Bilney
Human Resources. . . . . Tim Huval
Chief Financial Officer . . . . Brian Kane
Chief Information Officer . . . . Brian LeClaire
General Counsel . . . . Christopher M. Todoroff

396 Medical Center Healthnet Plan
529 Main Street
Suite 500
Charlestown, MA 02129
Toll-Free: 888-566-0008
Phone: 617-748-6000
memberquestions@bmchp.org
www.bmchp.org
Non-Profit Organization: Yes

Year Founded: 1997
Number of Affiliated Hospitals: 60
Number of Primary Care Physicians: 3,000
Number of Referral/Specialty Physicians: 12,000
Total Enrollment: 240,890
State Enrollment: 240,890

Healthplan and Services Defined
PLAN TYPE: HMO
Benefits Offered: Disease Management, Prescription, Wellness

Type of Coverage
Individual

Key Personnel
President . . . . Susan Coakley
Chief Financial Officer. . . . . Laurie Doran
Chief Actuary. . . . . Michael Guerriere
Chief Information Officer . . . . Kim Sinclair
Chief Medical Officer . . . . Jonathan Welch, MD
Chief Legal Officer. Matt Herndon

397 Minuteman Health
38 Chauncy Street
Boston, MA 02111
Toll-Free: 855-644-1776
Fax: 857-263-8951
info@minutemanhealth.org
minutemanhealth.org
Non-Profit Organization: Yes
Number of Affiliated Hospitals: 44

Healthplan and Services Defined
PLAN TYPE: HMO
Benefits Offered: Behavioral Health, Chiropractic, Physical Therapy, Prescription, Psychiatric, Wellness, Maternity; Pediatric; Chemotherapy & Radiology; Hearing; Short-Term Rehabilitation; Labs & Imaging; Speech Therapy

Type of Coverage
Coverage varies per plan

Geographic Areas Served
Massachusetts & New Hampshire

Key Personnel
General Counsel & COO . . . . Susan E. Brown
Chief Medical Officer. . . . . Jan Cook
Media Contact. . . . . Kevin Beagan
617-521-7347
kevin.beagan@state.ma.us

398 Neighborhood Health Plan
399 Revolution Drive
Somerville, MA 02145
Toll-Free: 866-414-5533
memberservices@nhp.org
www.nhp.org
Subsidiary of: Partners HealthCare
Non-Profit Organization: Yes
Year Founded: 1986

Owned by an Integrated Delivery Network (IDN): Yes
Number of Affiliated Hospitals: 41
Number of Primary Care Physicians: 2,800
Number of Referral/Specialty Physicians: 10,400
Total Enrollment: 430,000
State Enrollment: 430,000

Healthplan and Services Defined
  PLAN TYPE: HMO
  Model Type: Network
  Plan Specialty: ASO, Behavioral Health, Disease
    Management, Medicaid Focus
  Benefits Offered: Behavioral Health, Complementary
    Medicine, Dental, Disease Management, Home Care,
    Prescription, Vision, Wellness

Type of Coverage
  Commercial, Medicaid
  Catastrophic Illness Benefit: Covered

Geographic Areas Served
  Most of Massachusetts counties

Network Qualifications
  Pre-Admission Certification: Yes

Peer Review Type
  Utilization Review: Yes
  Second Surgical Opinion: Yes
  Case Management: Yes

Publishes and Distributes Report Card: Yes

Accreditation Certification
  State of Ma
  TJC Accreditation, Medicare Approved, Utilization Review,
    Pre-Admission Certification, State Licensure, Quality
    Assurance Program

Key Personnel
  President/CEO . . . . David Segal
  Chief Operating Officer . . . . Mark McCormick
  Chief Financial Officer . . . . Joseph C. Capezza
  Chief, Stategy/Marketing . . . . Dana Rashti
  Chief Medical Officer . . . . Anton B. Dodek, MD
  Media . . . . Jennifer Rosenberg
    781-854-2997
    jenn@howellcomm.com

Specialty Managed Care Partners
  Beacon Health Strategies
  Enters into Contracts with Regional Business Coalitions: No

---

399   Trinity Health of Massachusetts
Sisters of Providence Health System
271 Carew Street
Springfield, MA 01104
Phone: 734-343-1270
www.trinity-health.org
Subsidiary of: Trinity Health
Non-Profit Organization: Yes
Year Founded: 2013
Total Enrollment: 30,000,000

Healthplan and Services Defined
  PLAN TYPE: Other

Benefits Offered: Disease Management, Home Care,
    Long-Term Care, Psychiatric, Hospice programs, PACE
    (Program of All Inclusive Care for the Elderly)

Geographic Areas Served
  Western Massachusetts

Key Personnel
  Chief Executive Officer . . . . Richard J. Gilfillan
  Chief Financial Officer . . . . Benjamin R. Carter
  Human Resources . . . . Edmund F. Hodge
  General Counsel . . . . Paul G. Neumann
  Chief Clinical Officer . . . . Daniel J. Roth
  Chief Operating Officer . . . . Michael A. Slubowski

---

400   Tufts Health Medicare Plan
705 Mt Auburn Street
Watertown, MA 02472
Toll-Free: 800-890-6600
Phone: 617-972-9400
www.tuftshealthplan.com
Secondary Address: One Mercantile Street, Suite 130,
  Worcester, MA 01608
Non-Profit Organization: Yes
Year Founded: 1979

Healthplan and Services Defined
  PLAN TYPE: Medicare
  Benefits Offered: Chiropractic, Dental, Disease Management,
    Home Care, Inpatient SNF, Physical Therapy, Podiatry,
    Prescription, Psychiatric, Vision, Wellness

Type of Coverage
  Individual, Medicare

Geographic Areas Served
  Massachusetts, Connecticut, New Hampshire, Rhode Island
  and Vermont

Subscriber Information
  Average Monthly Fee Per Subscriber
    (Employee + Employer Contribution):
      Employee Only (Self): Varies
      Medicare: Varies
  Average Annual Deductible Per Subscriber:
      Employee Only (Self): Varies
      Medicare: Varies
  Average Subscriber Co-Payment:
      Primary Care Physician: Varies
      Non-Network Physician: Varies
      Prescription Drugs: Varies
      Hospital ER: Varies
      Home Health Care: Varies
      Home Health Care Max. Days/Visits Covered: Varies
      Nursing Home: Varies
      Nursing Home Max. Days/Visits Covered: Varies

Key Personnel
  President/CEO . . . . Thomas A. Crowsell
  Chief Operations Officer . . . . Tricia Terbino
  SVP/CIO . . . . Umesh Kurpad
  SVP/Senior Products . . . . Patty Blake
  Chief Medical Officer . . . . Pual Kasuba, MD
  Chief, Human Resources . . . . Lydia Greene

401 Tufts Health Plan

705 Mt Auburn Street
Watertown, MA 02472
Toll-Free: 800-462-0224
Phone: 617-972-9400
www.tuftshealthplan.com
Secondary Address: One Mercantile Street, Suite 130,
Worcester, MA 01608
Non-Profit Organization: Yes
Year Founded: 1979
Number of Affiliated Hospitals: 90
Number of Primary Care Physicians: 25,000
Number of Referral/Specialty Physicians: 12,500
Total Enrollment: 737,411

Healthplan and Services Defined
PLAN TYPE: Multiple
Other Type: POS
Model Type: IPA
Plan Specialty: ASO, Behavioral Health, Chiropractic,
Disease Management, EPO, Lab, PBM, Vision, Radiology,
UR, Pharmacy
Benefits Offered: Behavioral Health, Chiropractic,
Complementary Medicine, Disease Management, Home
Care, Inpatient SNF, Physical Therapy, Podiatry,
Prescription, Psychiatric, Transplant, Vision, Wellness

Type of Coverage
Commercial, Individual, Medicare, Supplemental Medicare,
Medicaid, HSA, HRA

Type of Payment Plans Offered
POS, DFFS, FFS, Combination FFS & DFFS

Geographic Areas Served
Massachusetts, New Hampshire and Rhode Island

Subscriber Information
Average Monthly Fee Per Subscriber
(Employee + Employer Contribution):
Employee Only (Self): $190.00-220.00
Employee & 2 Family Members: $800.00-950.00
Medicare: $150.00
Average Annual Deductible Per Subscriber:
Employee Only (Self): $1000.00
Employee & 1 Family Member: $500.00
Employee & 2 Family Members: $3000.00
Average Subscriber Co-Payment:
Primary Care Physician: $10.00
Non-Network Physician: 20%
Prescription Drugs: $10/20/35
Hospital ER: $50.00
Home Health Care: $0
Home Health Care Max. Days/Visits Covered: 120 days
Nursing Home: $0
Nursing Home Max. Days/Visits Covered: 120 days

Network Qualifications
Pre-Admission Certification: No

Peer Review Type
Utilization Review: Yes
Case Management: Yes

Publishes and Distributes Report Card: Yes

Accreditation Certification
TJC, AAPI, NCQA

Key Personnel
CEO/President . . . . Thomas A. Croswell
Chief Operations Officer. . . . . Tricia Terbino
Chief Financial Officer . . . . Umesh Kurpad
General Counsel . . . . Mary O'Toole Mahoney
Chief Medical Officer . . . . Paul Kasuba, MD
Chief, Human Resources . . . . Lydia Greene

Average Claim Compensation
Physician's Fees Charged: 75%
Hospital's Fees Charged: 70%

Specialty Managed Care Partners
Advance PCS, Private Healthe Care Systems

Employer References
Commonwealth of Massachuestts, Fleet Boston, Roman
Catholic Archdiocese of Boston, City of Boston, State
Street Corporation

402 UniCare Massachusetts

Brickstone Square
Eight Floor
Andover, MA 01810
Phone: 978-470-1795
www.unicare.com
Subsidiary of: Anthem, Inc.
Year Founded: 1985

Healthplan and Services Defined
PLAN TYPE: HMO/PPO
Model Type: Network
Benefits Offered: Behavioral Health, Chiropractic,
Complementary
Medicine, Dental, Disease Management, Home Care,
Inpatient SNF, Long-Term Care, Physical Therapy,
Podiatry, Prescription, Psychiatric, Transplant,
Vision, Wellness, Worker's Compensation, AD&D,
Life, LTD, STD

Type of Coverage
Commercial, Individual, Indemnity, Medicare

Geographic Areas Served
Massachusetts, Southern New Hampshire & Rhode Island

Subscriber Information
Average Monthly Fee Per Subscriber
(Employee + Employer Contribution):
Employee Only (Self): Varies
Employee & 1 Family Member: Varies
Employee & 2 Family Members: Varies
Medicare: Varies
Average Annual Deductible Per Subscriber:
Employee Only (Self): Varies
Employee & 1 Family Member: Varies
Employee & 2 Family Members: Varies
Medicare: Varies
Average Subscriber Co-Payment:
Primary Care Physician: Varies

Non-Network Physician: Varies
Prescription Drugs: Varies
Hospital ER: Varies
Home Health Care: Varies
Home Health Care Max. Days/Visits Covered: Varies
Nursing Home: Varies
Nursing Home Max. Days/Visits Covered: Varies

Network Qualifications
Pre-Admission Certification: Yes

Peer Review Type
Utilization Review: Yes
Second Surgical Opinion: Yes
Case Management: Yes

Publishes and Distributes Report Card: No

Accreditation Certification
URAC
TJC Accreditation, Medicare Approved, Utilization Review,
Pre-Admission Certification, State Licensure, Quality
Assurance Program

403   UnitedHealthcare of Massachusetts

475 Kilvert Street
Warwick, RI 02886
Toll-Free: 888-735-5842
www.uhc.com/contact-us/massachusetts
Subsidiary of: UnitedHealth Group
For Profit Organization: Yes

Healthplan and Services Defined
PLAN TYPE: HMO/PPO
Model Type: Network
Plan Specialty: Behavioral Health, Dental, Disease
Management, PBM, Vision
Benefits Offered: Behavioral Health, Dental, Disease
Management, Long-Term Care, Prescription, Vision,
Wellness, Life, LTD, STD
Offers Demand Management Patient Information Service:
Yes

Type of Coverage
Individual, Medicare, Supplemental Medicare, Medicaid,
Catastrophic, Family, Military, Veterans, Group,
Catastrophic Illness Benefit: None

Type of Payment Plans Offered
POS, FFS

Geographic Areas Served
Statewide. Massachusetts is covered by the Rhode Island
branch

Subscriber Information
Average Monthly Fee Per Subscriber
(Employee + Employer Contribution):
Employee Only (Self): $150.00
Employee & 2 Family Members: $300.00

Network Qualifications
Pre-Admission Certification: Yes

Peer Review Type
Utilization Review: Yes
Second Surgical Opinion: Yes

Case Management: Yes

Publishes and Distributes Report Card: Yes

Accreditation Certification
AAPI, NCQA
TJC Accreditation, Medicare Approved, Utilization Review,
Pre-Admission Certification, State Licensure, Quality
Assurance Program

Key Personnel
President . . . . David Wichmann
Chief Operating Officer . . . . Dan Schumacher
Chief Strategy Officer . . . . John Cosgriff
Communications Officer . . . . Kirsten Gorsuch
Chief Medical Officer. . . . . Sam Ho
Chief Legal Officer . . . . Thad Johnson
Chief Information Officer . . . . Phil McKoy
Chief Financial Officer. Jeff Putnam

Average Claim Compensation
Physician's Fees Charged: 70%
Hospital's Fees Charged: 80%

Specialty Managed Care Partners
Enters into Contracts with Regional Business Coalitions: Yes

Health Insurance Coverage Status and Type of Coverage by Age

Category	All Persons		Under 18 years		Under 65 years	
	Number	%	Number	%	Number	%
Total population	9,818	-	2,329	-	8,247	-
Covered by some type of health insurance	9,291 *(14)*	94.6 *(0.1)*	2,258 *(7)*	96.9 *(0.2)*	7,724 *(14)*	93.7 *(0.2)*
Covered by private health insurance	6,991 *(31)*	71.2 *(0.3)*	1,472 *(14)*	63.2 *(0.6)*	5,836 *(30)*	70.8 *(0.4)*
Employer-based	5,878 *(32)*	59.9 *(0.3)*	1,335 *(14)*	57.3 *(0.6)*	5,128 *(30)*	62.2 *(0.4)*
Direct purchase	1,340 *(22)*	13.7 *(0.2)*	147 *(9)*	6.3 *(0.4)*	801 *(21)*	9.7 *(0.2)*
TRICARE	124 *(7)*	1.3 *(0.1)*	19 *(3)*	0.8 *(0.1)*	74 *(5)*	0.9 *(0.1)*
Covered by public health insurance	3,795 *(28)*	38.7 *(0.3)*	906 *(14)*	38.9 *(0.6)*	2,258 *(29)*	27.4 *(0.3)*
Medicaid	2,240 *(28)*	22.8 *(0.3)*	900 *(14)*	38.7 *(0.6)*	2,050 *(28)*	24.9 *(0.3)*
Medicare	1,848 *(10)*	18.8 *(0.1)*	12 *(2)*	0.5 *(0.1)*	312 *(9)*	3.8 *(0.1)*
VA Care	202 *(6)*	2.1 *(0.1)*	2 *(1)*	0.1 *(Z)*	83 *(5)*	1.0 *(0.1)*
Not covered at any time during the year	527 *(14)*	5.4 *(0.1)*	71 *(5)*	3.1 *(0.2)*	523 *(14)*	6.3 *(0.2)*

Note: Numbers in thousands; Figures cover civilian noninstitutionalized population in 2016; N/A indicates that data was not available; Z represents or rounds to zero; Margin of error appears in parenthesis and is calculated using replicate weights.
Source: U.S. Census Bureau, American Community Survey, Table HIC-4_ACS. Health Insurance Coverage Status and Type of Coverage by State—All People: 2008 to 2016, Table HIC-5_ACS. Health Insurance Coverage Status and Type of Coverage by State—Children Under 18: 2008 to 2016, Table HIC-6_ACS. Health Insurance Coverage Status and Type of Coverage by State—Persons Under 65: 2008 to 2016

Michigan

404 Aetna Better Health of Michigan
1333 Gratiot Avenue
Suite 400
Detroit, MI 48207
Toll-Free: 866-316-3784
www.aetnabetterhealth.com/michigan
Subsidiary of: Aetna, Inc.
Non-Profit Organization: Yes
Year Founded: 1973

Healthplan and Services Defined
PLAN TYPE: HMO
Model Type: IPA
Benefits Offered: Disease Management, Prescription,
Wellness

Type of Coverage
Medicare, Supplemental Medicare, Medicaid
Catastrophic Illness Benefit: Varies per case

Type of Payment Plans Offered
POS, DFFS, Capitated, FFS, Combination FFS & DFFS

Geographic Areas Served
counties: Barry, Berrien, Branch, Calhoun, Cass, Kalamazoo,
St. Joseph, Van Buren, Wayne, Macomb

Subscriber Information
Average Monthly Fee Per Subscriber
(Employee + Employer Contribution):
Employee Only (Self): Varies by plan
Average Annual Deductible Per Subscriber:
Employee Only (Self): $0
Employee & 1 Family Member: $0
Employee & 2 Family Members: $0
Medicare: $0
Average Subscriber Co-Payment:
Home Health Care: $0
Home Health Care Max. Days/Visits Covered: Unlimited
Nursing Home: $0
Nursing Home Max. Days/Visits Covered: 30 days

Network Qualifications
Pre-Admission Certification: Yes

Peer Review Type
Utilization Review: Yes
Second Surgical Opinion: Yes
Case Management: Yes

Publishes and Distributes Report Card: Yes

Accreditation Certification
NCQA
TJC Accreditation, Medicare Approved, Utilization Review,
Pre-Admission Certification, State Licensure, Quality
Assurance Program

Key Personnel
Chief Executive Officer . . . . Mark T. Bertolini
President . . . . Karen S. Lynch
Chief Financial Officer . . . . Shawn M. Guertin
Operations & Technology . . . . Meg McCarthy
Chief Medical Officer . . . . Harold L. Paz

General Counsel . . . . Thomas Sabatino
Government Services . . . . Fran S. Soistman

Average Claim Compensation
Physician's Fees Charged: 1%
Hospital's Fees Charged: 1%

Specialty Managed Care Partners
Enters into Contracts with Regional Business Coalitions: Yes

405 Aetna Health of Michigan
151 Farmington Avenue
Hartford, CT 06156
Toll-Free: 800-872-3862
Phone: 860-273-0123
www.aetna.com
Subsidiary of: Aetna Inc.
For Profit Organization: Yes

Healthplan and Services Defined
PLAN TYPE: HMO/PPO
Other Type: POS
Model Type: Network
Plan Specialty: Behavioral Health, EPO, Lab, PBM,
Radiology
Benefits Offered: Behavioral Health, Dental, Disease
Management, Long-Term Care, Physical Therapy, Podiatry,
Prescription, Psychiatric, Vision, Wellness, Life, LTD, STD

Type of Coverage
Commercial, Catastrophic, Student health

Geographic Areas Served
Statewide

Key Personnel
CEO . . . . Mark Bertolini

406 Ascension At Home
Crittenton Home Care
2251 Squirrel Road, Suite 320
Auburn Hills, MI 48326
Phone: 248-656-6757
Fax: 248-656-6758
ascensionathome.com
Subsidiary of: Ascension
Non-Profit Organization: Yes

Healthplan and Services Defined
PLAN TYPE: Other
Plan Specialty: Disease Management
Benefits Offered: Dental, Disease Management, Home Care,
Wellness, Ambulance & Transportation; Nursing Service;
Short-and-long-term care management planning; Hospice

Geographic Areas Served
Texas, Alabama, Indiana, Kansas, Michigan, Mississippi,
Oklahoma, Wisconsin

Key Personnel
President . . . . Kirk Allen
Dir., Home Health Service . . . . Darcy Burthay

407 Blue Care Network of Michigan

20500 Civic Center Drive
Southfield, MI 48076
Toll-Free: 855-237-3501
www.bcbsm.com
Subsidiary of: Blue Cross Blue Shield of Michigan
Non-Profit Organization: Yes
Year Founded: 1998
Federally Qualified: Yes
Number of Primary Care Physicians: 5,000
Number of Referral/Specialty Physicians: 17,000
Total Enrollment: 807,000

Healthplan and Services Defined
PLAN TYPE: HMO
Model Type: IPA, Network
Plan Specialty: Lab, Radiology
Benefits Offered: Behavioral Health, Disease Management,
   Prescription, Psychiatric, Wellness

Type of Coverage
Commercial, Individual, Medicare, Medicaid
Catastrophic Illness Benefit: Covered

Geographic Areas Served
Statewide

Peer Review Type
Case Management: Yes

Publishes and Distributes Report Card: Yes

Accreditation Certification
NCQA

Key Personnel
President & CEO . . . . Daniel J. Loepp
EVP, Financial Officer. . . . . Mark R. Bartlett
SVP, Information Officer . . . . William M. Fandrich
SVP, Medical Officer . . . . Thomas L. Simmer, MD

Specialty Managed Care Partners
Enters into Contracts with Regional Business Coalitions: Yes

Employer References
General Motors, Ford Motor Company, State of Michigan,
   Federal Employee Program, Daimler Chrysler

408 Blue Care Network of Michigan

20500 Civic Center Drive
Southfield, MI 48076
www.bcbsm.com
Non-Profit Organization: Yes
Year Founded: 1998
Federally Qualified: Yes
Number of Primary Care Physicians: 5,000
Number of Referral/Specialty Physicians: 17,000
State Enrollment: 807,000

Healthplan and Services Defined
PLAN TYPE: HMO
Model Type: Network
Plan Specialty: Dental, Lab, Vision, Radiology
Benefits Offered: Behavioral Health, Dental, Disease
   Management, Physical Therapy, Prescription, Psychiatric,
   Vision, Wellness

Type of Coverage
Commercial, Individual
Catastrophic Illness Benefit: Varies per case

Type of Payment Plans Offered
POS, Capitated, Combination FFS & DFFS

Geographic Areas Served
Muskegon, Newago, Oceana & Ottawa counties

Peer Review Type
Utilization Review: Yes
Second Surgical Opinion: Yes

Publishes and Distributes Report Card: Yes

Key Personnel
President and CEO. . . . . Daniel Loepp
Chief Financial Officer . . . . Mark Bartlett
Chief Medical Officer . . . . Thomas Simmer, MD

409 Blue Cross Blue Shield of Michigan

500 E Lafayette Boulevard
Detroit, MI 48244
Toll-Free: 855-237-3501
www.bcbsm.com
Year Founded: 1939
Number of Affiliated Hospitals: 153
Number of Primary Care Physicians: 30,000
Total Enrollment: 5,800,000
State Enrollment: 4,500,000

Healthplan and Services Defined
PLAN TYPE: Multiple
Model Type: Network
Benefits Offered: Chiropractic, Disease Management, Home
   Care, Inpatient SNF, Physical Therapy, Podiatry,
   Prescription, Psychiatric, Wellness

Type of Coverage
Commercial, Individual, Medicare, Supplemental Medicare,
   Medicaid

Geographic Areas Served
Blue Care Network available in 26 counties in southeastern
   Michigan. PPO plans available statewide

Subscriber Information
Average Monthly Fee Per Subscriber
   (Employee + Employer Contribution):
      Employee Only (Self): Varies
      Medicare: Varies
Average Annual Deductible Per Subscriber:
      Employee Only (Self): Varies
      Medicare: Varies
Average Subscriber Co-Payment:
      Primary Care Physician: Varies
      Non-Network Physician: Varies
      Prescription Drugs: Varies
      Hospital ER: Varies
      Home Health Care: Varies
      Home Health Care Max. Days/Visits Covered: Varies
      Nursing Home: Varies
      Nursing Home Max. Days/Visits Covered: Varies

Key Personnel

President & CEO	Daniel J. Loepp
Chief Financial Officer	Mark R. Bartlett
Chief Operating Officer	Darrell E. Middleton
EVP, Group Business	Kenneth R. Dallafior
Chief Medical Officer	Thomas L. Simmer, MD
EVP, Strategy	Lynda M. Rossi
SVP, Corp. Secretary	Tricia A. Keith
Corporate Compliance	Michele A. Samuels

410   Cofinity

28588 Northwestern Highway
Southfield, MI 48034
Toll-Free: 800-831-1166
Fax: 888-499-3957
www.cofinity.net
Subsidiary of: Aetna
For Profit Organization: Yes
Year Founded: 1979
Physician Owned Organization: Yes
Total Enrollment: 2,500,000

Healthplan and Services Defined
PLAN TYPE: PPO
Other Type: TPA
Model Type: Network
Plan Specialty: Behavioral Health, Chiropractic, Disease
    Management, EPO, Lab, Vision, Radiology, Worker's
    Compensation, UR, Medical Management, Medical
    Networks, Out-of-Network Claims Mgmt, Fraud & Abuse
    Mgmt, Credentialing Services
Benefits Offered: Dental, Prescription, Transplant, Worker's
    Compensation

Type of Coverage
Catastrophic Illness Benefit: Varies per case

Type of Payment Plans Offered
FFS

Geographic Areas Served
Statewide

Network Qualifications
Pre-Admission Certification: Yes

Peer Review Type
Utilization Review: Yes
Second Surgical Opinion: Yes
Case Management: Yes

Publishes and Distributes Report Card: No

Accreditation Certification
TJC Accreditation, Medicare Approved, Utilization Review,
    Pre-Admission Certification, State Licensure, Quality
    Assurance Program

Key Personnel

President/CEO	Blaine Faulkner
VP, Business Development	Kara Dornig
VP, Operations	Kelly Wright
Director, Sales	John Bryan

Average Claim Compensation
Physician's Fees Charged: 1%

Hospital's Fees Charged: 1%

Specialty Managed Care Partners
Gentiva
Enters into Contracts with Regional Business Coalitions: No

411   ConnectCare

4000 Wellness Drive
Midland, MI 48670
Toll-Free: 888-646-2429
Phone: 989-839-1629
Fax: 989-389-1626
info@connectcare.com
www.connectcare.com
Subsidiary of: MidMichigan Health Network LLC
Non-Profit Organization: Yes
Year Founded: 1993
Physician Owned Organization: Yes
Owned by an Integrated Delivery Network (IDN): Yes
Federally Qualified: No
Number of Affiliated Hospitals: 5,000
Number of Referral/Specialty Physicians: 90,000
Total Enrollment: 17,000
State Enrollment: 36,000

Healthplan and Services Defined
PLAN TYPE: PPO
Model Type: Network
Benefits Offered: Behavioral Health, Dental, Home Care,
    Inpatient SNF, Long-Term Care, Physical Therapy,
    Podiatry, Prescription, Psychiatric, Wellness

Type of Coverage
Commercial, Indemnity

Type of Payment Plans Offered
POS, DFFS

Geographic Areas Served
Domiciled in central Michigan, with primary counties served
    including Clare, Gladwin, Gratiot, Isabella, Midland,
    Montcalm and Roscommon. Arrangement with national PPO's
    for coverage of downstate and those enrollees residing outside
    of Michigan

Subscriber Information
Average Annual Deductible Per Subscriber:
    Employee Only (Self): $275.00
    Employee & 2 Family Members: $550.00

Network Qualifications
Pre-Admission Certification: Yes

Peer Review Type
Utilization Review: Yes
Second Surgical Opinion: Yes
Case Management: Yes

Accreditation Certification
NCQA
Quality Assurance Program

412 Coventry Health Care of Michigan

1333 Gratiot Avenue
Suite 400
Detroit, MI 48207
Phone: 313-567-8619
www.coventryhealthcare.com
Subsidiary of: Aetna Inc.
For Profit Organization: Yes
Year Founded: 1975

Healthplan and Services Defined
PLAN TYPE: HMO/PPO
Model Type: Network
Plan Specialty: Behavioral Health, Dental, Worker's
    Compensation
Benefits Offered: Behavioral Health, Dental, Prescription,
    Wellness, Worker's Compensation

Type of Coverage
Commercial, Medicare, Medicaid

Geographic Areas Served
Statewide

Key Personnel
Chief Executive Officer . . . . Mark T. Bertolini
President . . . . Karen S. Lynch
Chief Financial Officer . . . . Shawn M. Guertin
Operations & Technology . . . . Meg McCarthy
Chief Medical Officer . . . . Harold L. Paz
General Counsel . . . . Thomas Sabatino Jr.
Government Services . . . . Fran S. Soistman

413 Delta Dental of Michigan

4100 Okemos Road
Okemos, MI 48864
Toll-Free: 800-524-0149
www.deltadentalmi.com
Subsidiary of: Delta Dental Plans Association
Number of Primary Care Physicians: 5,000
Total Enrollment: 14,100,000

Healthplan and Services Defined
PLAN TYPE: Dental
Plan Specialty: Dental
Benefits Offered: Dental

Type of Coverage
Commercial, Individual

Geographic Areas Served
Michigan, Ohio, Indiana and Tennessee

414 Dencap Dental Plans

45 E Milwaukee Street
Detroit, MI 48202
Toll-Free: 888-988-3384
Phone: 313-972-1400
Fax: 313-972-4662
info@dencap.com
www.dencap.com
Year Founded: 1984
Number of Primary Care Physicians: 200

State Enrollment: 20,000

Healthplan and Services Defined
PLAN TYPE: Dental
Model Type: Network
Plan Specialty: Dental
Benefits Offered: Dental

Type of Coverage
Commercial, Individual

Type of Payment Plans Offered
DFFS, FFS

Geographic Areas Served
Southeastern Michigan

Subscriber Information
Average Monthly Fee Per Subscriber
    (Employee + Employer Contribution):
        Employee Only (Self): Varies

Peer Review Type
Case Management: Yes

Publishes and Distributes Report Card: Yes

Accreditation Certification
Utilization Review, Quality Assurance Program

Key Personnel
CEO . . . . Joe Lentine, Jr
Provider Relations Dir . . . . Frank Berge

Specialty Managed Care Partners
Midwest and Dentals, Great Expression

415 DenteMax

25925 Telegraph Road
Suite 400
Southfield, MI 48033
Toll-Free: 800-752-1547
Fax: 888-586-0296
customerservices@dentemax.com
www.dentemax.com
Subsidiary of: Dental Network of America
For Profit Organization: Yes
Year Founded: 1985
Number of Primary Care Physicians: 113,000
Total Enrollment: 4,500,000

Healthplan and Services Defined
PLAN TYPE: Dental
Other Type: Dental PPO
Plan Specialty: Dental
Benefits Offered: Dental

Type of Coverage
Commercial, Individual
Catastrophic Illness Benefit: None

Type of Payment Plans Offered
DFFS

Geographic Areas Served
Nationwide

Subscriber Information
Average Monthly Fee Per Subscriber
(Employee + Employer Contribution):
Employee Only (Self): Varies by plan

Network Qualifications
Pre-Admission Certification: No

Peer Review Type
Utilization Review: Yes

Accreditation Certification
Quality Assurance Program

Key Personnel
President/CEO . . . . Melissa Wagner
VP, Dental Networks . . . . Mike Miller
Network Operations . . . . Andrea Garrett
Regulatory Oversight . . . . Kathy Larking
Dental Director . . . . Dr. Timothy Custer
Network Development . . . . Ignacio Quiaro von Thun
VP, Sales/Marketing . . . . Kim Sharbatz

416 Golden Dental Plans
29377 Hoover Road
Warren, MI 48093
Toll-Free: 800-451-5918
Phone: 586-573-8118
Fax: 586-573-8720
www.goldendentalplans.com
Secondary Address: 5671 Trumbell Street, Detroit, MI 48208
Year Founded: 1984
Number of Primary Care Physicians: 3,200
Total Enrollment: 130,000

Healthplan and Services Defined
PLAN TYPE: Dental
Other Type: Dental HMO
Model Type: Network
Plan Specialty: Dental
Benefits Offered: Dental

Type of Coverage
Individual

Type of Payment Plans Offered
DFFS

Geographic Areas Served
Statewide

Accreditation Certification
Utilization Review, Pre-Admission Certification

417 HAP-Health Alliance Plan: Flint
2050 S Linden Road
Flint, MI 48532
Toll-Free: 800-422-4641
www.hap.org
Secondary Address: 2850 W Grand Boulevard, Detroit, MI
48202, 313-872-8100
Non-Profit Organization: Yes
Year Founded: 1979
Federally Qualified: Yes
Number of Affiliated Hospitals: 29

Number of Primary Care Physicians: 900
Number of Referral/Specialty Physicians: 1,800
Total Enrollment: 650,000
State Enrollment: 650,000

Healthplan and Services Defined
PLAN TYPE: HMO/PPO
Model Type: Network
Plan Specialty: Lab, Radiology
Benefits Offered: Behavioral Health, Chiropractic,
Complementary Medicine, Disease Management, Home
Care, Inpatient SNF, Long-Term Care, Physical Therapy,
Podiatry, Prescription, Psychiatric, Transplant, Vision,
Wellness, Women's Health
Offers Demand Management Patient Information Service: Yes

Type of Coverage
Commercial, Individual, Medicare, Supplemental Medicare,
Medicaid, Catastrophic, TPA
Catastrophic Illness Benefit: Unlimited

Type of Payment Plans Offered
POS, DFFS, Capitated, Combination FFS & DFFS

Geographic Areas Served
Commercial Product: Bay, Genesee, Huron, Lapeer,
Livingston, Midland, Northern Oakland counties, Saginaw,
Sanilac, Shiawassee, Tuscola. Full counties: Arenac, Sanilac
and St Clair

Subscriber Information
Average Monthly Fee Per Subscriber
(Employee + Employer Contribution):
Employee Only (Self): Varies by plan

Network Qualifications
Pre-Admission Certification: Yes

Peer Review Type
Utilization Review: Yes
Second Surgical Opinion: Yes
Case Management: Yes

Publishes and Distributes Report Card: Yes

Accreditation Certification
NCQA
TJC Accreditation, Medicare Approved, Utilization Review,
Pre-Admission Certification, State Licensure, Quality
Assurance Program

Key Personnel
President/CEO . . . . Teresa Kline
Chief Financial Officer . . . . Richard Swift
VP, Human Resources . . . . Derek Adams
Chief Compliance Officer . . . . J. Douglas Clark
SVP, Chief of Marketing . . . . Mary Ann Tournoux
Chief Medical Officer . . . . Michael Genord, MD
VP, IT/CIO . . . . Annette M. Marcath

Specialty Managed Care Partners
American Healthways
Enters into Contracts with Regional Business Coalitions: No

Employer References
General Motors, Delphi, Covenant Health Partners

418 HAP-Health Alliance Plan: Senior Medicare Plan

2850 W Grand Boulevard
Detroit, MI 48202
Toll-Free: 800-422-4641
Phone: 313-872-8100
msweb1@hap.org
www.hap.org
Non-Profit Organization: Yes
Number of Affiliated Hospitals: 29
Number of Primary Care Physicians: 900
Number of Referral/Specialty Physicians: 1,800
Total Enrollment: 14,000
State Enrollment: 14,000

Healthplan and Services Defined
  PLAN TYPE: Medicare
  Benefits Offered: Chiropractic, Disease Management, Home Care, Inpatient SNF, Physical Therapy, Podiatry, Prescription, Psychiatric, Vision, Wellness

Type of Coverage
  Individual, Medicare, MIChild

Geographic Areas Served
  Health Plus Senior Medicare Coverage Plans available only within Michigan

Subscriber Information
  Average Monthly Fee Per Subscriber
    (Employee + Employer Contribution):
      Employee Only (Self): Varies
      Medicare: Varies
  Average Annual Deductible Per Subscriber:
      Employee Only (Self): Varies
      Medicare: Varies
  Average Subscriber Co-Payment:
      Primary Care Physician: Varies
      Non-Network Physician: Varies
      Prescription Drugs: Varies
      Hospital ER: Varies
      Home Health Care: Varies
      Home Health Care Max. Days/Visits Covered: Varies
      Nursing Home: Varies
      Nursing Home Max. Days/Visits Covered: Varies

Key Personnel
  President & CEO . . . . Teresa L. Kline
  Chief Financial Officer . . . . Richard Swift
  Chief Medical Officer . . . . Michael Genord, MD
  SVP, Marketing Officer . . . . Mary Ann Tournoux
  Human Resources . . . . Derick W. Adams
  Chief Compliance Officer. . . . . J. Douglas Clark
  Underwriting Officer . . . . Todd Hutchinson

419 Health Alliance Medicare

2850 W Grand Boulevard
Detroit, MI 48202
Toll-Free: 800-868-3153
Phone: 313-872-8100
msweb1@hap.org
www.hap.org/medicare
Non-Profit Organization: Yes
Total Enrollment: 383,000

Healthplan and Services Defined
  PLAN TYPE: Medicare
  Other Type: HMO/PPO, POS
  Benefits Offered: Chiropractic, Dental, Home Care, Inpatient SNF, Physical Therapy, Podiatry, Prescription, Psychiatric, Wellness, Worldwide Emergency, Fitness Benefits, Hearing Exams, Preventive Services, Eye Exams & Eyeglasses, Urgent Care, Hospice

Type of Coverage
  Individual, Medicare, Group Medicare Plans

Geographic Areas Served
  Statewide

Subscriber Information
  Average Monthly Fee Per Subscriber
    (Employee + Employer Contribution):
      Employee Only (Self): Varies
      Medicare: Varies
  Average Annual Deductible Per Subscriber:
      Employee Only (Self): Varies
      Medicare: Varies
  Average Subscriber Co-Payment:
      Primary Care Physician: Varies
      Non-Network Physician: Varies
      Prescription Drugs: Varies
      Hospital ER: Varies
      Home Health Care: Varies
      Home Health Care Max. Days/Visits Covered: Varies
      Nursing Home: Varies
      Nursing Home Max. Days/Visits Covered: Varies

Key Personnel
  President/CEO. . . . . Teresa Kline
  Chief Financial Officer . . . . Richard Swift
  VP, Human Resources . . . . Derek Adams
  Chief Compliance Officer. . . . . J. Douglas Clark
  SVP/Chief of Marketing . . . . Mary Ann Tournoux
  Chief Medical Officer . . . . Michael Genord, MD
  SVP, IT/CIO . . . . Annette M. Marcath

420 Health Alliance Plan

2850 W Grand Boulevard
Detroit, MI 48202
Toll-Free: 800-422-4641
Phone: 313-872-8100
msweb1@hap.org
www.hap.org
Non-Profit Organization: Yes
Year Founded: 1979
Number of Affiliated Hospitals: 157
Number of Primary Care Physicians: 18,000
Number of Referral/Specialty Physicians: 1,000
Total Enrollment: 650,000
State Enrollment: 650,000

Healthplan and Services Defined
  PLAN TYPE: HMO/PPO
  Other Type: EPO

Model Type: Staff
Benefits Offered: Dental, Disease Management, Prescription, Vision, Wellness, Alternative Medicine
Offers Demand Management Patient Information Service: Yes
DMPI Services Offered: Health Education Classes

Type of Coverage
Commercial, Individual, Medicare, Supplemental Medicare, Medicaid, Catastrophic

Type of Payment Plans Offered
POS, Capitated, FFS, Combination FFS & DFFS

Geographic Areas Served
Statewide

Network Qualifications
Pre-Admission Certification: Yes

Peer Review Type
Utilization Review: Yes
Second Surgical Opinion: No
Case Management: Yes

Publishes and Distributes Report Card: Yes

Accreditation Certification
NCQA
TJC Accreditation, Medicare Approved, Utilization Review, Pre-Admission Certification, State Licensure, Quality Assurance Program

Key Personnel
President/CEO . . . . Teresa Kline
Chief Financial Officer . . . . Richard Swift
VP, Human Resources . . . . Derek Adams
Chief Compliance Officer . . . . J. Douglas Clark
SVP, Chief of Marketing . . . . Mary Ann Tournoux
Chief Medical Officer . . . . Michael Genord, MD
VP, IT/CIO . . . . Annette M. Marcath

Specialty Managed Care Partners
Enters into Contracts with Regional Business Coalitions: Yes

---

421   Humana Health Insurance of Michigan
5555 Glenwood Hills Parkway
Suite 150
Grand Rapids, MI 49512
Toll-Free: 800-649-0059
Phone: 616-942-6701
Fax: 616-940-3655
www.humana.com
For Profit Organization: Yes

Healthplan and Services Defined
PLAN TYPE: HMO/PPO
Plan Specialty: ASO
Benefits Offered: Disease Management, Prescription, Wellness

Type of Coverage
Commercial, Individual

Geographic Areas Served
Michigan

Accreditation Certification
URAC, NCQA, CORE

Key Personnel
President & CEO . . . . Bruce D. Broussard
Chief Medical Officer . . . . Roy A. Beveridge
Chief Consumer Officer . . . . Jody L. Bilney
SVP, Human Resources . . . . Tim Huval
Chief Financial Officer . . . . Brian Kane
Chief Information Officer . . . . Brian LeClaire
SVP, General Counsel . . . . Christopher M. Todoroff

Specialty Managed Care Partners
Caremark Rx

Employer References
Tricare

---

422   Meridian Health Plan
1 Campus Martius
Suite 700
Detroit, MI 48226
Toll-Free: 888-437-0606
memberservices.mi@mhplan.com
www.mhplan.com
Total Enrollment: 750,000

Healthplan and Services Defined
PLAN TYPE: HMO

Geographic Areas Served
Michigan, Iowa, Illinois, Ohio, Indiana, Kentucky

Accreditation Certification
URAC, NCQA

Key Personnel
President . . . . Jon Cotton

---

423   Molina Healthcare of Michigan
880 West Long Lake Road
Troy, MI 48098
Toll-Free: 888-449-7969
Phone: 248-925-1700
www.molinahealthcare.com
Subsidiary of: Molina Healthcare, Inc.
For Profit Organization: Yes
Year Founded: 1980
Physician Owned Organization: Yes

Healthplan and Services Defined
PLAN TYPE: Medicare
Model Type: Network
Plan Specialty: Integrated Medicare/Medicaid (Duals)
Benefits Offered: Chiropractic, Dental, Home Care, Inpatient SNF, Long-Term Care, Podiatry, Vision

Type of Coverage
Commercial, Medicare, Supplemental Medicare, Medicaid

Accreditation Certification
URAC, NCQA

Key Personnel
Chief Executive Officer . . . . Joseph W. White
General Counsel . . . . Jeff D. Barlow

Chief Operating Officer . . . . Terry Bayer
SVP, Relations/Marketing . . . . Juan Jos, Orellana
Chief Information Officer . . . . Rick Hopfer

---

424   Paramount Care of Michigan

106 Park Place
Dundee, MI 48131
Toll-Free: 888-241-5604
Phone: 734-529-7800
www.paramounthealthcare.com
Subsidiary of: ProMedica Health System
For Profit Organization: Yes
Year Founded: 1988
Number of Affiliated Hospitals: 34
Number of Primary Care Physicians: 1,900
Total Enrollment: 187,000

Healthplan and Services Defined
  PLAN TYPE: HMO/PPO
  Benefits Offered: Disease Management, Prescription,
    Wellness

Type of Coverage
  Commercial, Medicare

Geographic Areas Served
  Southeast Michigan

Accreditation Certification
  NCQA

Key Personnel
  President. . . . . Jack Randolph

Specialty Managed Care Partners
  Express Scripts

---

425   Physicians Health Plan of Mid-Michigan

1400 East Michigan Avenue
Lansing, MI 48912
Toll-Free: 800-562-6197
Phone: 517-364-8400
www.phpmichigan.com
Mailing Address: PO Box 30377, Lansing, MI 48909-7877
Subsidiary of: Sparrow Health System
Non-Profit Organization: Yes
Year Founded: 1980
Owned by an Integrated Delivery Network (IDN): Yes
Number of Affiliated Hospitals: 31
Number of Primary Care Physicians: 3,100
Total Enrollment: 68,942
State Enrollment: 68,942

Healthplan and Services Defined
  PLAN TYPE: HMO/PPO
  Model Type: IPA
  Plan Specialty: Behavioral Health, Chiropractic, Dental,
    Disease Management, Lab, PBM, Vision, Radiology, UR
  Benefits Offered: Behavioral Health, Chiropractic, Dental,
    Disease Management, Home Care, Inpatient SNF, Physical
    Therapy, Podiatry, Prescription, Psychiatric, Transplant,
    Vision, Wellness, AD&D, Life, STD, FSA

Type of Coverage
  Commercial, Medicaid, Catastrophic, PPO, TPA
  Catastrophic Illness Benefit: Unlimited

Type of Payment Plans Offered
  POS, DFFS

Geographic Areas Served
  Clinton, Eaton, Gratiot, Ionia, Ingham, Isabella, Montcalm,
  Saginaw and Shiawassee counties

Subscriber Information
  Average Subscriber Co-Payment:
    Primary Care Physician: $10.00
    Non-Network Physician: 20%
    Prescription Drugs: $10.00/25.00/40.00
    Hospital ER: $50.00
    Home Health Care: $0
    Nursing Home: $0
    Nursing Home Max. Days/Visits Covered: 100

Network Qualifications
  Pre-Admission Certification: Yes

Peer Review Type
  Utilization Review: Yes
  Second Surgical Opinion: Yes
  Case Management: Yes

Publishes and Distributes Report Card: No

Accreditation Certification
  URAC, NCQA
  Medicare Approved, Utilization Review, Pre-Admission
    Certification, State Licensure, Quality Assurance Program

Key Personnel
  President/CEO. . . . . Dennis J Reese

Specialty Managed Care Partners
  United Behavioral Health
  Enters into Contracts with Regional Business Coalitions: No

---

426   Priority Health

1231 E Beltline Avenue NE
Grand Rapids, MI 49525-4501
Toll-Free: 800-318-2596
www.priorityhealth.com
Non-Profit Organization: Yes
Year Founded: 1985
Physician Owned Organization: Yes
Owned by an Integrated Delivery Network (IDN): Yes
Federally Qualified: No
Number of Affiliated Hospitals: 5,000
Number of Referral/Specialty Physicians: 617,000
Total Enrollment: 596,220

Healthplan and Services Defined
  PLAN TYPE: HMO
  Model Type: IPA
  Plan Specialty: ASO, Behavioral Health, Chiropractic, Dental,
    Disease Management, EPO, Lab, MSO, PBM, Vision,
    Radiology, UR
  Benefits Offered: Behavioral Health, Chiropractic,
    Complementary Medicine, Dental, Disease Management,
    Home Care, Inpatient SNF, Long-Term Care, Physical

Therapy, Podiatry, Prescription, Psychiatric, Transplant, Vision, Wellness, AD&D, Life, LTD, STD
Offers Demand Management Patient Information Service: No

Type of Coverage
Commercial, Individual, Indemnity, Medicare, Medicaid
Catastrophic Illness Benefit: Varies per case

Type of Payment Plans Offered
DFFS, Capitated, FFS, Combination FFS & DFFS

Geographic Areas Served
69 counties in Michigan

Subscriber Information
Average Monthly Fee Per Subscriber
(Employee + Employer Contribution):
Employee Only (Self): Varies
Employee & 1 Family Member: Varies
Employee & 2 Family Members: Varies
Medicare: Varies
Average Annual Deductible Per Subscriber:
Employee Only (Self): Varies
Employee & 1 Family Member: Varies
Employee & 2 Family Members: Varies
Medicare: Varies
Average Subscriber Co-Payment:
Primary Care Physician: Varies
Non-Network Physician: Varies
Prescription Drugs: Varies
Hospital ER: Varies
Home Health Care: Varies
Home Health Care Max. Days/Visits Covered: Varies
Nursing Home: Varies
Nursing Home Max. Days/Visits Covered: Varies

Network Qualifications
Pre-Admission Certification: No

Peer Review Type
Utilization Review: Yes
Case Management: Yes

Publishes and Distributes Report Card: No

Accreditation Certification
NCQA
Utilization Review, Pre-Admission Certification, State Licensure, Quality Assurance Program

Key Personnel
President and CEO . . . . Joan Budden
Chief Financial Officer . . . . Mary Anne Jones
Chief Operating Officer . . . . Michael Koziara
General Counsel . . . . Kimberly Thomas
Chief Medical Officer . . . . James D. Forshee, MD
VP Sales/Client Services . . . . Don Whitford

Specialty Managed Care Partners
Enters into Contracts with Regional Business Coalitions: Yes
National Federation of Independent Business

427 PriorityHealth Medicare Plans
1231 E Beltline NE
Grand Rapids, MI 49525-4501
Toll-Free: 800-942-0954
Phone: 616-942-0954
www.priorityhealth.com/medicare
Subsidiary of: PriorityHealth

Healthplan and Services Defined
PLAN TYPE: Medicare
Benefits Offered: Chiropractic, Dental, Disease Management, Home Care, Inpatient SNF, Physical Therapy, Podiatry, Prescription, Psychiatric, Vision, Wellness

Type of Coverage
Individual, Medicare

Geographic Areas Served
Statewide

Subscriber Information
Average Monthly Fee Per Subscriber
(Employee + Employer Contribution):
Employee Only (Self): Varies
Medicare: Varies
Average Annual Deductible Per Subscriber:
Employee Only (Self): Varies
Medicare: Varies
Average Subscriber Co-Payment:
Primary Care Physician: Varies
Non-Network Physician: Varies
Prescription Drugs: Varies
Hospital ER: Varies
Home Health Care: Varies
Home Health Care Max. Days/Visits Covered: Varies
Nursing Home: Varies
Nursing Home Max. Days/Visits Covered: Varies

Accreditation Certification
NCQA

Key Personnel
President and CEO . . . . Joan Budden
Chief Financial Officer . . . . Mary Anne Jones
Chief Operating Officer . . . . Michael Koziara
VP, General Counsel. . . . . Kimberly Thomas

428 SVS Vision
118 Cass Avenue
Mount Clemens, MI 48043
Toll-Free: 800-787-4600
Phone: 586-468-7612
customerservice@svsvision.com
www.svsvision.com
For Profit Organization: Yes
Year Founded: 1974
Total Enrollment: 390,000

Healthplan and Services Defined
PLAN TYPE: Vision
Other Type: Vision Plan
Plan Specialty: Vision
Benefits Offered: Vision, Services limited to vision care

Type of Payment Plans Offered
DFFS

Geographic Areas Served
Michigan; Illinois; Ohio; Indiana; Kentucky; Missouri; Georgia; New York

Subscriber Information
Average Monthly Fee Per Subscriber
(Employee + Employer Contribution):
Employee Only (Self): Varies by plan

Network Qualifications
Pre-Admission Certification: Yes

Peer Review Type
Utilization Review: Yes
Second Surgical Opinion: Yes
Case Management: Yes

Key Personnel
President/CFO .... Kenneth Stann
CEO .... Robert G. Farrell, Jr.
EVP/COO.............................. Lisa Stann
VP, Sales & Marketing.................. Seok Chung
586-464-1573
Media Contact .... Seok Chung
586-464-1573

429 Total Health Care
3011 W Grand Boulevard
Suite 1600
Detroit, MI 48202
Toll-Free: 800-826-2862
Phone: 313-871-2000
thc@thcmi.com
www.thcmi.com
Non-Profit Organization: Yes
Year Founded: 1973
Owned by an Integrated Delivery Network (IDN): Yes
Number of Affiliated Hospitals: 28
Total Enrollment: 90,000
State Enrollment: 90,000

Healthplan and Services Defined
PLAN TYPE: HMO
Other Type: PPN, POS
Model Type: Staff
Plan Specialty: Lab, Radiology
Benefits Offered: Behavioral Health, Chiropractic, Complementary
Medicine, Disease Management, Home Care, Inpatient
SNF, Long-Term Care, Physical Therapy, Podiatry,
Prescription, Psychiatric, Transplant, Vision,
Wellness, Worker's Compensation, Alternative
Treatments, Durable Medical Equipment, Speech, OT
24-hour Nurse Advice Line
Offers Demand Management Patient Information Service: Yes
DMPI Services Offered: Educational Classes and Programs

Type of Coverage
Commercial, Individual, Medicare, Medicaid

Type of Payment Plans Offered
Combination FFS & DFFS

Subscriber Information
Average Monthly Fee Per Subscriber
(Employee + Employer Contribution):
Employee Only (Self): $67.12
Employee & 2 Family Members: $164.88
Average Subscriber Co-Payment:
Primary Care Physician: $10.00
Hospital ER: $40.00

Accreditation Certification
TJC, NCQA

Key Personnel
Chief Executive Officer................ Randy Narowitz
Office Manager .... Nancy Kowal
Marketing Manager..................... Stephen Slaga
Medical Director .... Robyn James Arrington Jr, MD

Specialty Managed Care Partners
RxAmerica

Employer References
Federal Government, State of Michigan, American Airlines,
Detroit Board of Education, Wayne County Employees

430 Trinity Health
20555 Victor Parkway
Livonia, MI 48152-7018
Phone: 734-343-1000
www.trinity-health.org
Subsidiary of: Trinity Health
Non-Profit Organization: Yes
Year Founded: 2013
Number of Affiliated Hospitals: 86
Number of Primary Care Physicians: 3,600
Total Enrollment: 30,000,000

Healthplan and Services Defined
PLAN TYPE: Other
Benefits Offered: Disease Management, Home Care,
Long-Term Care, Psychiatric, Hospice programs, PACE
(Program of All Inclusive Care for the Elderly)

Geographic Areas Served
California, Connecticut, Delaware, Florida, Georgia, Idaho,
Illinois, Indiana, Iowa, Nebraska, Maryland, Massachusetts,
Michigan, New Jersey, New York, Ohio, and Pennsylvania

Key Personnel
Chief Executive Officer .... Richard Gilfillan
Chief Financial Officer.............. Benjamin R. Carter
Human Resources .... Edmund F. Hodge
General Counsel .... Paul G. Neumann
Chief Clinical Officer.................. Daniel J. Roth
Chief Operating Officer .... Michael A. Slubowski

431 Trinity Health of Michigan

Mercy Health Muskegon
1500 E Sherman Boulevard
Muskegon, MI 49444
Toll-Free: 800-825-4677
Phone: 231-861-2156
www.trinity-health.org
Secondary Address: St Mary Mercy Livonia, 36475 Five Mile
Road, Livonia, MI 48154, 734-655-4800
Subsidiary of: Trinity Health
Non-Profit Organization: Yes
Year Founded: 2013
Total Enrollment: 30,000,000

Healthplan and Services Defined
PLAN TYPE: Other
Benefits Offered: Disease Management, Home Care,
Long-Term Care, Psychiatric, Hospice programs, PACE
(Program of All Inclusive Care for the Elderly)

Geographic Areas Served
Statewide

Key Personnel
Chief Executive Officer . . . . Richard J. Gilfillan
Chief Financial Officer . . . . Benjamin R. Carter
Human Resources . . . . Edmund F. Hodge
General Counsel . . . . Paul G. Neumann
Chief Clinical Officer . . . . Daniel J. Roth
Chief Operating Officer . . . . Michael A. Slubowski

432 UniCare Michigan

3200 Greenfield Road
Dearborn, MI 48120
Phone: 313-336-5550
www.unicare.com
Subsidiary of: Anthem, Inc.
For Profit Organization: Yes ,
Year Founded: 1995

Healthplan and Services Defined
PLAN TYPE: HMO
Model Type: Network
Benefits Offered: Behavioral Health, Chiropractic,
Complementary Medicine, Dental, Disease Management,
Home Care, Inpatient SNF, Long-Term Care, Physical
Therapy, Podiatry, Prescription, Psychiatric, Transplant,
Vision, Wellness, Life

Type of Coverage
Commercial, Individual, Supplemental Medicare, Medicaid

Geographic Areas Served
Statewide

Network Qualifications
Pre-Admission Certification: Yes

Peer Review Type
Utilization Review: Yes
Second Surgical Opinion: Yes
Case Management: Yes

Publishes and Distributes Report Card: Yes

Accreditation Certification
URAC, NCQA
TJC Accreditation, Utilization Review, Pre-Admission
Certification, State Licensure, Quality Assurance Program

Specialty Managed Care Partners
WellPoint Pharmacy Management, WellPoint Dental Services,
WellPoint Behavioral Health
Enters into Contracts with Regional Business Coalitions: Yes

433 United Concordia of Michigan

4401 Deer Path Road
Harrisburg, PA 17110
Toll-Free: 800-332-0366
www.unitedconcordia.com
For Profit Organization: Yes
Year Founded: 1971
Total Enrollment: 7,800,000

Healthplan and Services Defined
PLAN TYPE: Dental
Plan Specialty: Dental
Benefits Offered: Dental

Type of Coverage
Commercial, Individual, Military personnel & families

Geographic Areas Served
Nationwide

Accreditation Certification
URAC

Key Personnel
President & COO . . . . Timothy J. Constantine
Contact . . . . Beth Rutherford
717-260-7659
beth.rutherford@ucci.com

434 UnitedHealthcare Great Lakes Health Plan

26957 Northwestern Highway
Suite 400
Southfield, MI 48033
www.glhp.com/mi.html
Subsidiary of: UnitedHealth Group
For Profit Organization: Yes
Year Founded: 1994
State Enrollment: 235,000

Healthplan and Services Defined
PLAN TYPE: HMO
Plan Specialty: Case Management
Benefits Offered: Disease Management, Home Care, Physical
Therapy, Prescription, Vision, Wellness, Hearing, Labs &
X-rays, Diabetic Support

Type of Coverage
Medicare, Medicaid, MIChild

Type of Payment Plans Offered
DFFS, Capitated

Geographic Areas Served
Allegan, Berrien, Branch, Calhoun, Cass, Hillsdale, Huron, Jackson, Kalamazoo, Kent, Lenawee, Livingston, Macomb, Monroe, Muskegon, Oakland, Oceana, Ottawa, Saginaw, Sanilac, St. Clair, St. Joseph, Tuscola, Van Buren and Wayne counties

Publishes and Distributes Report Card: No

Accreditation Certification
TJC
Utilization Review

Key Personnel
Chief Executive Officer . . . . David Wichmann
Chief Operating Officer . . . . Dan Schumacher
Chief Strategy Officer . . . . John Cosgriff
Communications Officer . . . . Kirsten Gorsuch
Chief Medical Officer. . . . . Sam Ho
Chief Legal Officer . . . . Thad Johnson
Chief Information. . . . . Phil McKoy

Specialty Managed Care Partners
Rx America
Enters into Contracts with Regional Business Coalitions: No

435 UnitedHealthcare of Michigan

26957 Northwestern Highway
Suite 400
Southfield, MI 48034
Toll-Free: 866-574-6088
www.uhc.com/contact-us/michigan
Subsidiary of: UnitedHealth Group
Year Founded: 1977

Healthplan and Services Defined
PLAN TYPE: HMO/PPO
Model Type: Network
Plan Specialty: Behavioral Health, Dental, Disease Management, Lab, PBM, Vision, Radiology
Benefits Offered: Behavioral Health, Chiropractic, Dental, Disease Management, Physical Therapy, Prescription, Vision, Wellness, AD&D, Life, LTD, STD

Type of Coverage
Commercial, Individual, Indemnity, Medicare, Supplemental Medicare, Medicaid, Catastrophic, Family, Military, Veterans, Group,

Geographic Areas Served
Statewide

Network Qualifications
Pre-Admission Certification: Yes

Peer Review Type
Utilization Review: Yes
Second Surgical Opinion: Yes
Case Management: Yes

Publishes and Distributes Report Card: Yes

Accreditation Certification
TJC, NCQA

Key Personnel
CEO. . . . . Stephen Hemsley

President & CFO . . . . David Wichmann

Specialty Managed Care Partners
Enters into Contracts with Regional Business Coalitions: Yes

436 Upper Peninsula Health Plan

853 W Washington Street
Marquette, MI 49855
Toll-Free: 800-835-2556
Phone: 906-225-7500
Fax: 906-225-7690
uphpwebmaster@uphp.com
www.uphp.com
Year Founded: 1998
Total Enrollment: 47,000
State Enrollment: 47,000

Healthplan and Services Defined
PLAN TYPE: HMO

Type of Coverage
Medicaid

Accreditation Certification
NCQA

Key Personnel
President & CEO . . . . Dennis Smith
Chief Quality Officer. . . . . Anne Levandoski
Corporate Communications . . . . Carly Harrington
906-225-7158
charrington@uphp.com

Health Insurance Coverage Status and Type of Coverage by Age

Category	All Persons		Under 18 years		Under 65 years	
	Number	%	Number	%	Number	%
Total population	5,462	-	1,364	-	4,662	-
Covered by some type of health insurance	5,237 *(10)*	95.9 *(0.2)*	1,318 *(6)*	96.6 *(0.4)*	4,438 *(10)*	95.2 *(0.2)*
Covered by private health insurance	4,196 *(20)*	76.8 *(0.4)*	976 *(9)*	71.6 *(0.7)*	3,617 *(20)*	77.6 *(0.4)*
Employer-based	3,377 *(25)*	61.8 *(0.5)*	876 *(10)*	64.3 *(0.8)*	3,163 *(23)*	67.8 *(0.5)*
Direct purchase	929 *(15)*	17.0 *(0.3)*	107 *(5)*	7.8 *(0.4)*	517 *(14)*	11.1 *(0.3)*
TRICARE	80 *(5)*	1.5 *(0.1)*	14 *(2)*	1.0 *(0.2)*	47 *(4)*	1.0 *(0.1)*
Covered by public health insurance	1,791 *(15)*	32.8 *(0.3)*	415 *(9)*	30.4 *(0.6)*	1,012 *(16)*	21.7 *(0.3)*
Medicaid	990 *(16)*	18.1 *(0.3)*	413 *(9)*	30.3 *(0.6)*	916 *(15)*	19.7 *(0.3)*
Medicare	882 *(5)*	16.2 *(0.1)*	4 *(1)*	0.3 *(0.1)*	104 *(4)*	2.2 *(0.1)*
VA Care	135 *(5)*	2.5 *(0.1)*	1 *(1)*	0.1 *(Z)*	45 *(3)*	1.0 *(0.1)*
Not covered at any time during the year	225 *(10)*	4.1 *(0.2)*	46 *(5)*	3.4 *(0.4)*	224 *(10)*	4.8 *(0.2)*

Note: Numbers in thousands; Figures cover civilian noninstitutionalized population in 2016; N/A indicates that data was not available; Z represents or rounds to zero; Margin of error appears in parenthesis and is calculated using replicate weights.
Source: U.S. Census Bureau, American Community Survey, Table HIC-4_ACS. Health Insurance Coverage Status and Type of Coverage by State—All People: 2008 to 2016, Table HIC-5_ACS. Health Insurance Coverage Status and Type of Coverage by State—Children Under 18: 2008 to 2016, Table HIC-6_ACS. Health Insurance Coverage Status and Type of Coverage by State—Persons Under 65: 2008 to 2016

Minnesota

437 Aetna Health of Minnesota

151 Farmington Avenue
Hartford, CT 06156
Toll-Free: 800-872-3862
Phone: 860-273-0123
www.aetna.com
Subsidiary of: Aetna Inc.
For Profit Organization: Yes

Healthplan and Services Defined
PLAN TYPE: PPO
Other Type: POS
Benefits Offered: Dental, Currently not marketing medical

Type of Coverage
Commercial, Student Health

Type of Payment Plans Offered
POS, DFFS, Combination FFS & DFFS

Geographic Areas Served
Statewide

Peer Review Type
Second Surgical Opinion: Yes
Case Management: Yes

Accreditation Certification
AAAHC, URAC
TJC Accreditation

Key Personnel
CEO . . . . Mark Bertolini

438 Americas PPO

7201 W 78th Street
Suite 100
Bloomington, MN 55439
Toll-Free: 800-948-9451
Phone: 952-896-1201
www.americasppo.com
Subsidiary of: Araz Group Inc
For Profit Organization: Yes
Year Founded: 1982
Physician Owned Organization: No
Number of Affiliated Hospitals: 260
Number of Primary Care Physicians: 18,000
Number of Referral/Specialty Physicians: 71,000
State Enrollment: 245,000

Healthplan and Services Defined
PLAN TYPE: PPO
Model Type: Staff, Group
Benefits Offered: Behavioral Health, Wellness, Worker's
Compensation, Maternity
Offers Demand Management Patient Information Service: No

Type of Coverage
Commercial, Individual, Medicaid
Catastrophic Illness Benefit: Maximum $1M

Type of Payment Plans Offered
DFFS, Capitated

Geographic Areas Served
Minnesota, South Dakota, North Dakota, Western Wisconsin

Subscriber Information
Average Monthly Fee Per Subscriber
(Employee + Employer Contribution):
Employee Only (Self): Varies by plan
Average Annual Deductible Per Subscriber:
Employee Only (Self): $500.00
Employee & 1 Family Member: $500.00
Employee & 2 Family Members: $750.00
Average Subscriber Co-Payment:
Primary Care Physician: $15.00
Non-Network Physician: $500.00-1000.00
Prescription Drugs: $10.00/15.00
Hospital ER: $150.00
Nursing Home: Varies

Network Qualifications
Pre-Admission Certification: Yes

Peer Review Type
Utilization Review: Yes
Case Management: Yes

Publishes and Distributes Report Card: No

Accreditation Certification
URAC
TJC Accreditation, Utilization Review, Pre-Admission
Certification, State Licensure, Quality Assurance Program

Key Personnel
President . . . . Amir Eftekhari
Founder and CEO . . . . Nazie Eftekhari

Specialty Managed Care Partners
Enters into Contracts with Regional Business Coalitions: Yes

439 Avesis: Minnesota

904 Oak Pond Court
Sartell, MN 56377
Toll-Free: 888-363-1377
www.avesis.com
Subsidiary of: Guardian Life Insurance Co.
Year Founded: 1978
Number of Primary Care Physicians: 25,000
Total Enrollment: 3,500,000

Healthplan and Services Defined
PLAN TYPE: PPO
Other Type: Vision, Dental
Model Type: Network
Plan Specialty: Dental, Vision, Hearing
Benefits Offered: Dental, Vision

Type of Coverage
Commercial

Type of Payment Plans Offered
POS, Capitated, Combination FFS & DFFS

Geographic Areas Served
Nationwide and Puerto Rico

Publishes and Distributes Report Card: Yes

Accreditation Certification
AAAHC
TJC Accreditation

Key Personnel
Chief Executive Officer . . . . Chris Swanker
Business Development . . . . Alan Cohn

440   Blue Cross & Blue Shield of Minnesota

P.O. Box 64560
St. Paul, MN 55164-0560
Toll-Free: 800-382-2000
Phone: 651-662-8000
www.bluecrossmn.com
Secondary Address: 3535 Blue Cross Road, Eagan, MN
55122-1154
Subsidiary of: Blue Cross Blue Shield
Non-Profit Organization: Yes
Year Founded: 1933
Owned by an Integrated Delivery Network (IDN): Yes
Number of Affiliated Hospitals: 30
Number of Primary Care Physicians: 8,000
Total Enrollment: 2,700,000
State Enrollment: 2,700,000

Healthplan and Services Defined
PLAN TYPE: HMO
Model Type: Network
Plan Specialty: Medical
Benefits Offered: Disease Management, Prescription,
Wellness, Life

Type of Coverage
Individual, Medicare, Supplemental Medicare

Geographic Areas Served
Statewide

Network Qualifications
Pre-Admission Certification: Yes

Peer Review Type
Utilization Review: Yes
Second Surgical Opinion: Yes

Publishes and Distributes Report Card: Yes

Accreditation Certification
URAC, NCQA

Key Personnel
President & CEO . . . . Michael J. Guyette
SVP, Health Services . . . . Garrett Black
SVP, Chief Legal Officer . . . . Scott Lynch
Director Public Relations . . . . Jim McManus
jim.mcmanus@bluecrossmn.com
SVP, Government Programs . . . . Kurt C. Small
SVP, Chief Financial Offc . . . . Jay Matushak
Chief Strategy Officer . . . . Rochelle Myers
SVP, Human Resources . . . . Paula Phillippe
SVP, Chief Tech Officer . . . . Ernie Franklin

Specialty Managed Care Partners
Enters into Contracts with Regional Business Coalitions: No

Employer References
General Mills/Pillsbury, Northwest Airlines, Target

441   Coventry Health Care of Minnesota

6720-B Rockledge Drive
Suite 700
Bethesda, MD 20817
Phone: 301-581-0600
www.coventryhealthcare.com
Subsidiary of: Aetna Inc.
For Profit Organization: Yes

Healthplan and Services Defined
PLAN TYPE: HMO/PPO
Model Type: Network
Plan Specialty: Behavioral Health, Dental, Worker's
Compensation
Benefits Offered: Behavioral Health, Dental, Prescription,
Wellness, Worker's Compensation

Type of Coverage
Commercial, Medicare, Medicaid

Geographic Areas Served
Statewide

Key Personnel
Chief Executive Officer . . . . Mark T. Bertolini
President . . . . Karen S. Lynch
Chief Financial Officer . . . . Shawn M. Guertin
Operations & Technology . . . . Meg McCarthy
Chief Medical Officer . . . . Harold L. Paz
General Counsel . . . . Thomas Sabatino Jr.
Government Services . . . . Fran S. Soistman

442   Delta Dental of Minnesota

500 Washington Avenue S
Suite 2060
Minneapolis, MN 55415
Toll-Free: 877-268-3384
www.deltadentalmn.org
Non-Profit Organization: Yes
Year Founded: 1969

Healthplan and Services Defined
PLAN TYPE: Dental
Other Type: Dental PPO
Model Type: Network
Plan Specialty: ASO, Dental
Benefits Offered: Dental

Type of Coverage
Commercial, Individual, Group
Catastrophic Illness Benefit: None

Geographic Areas Served
Minnesota and North Dakota

Key Personnel
President & CEO . . . . Rodney Young
Chief Financial Officer . . . . Tamera Robinson
Chief Operating Officer . . . . Michael McGuire
General Counsel . . . . Stephanie Albert
VP, Sales . . . . David Anderson

Underwring & Actuarial . . . . Jon Becker
VP, Marketing. . . . . Sarah Leeth
VP, Human Resources . . . . Judy Peterson

443 HealthPartners

8170 33rd Avenue S
Bloomington, MN 55425
Toll-Free: 800-883-2177
Phone: 952-883-6000
www.healthpartners.com
Non-Profit Organization: Yes
Year Founded: 1957
Owned by an Integrated Delivery Network (IDN): Yes

Healthplan and Services Defined
  PLAN TYPE: HMO
  Model Type: Staff, Network
  Benefits Offered: Behavioral Health, Chiropractic, Dental,
    Disease Management, Home Care, Inpatient SNF, Physical
    Therapy, Prescription, Psychiatric, Transplant, Vision,
    Worker's Compensation

Type of Coverage
  Commercial, Individual, Indemnity, Medicare, Supplemental
    Medicare, Medicaid
  Catastrophic Illness Benefit: Unlimited

Type of Payment Plans Offered
  POS, Combination FFS & DFFS

Geographic Areas Served
  Minnesota and 8 counties in Northwestern Wisconsin

Peer Review Type
  Utilization Review: Yes
  Case Management: Yes

Accreditation Certification
  URAC, NCQA

Key Personnel
  President & CEO. . . . . Andrea Walsh
  EVP, Chief Admin Officer . . . . Kathy Cooney
  SVP, General Counsel . . . . Barb Tretheway
  Chief Operating Officer . . . . Nance McClure
  Co-Medical Officer. . . . . Steven Connelly
  Co-Medical Officer . . . . Brian Rank
  SVP, Human Resources. . . . . Calvin Allen

Specialty Managed Care Partners
  Alere, Accordant, RMS
  Enters into Contracts with Regional Business Coalitions: Yes

Employer References
  University of MN, St Paul Public Schools, The College of St
    Catherine

444 Hennepin Health

Minneapolis Grain Exchange Building
400 South Fourth Street, Suite 201
Minneapolis, MN 55415
Toll-Free: 800-627-3529
Phone: 612-596-1036
hennepinhealth@hennepin.us
www.hennepinhealth.org

Non-Profit Organization: Yes
Year Founded: 2012
Total Enrollment: 10,500

Healthplan and Services Defined
  PLAN TYPE: HMO
  Model Type: Network
  Benefits Offered: Behavioral Health, Chiropractic, Dental,
    Disease Management, Home Care, Podiatry, Prescription,
    Psychiatric, Vision, Substance Abuse Care; Hearing;
    Durable Medical Equipment; Family Planning

Type of Coverage
  Medicaid

Type of Payment Plans Offered
  Combination FFS & DFFS

Geographic Areas Served
  Hennepin County

Subscriber Information
  Average Subscriber Co-Payment:
    Primary Care Physician: $0
    Non-Network Physician: $0
    Home Health Care: $0
    Nursing Home: $0

Peer Review Type
  Utilization Review: Yes
  Case Management: Yes

Key Personnel
  Chief Executive Officer . . . . Shannon Mayer
  Chief Financial Officer . . . . Abdirahman Abdi
  Medical Director . . . . Marc Manley

445 Humana Health Insurance of Minnesota

12600 Whitewater Drive
Suite 150
Minnetonka, MN 55343
Toll-Free: 877-367-6990
Phone: 952-253-3540
Fax: 952-938-2787
www.humana.com
Subsidiary of: Humana
For Profit Organization: Yes

Healthplan and Services Defined
  PLAN TYPE: HMO/PPO
  Model Type: Network
  Plan Specialty: Dental, Vision
  Benefits Offered: Dental, Vision, Life, LTD, STD

Type of Coverage
  Commercial, Individual

Geographic Areas Served
  Statewide

Accreditation Certification
  URAC, NCQA, CORE

Key Personnel
  President & CEO. Bruce Broussard
  Chief Medical Officer. . . . . Roy A. Beveridge
  Chief Consumer Officer. . . . . Jody L. Bilney

Human Resources. . . . . Tim Huval
Chief Financial Officer . . . . Brian Kane
Chief Information Officer . . . . Brian LeClaire
General Counsel . . . . Christopher M. Todoroff

446 Medica

401 Carlson Parkway
Minnetonka, MN 55305
Toll-Free: 800-952-3455
Phone: 952-992-2900
www.medica.com
Subsidiary of: Medica Holding Company
Non-Profit Organization: Yes
Year Founded: 1975
Total Enrollment: 1,700,000

Healthplan and Services Defined
PLAN TYPE: HMO
Model Type: IPA
Benefits Offered: Behavioral Health, Disease Management,
Prescription

Type of Coverage
Commercial, Individual, Medicare, Supplemental Medicare,
Pet insurance

Type of Payment Plans Offered
FFS

Geographic Areas Served
Iowa, Kansas, Minnesota, Nebraska, North Dakota, and
Wisconsin

Peer Review Type
Utilization Review: Yes
Second Surgical Opinion: Yes
Case Management: Yes

Publishes and Distributes Report Card: Yes

Accreditation Certification
NCQA
TJC Accreditation, Medicare Approved, Utilization Review,
Pre-Admission Certification, State Licensure, Quality
Assurance Program

Key Personnel
President & CEO . . . . John Naylor
SVP, Financial Officer . . . . Mark Baird
VP, Human Resources . . . . Lynn Altmann
SVP, General Counsel . . . . Jim Jacobson
SVP, General Manager. . . . . Paul Crowley
VP, General Manager . . . . Geoff Bartsh
SVP, Government Programs. . . . . Tom Lindquist
SVP, Marketing . . . . Rob Longendyke
Chief Information Officer . . . . Tim Thull

Average Claim Compensation
Physician's Fees Charged: 65%
Hospital's Fees Charged: 60%

447 National Imaging Associates

7805 Hudson Road
Suite 190
St Paul, MN 55125
Toll-Free: 877-NIA-9762
www.niahealthcare.com
Subsidiary of: Magellan Healthcare
For Profit Organization: Yes
Year Founded: 1995
Number of Referral/Specialty Physicians: 4,000

Healthplan and Services Defined
PLAN TYPE: PPO
Model Type: Network
Plan Specialty: Lab, Radiology
Benefits Offered: Disease Management

Type of Coverage
Commercial, Indemnity, Medicare, Medicaid

Type of Payment Plans Offered
POS, DFFS, Capitated, FFS, Combination FFS & DFFS

Geographic Areas Served
North Dakota, South Dakota, Minnesota, Wisconsin, Illinois,
Indiana, Ohio, Michigan, Kentucky, Iowa, Missouri, Montana,
Idaho, Nebraska, Tennessee, Kansas, Oklahoma, Utah,
Arkansas, Arizona, Georgia, Texas, Alabama

Peer Review Type
Utilization Review: Yes

Publishes and Distributes Report Card: Yes

Accreditation Certification
TJC, NCQA

Key Personnel
Chief Medical Officer. . . . . Michael J. Pentecost, MD
SVP, Clinical Services . . . . David Hodges
SVP, Sales . . . . Edie Jardine
Vice President, Finance . . . . William F. Henderson

Specialty Managed Care Partners
Enters into Contracts with Regional Business Coalitions: Yes

448 Optum Complex Medical Conditions

MN Office 102
11000 Optum Circle
Eden Prairie, MN 55344
Toll-Free: 877-801-3507
cmc_client_services@optum.com
www.myoptumhealthcomplexmedical.com
Subsidiary of: UnitedHealth Group
For Profit Organization: Yes
Year Founded: 1986

Healthplan and Services Defined
PLAN TYPE: Multiple
Model Type: Network
Plan Specialty: Complex medical conditions including
transplantation, cancer, kidney disease, congenital heart
disease and infertility.

Type of Payment Plans Offered
POS, Capitated, FFS

Geographic Areas Served
Nationwide

Peer Review Type
Utilization Review: Yes
Case Management: Yes

Publishes and Distributes Report Card: Yes

Accreditation Certification
URAC
Utilization Review, Quality Assurance Program

Key Personnel
Senior Vice President . . . . John DeSmet
SVP, Network Solutions . . . . Kevin O'Brien
VP, Transplant Solutions . . . . Heather Zick
Chief Medical Officer . . . . Jon Friedman, MD

Specialty Managed Care Partners
Enters into Contracts with Regional Business Coalitions: Yes

449 UCare

500 Stinson Boulevard NE
Minneapolis, MN 55413
Toll-Free: 866-457-7144
Phone: 612-676-6500
www.ucare.org
Secondary Address: 4310 Menard Drive, Hermantown, MN
55811, 218-336-4260
Non-Profit Organization: Yes
Year Founded: 1984
Owned by an Integrated Delivery Network (IDN): Yes
Number of Primary Care Physicians: 43,000
Total Enrollment: 147,000

Healthplan and Services Defined
PLAN TYPE: Multiple
Model Type: Network
Benefits Offered: Behavioral Health, Chiropractic, Dental,
Disease Management, Home Care, Inpatient SNF, Physical
Therapy, Podiatry, Prescription, Psychiatric, Transplant,
Vision, Wellness, Disability Plans available

Type of Coverage
Medicare, Supplemental Medicare, Medicaid
Catastrophic Illness Benefit: Unlimited

Type of Payment Plans Offered
POS

Geographic Areas Served
Statewide

Network Qualifications
Pre-Admission Certification: Yes

Peer Review Type
Utilization Review: Yes
Second Surgical Opinion: Yes
Case Management: Yes

Publishes and Distributes Report Card: Yes

Accreditation Certification
NCQA
Medicare Approved, Utilization Review, Pre-Admission
Certification, State Licensure, Quality Assurance Program

Key Personnel
Interim President & CEO . . . . Mark Traynor
Senior VP & CAO . . . . Hilary Marden-Resnik
Senior VP & CFO . . . . Beth Monsrud
SVP, Public Affairs/Mkt . . . . Ghita Worcester
Chief Medical Officer . . . . Lawrence (Larry) Lee

Specialty Managed Care Partners
Enters into Contracts with Regional Business Coalitions: Yes

450 UnitedHealth Group

P.O. Box 1459
Minneapolis, MN 55440-1459
Toll-Free: 800-328-5979
www.unitedhealthgroup.com
For Profit Organization: Yes
Year Founded: 1974
Total Enrollment: 70,000,000

Healthplan and Services Defined
PLAN TYPE: Medicare
Model Type: Network
Plan Specialty: Behavioral Health, Dental, Disease
Management, PBM, Vision
Benefits Offered: Behavioral Health, Dental, Disease
Management, Long-Term Care, Prescription, Vision,
Wellness, Life, LTD, STD

Type of Coverage
Individual, Medicare, Supplemental Medicare, Medicaid,
Catastrophic, Family, Military, Veterans, Group,

Geographic Areas Served
All 50 states, the District of Columbia, most U.S. territories &
125 countries

Key Personnel
Executive Chairman . . . . Stephen Hemsley
Chief Executive Officer . . . . David Wichmann
Vice-Chair . . . . Larry Renfro
Chief Financial Officer . . . . John Rex
Chief Legal Officer . . . . Marianna D. Short
Chief Marketing Officer . . . . Terry M. Clark
Chief Medical Officer . . . . Richard Migliori

451 UnitedHealthcare of Minnesota

9700 Health Care Lane
Minnetonka, MN 55343
Toll-Free: 800-842-3585
www.uhc.com/contact-us/minnesota
Subsidiary of: UnitedHealth Group
Year Founded: 1977

Healthplan and Services Defined
PLAN TYPE: HMO/PPO
Model Type: Network
Plan Specialty: Behavioral Health, Dental, Disease
Management, Lab, PBM, Vision, Radiology
Benefits Offered: Behavioral Health, Chiropractic, Dental,
Disease Management, Long-Term Care, Physical Therapy,
Prescription, Vision, Wellness, AD&D, Life, LTD, STD

Type of Coverage
Commercial, Individual, Indemnity, Medicare, Supplemental
Medicare, Medicaid, Catastrophic, Family, Military,
Veterans, Group,

Geographic Areas Served
Minnesota, North Dakota, South Dakota, Hawaii, and Puerto
Rico

Network Qualifications
Pre-Admission Certification: Yes

Peer Review Type
Utilization Review: Yes
Second Surgical Opinion: Yes
Case Management: Yes

Publishes and Distributes Report Card: Yes

Accreditation Certification
TJC, NCQA

Key Personnel
President . . . . David Wichmann
Chief Operating Officer . . . . Dan Schumacher
Chief Strategy Officer . . . . John Cosgriff
Communications Officer . . . . Kirsten Gorsuch
Chief Medical Officer. . . . . Sam Ho
Chief Legal Officer . . . . Thad Johnson
Chief Information Officer . . . . Phil McKoy
Chief Financial Officer. . . . . Jeff Putnam

Specialty Managed Care Partners
Enters into Contracts with Regional Business Coalitions: Yes

Health Insurance Coverage Status and Type of Coverage by Age

Category	All Persons		Under 18 years		Under 65 years	
	Number	%	Number	%	Number	%
Total population	2,924	-	771	-	2,488	-
Covered by some type of health insurance	2,578 *(13)*	88.2 *(0.4)*	734 *(7)*	95.2 *(0.6)*	2,143 *(13)*	86.1 *(0.5)*
Covered by private health insurance	1,759 *(18)*	60.2 *(0.6)*	362 *(10)*	46.9 *(1.2)*	1,524 *(18)*	61.3 *(0.7)*
Employer-based	1,368 *(17)*	46.8 *(0.6)*	300 *(8)*	38.9 *(1.0)*	1,272 *(18)*	51.1 *(0.7)*
Direct purchase	380 *(13)*	13.0 *(0.4)*	51 *(5)*	6.6 *(0.7)*	244 *(11)*	9.8 *(0.4)*
TRICARE	114 *(8)*	3.9 *(0.3)*	23 *(4)*	3.0 *(0.5)*	71 *(7)*	2.9 *(0.3)*
Covered by public health insurance	1,153 *(14)*	39.4 *(0.5)*	401 *(10)*	52.0 *(1.2)*	725 *(14)*	29.2 *(0.6)*
Medicaid	718 *(16)*	24.6 *(0.5)*	397 *(9)*	51.5 *(1.2)*	637 *(15)*	25.6 *(0.6)*
Medicare	544 *(5)*	18.6 *(0.2)*	4 *(1)*	0.6 *(0.2)*	116 *(5)*	4.7 *(0.2)*
VA Care	81 *(5)*	2.8 *(0.2)*	3 *(2)*	0.4 *(0.2)*	40 *(4)*	1.6 *(0.2)*
Not covered at any time during the year	346 *(12)*	11.8 *(0.4)*	37 *(4)*	4.8 *(0.6)*	345 *(12)*	13.9 *(0.5)*

Note: Numbers in thousands; Figures cover civilian noninstitutionalized population in 2016; N/A indicates that data was not available; Z represents or rounds to zero; Margin of error appears in parenthesis and is calculated using replicate weights.
Source: U.S. Census Bureau, American Community Survey, Table HIC-4_ACS. Health Insurance Coverage Status and Type of Coverage by State—All People: 2008 to 2016, Table HIC-5_ACS. Health Insurance Coverage Status and Type of Coverage by State—Children Under 18: 2008 to 2016, Table HIC-6_ACS. Health Insurance Coverage Status and Type of Coverage by State—Persons Under 65: 2008 to 2016

Mississippi

452　Aetna Health of Mississippi

151 Farmington Avenue
Hartford, CT 06156
Toll-Free: 800-872-3862
Phone: 860-273-0123
www.aetna.com
Subsidiary of: Aetna Inc.
For Profit Organization: Yes

Healthplan and Services Defined
PLAN TYPE: PPO
Other Type: POS
Model Type: Network
Plan Specialty: Behavioral Health, Dental, EPO, Lab, PBM, Vision, Radiology
Benefits Offered: Behavioral Health, Dental, Disease Management, Long-Term Care, Physical Therapy, Podiatry, Prescription, Psychiatric, Vision, Wellness, Life, LTD, STD

Type of Coverage
Commercial, Student health

Type of Payment Plans Offered
POS, FFS

Geographic Areas Served
Statewide

Key Personnel
CEO . . . . Mark Bertolini

453　Allegiance Life & Health Insurance Company

2806 S Garfield Street
P.O. Box 3507
Missoula, MT 59806-3507
Toll-Free: 800-737-3137
Phone: 406-523-3122
Fax: 406-523-3124
inquire@askallegiance.com
www.allegiancelifeandhealth.com
Subsidiary of: Cigna
For Profit Organization: Yes
Year Founded: 1981

Healthplan and Services Defined
PLAN TYPE: HMO
Benefits Offered: Dental, Vision, Wellness, Pharmacy

Type of Coverage
Commercial, Individual

Geographic Areas Served
Statewide

Key Personnel
President & Owner . . . . Dirk Visser

454　Health Link PPO

808 Varsity Drive
Tupelo, MS 38801
Toll-Free: 888-855-2740
Phone: 662-377-3868
Fax: 662-377-7599
www.healthlinkppo.com
Subsidiary of: North Mississippi Medical Center
Non-Profit Organization: Yes
Year Founded: 1986
Number of Affiliated Hospitals: 30
Number of Primary Care Physicians: 1,500
Total Enrollment: 155,070

Healthplan and Services Defined
PLAN TYPE: PPO
Benefits Offered: Dental, Long-Term Care, Prescription, Transplant, Vision, Life, LTD, STD, Major Medical

Type of Coverage
Commercial, Individual

Geographic Areas Served
Mississippi and northwest Alabama

Accreditation Certification
NCQA
Medicare Approved, Utilization Review, Pre-Admission Certification, State Licensure, Quality Assurance Program

Key Personnel
President . . . . Joe Reppert

455　Humana Health Insurance of Mississippi

772 Lake Harbour Drive
Suite 3
Ridgeland, MS 39157
Toll-Free: 866-945-4376
Phone: 601-605-5130
Fax: 601-856-5222
www.humana.com
Secondary Address: 2650 Beach Boulevard, Suite 31A, Biloxi, MS 39531, 228-271-6800
For Profit Organization: Yes

Healthplan and Services Defined
PLAN TYPE: HMO/PPO
Plan Specialty: ASO
Benefits Offered: Disease Management, Prescription, Wellness

Type of Coverage
Commercial, Individual, Medicare

Geographic Areas Served
Alabama, Mississippi

Accreditation Certification
URAC, NCQA

Key Personnel
President & CEO . . . . Bruce D. Broussard
Chief Medical Officer. . . . . Roy A. Beveridge
Chief Consumer Officer. . . . . Jody L. Bilney
SVP, Human Resources . . . . Tim Huval
Chief Financial Officer . . . . Brian Kane

Chief Information Officer . . . . Brian LeClaire
SVP, General Counsel . . . . Christopher M. Todoroff

Specialty Managed Care Partners
Caremark Rx

Employer References
Tricare

456   Magnolia Health

111 E Capitol Street
Suite 500
Jackson, MS 39201
Toll-Free: 866-912-6285
www.magnoliahealthplan.com
Subsidiary of: Centene Corporation

Healthplan and Services Defined
PLAN TYPE: Multiple
Plan Specialty: Medicaid, Mississippi Children's Health
Insurance Program (CHIP)
Benefits Offered: Behavioral Health, Disease Management,
Prescription, Wellness, Maternity & Newborn Care;
Transportation

Type of Coverage
Individual, Medicare, Medicaid

Geographic Areas Served
Statewide

Key Personnel
President & CEO . . . . Aaron Sisk

457   UnitedHealthcare of Mississippi

32 Milbranch Road
Suite 30
Hattiesburg, MS 39402
Toll-Free: 800-345-1520
www.uhc.com/contact-us/mississippi
Subsidiary of: UnitedHealth Group
For Profit Organization: Yes
Year Founded: 1992

Healthplan and Services Defined
PLAN TYPE: HMO/PPO
Model Type: Network
Plan Specialty: Behavioral Health, Dental, Disease
Management, PBM, Vision
Benefits Offered: Behavioral Health, Dental, Disease
Management, Long-Term Care, Prescription, Vision,
Wellness, Life, LTD, STD

Type of Coverage
Commercial, Individual, Indemnity, Medicare, Supplemental
Medicare, Medicaid, Catastrophic, Family, Military,
Veterans, Group,

Type of Payment Plans Offered
FFS

Geographic Areas Served
Statewide

Network Qualifications
Pre-Admission Certification: Yes

Peer Review Type
Utilization Review: Yes
Second Surgical Opinion: Yes
Case Management: Yes

Publishes and Distributes Report Card: Yes

Accreditation Certification
NCQA
TJC Accreditation, Medicare Approved, Utilization Review,
Pre-Admission Certification, State Licensure, Quality
Assurance Program

Key Personnel
President . . . . David Wichmann
Chief Operating Officer . . . . Dan Schumacher
Chief Strategy Officer . . . . John Cosgriff
Communications Officer . . . . Kirsten Gorsuch
Chief Medical Officer. . . . . Sam Ho
Chief Legal Officer . . . . Thad Johnson
Chief Information Officer . . . . Phil McKoy
Chief Financial Officer. . . . . Jeff Putnam

Specialty Managed Care Partners
Enters into Contracts with Regional Business Coalitions: Yes

Health Insurance Coverage Status and Type of Coverage by Age

Category	All Persons		Under 18 years		Under 65 years	
	Number	%	Number	%	Number	%
Total population	5,977	-	1,476	-	5,040	-
Covered by some type of health insurance	5,445 *(15)*	91.1 *(0.2)*	1,405 *(8)*	95.2 *(0.4)*	4,511 *(15)*	89.5 *(0.3)*
Covered by private health insurance	4,264 *(26)*	71.3 *(0.4)*	962 *(14)*	65.2 *(0.9)*	3,700 *(25)*	73.4 *(0.5)*
Employer-based	3,416 *(27)*	57.2 *(0.5)*	830 *(14)*	56.2 *(1.0)*	3,143 *(27)*	62.4 *(0.5)*
Direct purchase	907 *(19)*	15.2 *(0.3)*	124 *(8)*	8.4 *(0.5)*	580 *(18)*	11.5 *(0.4)*
TRICARE	148 *(8)*	2.5 *(0.1)*	30 *(3)*	2.0 *(0.2)*	97 *(7)*	1.9 *(0.1)*
Covered by public health insurance	1,885 *(18)*	31.5 *(0.3)*	483 *(13)*	32.7 *(0.9)*	972 *(18)*	19.3 *(0.3)*
Medicaid	882 *(19)*	14.7 *(0.3)*	476 *(13)*	32.2 *(0.8)*	790 *(18)*	15.7 *(0.4)*
Medicare	1,115 *(9)*	18.7 *(0.1)*	9 *(3)*	0.6 *(0.2)*	204 *(8)*	4.0 *(0.2)*
VA Care	165 *(5)*	2.8 *(0.1)*	2 *(1)*	0.1 *(0.1)*	71 *(4)*	1.4 *(0.1)*
Not covered at any time during the year	532 *(14)*	8.9 *(0.2)*	71 *(5)*	4.8 *(0.4)*	529 *(14)*	10.5 *(0.3)*

Note: Numbers in thousands; Figures cover civilian noninstitutionalized population in 2016; N/A indicates that data was not available; Z represents or rounds to zero; Margin of error appears in parenthesis and is calculated using replicate weights.
Source: U.S. Census Bureau, American Community Survey, Table HIC-4_ACS. Health Insurance Coverage Status and Type of Coverage by State—All People: 2008 to 2016, Table HIC-5_ACS. Health Insurance Coverage Status and Type of Coverage by State—Children Under 18: 2008 to 2016, Table HIC-6_ACS. Health Insurance Coverage Status and Type of Coverage by State—Persons Under 65: 2008 to 2016

Missouri

458 Aetna Health of Missouri

151 Farmington Avenue
Hartford, CT 06156
Toll-Free: 800-872-3862
Phone: 860-273-0123
www.aetna.com
Secondary Address: 6730-B Rockledge Drive, Suite 700,
 Bethesda, MD 20817, 301-581-0600
Subsidiary of: Aetna Inc.
For Profit Organization: Yes

Healthplan and Services Defined
 PLAN TYPE: HMO/PPO
 Other Type: POS
 Model Type: Network
 Plan Specialty: Behavioral Health, EPO, Lab, PBM,
  Radiology
 Benefits Offered: Behavioral Health, Dental, Disease
  Management, Long-Term Care, Physical Therapy,
  Podiatry, Prescription, Psychiatric, Vision, Wellness, Life,
  LTD, STD

Type of Coverage
 Commercial, Student health

Geographic Areas Served
 More than 50 counties

Key Personnel
 CEO . . . . Mark Bertolini

459 American Health Care Alliance

9229 Ward Parkway
Suite 300
Kansas City, MO 64114
Toll-Free: 800-870-6252
customerservice@ahappo.com
www.ahappo.com
Mailing Address: P.O. Box 8530, Kansas City, MO
 64114-0530
Year Founded: 1990
Number of Affiliated Hospitals: 5,745
Number of Primary Care Physicians: 190,736
Number of Referral/Specialty Physicians: 285,353
Total Enrollment: 942,000
State Enrollment: 860,000

Healthplan and Services Defined
 PLAN TYPE: PPO
 Model Type: Network of PPOs
 Benefits Offered: Behavioral Health, Chiropractic,
  Complementary Medicine, Dental, Home Care, Physical
  Therapy, Podiatry, Prescription, Psychiatric, Vision,
  Wellness
 Offers Demand Management Patient Information Service:
  Yes

Geographic Areas Served
 Nationwide

Subscriber Information
 Average Annual Deductible Per Subscriber:
  Employee Only (Self): Varies
  Employee & 1 Family Member: Varies
  Employee & 2 Family Members: Varies
  Medicare: Varies
 Average Subscriber Co-Payment:
  Primary Care Physician: Varies
  Non-Network Physician: Varies
  Prescription Drugs: Varies
  Hospital ER: Varies
  Home Health Care: Varies
  Nursing Home: Varies

Publishes and Distributes Report Card: Yes

Accreditation Certification
 AAAHC, URAC, AAPI, NCQA
 TJC Accreditation, Medicare Approved, Utilization Review,
  Pre-Admission Certification, State Licensure

Key Personnel
 Executive Vice President. . . . . Phil Mehelic
  pmehelic@ahappo.com
 Director Client Service . . . . Lisa Enslinger

460 Anthem Blue Cross & Blue Shield of Missouri

1831 Chestnut Street
St Louis, MO 63103
Phone: 314-923-4444
www.anthem.com
Subsidiary of: Anthem, Inc.
For Profit Organization: Yes

Healthplan and Services Defined
 PLAN TYPE: HMO/PPO
 Model Type: Network
 Plan Specialty: Behavioral Health, Dental, Disease
  Management, Lab, PBM, Vision, Radiology
 Benefits Offered: Behavioral Health, Dental, Disease
  Management, Inpatient SNF, Physical Therapy,
  Prescription, Psychiatric, Transplant, Vision, Wellness, Life

Type of Coverage
 Commercial, Individual, Medicare, Supplemental Medicare,
  Catastrophic

Geographic Areas Served
 All of Missouri, excluding 30 counties in the Kansas City area

Accreditation Certification
 URAC, NCQA

Key Personnel
 President & CEO . . . . Scott P. Serota
 Chief Financial Officer . . . . Robert Kolodgy
 Human Resources . . . . Maureen A. Cahill
 Chief Medical Officer. . . . . Trent Haywood
 General Counsel. . . . . Scott Nehs

461   Blue Cross Blue Shield of Kansas City

One Pershing Square
2301 Main Street
Kansas City, MO 64108
Toll-Free: 888-989-8842
Phone: 816-395-2583
www.bluekc.com
Non-Profit Organization: Yes
Year Founded: 1982

Healthplan and Services Defined
PLAN TYPE: PPO
Model Type: Network
Benefits Offered: Behavioral Health, Chiropractic, Dental,
  Physical Therapy, Podiatry, Prescription, Psychiatric

Type of Coverage
Commercial, Individual, Medicare, Supplemental Medicare,
  Travel Insurance
Catastrophic Illness Benefit: Maximum $2M

Type of Payment Plans Offered
POS, FFS

Geographic Areas Served
Serving 32 counties in greater Kansas City (including
  Johnson and Wyandotte) and northwestern Missouri

Network Qualifications
Pre-Admission Certification: Yes

Peer Review Type
Utilization Review: Yes

Publishes and Distributes Report Card: No

Accreditation Certification
URAC, NCQA

Key Personnel
President & CEO . . . . Danette Wilson
Chief Financial Officer . . . . David Mohr
VP, Human Resources . . . . Jill Beckman
Chief Information Officer. . . . . David Kaercher
General Counsel & Admin. . . . . Rick Kastner
VP, Chief Actuary. Tom Nightingale
SVP, Sales & Marketing . . . . Ron Rowe

Specialty Managed Care Partners
Enters into Contracts with Regional Business Coalitions: Yes

462   Centene Corporation

Centene Plaza
7700 Forsyth Blvd
St. Louis, MO 63105
Phone: 314-725-4477
www.centene.com
For Profit Organization: Yes
Year Founded: 1984
Total Enrollment: 11,000,000

Healthplan and Services Defined
PLAN TYPE: HMO/PPO
Model Type: Network
Plan Specialty: Behavioral Health, Dental, PBM, Vision

Benefits Offered: Behavioral Health, Dental, Vision,
  Wellness, Life, Correctional health services

Type of Coverage
Commercial, Individual, Medicare, Supplemental Medicare,
  Medicaid

Geographic Areas Served
Arizona, Arkansas, California, Florida, Georgia, Indiana,
  Illinois, Kansas, Louisiana, Massachusetts, Michigan,
  Mississippi, Missouri, Ohio, South Carolina, Texas,
  Washington, Wisconsin

Accreditation Certification
URAC, NCQA, CORE Phase III Certified

463   Children's Mercy Integrated Care Solutions

2400 Pershing Road
Suite 125
Kansas City, MO 64141
Toll-Free: 888-670-7261
www.cmics.org/pcn
Mailing Address: P.O. Box 411596, Kansas City, MO 64141
Subsidiary of: Children's Health Network
Non-Profit Organization: Yes
Year Founded: 1996
Owned by an Integrated Delivery Network (IDN): Yes
Number of Affiliated Hospitals: 31
Number of Primary Care Physicians: 200
Number of Referral/Specialty Physicians: 2,400
Total Enrollment: 49,976
State Enrollment: 49,976

Healthplan and Services Defined
PLAN TYPE: HMO
Model Type: Network, Medicaid
Benefits Offered: Behavioral Health, Dental, Disease
  Management, Home Care, Inpatient SNF, Physical Therapy,
  Podiatry, Prescription, Psychiatric, Vision, Wellness

Type of Coverage
Medicaid
Catastrophic Illness Benefit: None

Geographic Areas Served
Cass, Clay, Henry, Jackson, Johnson, Lafayette, Platte, Ray,
  St. Claire counties in Missouri

Subscriber Information
Average Monthly Fee Per Subscriber
  (Employee + Employer Contribution):
    Employee Only (Self): $0.00
    Employee & 1 Family Member: $0.00
    Employee & 2 Family Members: $0.00

Peer Review Type
Utilization Review: Yes
Second Surgical Opinion: Yes
Case Management: Yes

Publishes and Distributes Report Card: Yes

Key Personnel
VP/Executive Director . . . . Bob Finuf
Director, IT . . . . Bob Clark
Director, Finance . . . . Suzie Dunaway

Associate Medical Dir.. . . . . Julia Simmons, MD
Provider Relations Dir . . . . Pamela MK Johnson
Medical Director . . . . Doug Blowey, MD
Dir., Medical Economics. Kent Pack
Dir., Care Integration . . . . Candance Ramos

Average Claim Compensation
Physician's Fees Charged: 50%
Hospital's Fees Charged: 60%

Specialty Managed Care Partners
Enters into Contracts with Regional Business Coalitions: Yes

Employer References
State of Missouri, Division of Medical Services, State of
Kansas, SRS

464   Coventry Health Care of Missouri

550 Maryville Centre Drive
Suite 300
St. Louis, MO 63141
Toll-Free: 800-755-3901
marketingchcmo@cvty.com
chcmissouri.coventryhealthcare.com
Subsidiary of: Aetna Inc.
For Profit Organization: Yes
Year Founded: 1978

Healthplan and Services Defined
PLAN TYPE: HMO/PPO
Other Type: POS
Model Type: Network
Plan Specialty: Behavioral Health, Dental, Worker's
Compensation
Benefits Offered: Behavioral Health, Dental, Wellness,
Worker's Compensation

Type of Coverage
Commercial, Individual, Medicare, Supplemental Medicare,
Medicaid

Geographic Areas Served
All of Eastern Missouri including St. Louis, Jefferson City,
Columbia, Mexico, Kirksville, Hannibal, Rolla, West Plains
and Cape Girardeau

Accreditation Certification
URAC

Key Personnel
Chief Executive Officer. . . . . Mark T. Bertolini
President. . . . . Karen S. Lynch
Chief Financial Officer . . . . Shawn M. Guertin
Operations & Technology . . . . Meg McCarthy
Chief Medical Officer . . . . Harold L. Paz
General Counsel . . . . Thomas Sabatino Jr.
Government Services . . . . Fran S. Soistman

465   Cox Healthplans

Kelly Plaza
3200 S National, Building B
Springfield, MO 65807
Toll-Free: 800-664-1244
Phone: 417-269-4679
Fax: 417-269-2949
members@coxhealthplans.com
www.coxhealthplans.com
Mailing Address: P.O. Box 5750, Springfield, MO 65801-5750
Subsidiary of: CoxHealth
For Profit Organization: Yes
Number of Primary Care Physicians: 1,000
Number of Referral/Specialty Physicians: 5,000
Total Enrollment: 5,000
State Enrollment: 1,964

Healthplan and Services Defined
PLAN TYPE: HMO/PPO
Benefits Offered: Disease Management, Prescription,
Wellness

Type of Coverage
Commercial, Individual

Type of Payment Plans Offered
POS

Geographic Areas Served
Statewide

Key Personnel
President. . . . . Matt Aug
Chief Information Officer. . . . . Susan Butts
Chief Financial Officer . . . . Lisa Odom

Specialty Managed Care Partners
Caremark Rx

466   Delta Dental of Missouri

12399 Gravois Road
Suite 2
St. Louis, MO 63127
Toll-Free: 800-392-1167
Phone: 314-656-3000
service@deltadentalmo.com
www.deltadentalmo.com
Mailing Address: P.O. Box 8690, St. Louis, MO 63126-0690
Non-Profit Organization: Yes
Year Founded: 1958
Owned by an Integrated Delivery Network (IDN): Yes
State Enrollment: 1,700,000

Healthplan and Services Defined
PLAN TYPE: Dental
Other Type: Dental PPO
Model Type: Group
Plan Specialty: Dental, Vision
Benefits Offered: Dental, Vision

Type of Coverage
Commercial

Geographic Areas Served
Missouri and South Carolina

Publishes and Distributes Report Card: No

Specialty Managed Care Partners
Enters into Contracts with Regional Business Coalitions: No

467 Dental Health Alliance

2323 Grand Boulevard
Kansas City, MO 64108
Toll-Free: 800-522-1313
dha@sunlife.com
www.dha.com
Subsidiary of: Sunlife Financial
Year Founded: 1994
Number of Primary Care Physicians: 74,000
Total Enrollment: 1,700,000

Healthplan and Services Defined
PLAN TYPE: Dental
Other Type: Dental PPO Network
Model Type: Network, Dental PPO Network
Plan Specialty: Dental
Benefits Offered: Dental

Type of Coverage
Commercial

Type of Payment Plans Offered
POS, FFS, Combination FFS & DFFS

Geographic Areas Served
Nationwide

Network Qualifications
Pre-Admission Certification: No

Peer Review Type
Utilization Review: Yes

468 Essence Healthcare

13900 Riverport Drive
Maryland Heights, MO 63043
Toll-Free: 866-597-9560
Phone: 314-209-2700
Fax: 314-770-6096
customerservice@essencehealthcare.com
www.essencehealthcare.com
Secondary Address: 3354 S National, Suite F, Springfield, MO
  65807
Year Founded: 2004
Total Enrollment: 60,000

Healthplan and Services Defined
PLAN TYPE: Medicare
Benefits Offered: Chiropractic, Dental, Disease Management,
  Home Care, Inpatient SNF, Physical Therapy, Podiatry,
  Prescription, Psychiatric, Vision, Wellness

Type of Coverage
Individual, Medicare

Geographic Areas Served
Missouri: Boone, Christian, Greene, Jefferson, Stone, Saint
  Louis, Saint Louis City, Saint Charles, Saint Francois, and
  Taney counties. Illinois: Madison, Monroe, and Saint Clair
  counties

Subscriber Information
Average Monthly Fee Per Subscriber
  (Employee + Employer Contribution):
    Employee Only (Self): Varies
    Medicare: Varies
Average Annual Deductible Per Subscriber:
    Employee Only (Self): Varies
    Medicare: Varies
Average Subscriber Co-Payment:
    Primary Care Physician: Varies
    Non-Network Physician: Varies
    Prescription Drugs: Varies
    Hospital ER: Varies
    Home Health Care: Varies
    Home Health Care Max. Days/Visits Covered: Varies
    Nursing Home: Varies
    Nursing Home Max. Days/Visits Covered: Varies

Key Personnel
President & CEO. . . . . Richard Jones
Chief Operating Officer . . . . Martha Butler
Chief Medical Officer . . . . Deborah Zimmerman, MD
Claims & Customer Service . . . . Dawn Walter
VP, Sales & Marketing . . . . Joel Anderson

469 Government Employees Health Association (GEHA)

310 NE Mulberry Street
Lee's Summit, MO 64086
Toll-Free: 800-821-6136
www.geha.com
Non-Profit Organization: Yes
Year Founded: 1964

Healthplan and Services Defined
PLAN TYPE: Other
Plan Specialty: Dental, Vision, Federal employees
Benefits Offered: Dental, Disease Management, Prescription,
  Vision, Wellness, Life

Type of Coverage
Commercial, Medicare
Catastrophic Illness Maximum Benefit: $5,000

Type of Payment Plans Offered
FFS

Geographic Areas Served
Nationwide

Network Qualifications
Pre-Admission Certification: Yes

Accreditation Certification
URAC

Key Personnel
President & CEO . . . . Julie Browne

Average Claim Compensation
Hospital's Fees Charged: 85%

470   HealthLink HMO

1831 Chestnut Street
Suite 540
St. Louis, MO 63103
Toll-Free: 800-624-2356
Phone: 314-925-6000
www.healthlink.com
For Profit Organization: Yes
Year Founded: 1985

Healthplan and Services Defined
  PLAN TYPE: Multiple
  Benefits Offered: Dental, Vision, Wellness, Worker's
    Compensation, Life, LTD, STD, Reinsurance

Type of Coverage
  Catastrophic Illness Benefit: Varies per case

Geographic Areas Served
  Arkansas, Illinois, Missouri, Ohio, Kentucky, and Indiana

Network Qualifications
  Pre-Admission Certification: Yes

Peer Review Type
  Utilization Review: Yes
  Second Surgical Opinion: No
  Case Management: Yes

Accreditation Certification
  URAC
  Utilization Review, Pre-Admission Certification, Quality
    Assurance Program

Key Personnel
  President . . . . Graeme Stretch

Specialty Managed Care Partners
  WellPoint Pharmacy Management, Cigna Behavioral Health,
    Vision Service Plan
  Enters into Contracts with Regional Business Coalitions: Yes
  Gateway Purchases

Employer References
  Local fifty benefits service trust, Jefferson City Public
    Schools, ConAgra

471   Humana Health Insurance of Missouri

909 E Montclair
Suite 108
Springfield, MO 65807
Toll-Free: 800-951-0128
Phone: 417-882-3020
Fax: 417-882-2015
www.humana.com
Secondary Address: Creekwoods Commons, 215 NE
  Englewood Road, Suite A, Kansas City, MO 64118,
  816-459-7776
Subsidiary of: Humana
For Profit Organization: Yes

Healthplan and Services Defined
  PLAN TYPE: HMO/PPO
  Model Type: Network
  Plan Specialty: Dental, Vision
  Benefits Offered: Dental, Vision, Life, LTD, STD

Type of Coverage
  Commercial, Individual

Geographic Areas Served
  Statewide

Accreditation Certification
  URAC, NCQA, CORE

Key Personnel
  President & CEO. . . . . Bruce Broussard
  Chief Medical Officer. . . . . Roy A. Beveridge
  Chief Consumer Officer. . . . . Jody L. Bilney
  Human Resources. . . . . Tim Huval
  Chief Financial Officer . . . . Brian Kane
  Chief Information Officer . . . . Brian LeClaire
  General Counsel . . . . Christopher M. Todoroff

472   Liberty Dental Plan of Missouri

P.O. Box 26110
Santa Ana, CA 92799-6110
Toll-Free: 877-558-6489
www.libertydentalplan.com
For Profit Organization: Yes
Year Founded: 2001
Total Enrollment: 3,000,000

Healthplan and Services Defined
  PLAN TYPE: Dental
  Other Type: Dental HMO
  Plan Specialty: Dental
  Benefits Offered: Dental

Type of Coverage
  Commercial, Individual, Medicare, Medicaid, Unions

Geographic Areas Served
  Statewide

Accreditation Certification
  NCQA

Key Personnel
  Regional Manager, MO. . . . . John McCarthy
    314-489-7785
    jmccarthy@libertydentalplan.com

473   Med-Pay

1650 Battlefield
Suite 300
Springfield, MO 65804-3706
Toll-Free: 800-777-9087
Phone: 417-886-6886
Fax: 417-886-2276
www.med-pay.com
Year Founded: 1983
State Enrollment: 26,000

Healthplan and Services Defined
  PLAN TYPE: Other
  Other Type: TPA, HSA, HRA
  Model Type: Network
  Plan Specialty: ASO, Behavioral Health, Chiropractic, Dental,
    Disease Management, Lab, MSO, PBM, Vision, Radiology

Benefits Offered: Behavioral Health, Chiropractic, Dental, Disease Management, Home Care, Inpatient SNF, Long-Term Care, Physical Therapy, Prescription, Transplant, Vision

Offers Demand Management Patient Information Service: Yes

Type of Coverage
Commercial, Individual

Accreditation Certification
State of MO
Utilization Review

Specialty Managed Care Partners
HCC, BCBS, Healthlink
Enters into Contracts with Regional Business Coalitions: Yes

474 Mercy Clinic Missouri

615 S New Ballas Road
St Louis, MO 63141
Phone: 314-251-6000
mercy.net
Subsidiary of: IBM Watson Health
Non-Profit Organization: Yes
Number of Affiliated Hospitals: 44
Number of Primary Care Physicians: 700
Number of Referral/Specialty Physicians: 2,000

Healthplan and Services Defined
PLAN TYPE: HMO
Benefits Offered: Behavioral Health, Disease Management, Home Care, Physical Therapy, Vision, Wellness, Non-Surgical Weight Loss, Urgent Care, Dermatology, Rehabilitation, Breast Cancer, Orthopedics, Otosclerosis, Pediatrics

Type of Coverage
Commercial, Individual

Geographic Areas Served
Arkansas, Kansas, Missouri, Oklahoma

Key Personnel
President & CEO. . . . . Lynn Britton
EVP, COO. . . . . Michael McCurry
EVP, Strategy & CFO . . . . Shannon Sock

475 Sun Life Financial

2323 Grand Boulevard
Kansas City, MO 64108
Toll-Free: 816-474-2345
www.assurantemployeebenefits.com
For Profit Organization: Yes
Year Founded: 1865

Healthplan and Services Defined
PLAN TYPE: Multiple
Plan Specialty: Dental, Vision
Benefits Offered: Dental, Vision, Wellness, AD&D, Life, LTD, STD, Subject to regulatory approvals

Type of Coverage
Commercial, Individual

Geographic Areas Served
Nationwide

Subscriber Information
Average Monthly Fee Per Subscriber
(Employee + Employer Contribution):
Employee Only (Self): Varies by plan

Accreditation Certification
NCQA

Key Personnel
President. . . . . Dan Fishbein
SVP/CFO. . . . . Neil Haynes
SVP/General Counsel . . . . Scott Davis
VP, Dental/Vision. Stacia Almquist
VP, Marketing. . . . . Ed Milano
Head of Human Resources . . . . Kathy deCastro

476 UnitedHealthcare of Missouri

13655 Riverport Drive
Maryland Heights, MO 63043
Toll-Free: 800-627-0687
Phone: 314-592-7000
www.uhc.com/contact-us/missouri
Subsidiary of: UnitedHealth Group
For Profit Organization: Yes

Healthplan and Services Defined
PLAN TYPE: HMO/PPO
Model Type: Network
Plan Specialty: Behavioral Health, Dental, Disease Management, PBM, Vision
Benefits Offered: Behavioral Health, Dental, Disease Management, Long-Term Care, Prescription, Vision, Life, LTD, STD

Type of Coverage
Individual, Medicare, Supplemental Medicare, Medicaid, Catastrophic, Family, Military, Veterans, Group,

Geographic Areas Served
Statewide

Key Personnel
President . . . . David Wichmann
Chief Operating Officer . . . . Dan Schumacher
Chief Strategy Officer . . . . John Cosgriff
Communications Officer . . . . Kirsten Gorsuch
Chief Medical Officer. . . . . Sam Ho
Chief Legal Officer . . . . Thad Johnson
Chief Information Officer . . . . Phil McKoy
Chief Financial Officer. . . . . Jeff Putnam

Health Insurance Coverage Status and Type of Coverage by Age

Category	All Persons		Under 18 years		Under 65 years	
	Number	%	Number	%	Number	%
Total population	1,028	-	242	-	848	-
Covered by some type of health insurance	944 (6)	91.9 (0.5)	230 (3)	95.1 (0.9)	765 (6)	90.2 (0.7)
Covered by private health insurance	702 (9)	68.4 (0.9)	144 (5)	59.5 (1.9)	593 (9)	69.9 (1.0)
Employer-based	507 (9)	49.4 (0.9)	118 (4)	48.8 (1.8)	467 (9)	55.1 (1.1)
Direct purchase	195 (7)	19.0 (0.7)	21 (3)	8.8 (1.1)	122 (6)	14.4 (0.7)
TRICARE	40 (4)	3.9 (0.4)	8 (2)	3.4 (0.7)	27 (4)	3.2 (0.4)
Covered by public health insurance	388 (8)	37.8 (0.8)	96 (5)	39.6 (2.0)	212 (8)	24.9 (0.9)
Medicaid	203 (7)	19.8 (0.7)	95 (5)	39.3 (2.0)	182 (7)	21.5 (0.8)
Medicare	206 (3)	20.0 (0.3)	1 (Z)	0.4 (0.2)	29 (3)	3.5 (0.4)
VA Care	44 (3)	4.2 (0.3)	1 (Z)	0.2 (0.2)	20 (2)	2.4 (0.3)
Not covered at any time during the year	83 (6)	8.1 (0.5)	12 (2)	4.9 (0.9)	83 (6)	9.8 (0.7)

Note: Numbers in thousands; Figures cover civilian noninstitutionalized population in 2016; N/A indicates that data was not available; Z represents or rounds to zero; Margin of error appears in parenthesis and is calculated using replicate weights.
Source: U.S. Census Bureau, American Community Survey, Table HIC-4_ACS. Health Insurance Coverage Status and Type of Coverage by State—All People: 2008 to 2016, Table HIC-5_ACS. Health Insurance Coverage Status and Type of Coverage by State—Children Under 18: 2008 to 2016, Table HIC-6_ACS. Health Insurance Coverage Status and Type of Coverage by State—Persons Under 65: 2008 to 2016

Montana

477　Aetna Health of Montana

151 Farmington Avenue
Hartford, CT 06156
Toll-Free: 800-872-3862
Phone: 860-273-0123
www.aetna.com
Subsidiary of: Aetna Inc.
For Profit Organization: Yes

Healthplan and Services Defined
　PLAN TYPE: PPO
　Other Type: POS
　Model Type: Network
　Plan Specialty: Behavioral Health, EPO, Lab, PBM,
　　Radiology
　Benefits Offered: Behavioral Health, Disease Management,
　　Long-Term Care, Physical Therapy, Podiatry, Prescription,
　　Psychiatric, Vision, Wellness, Life, LTD, STD

Type of Coverage
　Commercial, Student health

Type of Payment Plans Offered
　POS, FFS

Geographic Areas Served
　Statewide

Key Personnel
　CEO. . . . . Mark Bertolini

478　Blue Cross & Blue Shield of Montana

3645 Alice Street
P.O. Box 4309
Helena, MT 59604-4309
Toll-Free: 800-447-7828
Phone: 406-437-6195
john_doran@bcbsmt.com
www.bcbsmt.com
Non-Profit Organization: Yes
Year Founded: 1986
Owned by an Integrated Delivery Network (IDN): Yes
Federally Qualified: Yes
Number of Affiliated Hospitals: 58
Number of Primary Care Physicians: 1,900
Number of Referral/Specialty Physicians: 2,800
Total Enrollment: 250,000
State Enrollment: 250,000

Healthplan and Services Defined
　PLAN TYPE: HMO
　Model Type: Network
　Plan Specialty: ASO, Behavioral Health, Chiropractic,
　　Dental, Disease Management, EPO, Lab, MSO, PBM,
　　Vision, Radiology, Worker's Compensation, UR
　Benefits Offered: Behavioral Health, Chiropractic,
　　Complementary
Medicine, Dental, Disease Management, Home Care,
Inpatient SNF, Long-Term Care, Physical Therapy,
Podiatry, Prescription, Psychiatric, Transplant,
Vision, Wellness, Worker's Compensation, AD&D,

Life, LTD, STD
　Offers Demand Management Patient Information Service: Yes

Type of Coverage
　Commercial, Individual, Indemnity, Medicare, Supplemental
　　Medicare, Catastrophic
　Catastrophic Illness Benefit: Varies per case

Type of Payment Plans Offered
　POS, DFFS, Capitated

Geographic Areas Served
　Beaverhead, Big Horn, Blaine, Broadwater, Carbon, Carter,
　　Cascade, Choteau, Custer, Deer Lodge, Flathead, Glacier,
　　Hill, Jefferson, Lake, Lewis and Clark, Liberty, Lincoln,
　　Madison, McCone, Meagher, Mineral, Missoula, Musselshell,
　　Pondera, Ravalli, Sanders, Silver Bow, Stillwater, Sweet
　　Grass, Teton, Wheatland, Yellowstone

Subscriber Information
　Average Subscriber Co-Payment:
　　Primary Care Physician: $15
　　Non-Network Physician: Deductible
　　Hospital ER: $75.00
　　Home Health Care: No deductible
　　Home Health Care Max. Days/Visits Covered: 180 days
　　Nursing Home: $300 per admit co-pay
　　Nursing Home Max. Days/Visits Covered: 60 days

Network Qualifications
　Pre-Admission Certification: Yes

Peer Review Type
　Utilization Review: Yes
　Second Surgical Opinion: Yes
　Case Management: Yes

Publishes and Distributes Report Card: Yes

Accreditation Certification
　URAC

Key Personnel
　President & CEO . . . . Michael Frank
　Chief Financial Officer . . . . Mark Burzynski
　Medical Director . . . . Fred Olson, MD

Specialty Managed Care Partners
　Behavioral Health, Chiropractic, Dental, Disease
　　Management, Home Care, Inpatient SNF, and more
　Enters into Contracts with Regional Business Coalitions: Yes

Employer References
　Montana University System, Evening Post Publishing
　　Company, Costco Wholesale, State of Montana, Huntley
　　Project Schools

479　Coventry Health Care of Montana

6720-B Rockledge Drive
Suite 700
Bethesda, MD 20817
Phone: 301-581-0600
www.coventryhealthcare.com
Subsidiary of: Aetna Inc.
For Profit Organization: Yes

Healthplan and Services Defined
  PLAN TYPE: HMO/PPO
  Model Type: Network
  Plan Specialty: Behavioral Health, Dental, Worker's
    Compensation
  Benefits Offered: Behavioral Health, Dental, Prescription,
    Wellness, Worker's Compensation

Type of Coverage
  Commercial, Medicare, Medicaid

Geographic Areas Served
  Statewide

Key Personnel
  Chief Executive Officer . . . . Mark T. Bertolini
  President . . . . Karen S. Lynch
  Chief Financial Officer . . . . Shawn M. Guertin
  Operations & Technology . . . . Meg McCarthy
  Chief Medical Officer . . . . Harold L. Paz
  General Counsel . . . . Thomas Sabatino Jr.
  Government Services . . . . Fran S. Soistman

480   First Choice Health

1156 16th Street W
Suite 18
Billings, MT 59102-4118
Toll-Free: 888-256-6556
Fax: 406-256-9466
contact@fchn.com
www.fchn.com
For Profit Organization: Yes
Year Founded: 1996
Number of Affiliated Hospitals: 94
Number of Primary Care Physicians: 980
Number of Referral/Specialty Physicians: 1,793
Total Enrollment: 80,000
State Enrollment: 56,000

Healthplan and Services Defined
  PLAN TYPE: PPO
  Model Type: Open Panel & GeoExclusive
  Benefits Offered: Wellness

Type of Coverage
  Commercial, Individual, Private & Public Plans, Geo-specifi

Geographic Areas Served
  Washington, Oregon, Alaska, Idaho, Montana, Wyoming, and
  select areas of North Dakota and South Dakota

Key Personnel
  Chief Executive Officer . . . . Robert L Hunter

Specialty Managed Care Partners
  Enters into Contracts with Regional Business Coalitions: Yes
  First Choice Health Network (Pacific NW)

481   HCSC Insurance Services Company

560 N Park Avenue
P.O. Box 4309
Helena, MT 59604-4309
Phone: 406-437-5000
hcsc.com

Subsidiary of: Blue Cross Blue Shield Association
Non-Profit Organization: Yes
Year Founded: 1936
Number of Primary Care Physicians: 8,000

Healthplan and Services Defined
  PLAN TYPE: HMO
  Benefits Offered: Behavioral Health, Dental, Disease
    Management, Psychiatric, Wellness

Geographic Areas Served
  Statewide

Key Personnel
  President & CEO . . . . Paula Steiner
  EVP, Plan Operations . . . . Colleen Reitan
  SVP, Clinical Officer . . . . Opella Ernest, MD
  SVP, Financial Officer . . . . Eric Feldstein
  SVP, Compliance Officer . . . . Thomas Lubben
  SVP, Human Resources . . . . Nazneen Razi
  SVP, Chief Legal Officer . . . . Blair Todt
  Media Contact . . . . Kristen Cunningham
    312-653-1686
    kristen_cunningham@hcsc.net
  Media Contact . . . . Greg Thompson
    312-653-7581
    greg_thompson@hcsc.net

482   Humana Health Insurance of Montana

12600 Whitewater Dirve
Suite 150
Minnetonka, MT 55343
Toll-Free: 877-367-6990
Fax: 952-938-2787
www.humana.com
Subsidiary of: Humana
For Profit Organization: Yes

Healthplan and Services Defined
  PLAN TYPE: HMO/PPO
  Model Type: Network
  Plan Specialty: Vision
  Benefits Offered: Dental, Vision, Life, LTD, STD

Type of Coverage
  Commercial

Geographic Areas Served
  Montana is covered by the Minnesota branch

Accreditation Certification
  URAC, NCQA, CORE

Key Personnel
  President & CEO . . . . Bruce Broussard
  Chief Medical Officer . . . . Roy A. Beveridge
  Chief Consumer Officer . . . . Jody L. Bilney
  Human Resources . . . . Tim Huval
  Chief Financial Officer . . . . Brian Kane
  Chief Information Officer . . . . Brian LeClaire
  General Counsel . . . . Christopher M. Todoroff

483   Montana Health Co-Op

5 & 6, 1005 Partridge Place
Helena, MT 59602
Toll-Free: 855-477-2900
memberservice@mhc.coop
mhc.coop
Mailing Address: P.O. Box 5358, Helena, MT 59604
Non-Profit Organization: Yes
Year Founded: 2013

Healthplan and Services Defined
   PLAN TYPE: HMO
   Benefits Offered: Chiropractic, Inpatient SNF, Physical
     Therapy, Prescription, Wellness, Labs & X-Ray; Maternity;
     Occupational & Speech Therapy

Geographic Areas Served
   Statewide

Key Personnel
   Chair.................................. Joan Miles
   Vice Chair .... Raymond Rogers
   Media Contact .... Karen Early
     208-917-1605
     kearly@mhc.coop

484   Mountain Health Co-Op

5 & 6, 1005 Partridge Place
Helena, ID 59602
Toll-Free: 855-477-2900
information@mhc.coop
mhc.coop
Non-Profit Organization: Yes
Year Founded: 2013

Healthplan and Services Defined
   PLAN TYPE: HMO
   Benefits Offered: Chiropractic, Inpatient SNF, Physical
     Therapy, Prescription, Wellness, Labs & X-Ray;
     Occupational & Speech Therapy; Maternity

Geographic Areas Served
   Statewide

Key Personnel
   Chair.................................. Joan Miles
   Vice-Chair .... Raymond Rogers
   Media Contact .... Karen Early
     208-917-1605
     kearly@mhc.com

485   UnitedHealthcare of Montana

1111 Third Avenue
Suite 1100
Seattle, WA 98101
Toll-Free: 800-842-8000
www.uhc.com/contact-us/montana
Subsidiary of: UnitedHealth Group
For Profit Organization: Yes
Year Founded: 1986

Healthplan and Services Defined
   PLAN TYPE: HMO/PPO

Model Type: Network
Plan Specialty: Behavioral Health, Dental, Disease
   Management, MSO, PBM, Vision
Benefits Offered: Behavioral Health, Chiropractic,
   Complementary Medicine, Dental, Disease Management,
   Home Care, Inpatient SNF, Long-Term Care, Physical
   Therapy, Podiatry, Prescription, Psychiatric, Transplant,
   Vision, Wellness, AD&D, Life

Type of Coverage
   Commercial, Individual, Medicare, Supplemental Medicare,
   Medicaid, Family, Military, Veterans, Group,

Type of Payment Plans Offered
   DFFS, FFS, Combination FFS & DFFS

Geographic Areas Served
   Statewide. Montana is covered by the Washington branch

Subscriber Information
   Average Monthly Fee Per Subscriber
    (Employee + Employer Contribution):
     Employee Only (Self): Varies
   Average Subscriber Co-Payment:
     Primary Care Physician: $10
     Prescription Drugs: $10/15/30
     Hospital ER: $50

Network Qualifications
   Pre-Admission Certification: Yes

Peer Review Type
   Case Management: Yes

Publishes and Distributes Report Card: Yes

Accreditation Certification
   URAC, NCQA
   State Licensure, Quality Assurance Program

Key Personnel
   Chief Executive Officer............... David Wichmann
   Chief Operating Officer .... Dan Schumacher
   Chief Strategy Officer .... John Cosgriff
   Communications Officer .... Kirsten Gorsuch
   Chief Medical Officer........................ Sam Ho
   Chief Legal Officer .... Thad Johnson
   Chief Information Officer .... Phil McKoy
   Chief Financial Officer................... Jeff Putnam

Average Claim Compensation
   Physician's Fees Charged: 70%
   Hospital's Fees Charged: 55%

Specialty Managed Care Partners
   United Behavioral Health
   Enters into Contracts with Regional Business Coalitions: No

Health Insurance Coverage Status and Type of Coverage by Age

Category	All Persons		Under 18 years		Under 65 years	
	Number	%	Number	%	Number	%
Total population	1,878	-	498	-	1,604	-
Covered by some type of health insurance	1,717 *(9)*	91.4 *(0.5)*	472 *(4)*	94.9 *(0.7)*	1,445 *(9)*	90.1 *(0.6)*
Covered by private health insurance	1,427 *(15)*	76.0 *(0.8)*	344 *(7)*	69.1 *(1.4)*	1,245 *(14)*	77.6 *(0.9)*
Employer-based	1,106 *(16)*	58.9 *(0.8)*	294 *(7)*	59.1 *(1.4)*	1,040 *(16)*	64.8 *(1.0)*
Direct purchase	339 *(9)*	18.1 *(0.5)*	50 *(4)*	10.0 *(0.8)*	217 *(8)*	13.5 *(0.5)*
TRICARE	59 *(5)*	3.1 *(0.2)*	14 *(2)*	2.7 *(0.4)*	41 *(4)*	2.5 *(0.3)*
Covered by public health insurance	513 *(9)*	27.3 *(0.5)*	142 *(7)*	28.5 *(1.3)*	247 *(9)*	15.4 *(0.6)*
Medicaid	243 *(9)*	13.0 *(0.5)*	140 *(6)*	28.2 *(1.3)*	213 *(9)*	13.3 *(0.6)*
Medicare	299 *(3)*	15.9 *(0.2)*	2 *(1)*	0.4 *(0.2)*	34 *(3)*	2.1 *(0.2)*
VA Care	54 *(2)*	2.9 *(0.1)*	1 *(1)*	0.2 *(0.1)*	22 *(2)*	1.4 *(0.1)*
Not covered at any time during the year	161 *(9)*	8.6 *(0.5)*	25 *(3)*	5.1 *(0.7)*	159 *(9)*	9.9 *(0.6)*

Note: Numbers in thousands; Figures cover civilian noninstitutionalized population in 2016; N/A indicates that data was not available; Z represents or rounds to zero; Margin of error appears in parenthesis and is calculated using replicate weights.
Source: U.S. Census Bureau, American Community Survey, Table HIC-4_ACS. Health Insurance Coverage Status and Type of Coverage by State—All People: 2008 to 2016, Table HIC-5_ACS. Health Insurance Coverage Status and Type of Coverage by State—Children Under 18: 2008 to 2016, Table HIC-6_ACS. Health Insurance Coverage Status and Type of Coverage by State—Persons Under 65: 2008 to 2016

Nebraska

486 Ameritas

5900 O Street
Lincoln, NE 68501-1889
Toll-Free: 800-311-7871
Fax: 402-325-4190
www.ameritas.com
For Profit Organization: Yes
Year Founded: 1990

Healthplan and Services Defined
PLAN TYPE: Multiple
Model Type: Staff
Plan Specialty: ASO, Dental, Vision
Benefits Offered: Dental, Vision, Life, Disability

Type of Coverage
Commercial, Individual

Type of Payment Plans Offered
POS, DFFS, Capitated, Combination FFS & DFFS

Geographic Areas Served
Nationwide

Peer Review Type
Utilization Review: Yes
Second Surgical Opinion: Yes
Case Management: Yes

Publishes and Distributes Report Card: Yes

Accreditation Certification
Medicare Approved

Key Personnel
President & CEO . . . . JoAnn M. Martin

487 Blue Cross & Blue Shield of Nebraska

1919 Aksarben Drive
P.O. Box 3248
Omaha, NE 68180
Toll-Free: 800-622-2763
Phone: 402-982-7000
sales@nebraskablue.com
www.nebraskablue.com
Secondary Address: 1233 Lincoln Mall, Lincoln, NE 68508,
402-458-4800
Year Founded: 1939
Total Enrollment: 717,000
State Enrollment: 717,000

Healthplan and Services Defined
PLAN TYPE: PPO
Model Type: Network
Benefits Offered: Behavioral Health, Chiropractic, Dental,
Disease Management, Home Care, Inpatient SNF,
Long-Term Care, Physical Therapy, Podiatry, Prescription,
Psychiatric, Vision

Type of Coverage
Commercial, Individual, Medicare, Supplemental Medicare

Geographic Areas Served
Statewide

Publishes and Distributes Report Card: No

Key Personnel
President/CEO . . . . Steve S Martin
402-982-7000
EVP, Finance/Admin. Dale Mackel
COO . . . . Steven H Grandfield
VP, Claims . . . . Barbara True
Chief Legal Officer . . . . Russell Collins
Chief Medical Officer . . . . Debra Esser
Chief Information Officer . . . . Rama Kolli

488 Coventry Health Care of Nebraska

15950 West Dodge Road
Omaha, NE 68118-4030
Toll-Free: 800-471-0240
chcnebraska.coventryhealthcare.com
Subsidiary of: Aetna Inc.
For Profit Organization: Yes
Year Founded: 1985
Number of Affiliated Hospitals: 264
Number of Primary Care Physicians: 15,000
Total Enrollment: 5,000,000

Healthplan and Services Defined
PLAN TYPE: HMO/PPO
Other Type: POS
Model Type: Network
Plan Specialty: Behavioral Health, Dental, Worker's
Compensation
Benefits Offered: Behavioral Health, Dental, Wellness,
Worker's Compensation

Type of Coverage
Commercial, Individual, Medicare, Supplemental Medicare,
Medicaid

Type of Payment Plans Offered
POS

Geographic Areas Served
Statewide

Accreditation Certification
URAC

Key Personnel
Chief Executive Officer . . . . Mark T. Bertolini
President . . . . Karen S. Lynch
Chief Financial Officer . . . . Shawn M. Guertin
Operations & Technology . . . . Meg McCarthy
Chief Medical Officer . . . . Harold L. Paz
General Counsel . . . . Thomas Sabatino Jr.
Government Services . . . . Fran S. Soistman

489 Delta Dental of Nebraska

Atrium Executive Square
11235 Davenport Street, Suite 113
Omaha, NE 68154
Toll-Free: 800-736-0710
Phone: 612-224-3341
www.deltadentalne.org
Non-Profit Organization: Yes

Year Founded: 1969

Healthplan and Services Defined
PLAN TYPE: Dental
Other Type: Dental PPO
Model Type: Network
Plan Specialty: ASO, Dental
Benefits Offered: Dental

Type of Coverage
Commercial, Individual
Catastrophic Illness Benefit: None

Geographic Areas Served
Statewide

Key Personnel
President . . . . Rodney Young

490   Humana Health Insurance of Nebraska

1415 Kimberly Road
Bettendorf, IA 52722
Toll-Free: 866-653-7275
Fax: 563-355-0730
www.humana.com
Subsidiary of: Humana
For Profit Organization: Yes

Healthplan and Services Defined
PLAN TYPE: HMO/PPO
Model Type: Network
Plan Specialty: Dental, Vision
Benefits Offered: Dental, Vision, Life, LTD, STD, Nebraska
is covered by the Iowa branch.

Geographic Areas Served
Statewide

Accreditation Certification
URAC, NCQA, CORE

Key Personnel
President & CEO. Bruce Broussard
Chief Medical Officer. . . . . Roy A. Beveridge
Chief Consumer Officer. . . . . Jody L. Bilney
Human Resources. . . . . Tim Huval
Chief Financial Officer . . . . Brian Kane
Chief Information Officer . . . . Brian LeClaire
General Counsel . . . . Christopher M. Todoroff

491   Medica with CHI Health

331 Village Point Plaza
Suite 304
Omaha, NE 68118
Toll-Free: 800-918-6892
www.medica.com
Subsidiary of: UniNet Health Care
Number of Affiliated Hospitals: 30
Number of Primary Care Physicians: 1,400

Healthplan and Services Defined
PLAN TYPE: HMO
Benefits Offered: Behavioral Health, Chiropractic, Dental,
Disease Management, Prescription, Wellness

Geographic Areas Served
Buffalo, Burt, Butler, Cass, Colfax, Cuming, Dodge, Douglas,
Fillmore, Hall, Johnson, Lancaster, Nance, Nemaha, Nuckolls,
Otoe, Pawnee, Saline, Sarpy, Saunders, Seward, Thayer or
Washington counties

Key Personnel
President & CEO . . . . John Naylor
VP, Human Resources . . . . Lynn Altmann
SVP, Financial Officer . . . . Mark Baird
VP, General Manager . . . . Geoff Bartsh
SVP, General Counsel . . . . Jim Jacobson
SVP, Government Programs. . . . . Tom Lindquist
Marketing/Communications. . . . . Rob Longendyke

492   Medica: Nebraska

331 Village Point Plaza
Suite 304
Omaha, NE 68118
Toll-Free: 800-918-6892
medica.com
Year Founded: 1974
Number of Affiliated Hospitals: 170
Number of Primary Care Physicians: 7,200

Healthplan and Services Defined
PLAN TYPE: HMO
Benefits Offered: Behavioral Health, Chiropractic, Dental,
Disease Management, Prescription, Wellness, AD&D, Life

Type of Coverage
Medicare

Geographic Areas Served
Statewide

Key Personnel
President & CEO . . . . John Naylor
VP, Human Resources . . . . Lynn Altmann
SVP, Financial Officer . . . . Mark Baird
VP, General Manager . . . . Geoff Bartsh
SVP, General Counsel . . . . Jim Jacobson
SVP, Government Programs. . . . . Tom Lindquist
Marketing/Communications. . . . . Rob Longendyke

493   Midlands Choice

8420 W Dodge Road
Suite 210
Omaha, NE 68114-3459
Phone: 402-390-8233
Fax: 402-390-7261
www.midlandschoice.com
For Profit Organization: Yes
Year Founded: 1993
Physician Owned Organization: Yes
Number of Affiliated Hospitals: 320
Number of Primary Care Physicians: 20,000
Total Enrollment: 615,000

Healthplan and Services Defined
PLAN TYPE: PPO
Model Type: PPO Network

Geographic Areas Served

Iowa, Nebraska, South Dakota, Colorado, and portions of Wyoming, Kansas, Missouri, Illinois, Wisconsin and Minnesota

Accreditation Certification

URAC

Key Personnel

President/CEO . . . . Greta Vaught
Vice President . . . . Daniel McCulley

Specialty Managed Care Partners

Enters into Contracts with Regional Business Coalitions: No

---

494 Mutual of Omaha Dental Insurance

3300 Mutual of Omaha Plaza
Omaha, NE 68175
www.mutualofomaha.com/dental
For Profit Organization: Yes
Year Founded: 1985

Healthplan and Services Defined
PLAN TYPE: Dental
Model Type: Network
Benefits Offered: Behavioral Health, Chiropractic, Complementary Medicine, Dental, Disease Management, Home Care, Inpatient SNF, Long-Term Care, Physical Therapy, Podiatry, Prescription, Psychiatric, Transplant, Vision, Wellness

Type of Coverage
Commercial, Individual

Peer Review Type
Utilization Review: Yes
Second Surgical Opinion: Yes
Case Management: Yes

Publishes and Distributes Report Card: Yes

Accreditation Certification
TJC Accreditation, Medicare Approved, Utilization Review, Pre-Admission Certification, State Licensure, Quality Assurance Program

Key Personnel
Chief Executive Officer . . . . James Blackledge
Chief Financial Officer . . . . Vibhu Sharma
General Counsel . . . . Richard Anderl
Chief Information Officer . . . . Michael Lechtenberger
Chief Marketing Officer . . . . Stephanie Pritchett

Specialty Managed Care Partners
Enters into Contracts with Regional Business Coalitions: No

---

495 Mutual of Omaha Health Plans

3300 Mutual of Omaha Plaza
Omaha, NE 68175
Toll-Free: 800-205-8193
www.mutualofomaha.com
For Profit Organization: Yes
Year Founded: 1909
Number of Affiliated Hospitals: 43
Number of Primary Care Physicians: 673

Number of Referral/Specialty Physicians: 1,718
Total Enrollment: 54,418
State Enrollment: 28,978

Healthplan and Services Defined
PLAN TYPE: HMO/PPO
Other Type: POS
Model Type: IPA
Plan Specialty: ASO, Behavioral Health, Chiropractic, Disease Management, Lab, Vision, Radiology, UR
Benefits Offered: Behavioral Health, Chiropractic, Disease Management, Home Care, Inpatient SNF, Long-Term Care, Physical Therapy, Podiatry, Prescription, Psychiatric, Transplant, Vision, Wellness, AD&D, Life, LTD, STD, Critical Illness, EAP

Type of Coverage
Commercial, Individual, Indemnity, Medicare, Supplemental Medicare, Medicaid
Catastrophic Illness Benefit: Covered

Type of Payment Plans Offered
POS, Combination FFS & DFFS

Geographic Areas Served
Iowa: Harrison, Mills & Pottawattamie counties; Nebraska: Burt, Butler, Cass, Colfas, Cuming, Oakota, Dixon, Filmore, Johnson, Lancaster, Madison, Otoe, Salone, Saunders, Seuard, Stanton, Dodge, Douglas, Sampy, Washington counties

Subscriber Information
Average Monthly Fee Per Subscriber
(Employee + Employer Contribution):
Employee Only (Self): Varies by plan
Average Annual Deductible Per Subscriber:
Employee Only (Self): $0.00
Average Subscriber Co-Payment:
Primary Care Physician: $15.00
Prescription Drugs: $15.00
Hospital ER: $50.00
Home Health Care: $25.00
Home Health Care Max. Days/Visits Covered: Unlimited
Nursing Home: $0.00
Nursing Home Max. Days/Visits Covered: 100 days

Network Qualifications
Pre-Admission Certification: Yes

Peer Review Type
Utilization Review: Yes
Second Surgical Opinion: No
Case Management: Yes

Publishes and Distributes Report Card: Yes

Accreditation Certification
URAC, NCQA
TJC Accreditation, Utilization Review, Pre-Admission Certification, State Licensure, Quality Assurance Program

Key Personnel
Chief Executive Officer . . . . James Blackledge
EVP/General Counsel . . . . Richard Anderl
EVP/CFO . . . . Vibhu Sharma
EVP, Corporate Services . . . . Stacy A Scholtz
EVP, Chief Investment Ofc. . . . . Richard Hrabchak
Chief Marketing Officer . . . . Stephanie Pritchett

EVP, Information Services . . . . Michael Lechtenberger

Average Claim Compensation
Physician's Fees Charged: 75%
Hospital's Fees Charged: 60%

Specialty Managed Care Partners
Enters into Contracts with Regional Business Coalitions: No

Employer References
Mutual of Omaha, Forest National Bank, Nebraska Furniture Mart, Saint Joseph Hospital

496   UnitedHealthcare of Nebraska

2717 North 118th Street
Suite 300
Omaha, NE 68164
Toll-Free: 800-284-0626
www.uhc.com/contact-us/nebraska
Subsidiary of: UnitedHealth Group
For Profit Organization: Yes
Year Founded: 1984

Healthplan and Services Defined
PLAN TYPE: HMO/PPO
Model Type: Network
Plan Specialty: ASO, Behavioral Health, Chiropractic, Dental, Disease Management, Lab, MSO, PBM, Vision, Radiology
Benefits Offered: Behavioral Health, Dental, Disease Management, Long-Term Care, Prescription, Vision, Wellness, Life, LTD, STD

Type of Coverage
Commercial, Individual, Medicare, Supplemental Medicare, Medicaid, Catastrophic, Family, Military, Veterans, Group,

Type of Payment Plans Offered
POS, DFFS, FFS

Geographic Areas Served
Iowa: Cass, Fremont, Harrison, Mills, Mononas, Page, Pottawattsmie, Shelby, Woodbury counties; Nebraska: Buffalo, Burt, Butler, Dodge, Douglas, Gage, Hale, Jefferson, Johnson, Lancaster, Madison, Nemaha, Otoe, Pierce, Platte, Saline, Sarpy, Seward, & Washington counties

Subscriber Information
Average Subscriber Co-Payment:
Primary Care Physician: $10.00
Non-Network Physician: Deductible
Prescription Drugs: $10.00
Hospital ER: $50.00

Network Qualifications
Pre-Admission Certification: Yes

Peer Review Type
Utilization Review: Yes
Second Surgical Opinion: Yes
Case Management: Yes

Publishes and Distributes Report Card: Yes

Accreditation Certification
TJC Accreditation, Medicare Approved, Utilization Review, Pre-Admission Certification, State Licensure, Quality Assurance Program

Key Personnel
President . . . . David Wichmann
Chief Operating Officer . . . . Dan Schumacher
Chief Strategy Officer . . . . John Cosgriff
Communications Officer . . . . Kirsten Gorsuch
Chief Medical Officer. . . . . Sam Ho
Chief Legal Officer . . . . Thad Johnson
Chief Information Officer . . . . Phil McKoy
Chief Financial Officer. . . . . Jeff Putnam

Health Insurance Coverage Status and Type of Coverage by Age

Category	All Persons		Under 18 years		Under 65 years	
	Number	%	Number	%	Number	%
Total population	2,906	-	712	-	2,468	-
Covered by some type of health insurance	2,575 (13)	88.6 (0.5)	662 (6)	93.0 (0.7)	2,145 (13)	86.9 (0.5)
Covered by private health insurance	1,881 (22)	64.7 (0.8)	426 (10)	59.8 (1.4)	1,650 (21)	66.9 (0.9)
Employer-based	1,529 (22)	52.6 (0.8)	368 (11)	51.7 (1.5)	1,408 (21)	57.1 (0.9)
Direct purchase	346 (14)	11.9 (0.5)	52 (6)	7.3 (0.8)	236 (13)	9.6 (0.5)
TRICARE	108 (7)	3.7 (0.2)	19 (3)	2.6 (0.4)	68 (6)	2.7 (0.2)
Covered by public health insurance	1,004 (20)	34.5 (0.7)	261 (10)	36.7 (1.5)	587 (19)	23.8 (0.8)
Medicaid	569 (19)	19.6 (0.6)	260 (10)	36.5 (1.5)	519 (19)	21.0 (0.8)
Medicare	476 (5)	16.4 (0.2)	3 (1)	0.4 (0.2)	61 (5)	2.5 (0.2)
VA Care	94 (4)	3.3 (0.1)	1 (Z)	0.1 (0.1)	44 (4)	1.8 (0.1)
Not covered at any time during the year	330 (13)	11.4 (0.5)	50 (5)	7.0 (0.7)	324 (13)	13.1 (0.5)

Note: Numbers in thousands; Figures cover civilian noninstitutionalized population in 2016; N/A indicates that data was not available; Z represents or rounds to zero; Margin of error appears in parenthesis and is calculated using replicate weights.
Source: U.S. Census Bureau, American Community Survey, Table HIC-4_ACS. Health Insurance Coverage Status and Type of Coverage by State—All People: 2008 to 2016, Table HIC-5_ACS. Health Insurance Coverage Status and Type of Coverage by State—Children Under 18: 2008 to 2016, Table HIC-6_ACS. Health Insurance Coverage Status and Type of Coverage by State—Persons Under 65: 2008 to 2016

Nevada

497   Aetna Health of Nevada

151 Farmington Avenue
Hartford, CT 06156
Toll-Free: 800-872-3862
Phone: 860-273-0123
www.aetna.com
Subsidiary of: Aetna Inc.
For Profit Organization: Yes

Healthplan and Services Defined
  PLAN TYPE: HMO/PPO
  Other Type: POS
  Model Type: Network
  Plan Specialty: Behavioral Health, EPO, Lab, PBM,
    Radiology
  Benefits Offered: Behavioral Health, Dental, Disease
    Management, Long-Term Care, Physical Therapy,
    Podiatry, Prescription, Psychiatric, Vision, Wellness, Life,
    LTD, STD

Type of Coverage
  Commercial, Medicare, Supplemental Medicare, Medicaid,
    Student health

Geographic Areas Served
  Statewide

Key Personnel
  CEO . . . . Mark Bertolini

498   Amerigroup Nevada

Desert Canyon Building 9
9133 W Russell Road
Las Vegas, NV 89148
Toll-Free: 800-600-4441
Phone: 702-228-1308
www.myamerigroup.com/nv
Subsidiary of: Anthem, Inc.
For Profit Organization: Yes
Year Founded: 2009

Healthplan and Services Defined
  PLAN TYPE: HMO

Type of Coverage
  Medicaid, Nevada Check Up, Taking Care of Bab

Accreditation Certification
  NCQA

Key Personnel
  EVP/Pres., Gov. Business . . . . Peter D. Haytaian

499   Anthem Blue Cross & Blue Shield of Nevada

9133 W Russell Road
Las Vegas, NV 89148
Phone: 317-488-6000
www.anthem.com
Secondary Address: 5250 S Virginia Street, Reno, NV 89502,
  775-448-4000
Subsidiary of: Anthem, Inc.

For Profit Organization: Yes

Healthplan and Services Defined
  PLAN TYPE: HMO/PPO
  Model Type: Network
  Plan Specialty: Behavioral Health, Dental, Disease
    Management, Lab, PBM, Vision, Radiology
  Benefits Offered: Behavioral Health, Dental, Disease
    Management, Inpatient SNF, Physical Therapy,
    Prescription, Psychiatric, Transplant, Vision, Wellness, Life

Type of Coverage
  Commercial, Individual, Medicare, Supplemental Medicare,
    Catastrophic

Geographic Areas Served
  Statewide

Accreditation Certification
  URAC, NCQA

Key Personnel
  President & CEO . . . . Scott P. Serota
  Chief Financial Officer . . . . Robert Kolodgy
  Human Resources . . . . Maureen A. Cahill
  Chief Medical Officer. . . . . Trent Haywood
  General Counsel . . . . Scott Nehs

500   Behavioral Healthcare Options, Inc.

2716 N Tenaya Way
Las Vegas, NV 89128
Toll-Free: 800-873-2246
www.bhoptions.com
Subsidiary of: UnitedHealthcare
Year Founded: 1991

Healthplan and Services Defined
  PLAN TYPE: PPO
  Model Type: Group
  Plan Specialty: Behavioral Health, Mental health, addiction
    treatment, employee assistance, work-life services
  Benefits Offered: Behavioral Health, Psychiatric

Accreditation Certification
  URAC

501   Coventry Health Care of Nevada

6730-B Rockledge Drive
Suite 700
Bethesda, MD 20817
Phone: 301-581-0600
www.coventryhealthcare.com
Subsidiary of: Aetna Inc.
For Profit Organization: Yes

Healthplan and Services Defined
  PLAN TYPE: HMO/PPO
  Model Type: Network
  Plan Specialty: Behavioral Health, Dental, Worker's
    Compensation
  Benefits Offered: Behavioral Health, Dental, Prescription,
    Wellness, Worker's Compensation

Type of Coverage
  Commercial, Medicare, Medicaid

Geographic Areas Served
Statewide

Key Personnel
Chief Executive Officer . . . . Mark T. Bertolini
President . . . . Karen S. Lynch
Chief Financial Officer . . . . Shawn M. Guertin
Operations & Technology . . . . Meg McCarthy
Chief Medical Officer . . . . Harold L. Paz
General Counsel . . . . Thomas Sabatino
Government Services . . . . Fran S. Soistman

502 Health Plan of Nevada

2720 N Tenaya Way
Las Vegas, NV 89128
Toll-Free: 800-777-1840
Phone: 702-242-7300
www.healthplanofnevada.com
Subsidiary of: United HealthCare Services, Inc.
For Profit Organization: Yes
Year Founded: 1982
Total Enrollment: 418,000
State Enrollment: 25,576

Healthplan and Services Defined
PLAN TYPE: HMO
Other Type: POS, Medicare
Model Type: Network
Benefits Offered: Disease Management, Prescription,
Wellness

Type of Coverage
Commercial, Individual, Medicare, Supplemental Medicare,
Medicaid

Geographic Areas Served
Statewide

Accreditation Certification
NCQA

Key Personnel
President/CEO . . . . Jonathan W Bunker
Chief Information Officer . . . . Robert Schaich
VP Network Development . . . . Scott Cassano

Specialty Managed Care Partners
Express Scripts

503 Hometown Health Plan

10315 Professional Circle
Reno, NV 89521
Toll-Free: 800-336-0123
Phone: 775-982-3232
Fax: 775-982-3741
customer_service@hometownhealth.com
www.hometownhealth.com
Subsidiary of: Renown Health
Non-Profit Organization: Yes
Year Founded: 1988
Owned by an Integrated Delivery Network (IDN): Yes
Number of Affiliated Hospitals: 19
Number of Primary Care Physicians: 256

Number of Referral/Specialty Physicians: 8,917
Total Enrollment: 32,000
State Enrollment: 10,000

Healthplan and Services Defined
PLAN TYPE: Multiple
Model Type: Network
Plan Specialty: ASO, Behavioral Health, Chiropractic, Dental,
Disease Management, EPO, Lab, PBM, Vision, Radiology,
Worker's Compensation, UR
Benefits Offered: Behavioral Health, Chiropractic,
Complementary Medicine, Dental, Disease Management,
Home Care, Inpatient SNF, Physical Therapy, Podiatry,
Prescription, Psychiatric, Transplant, Vision, Wellness,
Worker's Compensation, AD&D, Life, LTD, STD,
Accupuncture
Offers Demand Management Patient Information Service: Yes

Type of Coverage
Commercial, Individual, Medicare, Supplemental Medicare

Geographic Areas Served
Statewide

Subscriber Information
Average Monthly Fee Per Subscriber
(Employee + Employer Contribution):
Employee Only (Self): Varies
Employee & 1 Family Member: Varies
Employee & 2 Family Members: Varies
Medicare: Varies
Average Annual Deductible Per Subscriber:
Employee Only (Self): Varies
Employee & 1 Family Member: Varies
Employee & 2 Family Members: Varies
Medicare: Varies
Average Subscriber Co-Payment:
Primary Care Physician: Varies
Non-Network Physician: Varies
Prescription Drugs: Varies
Hospital ER: Varies
Home Health Care: Varies
Home Health Care Max. Days/Visits Covered: Varies
Nursing Home: Varies
Nursing Home Max. Days/Visits Covered: Varies

Accreditation Certification
TJC

Key Personnel
President/CEO . . . . Ty Windfeldt
VP/Chief Medical Officer . . . . Linda Ash-Jackson, MD

504 Humana Health Insurance of Nevada

770 E Warm Springs Road
Suite 340
Las Vegas, NV 89119
Phone: 702-837-4401
Fax: 702-562-0134
www.humana.com
Secondary Address: 1000 N Green Valley Parkway, Suite 720,
Henderson, NV 89074, 702-269-5200
Subsidiary of: Humana

For Profit Organization: Yes

Healthplan and Services Defined
PLAN TYPE: HMO/PPO
Model Type: Network
Plan Specialty: Dental, Vision
Benefits Offered: Dental, Vision, Life, LTD, STD

Type of Coverage
Commercial, Individual

Geographic Areas Served
Statewide

Accreditation Certification
URAC, NCQA, CORE

Key Personnel
President & CEO . . . . Bruce Broussard
Chief Medical Officer . . . . Roy A. Beveridge
Chief Consumer Officer . . . . Jody L. Binley
Human Resources . . . . Tim Huval
Chief Financial Officer . . . . Brian Kane
Chief Information Officer . . . . Brian LeClaire
General Counsel . . . . Christopher M. Todoroff

---

505   Liberty Dental Plan of Nevada

6385 S Rainbow Boulevard
Suite 200
Las Vegas, NV 89118
Toll-Free: 888-700-0643
www.libertydentalplan.com
For Profit Organization: Yes
Total Enrollment: 2,000,000

Healthplan and Services Defined
PLAN TYPE: Dental
Other Type: Dental HMO
Plan Specialty: Dental
Benefits Offered: Dental

Type of Coverage
Commercial, Medicare, Medicaid, Unions

Geographic Areas Served
Statewide

Accreditation Certification
NCQA

Key Personnel
President & CEO . . . . Amir Neshat
Executive Vice President . . . . John Carvelli
Chief Financial Officer . . . . Maja Kapic
General Counsel . . . . Lisa Wright
Chief Operating Officer . . . . Nico Alvarez
Chief Dental Officer . . . . Richard Goren
Dental Director . . . . Richard Hague

506   Nevada Preferred Healthcare Providers

1050 Meadow Wood Lane
Reno, NV 89502
Toll-Free: 800-776-6959
Phone: 775-356-1159
Fax: 775-356-5746
www.universalhealthnet.com
Subsidiary of: Universal Health Services, Inc.
Non-Profit Organization: Yes
Year Founded: 1991
Number of Affiliated Hospitals: 80
Number of Primary Care Physicians: 4,483
Total Enrollment: 150,000
State Enrollment: 150,000

Healthplan and Services Defined
PLAN TYPE: PPO
Other Type: EPO
Model Type: Network
Plan Specialty: EPO, Worker's Compensation
Benefits Offered: Behavioral Health, Chiropractic, Home
Care, Physical Therapy, Podiatry, Psychiatric, Transplant,
Wellness, Worker's Compensation

Type of Coverage
Commercial, Individual

Type of Payment Plans Offered
POS, DFFS, FFS, Combination FFS & DFFS

Geographic Areas Served
Nevada, and limited areas in Utah

Network Qualifications
Pre-Admission Certification: Yes

Peer Review Type
Utilization Review: Yes
Second Surgical Opinion: Yes
Case Management: Yes

Publishes and Distributes Report Card: No

Specialty Managed Care Partners
Enters into Contracts with Regional Business Coalitions: Yes

Employer References
State of Nevada, CCN, PPO USA GEHA, Valley Health
System, Pepperpill

---

507   Premier Access Insurance/Access Dental

P.O. Box 659010
Sacramento, CA 95865-9010
Toll-Free: 888-634-6074
Phone: 916-920-2500
Fax: 916-563-9000
info@premierlife.com
www.premierppo.com
Subsidiary of: Guardian Life Insurance Co.
For Profit Organization: Yes
Year Founded: 1989
Number of Primary Care Physicians: 1,000

Healthplan and Services Defined
PLAN TYPE: PPO
Other Type: Dental

Plan Specialty: Dental
Benefits Offered: Dental

Key Personnel
President & CEO . . . . Deanna M. Mulligan

508   Prominence Health Plan

1510 Meadow Wood Lane
Reno, NV 89502
Toll-Free: 800-433-3077
Phone: 775-770-9300
prominencehealthplan.com
Secondary Address: 2475 Village View Drive, Suite 100,
   Henderson, NV 89074
Subsidiary of: Universal Health Services, Inc.
For Profit Organization: Yes
Year Founded: 1993
Number of Affiliated Hospitals: 34
Number of Primary Care Physicians: 4,000
Number of Referral/Specialty Physicians: 1,500

Healthplan and Services Defined
   PLAN TYPE: HMO/PPO
   Other Type: POS
   Model Type: Group, Network
   Plan Specialty: ASO, Behavioral Health, Chiropractic,
      Dental, Disease Management, EPO, MSO, PBM, Vision,
      Radiology, Worker's Compensation
   Benefits Offered: Behavioral Health, Chiropractic,
      Complementary
Medicine, Dental, Disease Management, Home Care,
Inpatient SNF, Long-Term Care, Physical Therapy,
Podiatry, Prescription, Psychiatric, Transplant,
Vision, Wellness, Worker's Compensation, Routine
PE, pre and post-natal care, well baby/well child
care, mammography, GYN, prostate screenings

Type of Payment Plans Offered
   POS, DFFS, FFS, Combination FFS & DFFS

Geographic Areas Served
   Nevada and border communities in California and Arizona

Subscriber Information
   Average Monthly Fee Per Subscriber
      (Employee + Employer Contribution):
         Employee Only (Self): Varies by plan
   Average Subscriber Co-Payment:
      Nursing Home: Varies

Network Qualifications
   Pre-Admission Certification: Yes

Peer Review Type
   Utilization Review: Yes
   Second Surgical Opinion: Yes
   Case Management: Yes

Accreditation Certification
   NCQA
   TJC Accreditation, Medicare Approved, Pre-Admission
      Certification

Key Personnel
   President/CEO . . . . David Livingston

Director of Operations . . . . Majorie Henriksen

509   UnitedHealthcare of Nevada

2724 N Tenaya Way
Las Vegas, NV 89128
Phone: 702-821-2200
www.uhc.com/contact-us/nevada
Subsidiary of: UnitedHealth Group
For Profit Organization: Yes
Year Founded: 1984

Healthplan and Services Defined
   PLAN TYPE: HMO/PPO
   Other Type: POS
   Model Type: Network
   Plan Specialty: Behavioral Health, Dental, Disease
      Management, PBM, Vision
   Benefits Offered: Behavioral Health, Dental, Disease
      Management, Long-Term Care, Prescription, Vision,
      Wellness, Life, LTD, STD

Type of Coverage
   Individual, Medicare, Supplemental Medicare, Medicaid,
      Catastrophic, Family, Military, Veterans, Group,

Type of Payment Plans Offered
   POS, DFFS, Capitated, FFS

Geographic Areas Served
   Statewide

Subscriber Information
   Average Monthly Fee Per Subscriber
      (Employee + Employer Contribution):
         Employee Only (Self): $39.00
   Average Annual Deductible Per Subscriber:
         Employee Only (Self): $0
         Employee & 1 Family Member: $0
         Employee & 2 Family Members: $0
         Medicare: $0
   Average Subscriber Co-Payment:
         Primary Care Physician: $0.00
         Prescription Drugs: $10.00
         Hospital ER: $50.00
         Home Health Care: Varies
         Home Health Care Max. Days/Visits Covered: Unlimited
         Nursing Home: Varies
         Nursing Home Max. Days/Visits Covered: 100 days

Peer Review Type
   Case Management: Yes

Publishes and Distributes Report Card: Yes

Key Personnel
   President . . . . David Wichmann
   Chief Operating Officer . . . . Dan Schumacher
   Chief Strategy Officer . . . . John Cosgriff
   Communications Officer . . . . Kirsten Gorsuch
   Chief Medical Officer. . . . . Sam Ho
   Chief Legal Officer . . . . Thad Johnson
   Chief Information Officer . . . . Phil McKoy
   Chief Financial Officer. . . . . Jeff Putnam

Health Insurance Coverage Status and Type of Coverage by Age

Category	All Persons		Under 18 years		Under 65 years	
	Number	%	Number	%	Number	%
Total population	1,316	-	279	-	1,099	-
Covered by some type of health insurance	1,239 (6)	94.1 (0.4)	272 (3)	97.3 (0.6)	1,021 (6)	92.9 (0.5)
Covered by private health insurance	1,008 (12)	76.5 (0.9)	200 (5)	71.5 (1.8)	857 (11)	78.0 (1.0)
Employer-based	843 (13)	64.0 (1.0)	185 (5)	66.2 (1.8)	758 (12)	69.0 (1.1)
Direct purchase	181 (8)	13.7 (0.6)	16 (2)	5.6 (0.8)	107 (6)	9.8 (0.6)
TRICARE	32 (4)	2.4 (0.3)	3 (1)	1.2 (0.4)	15 (3)	1.4 (0.3)
Covered by public health insurance	412 (9)	31.3 (0.7)	81 (4)	28.9 (1.6)	200 (9)	18.2 (0.8)
Medicaid	181 (8)	13.8 (0.6)	80 (4)	28.5 (1.5)	164 (8)	15.0 (0.7)
Medicare	249 (4)	18.9 (0.3)	1 (1)	0.5 (0.2)	37 (3)	3.4 (0.3)
VA Care	39 (3)	3.0 (0.2)	1 (Z)	0.2 (0.2)	16 (2)	1.5 (0.2)
Not covered at any time during the year	78 (6)	5.9 (0.4)	8 (2)	2.7 (0.6)	78 (6)	7.1 (0.5)

Note: Numbers in thousands; Figures cover civilian noninstitutionalized population in 2016; N/A indicates that data was not available; Z represents or rounds to zero; Margin of error appears in parenthesis and is calculated using replicate weights.
Source: U.S. Census Bureau, American Community Survey, Table HIC-4_ACS. Health Insurance Coverage Status and Type of Coverage by State—All People: 2008 to 2016, Table HIC-5_ACS. Health Insurance Coverage Status and Type of Coverage by State—Children Under 18: 2008 to 2016, Table HIC-6_ACS. Health Insurance Coverage Status and Type of Coverage by State—Persons Under 65: 2008 to 2016

New Hampshire

510 Able Insurance Agency
130 Broadway
Concord, NH 03301
Phone: 603-225-6677
able2insure.com

Healthplan and Services Defined
PLAN TYPE: HMO
Benefits Offered: Wellness, Life

Geographic Areas Served
Greater Concord Area

Key Personnel
Principal .... PJ Cistulli
  pjcj@able2insure.com
Producer .... Angela Chicoine
  angela@able2insure.com
Agent .... Kathy Coleman
  kathy@able2insure.com
Marketing Coordinator .... Samantha Sharff
  samanthaleec@gmail.com

511 Anthem Blue Cross & Blue Shield of New Hampshire
1155 Elm Street
Suite 200
Manchester, NH 03101-1505
Phone: 603-541-2000
www.anthem.com
Subsidiary of: Anthem, Inc.
For Profit Organization: Yes

Healthplan and Services Defined
PLAN TYPE: HMO/PPO
Model Type: Network
Plan Specialty: Behavioral Health, Dental, Disease
  Management, Lab, PBM, Vision, Radiology
Benefits Offered: Behavioral Health, Dental, Disease
  Management, Inpatient SNF, Physical Therapy,
  Prescription, Psychiatric, Transplant, Vision, Wellness, Life

Type of Coverage
Commercial, Individual, Medicare, Supplemental Medicare,
Catastrophic

Geographic Areas Served
Statewide

Accreditation Certification
URAC, NCQA

Key Personnel
President & CEO .... Scott P. Serota
Chief Financial Officer .... Robert Kolodgy
Human Resources .... Maureen A. Cahill
Chief Medical Officer.................. Trent Haywood
General Counsel....................... Scott Nehs

512 Coventry Health Care of New Hampshire
1 Garside Way
Manchester, NH 03103
Phone: 603-670-2178
www.coventryhealthcare.com
Subsidiary of: Aetna Inc.
For Profit Organization: Yes

Healthplan and Services Defined
PLAN TYPE: HMO/PPO
Model Type: Network
Plan Specialty: Behavioral Health, Dental, Worker's
  Compensation
Benefits Offered: Behavioral Health, Dental, Prescription,
  Wellness, Worker's Compensation

Type of Coverage
Commercial, Medicare, Medicaid

Geographic Areas Served
Statewide

Key Personnel
Chief Executive Officer............... Mark T. Bertolini
President........................... Karen S. Lynch
Chief Financial Officer .... Shawn M. Guertin
Operations & Technology............... Meg McCarthy
Chief Medical Officer .... Harold L. Paz
General Counsel .... Thomas Sabatino Jr.
Government Services .... Fran S. Soistman

513 Harvard Pilgrim Health Care New Hampshire
650 Elm Street
Suite 700
Manchester, NH 03101-2596
Toll-Free: 888-888-4742
www.harvardpilgrim.org
Non-Profit Organization: Yes
Year Founded: 1977
Number of Affiliated Hospitals: 179
Number of Referral/Specialty Physicians: 53,000

Healthplan and Services Defined
PLAN TYPE: HMO/PPO
Benefits Offered: Wellness

Geographic Areas Served
Statewide

Accreditation Certification
NCQA

Key Personnel
President & CEO...................... Eric H. Schultz
Chief Financial Officer .... Charles Goheen
Chief Legal Officer .... Tisa Hughes
Chief Information Officer............. Deborah A. Norton
VP, Marketing .... Richard O'Connor
Human Resources...................... Cynthia Ring
Chief Medical Officer .... Michael Sherman
Senior VP, Sales & Mktg .... Beth Roberts

514 Humana Health Insurance of New Hampshire

1 New Hampshire Avenue
Suite 125
Portsmouth, NH 03801
Toll-Free: 800-967-2370
www.humana.com
Subsidiary of: Humana
For Profit Organization: Yes

Healthplan and Services Defined
PLAN TYPE: HMO/PPO
Model Type: Network
Plan Specialty: Dental, Vision
Benefits Offered: Dental, Vision, Life, LTD, STD

Type of Coverage
Commercial

Geographic Areas Served
Statewide

Accreditation Certification
URAC, NCQA, CORE

Key Personnel
President . . . . Bruce Broussard
Chief Medical Officer . . . . Roy A. Beveridge
Chief Consumer Officer . . . . Jody L. Bilney
Human Resources . . . . Tim Huval
Chief Financial Officer . . . . Brian Kane
Chief Information Officer . . . . Brian LeClaire
General Counsel . . . . Christopher M. Todoroff

515 Northeast Delta Dental

One Delta Dr
P.O. Box 2002
Concord, NH 03302-2002
Toll-Free: 800-537-1715
Phone: 603-223-1000
Fax: 603-223-1199
nedelta@nedelta.com
www.nedelta.com
Non-Profit Organization: Yes
Year Founded: 1961

Healthplan and Services Defined
PLAN TYPE: Dental
Other Type: Dental PPO
Model Type: Network
Plan Specialty: ASO, Dental
Benefits Offered: Dental

Type of Coverage
Commercial, Individual
Catastrophic Illness Benefit: None

Geographic Areas Served
Maine, New Hampshire and Vermont

Key Personnel
President & CEO . . . . Thomas Raffio
Chair . . . . Kathryn L. Yerkes

516 UnitedHealthcare of New Hampshire

475 Kilvert Street
Warwick, RI 02886
Toll-Free: 888-735-5842
www.uhc.com/contact-us/new-hampshire
Subsidiary of: UnitedHealth Group
For Profit Organization: Yes
Year Founded: 1986

Healthplan and Services Defined
PLAN TYPE: HMO/PPO
Model Type: Network
Plan Specialty: Behavioral Health, Dental, Disease
Management, MSO, PBM, Vision
Benefits Offered: Behavioral Health, Chiropractic,
Complementary Medicine, Dental, Disease Management,
Home Care, Inpatient SNF, Long-Term Care, Physical
Therapy, Podiatry, Prescription, Psychiatric, Transplant,
Vision, Wellness, AD&D, Life, LTD, STD

Type of Coverage
Commercial, Individual, Medicare, Supplemental Medicare,
Medicaid, Catastrophic, Family, Military, Veterans, Group,

Type of Payment Plans Offered
DFFS, FFS, Combination FFS & DFFS

Geographic Areas Served
Statewide. New Hampshire is covered by the Rhode Island
branch

Subscriber Information
Average Monthly Fee Per Subscriber
(Employee + Employer Contribution):
Employee Only (Self): Varies
Average Subscriber Co-Payment:
Primary Care Physician: $10
Prescription Drugs: $10/15/30
Hospital ER: $50

Network Qualifications
Pre-Admission Certification: Yes

Peer Review Type
Case Management: Yes

Publishes and Distributes Report Card: Yes

Accreditation Certification
URAC, NCQA, State Licensure, Quality Assurance Program

Key Personnel
President . . . . David Wichmann
Chief Operating Officer . . . . Dan Schumacher
Chief Strategy Officer . . . . John Cosgriff
Communications Officer . . . . Kirsten Gorsuch
Chief Medical Officer . . . . Sam Ho
Chief Legal Officer . . . . Thad Johnson
Chief Information Officer . . . . Phil McKoy
Chief Financial Officer . . . . Jeff Putnam

Average Claim Compensation
Physician's Fees Charged: 70%
Hospital's Fees Charged: 55%

Specialty Managed Care Partners
United Behavioral Health
Enters into Contracts with Regional Business Coalitions: No

Health Insurance Coverage Status and Type of Coverage by Age

Category	All Persons		Under 18 years		Under 65 years	
	Number	%	Number	%	Number	%
Total population	8,838	-	2,094	-	7,505	-
Covered by some type of health insurance	8,133 (19)	92.0 (0.2)	2,016 (7)	96.3 (0.3)	6,817 (18)	90.8 (0.2)
Covered by private health insurance	6,388 (32)	72.3 (0.4)	1,411 (16)	67.4 (0.7)	5,547 (32)	73.9 (0.4)
Employer-based	5,483 (34)	62.0 (0.4)	1,278 (17)	61.1 (0.8)	4,952 (33)	66.0 (0.4)
Direct purchase	1,093 (18)	12.4 (0.2)	144 (8)	6.9 (0.4)	687 (18)	9.2 (0.2)
TRICARE	86 (6)	1.0 (0.1)	18 (3)	0.9 (0.1)	53 (5)	0.7 (0.1)
Covered by public health insurance	2,747 (26)	31.1 (0.3)	670 (15)	32.0 (0.7)	1,479 (25)	19.7 (0.3)
Medicaid	1,516 (25)	17.2 (0.3)	663 (15)	31.7 (0.7)	1,351 (24)	18.0 (0.3)
Medicare	1,450 (10)	16.4 (0.1)	10 (2)	0.5 (0.1)	183 (8)	2.4 (0.1)
VA Care	94 (4)	1.1 (0.1)	1 (1)	0.1 (0.1)	30 (4)	0.4 (Z)
Not covered at any time during the year	705 (19)	8.0 (0.2)	78 (7)	3.7 (0.3)	688 (18)	9.2 (0.2)

Note: Numbers in thousands; Figures cover civilian noninstitutionalized population in 2016; N/A indicates that data was not available; Z represents or rounds to zero; Margin of error appears in parenthesis and is calculated using replicate weights.
Source: U.S. Census Bureau, American Community Survey, Table HIC-4_ACS. Health Insurance Coverage Status and Type of Coverage by State—All People: 2008 to 2016, Table HIC-5_ACS. Health Insurance Coverage Status and Type of Coverage by State—Children Under 18: 2008 to 2016, Table HIC-6_ACS. Health Insurance Coverage Status and Type of Coverage by State—Persons Under 65: 2008 to 2016

New Jersey

517 Aetna Health of New Jersey

151 Farmington Avenue
Hartford, CT 06156
Toll-Free: 800-872-3862
Phone: 860-273-0123
www.aetna.com
Subsidiary of: Aetna Inc.
For Profit Organization: Yes

Healthplan and Services Defined
  PLAN TYPE: HMO/PPO
  Other Type: POS
  Model Type: Network
  Plan Specialty: Behavioral Health, EPO, Lab, PBM,
    Radiology
  Benefits Offered: Behavioral Health, Dental, Disease
    Management, Long-Term Care, Physical Therapy,
    Podiatry, Prescription, Psychiatric, Vision, Wellness, Life,
    LTD, STD

Type of Coverage
  Commercial, Medicare, Supplemental Medicare, Student
  health

Geographic Areas Served
  Statewide

Key Personnel
  CEO . . . . Mark Bertolini

518 AmeriHealth New Jersey

259 Prospect Plains Road
Cranbury, NJ 08512-3706
Toll-Free: 877-744-5422
www.amerihealthnj.com
Total Enrollment: 265,000

Healthplan and Services Defined
  PLAN TYPE: HMO/PPO
  Benefits Offered: Dental, Disease Management, Prescription,
    Vision, Wellness

Type of Coverage
  Commercial, Individual

Geographic Areas Served
  New Jersey

Key Personnel
  Market President . . . . Mike Munoz
  Networking Operations . . . . Ken Kobylowski
  Vice President of Sales . . . . Ryan J. Petrizzi
  Senior Medical Director . . . . Frank L. Urbano

519 Atlanticare Health Plans

2500 English Creek Avenue
Egg Harbor Township, NJ 08234
Toll-Free: 888-569-1000
Phone: 609-407-2300
webmaster@atlanticare.org
www.atlanticare.org

Non-Profit Organization: Yes
Year Founded: 1993
Number of Affiliated Hospitals: 36
Number of Primary Care Physicians: 600
Number of Referral/Specialty Physicians: 4,000
Total Enrollment: 150,000
State Enrollment: 150,000

Healthplan and Services Defined
  PLAN TYPE: HMO/PPO
  Model Type: IPA
  Plan Specialty: ASO, Behavioral Health, Worker's
    Compensation, UR

Type of Payment Plans Offered
  Combination FFS & DFFS

Geographic Areas Served
  Southeastern New Jersey

Subscriber Information
  Average Subscriber Co-Payment:
    Primary Care Physician: $10.00
    Non-Network Physician: $20.00
    Prescription Drugs: $15.00
    Hospital ER: $50.00
    Home Health Care: $60
    Nursing Home: $120

Network Qualifications
  Pre-Admission Certification: Yes

Peer Review Type
  Utilization Review: Yes
  Second Surgical Opinion: Yes
  Case Management: Yes

Accreditation Certification
  TJC, URAC, NCQA

Specialty Managed Care Partners
  Horizon BC/BS of NJ

520 CHN PPO

300 American Metro Boulevard
Suite 170
Hamilton, NJ 08619
Toll-Free: 800-225-4246
www.chn.com
Secondary Address: Towamencin Corporate Center, Building
  1, 1555 Bustard Road, Suite 100, Lansdale, PA 19446,
  215-661-0500
Subsidiary of: Consolidated Services Group
For Profit Organization: Yes
Year Founded: 1986
Number of Affiliated Hospitals: 165
Number of Primary Care Physicians: 116,000
Number of Referral/Specialty Physicians: 57,550
Total Enrollment: 975,000

Healthplan and Services Defined
  PLAN TYPE: PPO
  Model Type: Network
  Plan Specialty: Behavioral Health, Chiropractic, EPO, Lab,
    Vision, Radiology, Worker's Compensation, UR

Benefits Offered: Behavioral Health, Chiropractic, Disease
Management, Home Care, Inpatient SNF, Long-Term Care,
Physical Therapy, Podiatry, Psychiatric, Transplant, Vision,
Wellness, Worker's Compensation

Type of Coverage
Catastrophic Illness Benefit: Varies per case

Type of Payment Plans Offered
POS, DFFS, FFS

Geographic Areas Served
Connecticut, New Jersey & New York

Subscriber Information
Average Monthly Fee Per Subscriber
(Employee + Employer Contribution):
Employee Only (Self): Varies
Employee & 1 Family Member: Varies
Employee & 2 Family Members: Varies
Medicare: Varies
Average Annual Deductible Per Subscriber:
Employee Only (Self): Varies
Employee & 1 Family Member: Varies
Employee & 2 Family Members: Varies
Medicare: Varies
Average Subscriber Co-Payment:
Primary Care Physician: Varies
Non-Network Physician: Varies
Prescription Drugs: Varies
Hospital ER: Varies
Home Health Care: Varies
Home Health Care Max. Days/Visits Covered: Varies
Nursing Home: Varies
Nursing Home Max. Days/Visits Covered: Varies

Network Qualifications
Pre-Admission Certification: Yes

Peer Review Type
Utilization Review: Yes
Second Surgical Opinion: Yes
Case Management: Yes

Accreditation Certification
URAC, AAPI
TJC Accreditation, Medicare Approved, Utilization Review,
Pre-Admission Certification, State Licensure, Quality
Assurance Program

Key Personnel
President/CEO . . . . Craig Goldstein
SVP/Director of Operation . . . . Mark Hepperlen
SVP, Financial Operations . . . . Lee Ann Iannelli
SVP, Network Operations . . . . Cara Ianniello
SVP, Medical Case Mgmt . . . . Maria Longworth
VP Strategic Partnerships . . . . Missy Pudimott
Chief Medical Officer . . . . William P. Anthony, MD
SVP, Chief Info Officer . . . . Stan Tomasevich
Vice President, Sales . . . . Steve Armenti

Average Claim Compensation
Physician's Fees Charged: 33%
Hospital's Fees Charged: 40%

Specialty Managed Care Partners
Enters into Contracts with Regional Business Coalitions: Yes

---

521 **Coventry Health Care of New Jersey**
601 Jack Stephan Way
Trenton, NJ 08628
Phone: 609-323-7867
www.coventryhealthcare.com
Subsidiary of: Aetna Inc.
For Profit Organization: Yes

Healthplan and Services Defined
PLAN TYPE: HMO/PPO
Model Type: Network
Plan Specialty: Behavioral Health, Dental, Worker's
Compensation
Benefits Offered: Behavioral Health, Dental, Prescription,
Wellness, Worker's Compensation

Type of Coverage
Commercial, Medicare, Medicaid

Geographic Areas Served
Statewide

Key Personnel
Chief Executive Officer . . . . Mark T. Bertolini
President . . . . Karen S. Lynch
Chief Financial Officer . . . . Shawn M. Guertin
Operations & Technology . . . . Meg McCarthy
Chief Medical Officer . . . . Harold L. Paz
General Counsel . . . . Thomas Sabatino Jr.
Government Services . . . . Fran S. Soistman

---

522 **Delta Dental of New Jersey**
1639 Route 10
Parsippany, NJ 07054
Toll-Free: 800-452-9310
service@deltadentalnj.com
www.deltadentalnj.com
Non-Profit Organization: Yes
Year Founded: 1969

Healthplan and Services Defined
PLAN TYPE: Dental
Other Type: Dental HMO/PPO/POS
Model Type: Staff
Plan Specialty: Dental
Benefits Offered: Dental

Type of Coverage
Commercial

Type of Payment Plans Offered
POS, DFFS, Capitated, FFS, Combination FFS & DFFS

Geographic Areas Served
New Jersey and Connecticut

Key Personnel
President & CEO . . . . Dennis G. Wilson

523 **Horizon Blue Cross Blue Shield of New Jersey**

P.O. Box 820
Newark, NJ 07101
Toll-Free: 800-355-2583
www.horizonblue.com
Non-Profit Organization: Yes
Year Founded: 1932
State Enrollment: 3,800,000

Healthplan and Services Defined
PLAN TYPE: HMO/PPO
Other Type: POS
Model Type: Staff, Network
Benefits Offered: Behavioral Health, Dental, Prescription, Psychiatric, Worker's Compensation
Offers Demand Management Patient Information Service: Yes

Type of Coverage
Commercial, Individual, Indemnity, Medicare
Catastrophic Illness Benefit: None

Geographic Areas Served
Statewide

Peer Review Type
Utilization Review: Yes
Second Surgical Opinion: Yes
Case Management: Yes

Accreditation Certification
AAAHC, URAC, NCQA
TJC Accreditation, Medicare Approved, Utilization Review, Pre-Admission Certification, State Licensure, Quality Assurance Program

Key Personnel
President & CEO . . . . Robert A. Marino
Chief Operating Officer . . . . Kevin P. Conlin
Chief Information Officer . . . . Douglas E. Blackwell
Human Resources . . . . Margaret M. Coons
Chief Financial Officer . . . . Dave R. Huber

Specialty Managed Care Partners
Enters into Contracts with Regional Business Coalitions: Yes

524 **Horizon NJ Health**

210 Silvia Street
West Trenton, NJ 08628
Toll-Free: 800-682-9090
www.horizonnjhealth.com
Subsidiary of: Horizon Blue Cross Blue Shield of NJ
Year Founded: 1993
Total Enrollment: 467,000
State Enrollment: 467,000

Healthplan and Services Defined
PLAN TYPE: PPO
Model Type: Network
Benefits Offered: Dental, Disease Management, Prescription, Vision, Wellness

Type of Coverage
Individual, Medicaid

Geographic Areas Served
Statewide

Accreditation Certification
URAC

Key Personnel
President & COO . . . . Karen L Clark
Controller . . . . James D'Alessio
Dir, Marketing & Comm . . . . Len Kudgis
Chief Medical Officer . . . . Philip M Bonaparte, MD
Media Contact . . . . Carol Chernack
     609-718-9290
     carol_chernack@horizonnjhealth.com

525 **Humana Health Insurance of New Jersey**

1 International Boulevard
Suite 904
Mahwah, NJ 07495
Toll-Free: 800-967-2370
Fax: 201-934-1369
www.humana.com
Subsidiary of: Humana
For Profit Organization: Yes

Healthplan and Services Defined
PLAN TYPE: HMO/PPO
Model Type: Network
Plan Specialty: Dental, Vision
Benefits Offered: Dental, Vision, Life, LTD, STD

Type of Coverage
Commercial

Geographic Areas Served
New Jersey, Massachusetts, Connecticut, and Rhode Island

Accreditation Certification
URAC, NCQA, CORE

Key Personnel
President & CEO . . . . Bruce Broussard
Chief Medical Officer . . . . Roy A. Beveridge
Chief Consumer Officer . . . . Jody L. Bilney
Human Resources . . . . Tim Huval
Chief Financial Officer . . . . Brian Kane
Chief Information Officer . . . . Brian LeClaire
General Counsel . . . . Christopher M. Todoroff

526 **Liberty Dental Plan of New Jersey**

P.O. Box 26110
Santa Ana, CA 92799-6110
Toll-Free: 877-558-6489
www.libertydentalplan.com
For Profit Organization: Yes
Year Founded: 2001
Total Enrollment: 3,000,000

Healthplan and Services Defined
PLAN TYPE: Dental
Other Type: Dental HMO
Plan Specialty: Dental
Benefits Offered: Dental

Type of Coverage
Commercial, Individual, Medicare, Medicaid, Unions

Geographic Areas Served
Statewide

Accreditation Certification
NCQA

Key Personnel
Dental Director . . . . Peter Fuentes, DMD

---

527 Molina Medicaid Solutions
3705 Quakerbridge Road
Trenton, NJ 08619
Toll-Free: 800-776-6334
www.molinahealthcare.com
Subsidiary of: Molina Healthcare, Inc.
For Profit Organization: Yes

Healthplan and Services Defined
PLAN TYPE: Medicare

Type of Coverage
Medicaid information management sys

Geographic Areas Served
Statewide

Key Personnel
Chief Executive Officer . . . . Joseph W. White
Chief Operating Officer . . . . Terry Bayer
General Counsel. . . . . Jeff D. Barlow
SVP, Relations/Marketing . . . . Juan Jos, Orellana
Chief Information Officer . . . . Rick Hopfer

---

528 QualCare
30 Knightsbridge Road
Piscataway, NJ 08854
Toll-Free: 800-992-6613
Phone: 732-562-0833
info@qualcareinc.com
www.qualcareinc.com
Subsidiary of: QualCare Alliance Networks, Inc.
For Profit Organization: Yes
Year Founded: 1993
Federally Qualified: Yes
Number of Affiliated Hospitals: 100
Number of Primary Care Physicians: 9,000
Number of Referral/Specialty Physicians: 14,000
Total Enrollment: 750,000
State Enrollment: 750,000

Healthplan and Services Defined
PLAN TYPE: Multiple
Other Type: POS, TPA
Model Type: Network
Plan Specialty: ASO, Behavioral Health, Chiropractic,
    Dental, Disease Management, EPO, Lab, MSO, PBM,
    Vision, Radiology, Worker's Compensation, UR
Benefits Offered: Behavioral Health, Chiropractic,
    Complementary
Medicine, Dental, Disease Management, Home Care,
Inpatient SNF, Long-Term Care, Physical Therapy,

Podiatry, Prescription, Psychiatric, Transplant,
Vision, Wellness, Worker's Compensation, AD&D,
Life, LTD, STD
    Offers Demand Management Patient Information Service: Yes

Type of Coverage
Commercial

Type of Payment Plans Offered
FFS

Geographic Areas Served
New Jersey, Pennsylvania, New York

Peer Review Type
Utilization Review: Yes
Second Surgical Opinion: Yes
Case Management: Yes

Publishes and Distributes Report Card: Yes

Accreditation Certification
AAAHC, TJC, AAPI, NCQA
Medicare Approved, Utilization Review, State Licensure,
    Quality Assurance Program

Key Personnel
CEO. . . . . Annette Catino
Chief Financial Officer . . . . Janet Buggle
Chief Operating Officer . . . . Kevin Joyce
VP, Network/Delivery. . . . . Jennifer Lagasca
Medical Director . . . . Michael McNeil, MD
EVP, CIO . . . . Vivek Dabke
VP, Sales & Insurance . . . . Bridget Gielis

Specialty Managed Care Partners
Multiplan

---

529 Trinity Health of New Jersey
Lourdes Health System
1600 Haddon Avenue
Camden, NJ 08103
Phone: 856-757-3500
www.trinity-health.org
Secondary Address: St Francis Medical Center, 601 Hamilton
    Avenue, Trenton, NJ 08629, 609-599-5000
Subsidiary of: Trinity Health
Non-Profit Organization: Yes
Year Founded: 2013
Total Enrollment: 30,000,000

Healthplan and Services Defined
PLAN TYPE: Other
Benefits Offered: Disease Management, Home Care,
    Long-Term Care, Psychiatric, Hospice programs, PACE
    (Program of All Inclusive Care for the Elderly)

Geographic Areas Served
Southern New Jersey

Key Personnel
Chief Executive Officer . . . . Richard J. Gilfillan
Chief Financial Officer. . . . . Benjamin R. Carter
Human Resources . . . . Edmund F. Hodge
General Counsel . . . . Paul G. Neumann
Chief Clinical Officer . . . . Daniel J. Roth
Chief Operating Officer . . . . Michael A. Slubowski

530   UnitedHealthcare of New Jersey

170 Wood Avenue South
3rd Floor
Iselin, NJ 08830
Toll-Free: 866-223-5802
Phone: 732-623-1000
www.uhc.com/contact-us/new-jersey
Subsidiary of: UnitedHealth Group
For Profit Organization: Yes

Healthplan and Services Defined
  PLAN TYPE: HMO/PPO
  Model Type: Network
  Plan Specialty: Behavioral Health, Dental, Disease
    Management, PBM, Vision
  Benefits Offered: Behavioral Health, Dental, Disease
    Management, Long-Term Care, Prescription, Vision,
    Wellness, Life, LTD, STD

Type of Coverage
  Individual, Medicare, Supplemental Medicare, Medicaid,
    Catastrophic, Family, Military, Veterans, Group,

Geographic Areas Served
  Statewide

Key Personnel
  President . . . . David Wichmann
  Chief Operating Officer . . . . Dan Schumacher
  Chief Strategy Officer . . . . John Cosgriff
  Communications Officer . . . . Kirsten Gorsuch
  Chief Medical Officer. . . . . Sam Ho
  Cheif Legal Officer . . . . Thad Johnson
  Chief Information Officer . . . . Phil McKoy
  Chief Financial Officer. . . . . Jeff Putnam

531   Zelis Healthcare

2 Crossroads Drive
Bedminster, NJ 07921
Phone: 888-311-3505
www.zelis.com
Subsidiary of: Zelis Healthcare
For Profit Organization: Yes
Year Founded: 2016
Owned by an Integrated Delivery Network (IDN): Yes

Healthplan and Services Defined
  PLAN TYPE: PPO
  Plan Specialty: Dental, Worker's Compensation
  Benefits Offered: Dental, Worker's Compensation

Type of Coverage
  Individual

Health Insurance Coverage Status and Type of Coverage by Age

Category	All Persons		Under 18 years		Under 65 years	
	Number	%	Number	%	Number	%
Total population	2,046	-	519	-	1,709	-
Covered by some type of health insurance	1,858 (11)	90.8 (0.5)	491 (5)	94.7 (0.7)	1,524 (11)	89.2 (0.6)
Covered by private health insurance	1,127 (18)	55.1 (0.9)	219 (9)	42.2 (1.6)	941 (17)	55.0 (1.0)
Employer-based	894 (20)	43.7 (1.0)	185 (9)	35.7 (1.7)	784 (19)	45.9 (1.1)
Direct purchase	220 (9)	10.8 (0.4)	25 (3)	4.8 (0.6)	142 (8)	8.3 (0.5)
TRICARE	84 (7)	4.1 (0.4)	17 (3)	3.3 (0.6)	54 (6)	3.2 (0.4)
Covered by public health insurance	985 (17)	48.2 (0.9)	295 (8)	56.8 (1.5)	662 (17)	38.7 (1.0)
Medicaid	665 (16)	32.5 (0.8)	294 (8)	56.6 (1.5)	612 (16)	35.8 (0.9)
Medicare	384 (6)	18.7 (0.3)	3 (1)	0.5 (0.2)	61 (5)	3.6 (0.3)
VA Care	62 (4)	3.0 (0.2)	1 (1)	0.2 (0.1)	28 (3)	1.6 (0.2)
Not covered at any time during the year	188 (10)	9.2 (0.5)	28 (3)	5.3 (0.7)	185 (10)	10.8 (0.6)

Note: Numbers in thousands; Figures cover civilian noninstitutionalized population in 2016; N/A indicates that data was not available; Z represents or rounds to zero; Margin of error appears in parenthesis and is calculated using replicate weights.
Source: U.S. Census Bureau, American Community Survey, Table HIC-4_ACS. Health Insurance Coverage Status and Type of Coverage by State—All People: 2008 to 2016, Table HIC-5_ACS. Health Insurance Coverage Status and Type of Coverage by State—Children Under 18: 2008 to 2016, Table HIC-6_ACS. Health Insurance Coverage Status and Type of Coverage by State—Persons Under 65: 2008 to 2016

New Mexico

532 Blue Cross & Blue Shield of New Mexico

5701 Balloon Fiesta Parkway NE
Albuquerque, NM 87113
Toll-Free: 800-835-8699
Phone: 505-291-3500
www.bcbsnm.com
Mailing Address: P.O. Box 27630, Albuquerque, NM
   87125-7630
Subsidiary of: Health Care Service Corporation
Non-Profit Organization: Yes
Year Founded: 1940
Owned by an Integrated Delivery Network (IDN): Yes
Number of Affiliated Hospitals: 54
Number of Primary Care Physicians: 3,322
Number of Referral/Specialty Physicians: 6,742
Total Enrollment: 367,000
State Enrollment: 367,000

Healthplan and Services Defined
   PLAN TYPE: HMO/PPO
   Other Type: EPO, CDHP
   Model Type: Network
   Plan Specialty: ASO, Behavioral Health
   Benefits Offered: Dental, Disease Management, Vision,
      Wellness, Medical, Case Management
   Offers Demand Management Patient Information Service:
      Yes
   DMPI Services Offered: Fully Insured

Type of Coverage
   Commercial, Individual, Indemnity, Supplemental Medicare

Geographic Areas Served
   Statewide

Network Qualifications
   Pre-Admission Certification: Yes

Peer Review Type
   Utilization Review: Yes
   Second Surgical Opinion: Yes

Publishes and Distributes Report Card: Yes

Accreditation Certification
   NCQA

Key Personnel
   President/CEO. . . . . Kurt Shipley
   Media Contact . . . . Becky Kenny
      505-816-2012
      becky_kenny@bcbsnm.com

Specialty Managed Care Partners
   Pharmacy Manager, Prime Theraputics

533 Coventry Health Care of New Mexico

6720-B Rockledge Drive
Suite 700
Bethesda, MD 20817
Phone: 301-581-0600
www.coventryhealthcare.com
Subsidiary of: Aetna Inc.

For Profit Organization: Yes

Healthplan and Services Defined
   PLAN TYPE: HMO/PPO
   Model Type: Network
   Plan Specialty: Behavioral Health, Dental, Worker's
      Compensation
   Benefits Offered: Behavioral Health, Dental, Prescription,
      Wellness, Worker's Compensation

Type of Coverage
   Commercial, Medicare, Medicaid

Geographic Areas Served
   Statewide

Key Personnel
   Chief Executive Officer. . . . . Mark T. Bertolini
   President. . . . . Karen S. Lynch
   Chief Financial Officer . . . . Shawn M. Guertin
   Operations & Technology . . . . Meg McCarthy
   Chief Medical Officer . . . . Harold L. Paz
   General Counsel . . . . Thomas Sabatino Jr.
   Government Services . . . . Fran S. Soistman

534 Delta Dental of New Mexico

2500 Louisiana Boulevard NE
Suite 600
Albuquerque, NM 87110
Toll-Free: 877-395-9420
Phone: 505-883-4777
Fax: 505-883-7444
www.deltadentalnm.com
Non-Profit Organization: Yes
Year Founded: 1971
Number of Primary Care Physicians: 979
State Enrollment: 390,000

Healthplan and Services Defined
   PLAN TYPE: Dental
   Other Type: Dental PPO
   Model Type: Group
   Plan Specialty: ASO, Dental, Vision
   Benefits Offered: Dental, Vision
   Offers Demand Management Patient Information Service: Yes

Type of Coverage
   Commercial

Geographic Areas Served
   Statewide

Network Qualifications
   Pre-Admission Certification: Yes

Publishes and Distributes Report Card: Yes

Key Personnel
   President & CEO . . . . Edward Lopez Jr.
   Chief Financial Officer . . . . Goran Jurkovic
   Chief Operating Officer . . . . Cynthia Lucero-Ali
   VP of Marketing . . . . JoLou Trujillo-Ottino

Specialty Managed Care Partners
   Enters into Contracts with Regional Business Coalitions: Yes

535 HCSC Insurance Services Company

5701 Balloon Fiesta Pkwy NE
Albuquerque, NM 87113
Toll-Free: 800-835-8699
hcsc.com
Subsidiary of: Blue Cross Blue Shield Association
Non-Profit Organization: Yes
Year Founded: 1936
Number of Primary Care Physicians: 14,400

Healthplan and Services Defined
PLAN TYPE: HMO
Benefits Offered: Behavioral Health, Dental, Disease Management, Psychiatric, Wellness

Geographic Areas Served
Statewide

Key Personnel
President & CEO . . . . Paula Steiner
EVP, Plan Operations. . . . . Colleen Reitan
SVP, Clinical Officer. . . . . Opella Ernest, MD
SVP, Financial Officer. . . . . Eric Feldstein
SVP, Compliance Officer. . . . . Thomas Lubben
SVP, Human Resources. . . . . Nazneen Razi
SVP, Chief Legal Officer. . . . . Blair Todt
Media Contact . . . . Kristen Cunningham
   312-653-1686
   kristen_cunningham@hcsc.net
Media Contact . . . . Greg Thompson
   312-653-7581
   greg_thompson@hcsc.net

536 Humana Health Insurance of New Mexico

4904 Alameda Boulevard NE
Suite A
Albuquerque, NM 87113
Toll-Free: 800-681-0680
Phone: 505-468-0500
Fax: 505-468-0554
www.humana.com
Subsidiary of: Humana
For Profit Organization: Yes

Healthplan and Services Defined
PLAN TYPE: HMO/PPO

Type of Coverage
Commercial, Individual

Geographic Areas Served
Statewide

Accreditation Certification
URAC, NCQA, CORE

Key Personnel
President & CEO. . . . . Bruce Broussard
Chief Medical Officer. . . . . Roy A. Beveridge
Chief Consumer Officer. . . . . Jody L. Bilney
Human Resources. . . . . Tim Huval
Chief Financial Officer . . . . Brian Kane
Chief Information Officer . . . . Brian LeClaire
General Counsel. . . . . Christopher M. Todoroff

537 Molina Healthcare of New Mexico

400 Tijeras Avenue NW
Suite 200
Albuquerque, NM 87102
Toll-Free: 800-377-9594
Phone: 505-342-4660
www.molinahealthcare.com
Subsidiary of: Molina Healthcare, Inc.
For Profit Organization: Yes

Healthplan and Services Defined
PLAN TYPE: Medicare
Model Type: Network
Plan Specialty: Dental, PBM, Vision, Integrated Medicare/Medicaid (Duals)
Benefits Offered: Dental, Prescription, Vision, Wellness, Life

Type of Coverage
Individual, Medicare, Supplemental Medicare, Medicaid

Geographic Areas Served
Statewide

Key Personnel
Chief Executive Officer . . . . Joseph W. White
Chief Operating Officer . . . . Terry Bayer
General Counsel. . . . . Jeff D. Barlow
SVP, Relations/Marketing . . . . Juan Jos, Orellana
Chief Information Officer . . . . Rick Hopfer

538 New Mexico Health Connections

2440 Louisiana Boulevard
Suite 601
Albuquerque, NM 87110
Toll-Free: 855-769-6642
Phone: 505-633-8020
Fax: 866-231-1344
mynmhc.org

Healthplan and Services Defined
PLAN TYPE: HMO
Benefits Offered: Behavioral Health, Disease Management, Wellness

Geographic Areas Served
Statewide

Key Personnel
Chief Executive Officer . . . . Martin Hickey
Chief Operating Officer. . . . . Anne Brennan Sapon
Chief Medical Officer . . . . Mark Epstein, MD
Chief Compliance Officer. . . . . Angela Vigil
Chief Information Officer . . . . Richard Hilliard
Chief Financial Officer . . . . Nathan Johns

539 Presbyterian Health Plan

9521 San Mateo Boulevard NE
Albuquerque, NM 87113
Toll-Free: 800-356-2219
Phone: 505-923-5700
info@phs.org
www.phs.org
Non-Profit Organization: Yes

Year Founded: 1908
Number of Affiliated Hospitals: 28
Number of Primary Care Physicians: 18,843
Number of Referral/Specialty Physicians: 4,850
Total Enrollment: 400,000
State Enrollment: 400,000

Healthplan and Services Defined
  PLAN TYPE: HMO
  Other Type: POS
  Model Type: Contracted Network
  Benefits Offered: Disease Management, Inpatient SNF,
    Prescription

Type of Coverage
  Commercial, Medicare, Medicaid

Type of Payment Plans Offered
  POS, DFFS, Capitated, FFS

Geographic Areas Served
  Statewide

Subscriber Information
  Average Monthly Fee Per Subscriber
    (Employee + Employer Contribution):
      Employee Only (Self): Varies by plan
  Average Subscriber Co-Payment:
    Primary Care Physician: $10.00
    Prescription Drugs: $0
    Hospital ER: $50.00

Accreditation Certification
  NCQA

Key Personnel
  Chair . . . . Katharine Winograd, PhD
  Vice Chair . . . . Brian Burnett
  Board Member. . . . . Sandra Begay
  Baord Member . . . . Larry Clevenger, MD
  Board Member . . . . Frank Figueroa
  VP, Sales & Marketing. . . . . Neal Spero

Employer References
  State of New Mexico, Albuquerque Public Schools, Intel
    Corporation

---

540   Presbyterian Medicare Advantage Plans
The Cooper Center
9521 San Mateo Boulevard NE
Albuquerque, NM 87113
Toll-Free: 800-979-5343
Phone: 505-923-6060
info@phs.org
www.phs.org

Healthplan and Services Defined
  PLAN TYPE: Medicare
  Benefits Offered: Chiropractic, Dental, Disease Management,
    Home Care, Inpatient SNF, Physical Therapy, Podiatry,
    Prescription, Psychiatric, Vision, Wellness, Hearing;
    Rehabilitation; Durable Medical Equipment;
    Transportation

Type of Coverage
  Individual, Medicare

Geographic Areas Served
  Bernalillo, Cibola, Rio Arriba, Sandoval, Santa Fe, Socorro,
    Torrance and Valencia

Key Personnel
  Chair . . . . Katharine Winograd
  Vice Chair . . . . Brian Burnett

---

541   United Concordia of New Mexico
4401 Deer Path Road
Harrisburg, PA 17110
Toll-Free: 800-232-0366
www.unitedconcordia.com
For Profit Organization: Yes
Year Founded: 1971
Total Enrollment: 7,800,000

Healthplan and Services Defined
  PLAN TYPE: Dental
  Plan Specialty: Dental
  Benefits Offered: Dental

Type of Coverage
  Commercial, Individual, Military personnel & families

Geographic Areas Served
  Nationwide

Accreditation Certification
  URAC

Key Personnel
  President & COO . . . . Timohty J. Constantine
  Contact. . . . . Beth Rutherford
    717-260-7659
    beth.rutherford@ucci.com

---

542   UnitedHealthcare of New Mexico
8801 Horizon Blvd NE
Suite 260
Albuquerque, NM 87113
Toll-Free: 866-573-2458
Phone: 505-449-4100
www.uhc.com/contact-us/new-mexico
Subsidiary of: UnitedHealth Group
For Profit Organization: Yes

Healthplan and Services Defined
  PLAN TYPE: HMO/PPO
  Model Type: Network
  Plan Specialty: Behavioral Health, Dental, Disease
    Management, PBM, Vision
  Benefits Offered: Behavioral Health, Dental, Disease
    Management, Long-Term Care, Prescription, Vision,
    Wellness, Life, LTD, STD

Type of Coverage
  Individual, Medicare, Supplemental Medicare, Medicaid,
    Catastrophic, Family, Military, Veterans, Group,

Geographic Areas Served
  Statewide

Key Personnel
  President . . . . David Wichmann

Chief Operating Officer . . . . Dan Schumacher
Chief Strategy Officer . . . . John Cosgriff
Communications Officer . . . . Kirsten Gorsuch
Chief Medical Officer. Sam Ho
Chief Legal Officer . . . . Thad Johnson
Chief Information Officer . . . . Phil McKoy
Chief Financial Officer. . . . . Jeff Putnam

Health Insurance Coverage Status and Type of Coverage by Age

Category	All Persons		Under 18 years		Under 65 years	
	Number	%	Number	%	Number	%
Total population	19,506	-	4,433	-	16,570	-
Covered by some type of health insurance	18,323 *(26)*	93.9 *(0.1)*	4,321 *(9)*	97.5 *(0.2)*	15,412 *(27)*	93.0 *(0.2)*
Covered by private health insurance	12,993 *(50)*	66.6 *(0.3)*	2,716 *(24)*	61.3 *(0.5)*	11,275 *(47)*	68.0 *(0.3)*
Employer-based	10,880 *(48)*	55.8 *(0.2)*	2,294 *(20)*	51.7 *(0.5)*	9,726 *(45)*	58.7 *(0.3)*
Direct purchase	2,530 *(32)*	13.0 *(0.2)*	460 *(15)*	10.4 *(0.3)*	1,790 *(30)*	10.8 *(0.2)*
TRICARE	177 *(7)*	0.9 *(Z)*	36 *(3)*	0.8 *(0.1)*	119 *(7)*	0.7 *(Z)*
Covered by public health insurance	7,654 *(47)*	39.2 *(0.2)*	1,854 *(24)*	41.8 *(0.5)*	4,850 *(47)*	29.3 *(0.3)*
Medicaid	5,128 *(48)*	26.3 *(0.2)*	1,838 *(24)*	41.5 *(0.5)*	4,554 *(47)*	27.5 *(0.3)*
Medicare	3,272 *(13)*	16.8 *(0.1)*	29 *(4)*	0.7 *(0.1)*	471 *(12)*	2.8 *(0.1)*
VA Care	281 *(7)*	1.4 *(Z)*	4 *(1)*	0.1 *(Z)*	113 *(5)*	0.7 *(Z)*
Not covered at any time during the year	1,183 *(26)*	6.1 *(0.1)*	113 *(8)*	2.5 *(0.2)*	1,158 *(27)*	7.0 *(0.2)*

Note: Numbers in thousands; Figures cover civilian noninstitutionalized population in 2016; N/A indicates that data was not available; Z represents or rounds to zero; Margin of error appears in parenthesis and is calculated using replicate weights.
Source: U.S. Census Bureau, American Community Survey, Table HIC-4_ACS. Health Insurance Coverage Status and Type of Coverage by State—All People: 2008 to 2016, Table HIC-5_ACS. Health Insurance Coverage Status and Type of Coverage by State—Children Under 18: 2008 to 2016, Table HIC-6_ACS. Health Insurance Coverage Status and Type of Coverage by State—Persons Under 65: 2008 to 2016

New York

543   Aetna Health of New York

151 Farmington Avenue
Hartford, CT 06156
Toll-Free: 800-872-3862
Phone: 860-273-0123
www.aetna.com
Subsidiary of: Aetna Inc.
For Profit Organization: Yes
Year Founded: 1986
Number of Affiliated Hospitals: 61
Number of Primary Care Physicians: 2,691
Total Enrollment: 154,162
State Enrollment: 154,162

Healthplan and Services Defined
  PLAN TYPE: HMO/PPO
  Model Type: Network
  Plan Specialty: Behavioral Health, Dental, EPO, Lab, PBM,
    Vision, Radiology
  Benefits Offered: Behavioral Health, Dental, Disease
    Management, Long-Term Care, Physical Therapy,
    Podiatry, Prescription, Psychiatric, Vision, Wellness, Life,
    LTD, STD

Type of Coverage
  Commercial, Supplemental Medicare, Medicaid, Student
  health
  Catastrophic Illness Benefit: Varies per case

Type of Payment Plans Offered
  POS, Capitated

Geographic Areas Served
  Statewide

Network Qualifications
  Pre-Admission Certification: Yes

Peer Review Type
  Utilization Review: Yes
  Second Surgical Opinion: No
  Case Management: Yes

Publishes and Distributes Report Card: Yes

Accreditation Certification
  NCQA
  TJC Accreditation, Medicare Approved, Utilization Review,
    Pre-Admission Certification, State Licensure, Quality
    Assurance Program

Key Personnel
  CEO . . . . Mark Bertolini

Specialty Managed Care Partners
  Enters into Contracts with Regional Business Coalitions: Yes

544   Affinity Health Plan

1250 Waters Place
Bronx, NY 10461
Toll-Free: 866-247-5678
Fax: 718-794-7804
mainoffice@affinityplan.org

www.affinityplan.org
Non-Profit Organization: Yes
Year Founded: 1986
Number of Affiliated Hospitals: 60
Number of Primary Care Physicians: 1,400
Number of Referral/Specialty Physicians: 5,000
Total Enrollment: 134,837
State Enrollment: 134,837

Healthplan and Services Defined
  PLAN TYPE: HMO
  Model Type: Staff

Type of Coverage
  Medicaid

Geographic Areas Served
  NY Metropolitan Area

Accreditation Certification
  TJC Accreditation, Medicare Approved, Utilization Review,
    State Licensure

Key Personnel
  President/CEO . . . . Michael G. Murphy
  SVP, Operations . . . . Anita Wilenkin
  Chief Marketing Officer . . . . Denise J. Pesich
  Director, Medicaid . . . . Adrian Robert
  Chief Financial Officer . . . . Steve Giasi

545   AlphaCare

335 Adams Street
Suite 2600
Brooklyn, NY 11201
Toll-Free: 855-363-6110
www.alphacare.com
Subsidiary of: Magellan Health
For Profit Organization: Yes

Healthplan and Services Defined
  PLAN TYPE: Multiple
  Plan Specialty: Chronic illness and long-term care.
  Benefits Offered: Long-Term Care

Type of Coverage
  Medicare, Medicaid

Geographic Areas Served
  Bronx, Brooklyn, Manhattan, Queens and Westchester
  counties

Key Personnel
  CEO . . . . Daniel M. Parietti

546   BlueCross BlueShield of Western New York

257 W Genesee Street
Buffalo, NY 14202-2657
Toll-Free: 800-544-2583
Phone: 716-884-2800
customerservice@bcbswny.com
www.bcbswny.com
Mailing Address: P.O. Box 80, Buffalo, NY 14240-0080
Non-Profit Organization: Yes
Year Founded: 1936

Total Enrollment: 555,405
State Enrollment: 197,194

Healthplan and Services Defined
 PLAN TYPE: HMO/PPO
 Other Type: POS, EPO
 Plan Specialty: Dental, Lab, Vision
 Benefits Offered: Dental, Disease Management, Prescription, Vision, Wellness

Type of Coverage
 Commercial, Medicare, Supplemental Medicare, Medicaid

Geographic Areas Served
 Statewide

Key Personnel
 President & CEO . . . . David W. Anderson
 Chief Financial Officer . . . . Stephen T. Swift
 Senior VP, Operations. . . . . Christopher M. Leardini
 SVP, Chief Sales Officer. . . . . David Busch
 SVP, Network Officer . . . . Ronald Mornelli
 SVP, Human Resources . . . . Douglas Parks
 SVP, Medical Officer . . . . Thomas E. Schenk, MD

Specialty Managed Care Partners
 Wellpoint Pharmacy Management

547 BlueShield of Northeastern New York
40 Century Hill Drive
Latham, NY 12110
Toll-Free: 800-888-1238
Phone: 518-220-4600
customerservice@bsneny.com
www.bsneny.com
Mailing Address: P.O. Box 15013, Albany, NY 12212
Non-Profit Organization: Yes
Year Founded: 1946
Total Enrollment: 193,498
State Enrollment: 72,563

Healthplan and Services Defined
 PLAN TYPE: HMO/PPO
 Other Type: POS, EPO
 Plan Specialty: Dental
 Benefits Offered: Dental, Disease Management, Prescription, Wellness

Type of Coverage
 Commercial, Medicare, Supplemental Medicare, Medicaid

Type of Payment Plans Offered
 POS, FFS

Geographic Areas Served
 Albany, Clinton, Columbia, Essex, Fulton, Green, Montgomery, Schoharie, Schenectedy, Warren and Washington counties

Accreditation Certification
 NCQA

Key Personnel
 President & CEO . . . . David W. Anderson
 Chief Financial Officer . . . . Stephen T. Swift
 VP, Medical Director . . . . Kirk Panneton
 SVP, Chief Sales Officer. . . . . David Busch

 SVP, Operations . . . . Christopher Leardini
 SVP, Network Officer . . . . Ronald Mornelli
 Chief Medical Officer . . . . Thomas E. Schenk, MD

Specialty Managed Care Partners
 Wellpoint Pharmacy Management

548 CareCentrix: New York
3 Huntington Quadrangle
Suite 200S
Melville, NY 11747
Toll-Free: 800-808-1902
carecentrix.com
Year Founded: 1996
Number of Primary Care Physicians: 8,000

Healthplan and Services Defined
 PLAN TYPE: HMO
 Benefits Offered: Home Care, Physical Therapy, Durable Medical Equipment; Occupational & Respiratory Theraoy; Orthotics; Prosthetics

Key Personnel
 Chief Executive Officer . . . . John Driscoll
 Chief Data Officer. . . . . Tej Anand
 Chief Medical Officer. . . . . Michael Cantor
 Chief Operating Officer . . . . Mary Daschner
 Chief Customer Officer . . . . Tom Gaffney

549 CDPHP Medicare Plan
500 Patroon Creek Boulevard
Albany, NY 12206-1057
Toll-Free: 888-248-6522
Phone: 518-641-3950
www.cdphp.com
Year Founded: 1984
Total Enrollment: 400,000

Healthplan and Services Defined
 PLAN TYPE: Medicare
 Benefits Offered: Chiropractic, Dental, Disease Management, Home Care, Inpatient SNF, Physical Therapy, Podiatry, Prescription, Psychiatric, Vision, Wellness

Type of Coverage
 Individual, Medicare

Geographic Areas Served
 Statewide

Subscriber Information
 Average Monthly Fee Per Subscriber
  (Employee + Employer Contribution):
   Employee Only (Self): Varies
   Medicare: Varies
 Average Annual Deductible Per Subscriber:
   Employee Only (Self): Varies
   Medicare: Varies
 Average Subscriber Co-Payment:
   Primary Care Physician: Varies
   Non-Network Physician: Varies
   Prescription Drugs: Varies
   Hospital ER: Varies

Home Health Care: Varies
Home Health Care Max. Days/Visits Covered: Varies
Nursing Home: Varies
Nursing Home Max. Days/Visits Covered: Varies

Key Personnel

President & CEO . . . . John D. Bennett
Chief Operating Officer . . . . Barbara A. Downs
SVP, General Counsel . . . . Frederick B. Galt
Chief Strategy Officer . . . . Robert R. Hinckley
Chief Marketing Officer. . . . . Brian J. Morrissey
Chief Information Officer . . . . Neil Brandmaier
Chief Financial Officer . . . . Bethany R. Smith

550　CDPHP: Capital District Physicians' Health Plan

500 Patroon Creek Boulevard
Albany, NY 12206-1057
Toll-Free: 800-777-2273
Phone: 518-729-4732
www.cdphp.com
Non-Profit Organization: Yes
Year Founded: 1984
Number of Primary Care Physicians: 5,000
Total Enrollment: 350,000
State Enrollment: 350,000

Healthplan and Services Defined
PLAN TYPE: HMO/PPO
Other Type: POS, ASO
Model Type: IPA
Benefits Offered: Dental, Disease Management, Prescription, Wellness

Type of Coverage
Commercial, Individual, Medicare, Medicaid

Geographic Areas Served
Albany, Broome, Chenango, Columbia, Delaware, Dutchess, Essex, Fulton, Greene, Hamilton, Herkimer, Madison, Montgomery, Oneida, Orange, Ostego, Rensselaer, Saratoga, Schenectady, Schoharie, Tioga, Ulster, Warren, and Washington counties

Subscriber Information
Average Monthly Fee Per Subscriber
(Employee + Employer Contribution):
Employee Only (Self): $64.41
Employee & 2 Family Members: $175.47
Average Subscriber Co-Payment:
Primary Care Physician: $10
Prescription Drugs: $5-20

Accreditation Certification
NCQA

Key Personnel
President & CEO . . . . John D Bennett, MD
Chief Operating Officer . . . . Barbara A. Downs
SVP, General Counsel . . . . Frederick B. Galt
SVP, Strategy Officer . . . . Robert R. Hinckley
SVP, Financial Officer. . . . . Bethany R. Smith
SVP, Marketing . . . . Brian J. Morrissey

551　Coventry Health Care of New York

6720-B Rockledge Drive
Suite 700
Bethesda, MD 20817
Phone: 301-581-0600
www.coventryhealthcare.com
Subsidiary of: Aetna Inc.
For Profit Organization: Yes

Healthplan and Services Defined
PLAN TYPE: HMO/PPO
Model Type: Network
Plan Specialty: Behavioral Health, Dental, Worker's Compensation
Benefits Offered: Behavioral Health, Dental, Prescription, Wellness, Worker's Compensation

Type of Coverage
Commercial, Medicare, Medicaid

Geographic Areas Served
Statewide

Key Personnel
Chief Executive Officer . . . . Mark T. Bertolini
President . . . . Karen S. Lynch
Chief Financial Officer . . . . Shawn M. Guertin
Operations & Technology . . . . Meg McCarthy
Chief Medical Officer . . . . Harold L. Paz
General Counsel . . . . Thomas Sabatino Jr.
Government Services . . . . Fran S. Soistman

552　Davis Vision

Capital Region Health Park, Suite 301
711 Troy-Schenectady Road
Latham, NY 12110
Toll-Free: 800-999-5431
www.davisvision.com
Secondary Address: Davis Vision Corporate Headquarters, 175 E Houston Street, San Antonio, TX 78205
Subsidiary of: HVHC Inc.
For Profit Organization: Yes
Year Founded: 1964
Number of Primary Care Physicians: 30,000
Total Enrollment: 55,000,000

Healthplan and Services Defined
PLAN TYPE: Vision
Model Type: Network
Plan Specialty: Vision
Benefits Offered: Vision
Offers Demand Management Patient Information Service: Yes

Type of Payment Plans Offered
DFFS, Capitated, FFS

Geographic Areas Served
National & Puerto Rico, Guam, Saipan, Dominican Republic

Subscriber Information
Average Monthly Fee Per Subscriber
(Employee + Employer Contribution):
Employee Only (Self): Varies by plan
Medicare: Varies

Network Qualifications
Pre-Admission Certification: No

Peer Review Type
Utilization Review: Yes
Second Surgical Opinion: Yes
Case Management: Yes

Publishes and Distributes Report Card: Yes

Accreditation Certification
NCQA, COLTS Certification
TJC Accreditation

Key Personnel
President . . . . Danny Bentley
Chief Financial Officer . . . . Scott Hamey
VP, Operations . . . . Sue Ann Brown
Chief Information Officer . . . . Walt Meffert
Chief Medical Officer . . . . Jeff Smith

Average Claim Compensation
Physician's Fees Charged: 75%

Specialty Managed Care Partners
Enters into Contracts with Regional Business Coalitions: Yes

553 Delta Dental of New York

One Delta Drive
Mechanicsburg, PA 17055-6999
Toll-Free: 800-932-0783
www.deltadentalins.com
Non-Profit Organization: Yes

Healthplan and Services Defined
PLAN TYPE: Dental
Other Type: Dental PPO
Plan Specialty: Dental
Benefits Offered: Dental

Type of Coverage
Commercial, Individual

Geographic Areas Served
Statewide

Key Personnel
President & CEO . . . . Tony Barth
Chief Financial Officer . . . . Michael Castro
Chief Legal Officer . . . . Michael Hankinson
EVP, Sales & Marketing . . . . Belinda Martinez
Chief Operating Officer . . . . Nilesh Patel

554 Dentcare Delivery Systems

333 Earle Ovington Boulevard
Uniondale, NY 11553-3608
Toll-Free: 800-468-0608
Phone: 516-542-2200
Fax: 516-794-3186
www.dentcaredeliverysystems.org
Subsidiary of: Healthplex
Non-Profit Organization: Yes
Year Founded: 1978

Healthplan and Services Defined
PLAN TYPE: Dental

Model Type: IPA
Plan Specialty: Dental
Benefits Offered: Dental

Type of Coverage
Commercial, Individual
Catastrophic Illness Benefit: None

Type of Payment Plans Offered
FFS

Geographic Areas Served
Statewide

Accreditation Certification
NCQA
Utilization Review, Quality Assurance Program

Key Personnel
Treasurer . . . . Deborah Wissing

555 Elderplan

6323 Seventh Avenue
Brooklyn, NY 11220
Toll-Free: 800-353-3765
Phone: 718-921-7979
Fax: 718-630-2624
www.elderplan.org
Subsidiary of: MJHS
Non-Profit Organization: Yes
Year Founded: 1985
Number of Affiliated Hospitals: 35
Number of Primary Care Physicians: 1,200
Number of Referral/Specialty Physicians: 3,800
Total Enrollment: 16,000
State Enrollment: 15,000

Healthplan and Services Defined
PLAN TYPE: Medicare
Other Type: Medicare Advantage
Model Type: Network
Plan Specialty: ASO, Behavioral Health, Chiropractic, Dental,
Disease Management, EPO, Lab, Vision, Radiology
Benefits Offered: Behavioral Health, Chiropractic,
Complementary
Medicine, Dental, Disease Management, Home Care,
Inpatient SNF, Long-Term Care, Physical Therapy,
Podiatry, Prescription, Psychiatric, Transplant,
Vision, Hearing; Durable Medical Equipment; Speech
Therapy; Transportation

Type of Coverage
Medicare

Type of Payment Plans Offered
FFS

Geographic Areas Served
Brooklyn, Bronx, Manhattan, Queens and Staten Island

Subscriber Information
Average Monthly Fee Per Subscriber
(Employee + Employer Contribution):
Medicare: No premium
Average Annual Deductible Per Subscriber:
Medicare: $0.00

Average Subscriber Co-Payment:
    Primary Care Physician: $0.00 co-pay
    Prescription Drugs: $5.00/9.00
    Hospital ER: $50.00
    Home Health Care: $0.00
    Home Health Care Max. Days/Visits Covered: 365 days
    Nursing Home Max. Days/Visits Covered: 200 days

Network Qualifications
Pre-Admission Certification: Yes

Peer Review Type
Utilization Review: Yes
Second Surgical Opinion: Yes
Case Management: Yes

Publishes and Distributes Report Card: No

Accreditation Certification
TJC Accreditation, Medicare Approved, Utilization Review,
    State Licensure, Quality Assurance Program

Specialty Managed Care Partners
HomeFirst, Maxore
Enters into Contracts with Regional Business Coalitions: Yes

556 EmblemHealth

55 Water Street
New York, NY 10041-8190
Toll-Free: 877-411-3625
www.emblemhealth.com
Non-Profit Organization: Yes
Year Founded: 1985

Healthplan and Services Defined
    PLAN TYPE: Other
Model Type: IPA
Plan Specialty: ASO, Chiropractic, Dental, Disease
    Management, EPO, Vision, Radiology
Benefits Offered: Behavioral Health, Chiropractic,
    Complementary Medicine, Dental, Disease Management,
    Home Care, Inpatient SNF, Physical Therapy, Podiatry,
    Prescription, Psychiatric, Transplant, Vision, Wellness

Type of Payment Plans Offered
Capitated

Geographic Areas Served
City employees and retirees under 65: Queens, Nassau,
Suffolk

Accreditation Certification
URAC, NCQA
TJC Accreditation, Medicare Approved, Utilization Review,
    Pre-Admission Certification, State Licensure, Quality
    Assurance Program

Key Personnel
President & CEO. Karen M. Ignagni
Administrative Officer. . . . . Michael Palmateer
Chief Legal Officer. . . . . Jeffrey D. Chansler
Human Resources. . . . . Mariann E. Drohan
Chief Marketing Officer . . . . Beth A. Leonard
Chief Compliance Officer . . . . Debra M. Lightner
Chief Medical Officer. . . . . Navarra Rodriguez, MD

557 EmblemHealth Enhanced Care Plus (HARP)

55 Water Street
New York, NY 10041-8190
Toll-Free: 855-283-2146
www.emblemhealth.com
Subsidiary of: EmblemHealth
Non-Profit Organization: Yes

Healthplan and Services Defined
    PLAN TYPE: Other
Benefits Offered: Behavioral Health, Dental, Home Care,
    Inpatient SNF, Prescription, Psychiatric, Vision, Wellness,
    Maternity care; Therapy for TB; Hospice; Labs & X-Ray;
    Substance Abuse services; Durable Medical Equipment;
    HIV testing

Geographic Areas Served
Bronx, Queens, Brooklyn, Manhattan, Staten Island, Nassau,
Suffolk and Westchester

Key Personnel
President & CEO. Karen M. Ignagni
Administrative Officer. . . . . Michael Palmateer
Chief Legal Officer. . . . . Jeffrey D. Chansler
Human Resources. . . . . Mariann E. Drohan
Chief Marketing Officer . . . . Beth A. Leonard
Chief Compliance Officer . . . . Debra M. Lightner
Chief Medical Officer. . . . . Navarra Rodriguez, MD

558 Empire BlueCross BlueShield

15 MetroTech Center
Brooklyn, NY 11201
Toll-Free: 888-519-8849
www.empireblue.com
Subsidiary of: Anthem, Inc.

Healthplan and Services Defined
    PLAN TYPE: HMO/PPO
Model Type: Network
Plan Specialty: Behavioral Health, Dental, Disease
    Management, Lab, PBM, Vision, Radiology
Benefits Offered: Behavioral Health, Dental, Disease
    Management, Inpatient SNF, Physical Therapy,
    Prescription, Psychiatric, Transplant, Vision, Wellness, Life

Type of Coverage
Commercial, Individual, Medicare, Supplemental Medicare,
Catastrophic

Geographic Areas Served
Serving the 28 eastern and southeastern counties of New York
State

Accreditation Certification
URAC

Key Personnel
President & CEO . . . . Scott P. Serota
Chief Financial Officer . . . . Robert Kolodgy
Human Resources . . . . Maureen A. Cahill
Chief Medical Officer. . . . . Trent Haywood
General Counsel. . . . . Scott Nehs

559 Excellus BlueCross BlueShield

165 Court Street
Rochester, NY 14647
Toll-Free: 877-883-9577
www.excellusbcbs.com
Non-Profit Organization: Yes
Year Founded: 1985
Total Enrollment: 1,500,000

Healthplan and Services Defined
PLAN TYPE: HMO
Model Type: IPA
Benefits Offered: Disease Management, Prescription,
Wellness

Type of Payment Plans Offered
POS, Combination FFS & DFFS

Geographic Areas Served
Central New York, the Rochester area and Utica-Watertown

Publishes and Distributes Report Card: Yes

Accreditation Certification
NCQA
TJC Accreditation, Medicare Approved, Utilization Review,
State Licensure, Quality Assurance Program

Key Personnel
President . . . . Arthur Vercillo

560 Fidelis Care

95-25 Queens Boulevard
Rego Park, NY 11374
Toll-Free: 888-343-3547
Fax: 718-896-6832
www.fideliscare.org
Secondary Address: 480 CrossPoint Parkway, Getzville, NY
14068, 716-564-3630
For Profit Organization: Yes
Year Founded: 1993
Number of Primary Care Physicians: 42,000
Total Enrollment: 625,000
State Enrollment: 625,000

Healthplan and Services Defined
PLAN TYPE: Multiple
Model Type: Network
Benefits Offered: Behavioral Health, Chiropractic, Dental,
Disease Management, Home Care, Inpatient SNF, Physical
Therapy, Podiatry, Prescription, Psychiatric, Vision,
Wellness

Type of Coverage
Individual, Medicare, Medicaid

Geographic Areas Served
53 counties in New York State

Subscriber Information
Average Monthly Fee Per Subscriber
(Employee + Employer Contribution):
Employee Only (Self): Varies
Medicare: Varies
Average Annual Deductible Per Subscriber:
Employee Only (Self): Varies

Medicare: Varies
Average Subscriber Co-Payment:
Primary Care Physician: Varies
Non-Network Physician: Varies
Prescription Drugs: Varies
Hospital ER: Varies
Home Health Care: Varies
Home Health Care Max. Days/Visits Covered: Varies
Nursing Home: Varies
Nursing Home Max. Days/Visits Covered: Varies

Key Personnel
CEO . . . . Patrick Frawley
President/COO . . . . David Thomas
Director, IT . . . . Gary Crane
Chief Medical Officer . . . . Sanjiv Shah, MD
VP, Communications . . . . Darla Skiermont

561 GHI Medicare Plan

55 Water Street Lobby
New York, NY 10041-8190
Toll-Free: 800-477-9169
Phone: 212-501-4444
www.emblemhealth.com
Mailing Address: P.O. Box 3000, New York, NY 10116-3000
Subsidiary of: EmblemHealth
Year Founded: 1931
Total Enrollment: 53,000

Healthplan and Services Defined
PLAN TYPE: Medicare
Benefits Offered: Chiropractic, Dental, Disease Management,
Home Care, Inpatient SNF, Physical Therapy, Podiatry,
Prescription, Psychiatric, Vision, Wellness

Type of Coverage
Individual, Medicare

Geographic Areas Served
Statwide

Subscriber Information
Average Monthly Fee Per Subscriber
(Employee + Employer Contribution):
Employee Only (Self): Varies
Medicare: Varies
Average Annual Deductible Per Subscriber:
Employee Only (Self): Varies
Medicare: Varies
Average Subscriber Co-Payment:
Primary Care Physician: Varies
Non-Network Physician: Varies
Prescription Drugs: Varies
Hospital ER: Varies
Home Health Care: Varies
Home Health Care Max. Days/Visits Covered: Varies
Nursing Home: Varies
Nursing Home Max. Days/Visits Covered: Varies

Key Personnel
President/CEO . . . . Karen M. Ignagni
EVP/Chief Admin Officer . . . . Michael . Palmateer
Chief Legal Officer . . . . Jeffrey D. Chansler

Chief, Human Resources . . . . Mariann E. Drohan
Chief Marketing Officer . . . . Beth A. Leonard
Chief Compliance Officer . . . . Debra M. Lightner

562 Group Health Insurance

55 Water Street Lobby
New York, NY 10041-8190
Toll-Free: 800-624-2414
Phone: 212-501-4444
www.emblemhealth.com
Mailing Address: P.O. Box 3000, New York, NY 10116-3000
Subsidiary of: EmblemHealth
Non-Profit Organization: Yes
Year Founded: 1937
Number of Affiliated Hospitals: 230
Number of Primary Care Physicians: 15,529
Number of Referral/Specialty Physicians: 25,173
Total Enrollment: 3,100,000
State Enrollment: 3,100,000

Healthplan and Services Defined
PLAN TYPE: HMO/PPO
Model Type: Network
Plan Specialty: ASO, Behavioral Health, Dental, EPO
Benefits Offered: Behavioral Health, Chiropractic,
Complementary Medicine, Dental, Disease Management,
Home Care, Inpatient SNF, Physical Therapy, Podiatry,
Prescription, Psychiatric, Transplant, Vision, Wellness

Type of Coverage
Commercial, Individual, Indemnity, Medicare, Supplemental
Medicare, Medicaid

Type of Payment Plans Offered
DFFS

Geographic Areas Served
GHI operates statewide in New York. GHI HMO serves 26
eastern New York counties, including five New York City
boroughs

Subscriber Information
Average Monthly Fee Per Subscriber
(Employee + Employer Contribution):
Employee Only (Self): $69.44
Average Annual Deductible Per Subscriber:
Employee & 2 Family Members: $214.30
Average Subscriber Co-Payment:
Primary Care Physician: $10.00
Prescription Drugs: $10.00/20.00/30.00

Peer Review Type
Utilization Review: Yes
Second Surgical Opinion: Yes
Case Management: Yes

Accreditation Certification
NCQA

Key Personnel
Chairman/CEO . . . . Karen M. Ignagni
EVP, Chief Admin Officer. . . . . Michael Palmateer
Chief Legal Officer. . . . . Jeffrey D. Chansler
Chief, Human Resources . . . . Mariann E. Drohan
Chief Marketing Officer . . . . Beth A. Leonard

Chief Compliance Officer . . . . Debra M. Lightner

Specialty Managed Care Partners
Value Options, Express Scrips, Davis Vision, New York
Medical Imaging, Multi-Plan, CCN

563 Guardian Life Insurance Company of America

7 Hanover Square
H-6-D
New York, NY 10004
Toll-Free: 888-482-7342
Phone: 212-598-8000
www.guardianlife.com
Subsidiary of: Guardian
For Profit Organization: Yes
Year Founded: 1860
Owned by an Integrated Delivery Network (IDN): Yes
Number of Affiliated Hospitals: 2,966
Number of Primary Care Physicians: 121,815
Number of Referral/Specialty Physicians: 193,137
Total Enrollment: 205,677

Healthplan and Services Defined
PLAN TYPE: HMO/PPO
Model Type: Network
Plan Specialty: Chiropractic, Dental, Disease Management,
Lab, PBM, Vision, Radiology, UR
Benefits Offered: Behavioral Health, Chiropractic,
Complementary Medicine, Dental, Disease Management,
Home Care, Physical Therapy, Podiatry, Prescription,
Psychiatric, Vision, Wellness, AD&D, Life, LTD, STD

Type of Coverage
Commercial, Individual, Indemnity

Type of Payment Plans Offered
Combination FFS & DFFS

Geographic Areas Served
Nationwide

Subscriber Information
Average Monthly Fee Per Subscriber
(Employee + Employer Contribution):
Employee Only (Self): Varies by plan

Peer Review Type
Utilization Review: Yes
Second Surgical Opinion: Yes
Case Management: Yes

Publishes and Distributes Report Card: Yes

Accreditation Certification
URAC, NCQA

Key Personnel
EVP, Chief Financial Offi . . . . Michael Ferik
EVP, General Counsel . . . . Tracy L. Rich
President/CEO . . . . Deanna M. Mulligan
Chief Investment Officer . . . . Thomas G Sorell
EVP, Individual Markets . . . . Chris Dyrhaug
SVP, Chief Human Resource. . . . . Jay Rosenblum
EVP, CIO . . . . Dean Del Vecchio

Specialty Managed Care Partners
Health Net
Enters into Contracts with Regional Business Coalitions: Yes

564   Healthfirst

100 Church Street
New York, NY 10007
Toll-Free: 888-260-1010
healthfirst.org
Non-Profit Organization: Yes
Number of Affiliated Hospitals: 6

Healthplan and Services Defined
PLAN TYPE: Multiple
Benefits Offered: Dental, Inpatient SNF, Physical Therapy,
Vision, Wellness

Type of Coverage
Medicare, Medicaid, Child Health Plus; Managed Long Ter

Key Personnel
President & CEO . . . . Pat Wang
Chief Operating Officer . . . . Steve Black
Cheif Financial Officer . . . . John J. Bermel
Chief Clinical Officer . . . . Jay Schechtman, MD
Chief Legal Officer . . . . Linda Tiano
Human Resources. . . . . Sean Kane
Chief Information Officer . . . . G.T. Sweeney

565   Healthplex

333 Earle Ovington Boulevard
Suite 300
Uniondale, NY 11553
Toll-Free: 800-468-0608
info@healthplex.com
www.healthplex.com
For Profit Organization: Yes
Year Founded: 1977
Number of Primary Care Physicians: 2,855
Number of Referral/Specialty Physicians: 448
Total Enrollment: 3,500,000

Healthplan and Services Defined
PLAN TYPE: Dental
Other Type: Dental HMO/PPO
Model Type: IPA
Plan Specialty: Dental
Benefits Offered: Dental

Type of Coverage
Commercial, Individual, Indemnity

Type of Payment Plans Offered
POS, DFFS, Capitated, FFS, Combination FFS & DFFS

Geographic Areas Served
New Jersey & New York

Subscriber Information
Average Monthly Fee Per Subscriber
(Employee + Employer Contribution):
Employee Only (Self): $159.00
Employee & 1 Family Member: $264.00
Employee & 2 Family Members: $350.00

Average Annual Deductible Per Subscriber:
Employee Only (Self): $0
Employee & 1 Family Member: $0
Employee & 2 Family Members: $0

Network Qualifications
Pre-Admission Certification: No

Peer Review Type
Utilization Review: Yes
Second Surgical Opinion: Yes
Case Management: Yes

Accreditation Certification
NCQA
Utilization Review, Quality Assurance Program

Key Personnel
President/Co-CEO . . . . Sharon Zelkind
Controller . . . . Mary Jean Kelly
Human Resources . . . . Eileen Scaturro

Specialty Managed Care Partners
Enters into Contracts with Regional Business Coalitions: Yes

566   Humana Health Insurance of New York

125 Wolf Road
Suite 501
Albany, NY 12205
Toll-Free: 800-967-2370
Fax: 518-435-0412
www.humana.com
Secondary Address: 290 Elwood Davis Road, Suite 225,
Liverpool, NY 13088
Subsidiary of: Humana
For Profit Organization: Yes

Healthplan and Services Defined
PLAN TYPE: HMO/PPO
Model Type: Network
Plan Specialty: Dental, Vision
Benefits Offered: Dental, Vision, Life, LTD, STD

Type of Coverage
Commercial

Accreditation Certification
URAC, NCQA, CORE

Key Personnel
President & CEO. . . . . Bruce Broussard
Chief Medical Officer. . . . . Roy A. Beveridge
Chief Consumer Officer. . . . . Jody L. Bilney
Human Resources. . . . . Tim Huval
Chief Financial Officer . . . . Brian Kane
Chief Information Officer . . . . Brian LeClaire
General Counsel . . . . Christopher M. Todoroff

567   Independent Health

511 Farber Lakes Drive
Buffalo, NY 14221
Toll-Free: 800-501-3439
Phone: 716-631-3001
www.independenthealth.com
Non-Profit Organization: Yes

Year Founded: 1980
Number of Affiliated Hospitals: 35
Number of Primary Care Physicians: 1,125
Number of Referral/Specialty Physicians: 1,626
Total Enrollment: 365,000
State Enrollment: 365,000

Healthplan and Services Defined
PLAN TYPE: HMO/PPO
Model Type: IPA
Plan Specialty: EPO
Benefits Offered: Behavioral Health, Chiropractic, Dental, Disease Management, Home Care, Inpatient SNF, Physical Therapy, Podiatry, Prescription, Psychiatric, Transplant, Vision, Wellness

Type of Coverage
Commercial, Individual, Indemnity, Medicare, Medicaid, Choice
Catastrophic Illness Benefit: Varies per case

Type of Payment Plans Offered
POS, Combination FFS & DFFS

Geographic Areas Served
Allegany, Cattaraugus, Chautauqua, Erie, Genesee, Niagara, Orleans & Wyoming counties of western New York

Subscriber Information
Average Monthly Fee Per Subscriber
(Employee + Employer Contribution):
Employee Only (Self): Varies by plan

Network Qualifications
Pre-Admission Certification: Yes

Peer Review Type
Utilization Review: Yes
Second Surgical Opinion: Yes
Case Management: Yes

Publishes and Distributes Report Card: No

Accreditation Certification
TJC, NCQA
Utilization Review, Pre-Admission Certification, State Licensure, Quality Assurance Program

Key Personnel
President and CEO . . . . Michael W Cropp, MD
EVP/COO . . . . John Rodgers
EVP/CFO . . . . Mark Johnson
EVP, General Counsel . . . . John Mineo
Chief Medical Officer . . . . Thomas J. Foels, MD
EVP, Human Resources. . . . . Patricia Clabeaux

Specialty Managed Care Partners
Enters into Contracts with Regional Business Coalitions: No

---

568 Independent Health Medicare Plan
511 Farber Lakes Drive
Buffalo, NY 14221
Toll-Free: 800-501-3439
Phone: 716-631-3001
www.independenthealth.com
Non-Profit Organization: Yes
Year Founded: 1980

Healthplan and Services Defined
PLAN TYPE: Medicare
Benefits Offered: Chiropractic, Dental, Disease Management, Home Care, Inpatient SNF, Physical Therapy, Podiatry, Prescription, Psychiatric, Vision, Wellness

Type of Coverage
Individual, Medicare

Geographic Areas Served
Statewide

Subscriber Information
Average Monthly Fee Per Subscriber
(Employee + Employer Contribution):
Employee Only (Self): Varies
Medicare: Varies
Average Annual Deductible Per Subscriber:
Employee Only (Self): Varies
Medicare: Varies
Average Subscriber Co-Payment:
Primary Care Physician: Varies
Non-Network Physician: Varies
Prescription Drugs: Varies
Hospital ER: Varies
Home Health Care: Varies
Home Health Care Max. Days/Visits Covered: Varies
Nursing Home: Varies
Nursing Home Max. Days/Visits Covered: Varies

Key Personnel
President and CEO . . . . Michael W Cropp, MD
EVP/COO . . . . John Rodgers
EVP/CFO . . . . Mark Johnson
EVP, General Counsel . . . . John Mineo
Chief Medical Officer . . . . Thomas J. Foels, MD
EVP, Human Resources. . . . . Patricia Clabeaux

---

569 Island Group Administration, Inc.
3 Toilsome Lane
East Hampton, NY 11937
Toll-Free: 800-926-2306
Phone: 631-324-2306
Fax: 631-324-7021
www.islandgroupadmin.com
For Profit Organization: Yes
Year Founded: 1990
Federally Qualified: No
Number of Affiliated Hospitals: 9,055
Number of Primary Care Physicians: 21,010
Total Enrollment: 52,000

Healthplan and Services Defined
PLAN TYPE: PPO
Model Type: TPA
Plan Specialty: Dental, Vision, Radiology, Worker's Compensation, UR, Medical
Benefits Offered: Chiropractic, Dental, Disease Management, Home Care, Podiatry, Prescription, Psychiatric, Transplant, Vision, Wellness, Worker's Compensation, Medical, Hospital

Type of Coverage
Commercial, Individual, Varies

Geographic Areas Served
Nationwide

Subscriber Information
Average Monthly Fee Per Subscriber
(Employee + Employer Contribution):
Employee Only (Self): Varies by plan

Peer Review Type
Utilization Review: Yes
Second Surgical Opinion: Yes
Case Management: Yes

Accreditation Certification
Utilization Review, Pre-Admission Certification, State
Licensure

Key Personnel
President . . . . Alan Kaplan
VP, Operations . . . . Rosemarie Nuzzi
EVP & Provider Relations . . . . Lynn Kaplan
Supervisor, Plan Mngmnt. . . . . Cindy Bacon
Case Review . . . . Lucille Dunn, RN

Specialty Managed Care Partners
Standard Security; CareMark PBM

570   Liberty Dental Plan of New York
One Rockefeller Plaza
11th Floor
New York, NY 10020
Toll-Free: 888-352-7924
www.libertydentalplan.com
For Profit Organization: Yes
Total Enrollment: 2,000,000

Healthplan and Services Defined
PLAN TYPE: Dental
Other Type: Dental HMO
Plan Specialty: Dental
Benefits Offered: Dental

Type of Coverage
Commercial, Medicare, Medicaid, Unions

Geographic Areas Served
Statewide

Accreditation Certification
NCQA

Key Personnel
President & CEO. . . . . Amir Neshat
Executive Vice President . . . . John Carvelli
Chief Financial Officer . . . . Maja Kapic
General Counsel . . . . Lisa Wright
Chief Operating Officer . . . . Nico Alvarez
Chief Dental Officer. . . . . Richard Goren
Dental Director . . . . Richard Hague

571   Liberty Health Advantage HMO
1 Huntington Quadrangle
Suite 3N01
Melville, NY 11747
Toll-Free: 866-542-4269
Fax: 631-227-3484
www.lhany.com

Healthplan and Services Defined
PLAN TYPE: HMO
Plan Specialty: Integrated Medicare/Medicaid (Duals)
Benefits Offered: Chiropractic, Dental, Disease Management,
Home Care, Inpatient SNF, Physical Therapy, Podiatry,
Prescription, Psychiatric, Vision, Wellness

Type of Coverage
Individual, Medicare, Supplemental Medicare, Medicaid

Geographic Areas Served
New York City and Nassau County

Subscriber Information
Average Monthly Fee Per Subscriber
(Employee + Employer Contribution):
Employee Only (Self): Varies
Medicare: Varies
Average Annual Deductible Per Subscriber:
Employee Only (Self): Varies
Medicare: Varies
Average Subscriber Co-Payment:
Primary Care Physician: Varies
Non-Network Physician: Varies
Prescription Drugs: Varies
Hospital ER: Varies
Home Health Care: Varies
Home Health Care Max. Days/Visits Covered: Varies
Nursing Home: Varies
Nursing Home Max. Days/Visits Covered: Varies

Key Personnel
VP of Operations . . . . Lucy Oliva

572   MagnaCare
One Penn Plaza
46th Floor
New York, NY 10119
Toll-Free: 800-235-7267
Phone: 516-282-8000
www.magnacare.com
Secondary Address: 1600 Stewart Avenue, Suite 700,
Westbury, NY 11590
For Profit Organization: Yes
Year Founded: 1990
Number of Affiliated Hospitals: 260
Number of Primary Care Physicians: 70,000
Number of Referral/Specialty Physicians: 58,000
Total Enrollment: 1,326,000
State Enrollment: 928,200

Healthplan and Services Defined
PLAN TYPE: PPO
Model Type: Network

Plan Specialty: ASO, Behavioral Health, Chiropractic, Dental, Lab, Radiology, Worker's Compensation, UR
Benefits Offered: Behavioral Health, Chiropractic, Dental, Home Care, Inpatient SNF, Physical Therapy, Podiatry, Prescription, Psychiatric, Worker's Compensation, Correctional health services

Type of Coverage
Commercial, Individual, Leased Network Arrangement

Type of Payment Plans Offered
DFFS

Geographic Areas Served
New Jersey and New York

Subscriber Information
Average Monthly Fee Per Subscriber
(Employee + Employer Contribution):
Employee Only (Self): Varies
Average Subscriber Co-Payment:
Home Health Care: Varies
Home Health Care Max. Days/Visits Covered: Varies
Nursing Home: Varies
Nursing Home Max. Days/Visits Covered: Varies

Network Qualifications
Pre-Admission Certification: Yes

Peer Review Type
Utilization Review: Yes
Second Surgical Opinion: No
Case Management: Yes

Accreditation Certification
TJC Accreditation, Utilization Review, Pre-Admission Certification, State Licensure, Quality Assurance Program

Key Personnel
President & CEO . . . . Simeon Schindelman
VP of Finance . . . . Vanessa Hargrave
Chairman . . . . Joseph Berardo, Jr
Chief Legal Officer. Adam Young
Chief Compliance Officer . . . . Joseph Brennan
SVP, Human Resources . . . . Julie Bank

Average Claim Compensation
Physician's Fees Charged: 50%
Hospital's Fees Charged: 60%

Specialty Managed Care Partners
American Psych Systems, Intra State Choice Management Chiropractic

Employer References
Local 947, District Council of Painters #9

---

573   Meritain Health
300 Corporate Parkway
Amherst, NY 14226
Toll-Free: 888-324-5789
service@meritain.com
www.meritain.com
Subsidiary of: Aetna
For Profit Organization: Yes

Healthplan and Services Defined
PLAN TYPE: Multiple
Model Type: Network
Plan Specialty: Dental, Disease Management, Vision, Radiology, UR
Benefits Offered: Dental, Prescription, Vision
Offers Demand Management Patient Information Service: Yes

Type of Coverage
Commercial

Geographic Areas Served
Nationwide

Accreditation Certification
URAC
TJC Accreditation, Medicare Approved, Utilization Review, Pre-Admission Certification, State Licensure, Quality Assurance Program

Key Personnel
Cheief Executive Officer . . . . Mark T. Bertolini
President . . . . Karen S. Lynch

Average Claim Compensation
Physician's Fees Charged: 78%
Hospital's Fees Charged: 90%

---

574   MetroPlus Health Plan
160 Water Street
3rd Floor
New York, NY 10038
Toll-Free: 800-303-9626
Phone: 212-908-8600
Fax: 212-908-8601
www.metroplus.org
Subsidiary of: New York City Health Hospitals Corporation
Non-Profit Organization: Yes
Year Founded: 1985
Owned by an Integrated Delivery Network (IDN): Yes
Number of Affiliated Hospitals: 11
Number of Primary Care Physicians: 12,000
Total Enrollment: 332,128
State Enrollment: 332,128

Healthplan and Services Defined
PLAN TYPE: Medicare
Model Type: Network
Benefits Offered: Dental, Disease Management, Prescription, Vision, Wellness, Nurse management line, TeleHealth

Type of Coverage
Medicare, Medicaid, Child Health Plus, Family Health Pl

Geographic Areas Served
Brooklyn, Bronx, Manhattan and Queens

Accreditation Certification
TJC Accreditation

Key Personnel
Chief Financial Officer. John Cuda
President/CEO . . . . Arnold Saperstein, MD
Chief Operating Officer . . . . Seth Diamond
Chief, Human Resources . . . . Ryan Harris
Chief Customer Officer . . . . Gail L. Smith

CIO . . . . Susan Sun

Specialty Managed Care Partners
Enters into Contracts with Regional Business Coalitions: Yes

575 Molina Healthcare of New York

5232 Witz Drive
North Syracuse, NY 13212
Toll-Free: 800-223-7242
molinahealthcare.com
For Profit Organization: Yes
Year Founded: 1980

Healthplan and Services Defined
PLAN TYPE: Medicare
Plan Specialty: Dental, PBM, Vision, Integrated
Medicare/Medicaid (Duals)
Benefits Offered: Dental, Prescription, Vision, Wellness, Life

Geographic Areas Served
Statewide

Key Personnel
Chief Executive Officer . . . . Joseph W. White
Chief Operating Officer . . . . Terry Bayer
SVP, General Counsel . . . . Jeff D. Barlow
Investor Relations. . . . . Juan Jos, Orellana
Chief Information Officer . . . . Rick Hopfer

576 MVP Health Care

625 State Street
P.O. Box 2207
Schenectady, NY 12301-2207
Toll-Free: 800-777-4793
Phone: 518-370-4793
Fax: 518-370-0830
mvphealthcare.com
Secondary Address: 62 Merchants Row, Williston, VT 05495,
802-264-6500
Non-Profit Organization: Yes
Total Enrollment: 700,000

Healthplan and Services Defined
PLAN TYPE: Multiple
Benefits Offered: Chiropractic, Dental, Disease Management,
Home Care, Inpatient SNF, Physical Therapy, Podiatry,
Prescription, Psychiatric, Vision, Wellness

Type of Coverage
Commercial, Individual, Medicare

Geographic Areas Served
New York, Vermont

Accreditation Certification
NCQA

Key Personnel
President & CEO . . . . Denise Gonick
Chief Operating Officer . . . . Christopher Del Vecchio
EVP, Financial Officer. . . . . Karla A. Austen
Chief Medical Officer. . . . . Elizabeth Malko, MD
EVP, General Counsel . . . . Dawn Jablonski
VP, Human Resources . . . . Lynn Manning
Chief Information Officer . . . . Michael Della Villa

577 Nova Healthcare Administrators

6400 Main Street
Suite 210
Williamsville, NY 14221
Toll-Free: 800-999-5703
Phone: 716-773-2122
sales@novahealthcare.com
www.novahealthcare.com
Subsidiary of: Independent Health Association, Inc.
For Profit Organization: Yes
Year Founded: 1982
Total Enrollment: 210,000

Healthplan and Services Defined
PLAN TYPE: Multiple
Plan Specialty: ASO, Dental
Benefits Offered: Dental, Disease Management, Prescription,
Wellness

Type of Coverage
Commercial, Indemnity

Geographic Areas Served
Nationwide

Network Qualifications
Pre-Admission Certification: Yes

Peer Review Type
Utilization Review: Yes
Second Surgical Opinion: Yes
Case Management: Yes

Key Personnel
President. . . . . Larry Thompson

Specialty Managed Care Partners
Express Scripts

578 Oscar Health

295 Lafayette Street
New York, NY 10012
Toll-Free: 855-672-2788
guides@hioscar.com
www.hioscar.com
Subsidiary of: Mulberry Health, Inc.
For Profit Organization: Yes
Year Founded: 2012

Healthplan and Services Defined
PLAN TYPE: PPO
Benefits Offered: Inpatient SNF, Physical Therapy,
Prescription, Psychiatric, Wellness, Labs & Imaging;
Occupational & Speech Therapy

Geographic Areas Served
New York, California, and Texas

Key Personnel
Co-Founder . . . . Joshua Kushner
Co-Founder . . . . Mario Schlosser
Co-Founder. . . . . Kevin Nazemi

579   Quality Health Plans of New York

2805 Veterans Memorial Highway
Suite 17
Ronkonkoma, NY 11779
Toll-Free: 877-233-7058
Fax: 631-403-4266
www.qhpny.com
Secondary Address: Quality Health Plans of New York
    Claims, P.O. Box 340397, Tampa, FL 33694-0397
Year Founded: 2003
Physician Owned Organization: Yes
Total Enrollment: 19,000

Healthplan and Services Defined
    PLAN TYPE: Medicare
    Other Type: Medicare HMO

Type of Coverage
    Supplemental Medicare

Geographic Areas Served
    13 counties in Florida

Key Personnel
    Chief Executive Officer . . . . Frank Olsen
    Compliance Officer. . . . . Monique Slater

580   Trinity Health of New York

St James Mercy Health System
411 Canisteo Street
Hornell, NY 14843
Phone: 607-324-8000
www.trinity-health.org
Secondary Address: St. Peter's Health Partners, 315 S
    Manning Boulevard, Albany, NY 12208, 518-525-1111
Subsidiary of: Trinity Health
Non-Profit Organization: Yes
Year Founded: 2013
Total Enrollment: 30,000,000

Healthplan and Services Defined
    PLAN TYPE: Other
    Benefits Offered: Disease Management, Home Care,
      Long-Term Care, Psychiatric, Hospice programs, PACE
      (Program of All Inclusive Care for the Elderly)

Geographic Areas Served
    Western New York and Albany

Key Personnel
    Chief Executive Officer . . . . Richard J. Gilfillan
    Chief Financial Officer. . . . . Benjamin R. Carter
    Human Resources. . . . . Edmund F. Hodge
    General Counsel . . . . Paul G. Neumann
    Chief Clinical Officer. . . . . Daniel J. Roth
    Chief Operating Officer . . . . Michael A. Slubowski

581   United Concordia of New York

4401 Deer Path Road
Harrisburg, PA 17110
Toll-Free: 800-232-0366
www.unitedconcordia.com
For Profit Organization: Yes

Year Founded: 1971
Total Enrollment: 7,800,000

Healthplan and Services Defined
    PLAN TYPE: Dental
    Plan Specialty: Dental
    Benefits Offered: Dental

Type of Coverage
    Commercial, Individual, Military personnel & families

Geographic Areas Served
    Nationwide

Accreditation Certification
    URAC

Key Personnel
    President & COO . . . . Timothy J. Constantine
    Contact. . . . . Beth Rutherford
      717-260-7659
      beth.rutherford@ucci.com

582   UnitedHealthcare of New York

1 Pennsylvania Plaza
New York, NY 10119
Toll-Free: 877-769-7447
newyork_nm_team@uhc.com
www.uhc.com/contact-us/new-york
Subsidiary of: UnitedHealth Group
For Profit Organization: Yes
Year Founded: 1987
Federally Qualified: Yes

Healthplan and Services Defined
    PLAN TYPE: HMO/PPO
    Model Type: Network
    Plan Specialty: Behavioral Health, Dental, Disease
      Management, PBM, Vision
    Benefits Offered: Behavioral Health, Dental, Disease
      Management, Long-Term Care, Prescription, Vision,
      Wellness, Life, LTD, STD

Type of Coverage
    Individual, Medicare, Supplemental Medicare, Medicaid,
      Catastrophic, Family, Military, Veterans, Group,

Type of Payment Plans Offered
    DFFS, Capitated

Geographic Areas Served
    Statewide

Network Qualifications
    Pre-Admission Certification: Yes

Peer Review Type
    Utilization Review: Yes
    Second Surgical Opinion: Yes
    Case Management: Yes

Publishes and Distributes Report Card: Yes

Accreditation Certification
    TJC Accreditation, Medicare Approved, Utilization Review,
      Pre-Admission Certification, State Licensure, Quality
      Assurance Program

Key Personnel

President	David Wichmann
Chief Operating Officer	Dan Schumacher
Chief Strategy Officer	John Cosgriff
Communications Officer	Kirsten Gorsuch
Chief Medical Officer	Sam Ho
Chief Legal Officer	Thad Johnson
Chief Information Officer	Phil McKoy
Chief Financial Officer	Jeff Putnam

Specialty Managed Care Partners

Enters into Contracts with Regional Business Coalitions: Yes

583 Univera Healthcare

205 Park Club Lane
Buffalo, NY 14221
Toll-Free: 800-499-1275
www.univerahealthcare.com
Subsidiary of: The Lifetime Healthcare Companies
Non-Profit Organization: Yes
Number of Affiliated Hospitals: 35
Number of Primary Care Physicians: 5,700
Total Enrollment: 1,500,000
State Enrollment: 1,500,000

Healthplan and Services Defined
PLAN TYPE: HMO
Model Type: Network
Plan Specialty: ASO, Behavioral Health, Chiropractic,
    Dental, Disease Management, EPO, Lab, MSO, PBM,
    Vision, Radiology, Worker's Compensation, UR
Benefits Offered: Behavioral Health, Chiropractic,
    Complementary Medicine, Dental, Disease Management,
    Home Care, Inpatient SNF, Long-Term Care, Physical
    Therapy, Podiatry, Prescription, Psychiatric, Transplant,
    Vision, Wellness, Worker's Compensation, Life

Type of Coverage
Commercial, Individual, Medicare

Geographic Areas Served
Allegany, Cattaraugus, Chautauqua, Erie, Genesee, Niagara,
Orleans and Wyoming counties

Subscriber Information
Average Monthly Fee Per Subscriber
    (Employee + Employer Contribution):
        Employee Only (Self): Varies by plan
Average Subscriber Co-Payment:
    Primary Care Physician: Varies
    Prescription Drugs: Varies

Publishes and Distributes Report Card: Yes

Accreditation Certification
NCQA

Key Personnel

President	Arthur Wingerter
Chief Executive Officer	Christopher C. Booth
Chief Financial Officer	Dorothy Coleman
Chief Medical Officer	Richard Vienne
VP, Sales	Pamela J. Pawenski

VP, Communications	Peter B Kates

716-857-4495
peter.kates@univerahealthcare.com

584 Universal American Medicare Plans

44 S Broadway
Suite 1200
White Plains, NY 10601-4411
Phone: 914-934-5200
Fax: 914-934-0700
www.universalamerican.com
Subsidiary of: Wellcare Health Plans
Number of Primary Care Physicians: 4,200
Total Enrollment: 2,000,000

Healthplan and Services Defined
PLAN TYPE: Medicare
Other Type: HMO-POS, PPO, PFFS
Benefits Offered: Prescription

Type of Coverage
Individual, Medicare

Geographic Areas Served
Texas, New York, Maine

Subscriber Information
Average Monthly Fee Per Subscriber
    (Employee + Employer Contribution):
        Employee Only (Self): Varies
        Medicare: Varies
Average Annual Deductible Per Subscriber:
        Employee Only (Self): Varies
        Medicare: Varies
Average Subscriber Co-Payment:
    Primary Care Physician: Varies
    Non-Network Physician: Varies
    Prescription Drugs: Varies
    Hospital ER: Varies

Key Personnel

Chairman & CEO	Richard A Barasch
Chief Financial Officer	Adam C. Thackery
Administrative Officer	Steven H. Black
President, Medicare	Erin Page
EVP, Health Care Services	Theodore M. Carpenter Jr.
EVP, General Counsel	Anthony L. Wolk

Health Insurance Coverage Status and Type of Coverage by Age

Category	All Persons		Under 18 years		Under 65 years	
	Number	%	Number	%	Number	%
Total population	9,958	-	2,440	-	8,431	-
Covered by some type of health insurance	8,919 *(21)*	89.6 *(0.2)*	2,325 *(9)*	95.3 *(0.3)*	7,400 *(21)*	87.8 *(0.2)*
Covered by private health insurance	6,727 *(39)*	67.6 *(0.4)*	1,366 *(18)*	56.0 *(0.8)*	5,770 *(36)*	68.4 *(0.4)*
Employer-based	5,104 *(37)*	51.3 *(0.4)*	1,095 *(18)*	44.9 *(0.8)*	4,626 *(34)*	54.9 *(0.4)*
Direct purchase	1,600 *(22)*	16.1 *(0.2)*	196 *(9)*	8.0 *(0.4)*	1,057 *(20)*	12.5 *(0.2)*
TRICARE	459 *(15)*	4.6 *(0.1)*	121 *(8)*	4.9 *(0.3)*	330 *(14)*	3.9 *(0.2)*
Covered by public health insurance	3,459 *(29)*	34.7 *(0.3)*	1,043 *(20)*	42.8 *(0.8)*	1,970 *(29)*	23.4 *(0.3)*
Medicaid	1,865 *(28)*	18.7 *(0.3)*	1,030 *(20)*	42.2 *(0.8)*	1,673 *(26)*	19.8 *(0.3)*
Medicare	1,803 *(11)*	18.1 *(0.1)*	15 *(3)*	0.6 *(0.1)*	316 *(10)*	3.7 *(0.1)*
VA Care	289 *(8)*	2.9 *(0.1)*	6 *(2)*	0.3 *(0.1)*	146 *(7)*	1.7 *(0.1)*
Not covered at any time during the year	1,038 *(21)*	10.4 *(0.2)*	115 *(6)*	4.7 *(0.3)*	1,031 *(21)*	12.2 *(0.2)*

Note: Numbers in thousands; Figures cover civilian noninstitutionalized population in 2016; N/A indicates that data was not available; Z represents or rounds to zero; Margin of error appears in parenthesis and is calculated using replicate weights.
Source: U.S. Census Bureau, American Community Survey, Table HIC-4_ACS. Health Insurance Coverage Status and Type of Coverage by State—All People: 2008 to 2016, Table HIC-5_ACS. Health Insurance Coverage Status and Type of Coverage by State—Children Under 18: 2008 to 2016, Table HIC-6_ACS. Health Insurance Coverage Status and Type of Coverage by State—Persons Under 65: 2008 to 2016

North Carolina

585 Aetna Health of North Carolina

151 Farmington Avenue
Hartford, CT 06156
Toll-Free: 800-872-3862
Phone: 860-273-0123
www.aetna.com
Subsidiary of: Aetna Inc.
For Profit Organization: Yes

Healthplan and Services Defined
PLAN TYPE: HMO/PPO
Other Type: POS
Model Type: Network
Plan Specialty: Behavioral Health, EPO, Lab, PBM,
 Radiology
Benefits Offered: Behavioral Health, Dental, Disease
 Management, Long-Term Care, Physical Therapy,
 Podiatry, Prescription, Psychiatric, Vision, Wellness, Life,
 LTD, STD

Type of Coverage
Commercial, Student health

Geographic Areas Served
Statewide

Key Personnel
CEO . . . . Mark Bertolini

586 Blue Cross Blue Shield of North Carolina

4615 Univerisity Drive
Durham, NC 27707
Toll-Free: 800-324-4973
www.bcbsnc.com
Mailing Address: P.O. Box 2291, DurhamNC 27702-2291
Non-Profit Organization: Yes
Year Founded: 1933
Total Enrollment: 3,890,000

Healthplan and Services Defined
PLAN TYPE: HMO/PPO
Model Type: Network
Plan Specialty: ASO, Behavioral Health, Chiropractic,
 Dental, Disease Management, Lab, PBM, Vision,
 Radiology, UR
Benefits Offered: Behavioral Health, Chiropractic,
 Complementary Medicine, Dental, Disease Management,
 Home Care, Inpatient SNF, Long-Term Care, Physical
 Therapy, Podiatry, Prescription, Psychiatric, Transplant,
 Vision, Wellness, AD&D, Life, LTD, STD

Type of Coverage
Commercial, Individual, Supplemental Medicare

Type of Payment Plans Offered
POS, DFFS, FFS, Combination FFS & DFFS

Geographic Areas Served
Statewide

Peer Review Type
Utilization Review: Yes
Second Surgical Opinion: Yes

Case Management: Yes

Accreditation Certification
NCQA
State Licensure

Key Personnel
President & CEO . . . . J. Bradley Wilson
SVP, Operating Officer . . . . Gerald Petkau
SVP, Financial Officer . . . . Mitch Perry
SVP, Human Resources . . . . Fara M. Palumbo
SVP, General Counsel . . . . N. King Prather
SVP, Sales & Marketing . . . . John T. Roos
Chief Medical Officer . . . . Brian Caveney

Average Claim Compensation
Physician's Fees Charged: 43%
Hospital's Fees Charged: 35%

587 Coventry Health Care of the Carolinas

2815 Coliseum Centre Drive
Suite 550
Charlotte, NC 28217
Toll-Free: 800-470-4523
chccarolinas.coventryhealthcare.com
Secondary Address: 221 Dawson Road, Columbia, SC 29223,
 803-333-1000
Subsidiary of: Aetna Inc.
For Profit Organization: Yes
Total Enrollment: 5,000,000
State Enrollment: 187,000

Healthplan and Services Defined
PLAN TYPE: HMO/PPO
Model Type: Network
Plan Specialty: Behavioral Health, Dental, Worker's
 Compensation
Benefits Offered: Behavioral Health, Dental, Prescription,
 Wellness, Worker's Compensation

Type of Coverage
Commercial, Individual, Medicare, Medicaid

Geographic Areas Served
North and South Carolina

Key Personnel
Chief Executive Officer . . . . Mark T. Bertolini
President . . . . Karen S. Lynch
Chief Financial Officer . . . . Shawn M. Guertin
Operations & Technology . . . . Meg McCarthy
Chief Medical Officer . . . . Harold L. Paz
General Counsel . . . . Thomas Sabatino Jr.
Government Services . . . . Fran S. Soistman

588 Crescent Health Solutions

1200 Ridgefield Boulevard
Suite 215
Asheville, NC 28806
Toll-Free: 800-707-7726
Phone: 828-670-9145
Fax: 828-670-9155
www.crescenths.com

Year Founded: 1999
Physician Owned Organization: Yes
Number of Affiliated Hospitals: 15
Number of Primary Care Physicians: 1,900
Number of Referral/Specialty Physicians: 2,400
Total Enrollment: 40,000
State Enrollment: 40,000

Healthplan and Services Defined
PLAN TYPE: PPO
Benefits Offered: Disease Management, Prescription, Wellness, Case Management, UR, TPA Services

Type of Coverage
Commercial, Individual

Geographic Areas Served
North Carolina, South Carolina, Georgia, and Oklahoma

Peer Review Type
Utilization Review: Yes
Case Management: Yes

Key Personnel
CEO . . . . Andrew L. Wilson
VP, Operations/Business . . . . Desiree Greene
CFO . . . . Tara Pressley
TPA Claims Manager . . . . Cindy Beaver
Dir., Provider Relations . . . . Deana Gardner
Chief Medical Officer . . . . W. Virgil Thrash, MD
Director of Sales . . . . Blake Spell

---

589   Delta Dental of North Carolina
4208 Six Forks Road
Suite 970
Raleigh, NC 27609
Toll-Free: 800-662-8856
www.deltadentalnc.org
Non-Profit Organization: Yes

Healthplan and Services Defined
PLAN TYPE: Dental
Other Type: Dental PPO
Plan Specialty: Dental
Benefits Offered: Dental

Type of Coverage
Commercial, Individual

Type of Payment Plans Offered
POS, DFFS, FFS

Geographic Areas Served
Statewide

Key Personnel
President & CEO . . . . Curtis Ladig

---

590   Envolve Vision
112 Zebulon Court
P.O. Box 7548
Rocky Mount, NC 27804
Toll-Free: 800-334-3937
Fax: 877-940-9243
visionbenefits.envolvehealth.com

For Profit Organization: Yes
Number of Primary Care Physicians: 20,000

Healthplan and Services Defined
PLAN TYPE: Vision
Model Type: Network
Plan Specialty: Vision
Benefits Offered: Vision

Type of Coverage
Commercial, Medicare, Supplemental Medicare, Medicaid

Type of Payment Plans Offered
POS, DFFS, Capitated, FFS, Combination FFS & DFFS

Geographic Areas Served
Nationwide

Peer Review Type
Utilization Review: Yes
Case Management: Yes

Accreditation Certification
AAAHC, NCQA, State Licensure

Key Personnel
President/CEO . . . . David Lavely
SVP, Information Systems . . . . Juan Marrero
SVP, Regulatory Affairs . . . . Larry Keeley
SVP, Finance . . . . George Verrastro
Chief Operating Officer . . . . Michael Grover

Employer References
Wilmer-Hutchins Independent School D+strict

---

591   FirstCarolinaCare
42 Memorial Drive
Pinehurst, NC 28374
Toll-Free: 800-811-3298
Phone: 910-715-8100
www.firstcarolinacare.com
Subsidiary of: FirstHealth of the Carolinas
Non-Profit Organization: Yes
Total Enrollment: 13,000
State Enrollment: 13,000

Healthplan and Services Defined
PLAN TYPE: HMO
Offers Demand Management Patient Information Service: Yes
DMPI Services Offered: Nurse Helpline

Type of Coverage
Individual

Key Personnel
President . . . . Craig Humphrey

---

592   Humana Health Insurance of North Carolina
5955 Carnegie Boulevard
Suite 100
Charlotte, NC 28209
Toll-Free: 800-211-2389
Phone: 704-643-1009
www.humana.com
Secondary Address: Harvest Plaza, 8800 Harvest Oaks Drive, Suite 100, Raleigh, NC 27615, 919-870-4992

For Profit Organization: Yes

Healthplan and Services Defined
PLAN TYPE: HMO/PPO
Plan Specialty: ASO
Benefits Offered: Disease Management, Prescription,
Wellness

Type of Coverage
Commercial, Individual

Geographic Areas Served
North Carolina, South Carolina, Virginia

Accreditation Certification
URAC, NCQA, CORE

Key Personnel
President & CEO . . . . Bruce D. Broussard
Chief Medical Officer . . . . Roy A. Beveridge
Chief Consumer Officer . . . . Jody L. Bilney
SVP, Human Resources . . . . Tim Huval
Chief Financial Officer . . . . Brian Kane
Chief Information Officer . . . . Brian LeClaire
SVP, General Counsel . . . . Christopher M. Todoroff

Specialty Managed Care Partners
Caremark Rx

Employer References
Tricare

---

593 MedCost

165 Kimel Park Drive
Winston Salem, NC 27103
Toll-Free: 800-433-9178
www.medcost.com
Secondary Address: 1915 Rexford Road, Suite 120, Charlotte,
NC 28211
Subsidiary of: Carolinas HealthCare System
For Profit Organization: Yes
Year Founded: 1983
Number of Affiliated Hospitals: 191
Number of Primary Care Physicians: 12,349
Number of Referral/Specialty Physicians: 21,295
Total Enrollment: 670,000
State Enrollment: 670,000

Healthplan and Services Defined
PLAN TYPE: PPO
Model Type: Network
Plan Specialty: UR, PPO Network, Maternity Management,
Case Management, Nurse Coaching
Benefits Offered: Behavioral Health, Dental, Home Care,
Inpatient SNF, Long-Term Care, Physical Therapy,
Podiatry, Psychiatric, Transplant, Vision, Wellness,
Medical, Hospice, Durable Medical Equipment

Type of Coverage
Commercial

Type of Payment Plans Offered
FFS

Geographic Areas Served
North Carolina, South Carolina, and Virginia

Subscriber Information
Average Subscriber Co-Payment:
Primary Care Physician: Varies
Non-Network Physician: Varies
Prescription Drugs: Varies
Hospital ER: Varies
Home Health Care: Varies
Home Health Care Max. Days/Visits Covered: Varies
Nursing Home: Varies
Nursing Home Max. Days/Visits Covered: Varies

Peer Review Type
Utilization Review: Yes
Second Surgical Opinion: Yes
Case Management: Yes

Publishes and Distributes Report Card: Yes

Accreditation Certification
URAC

Key Personnel
President . . . . Kathryn Showalter
Chief Financial Officer . . . . Greg Bray

---

594 United Concordia of North Carolina

10700 Sikes Place
Suite 331
Charlotte, NC 28277
Phone: 704-845-8224
www.unitedconcordia.com
For Profit Organization: Yes
Year Founded: 1971
Total Enrollment: 7,800,000

Healthplan and Services Defined
PLAN TYPE: Dental
Plan Specialty: Dental
Benefits Offered: Dental

Type of Coverage
Commercial, Individual, Military personnel & families

Geographic Areas Served
Nationwide

Accreditation Certification
URAC

Key Personnel
President & COO . . . . Timothy J. Constantine
Contact. . . . . Beth Rutherford
717-260-7659
beth.rutherford@ucci.com

---

595 UnitedHealthcare of North Carolina

1001 Winstead Drive
Suite 200
Cary, NC 27615
Toll-Free: 800-362-0655
Fax: 803-454-1340
www.uhc.com/contact-us/north-carolina
Subsidiary of: UnitedHealth Group
For Profit Organization: Yes
Year Founded: 1985

Healthplan and Services Defined
PLAN TYPE: HMO/PPO
Model Type: Network
Plan Specialty: Behavioral Health, Dental, Disease
    Management, PBM, Vision
Benefits Offered: Behavioral Health, Dental, Disease
    Management, Long-Term Care, Prescription, Vision,
    Wellness, Life, LTD, STD

Type of Coverage
Individual, Medicare, Supplemental Medicare, Medicaid,
    Catastrophic, Family, Military, Veterans, Group,
Catastrophic Illness Benefit: Maximum $2M

Type of Payment Plans Offered
POS, DFFS, FFS, Combination FFS & DFFS

Geographic Areas Served
Statewide

Subscriber Information
Average Subscriber Co-Payment:
    Primary Care Physician: $10.00
    Non-Network Physician: 20%
    Prescription Drugs: $10.00
    Hospital ER: $35.00
    Home Health Care: $0
    Home Health Care Max. Days/Visits Covered: 30 days
    Nursing Home: 20%
    Nursing Home Max. Days/Visits Covered: 30 days

Network Qualifications
Pre-Admission Certification: Yes

Peer Review Type
Utilization Review: Yes
Second Surgical Opinion: No
Case Management: Yes

Publishes and Distributes Report Card: Yes

Accreditation Certification
TJC Accreditation, Utilization Review, Pre-Admission
    Certification, State Licensure, Quality Assurance Program

Key Personnel
President . . . . David Wichmann
Chief Operating Officer . . . . Dan Schumacher
Chief Strategy Officer . . . . John Cosgriff
Communications Officer . . . . Kirsten Gorsuch
Chief Medical Officer. . . . . Sam Ho
Chief Legal Officer . . . . Thad Johnson
Chief Information Officer . . . . Phil McKoy
Chief Financial Officer. . . . . Jeff Putnam

Health Insurance Coverage Status and Type of Coverage by Age

Category	All Persons		Under 18 years		Under 65 years	
	Number	%	Number	%	Number	%
Total population	741	-	186	-	638	-
Covered by some type of health insurance	689 (5)	93.0 (0.6)	171 (3)	92.0 (1.2)	586 (5)	91.9 (0.7)
Covered by private health insurance	597 (7)	80.5 (1.0)	141 (3)	75.6 (1.7)	518 (7)	81.3 (1.1)
Employer-based	456 (10)	61.5 (1.3)	115 (4)	61.7 (2.2)	426 (9)	66.9 (1.4)
Direct purchase	151 (6)	20.4 (0.8)	24 (3)	12.9 (1.5)	97 (5)	15.3 (0.8)
TRICARE	28 (4)	3.7 (0.6)	8 (2)	4.2 (1.1)	21 (4)	3.4 (0.6)
Covered by public health insurance	193 (6)	26.0 (0.8)	39 (3)	21.2 (1.8)	91 (6)	14.3 (0.9)
Medicaid	86 (6)	11.6 (0.7)	39 (3)	20.8 (1.8)	77 (6)	12.0 (0.9)
Medicare	116 (2)	15.6 (0.3)	1 (1)	0.8 (0.4)	14 (2)	2.3 (0.3)
VA Care	21 (2)	2.8 (0.2)	Z (Z)	0.2 (0.2)	9 (2)	1.4 (0.2)
Not covered at any time during the year	52 (5)	7.0 (0.6)	15 (2)	8.0 (1.2)	52 (5)	8.1 (0.7)

Note: Numbers in thousands; Figures cover civilian noninstitutionalized population in 2016; N/A indicates that data was not available; Z represents or rounds to zero; Margin of error appears in parenthesis and is calculated using replicate weights.

Source: U.S. Census Bureau, American Community Survey, Table HIC-4_ACS. Health Insurance Coverage Status and Type of Coverage by State—All People: 2008 to 2016, Table HIC-5_ACS. Health Insurance Coverage Status and Type of Coverage by State—Children Under 18: 2008 to 2016, Table HIC-6_ACS. Health Insurance Coverage Status and Type of Coverage by State—Persons Under 65: 2008 to 2016

North Dakota

596 Aetna Health of North Dakota

151 Farmington Avenue
Hartford, CT 06156
Toll-Free: 800-872-3862
Phone: 860-273-0123
www.aetna.com
Subsidiary of: Aetna Inc.
For Profit Organization: Yes

Healthplan and Services Defined
PLAN TYPE: PPO
Other Type: POS
Model Type: Network
Plan Specialty: Behavioral Health, EPO, Lab, PBM, Radiology
Benefits Offered: Behavioral Health, Disease Management, Long-Term Care, Physical Therapy, Podiatry, Prescription, Psychiatric, Wellness, Life, LTD, STD

Type of Coverage
Commercial, Student health

Type of Payment Plans Offered
POS, FFS

Geographic Areas Served
Statewide

Key Personnel
CEO . . . . Mark Bertolini

597 Coventry Health Care of North Dakota

521 N 10th Street
Bismarck, ND 58501
Phone: 701-250-5380
www.coventryhealthcare.com
Subsidiary of: Aetna Inc.
For Profit Organization: Yes

Healthplan and Services Defined
PLAN TYPE: HMO/PPO
Model Type: Network
Plan Specialty: Behavioral Health, Dental, Worker's Compensation
Benefits Offered: Behavioral Health, Dental, Prescription, Wellness, Worker's Compensation

Type of Coverage
Commercial, Medicare, Medicaid

Geographic Areas Served
Statewide

Key Personnel
Chief Executive Officer . . . . Mark T. Bertolini
President . . . . Karen S. Lynch
Chief Financial Officer . . . . Shawn M. Guertin
Operations & Technology . . . . Meg McCarthy
Chief Medical Officer . . . . Harold L. Paz
General Counsel . . . . Thomas Sabatino Jr.
Government Services . . . . Fran S. Soistman

598 Heart of America Health Plan

810 South Main Avenue
Rugby, ND 58368
Toll-Free: 877-652-1845
Phone: 701-776-5848
Fax: 605-328-6811
www.hoahp.com
Mailing Address: P.O. Box 1999, Fargo, ND 58107
Non-Profit Organization: Yes
Year Founded: 1982
Number of Affiliated Hospitals: 1
Number of Primary Care Physicians: 15
Number of Referral/Specialty Physicians: 500
Total Enrollment: 1,000
State Enrollment: 2,049

Healthplan and Services Defined
PLAN TYPE: HMO
Model Type: Group
Benefits Offered: Behavioral Health, Disease Management, Podiatry, Psychiatric, Wellness, LTD, Substance Abuse, Maternity

Type of Coverage
Medicare, Supplemental Medicare

Type of Payment Plans Offered
POS, DFFS

Geographic Areas Served
North Central North Dakota: Pierce, Rolette, Bottineau, McHenry, Towner, Ward and Renville counties in North Dakota and portions of Benson, Wells, Sheridan, McLean, Mountrail and Burke counties

Subscriber Information
Average Annual Deductible Per Subscriber:
Employee Only (Self): $600
Employee & 1 Family Member: $0
Employee & 2 Family Members: $0
Medicare: $0
Average Subscriber Co-Payment:
Primary Care Physician: $10.00
Non-Network Physician: 20%
Prescription Drugs: $0.00
Hospital ER: $30.00

Accreditation Certification
TJC Accreditation

Average Claim Compensation
Physician's Fees Charged: 1%
Hospital's Fees Charged: 1%

Employer References
Federal Employee Plan

599 Humana Health Insurance of North Dakota

12600 Whitewater Drive
Suite 150
Minnetonka, MT 55343
Toll-Free: 877-367-6990
Fax: 952-938-2787
www.humana.com

Subsidiary of: Humana

For Profit Organization: Yes

Healthplan and Services Defined
  PLAN TYPE: HMO/PPO
  Model Type: Network
  Plan Specialty: Dental, Vision
  Benefits Offered: Dental, Vision, Life, LTD, STD

Type of Coverage
  Commercial

Geographic Areas Served
  North Dakota is covered by the Minnesota branch

Accreditation Certification
  URAC, NCQA, CORE

Key Personnel
  President & CEO. . . . . Bruce Broussard
  Chief Medical Officer. . . . . Roy A. Beveridge
  Chief Consumer Officer. . . . . Jody L. Bilney
  Human Resources. . . . . Tim Huval
  Chief Financial Officer . . . . Brian Kane
  Chief Information Officer . . . . Brian LeClaire
  General Counsel. . . . . Christopher M. Todoroff

---

600 Medica: North Dakota

1711 Gold Drive South
Suite 210
Fargo, ND 58103
Phone: 701-293-4700
www.medica.com
Non-Profit Organization: Yes
Year Founded: 1974
Number of Affiliated Hospitals: 158
Number of Primary Care Physicians: 24,000
Total Enrollment: 1,600,000

Healthplan and Services Defined
  PLAN TYPE: HMO
  Model Type: IPA
  Benefits Offered: Behavioral Health, Chiropractic, Dental,
    Disease Management, Prescription, Wellness, AD&D, Life,
    LTD, STD
  Offers Demand Management Patient Information Service:
    Yes

Type of Coverage
  Medicare
  Catastrophic Illness Benefit: Covered

Type of Payment Plans Offered
  Capitated, FFS, Combination FFS & DFFS

Geographic Areas Served
  Aitkin, Anoka, Becker, Beltrami, Benton, Big Stone, Blue
  Earth, Brown, Carlton, Carver, Cass, Chisago, Clay,
  Clearwater, Cottonwood, Crow Wing, Dakota, Dodge,
  Douglas, Fillmore, Goodhue, Grant, Hennepin, Hubbard,
  Isanti, Itaska, Kanabec, Kandiyohi, Koochiching, Jackson,
  Lac Qui Parle, Lake, Le Sueur, Lincoln, Lyon, Mahnomen,
  McLeod, Meeker, Mille Lacs, Morrison, Murray, Nicollet,
  Norman, Olnsted, Otter Tail, Pine, Polk, Pope, Ramsey,
  Renville, Rice, Rock, Scott

Subscriber Information
  Average Monthly Fee Per Subscriber
    (Employee + Employer Contribution):
      Employee Only (Self): Varies by plan
  Average Subscriber Co-Payment:
    Primary Care Physician: $15.00
    Non-Network Physician: Deductible + 20%
    Prescription Drugs: $11.00
    Hospital ER: $60.00
    Home Health Care: 20%
    Nursing Home: 20%

Network Qualifications
  Pre-Admission Certification: Yes

Peer Review Type
  Utilization Review: Yes
  Second Surgical Opinion: Yes
  Case Management: Yes

Publishes and Distributes Report Card: Yes

Accreditation Certification
  NCQA
  TJC Accreditation, Medicare Approved, Utilization Review,
    Pre-Admission Certification, State Licensure, Quality
    Assurance Program

Key Personnel
  President/CEO . . . . John Naylor
  SVP, Government Programs. . . . . Tom Lindquist
  SVP, Marketing & Comm . . . . Rob Longendyke
  SVP/CFO . . . . Mark Baird
  SVP/General Manager . . . . Geoff Bartsh
  SVP, General Counsel . . . . Jim Jacobson
  VP, Human Resources . . . . Lynn Altmann

Average Claim Compensation
  Physician's Fees Charged: 65%
  Hospital's Fees Charged: 60%

Specialty Managed Care Partners
  Express Scrips, Vision Service Plan, National Healthcare
    Resources, Cigna Behavioral Resources
  Enters into Contracts with Regional Business Coalitions: Yes

Employer References
  Construction Industry Laborers Welfare Fund-Jefferson City,
    District 9 Machinists (Missouri/Welfare Plan), Government
    Employees Hospital Association/GEHA, Missouri Highway
    & Transportation Department/Highway Patrol

---

601 Noridian Insurance Services Inc.

4510 13th Avenue S
Fargo, ND 58121
Toll-Free: 800-575-9643
www.mynisi.com
For Profit Organization: Yes

Healthplan and Services Defined
  PLAN TYPE: PPO
  Plan Specialty: Dental, Vision
  Benefits Offered: Dental, Long-Term Care, Vision, AD&D,
    Life, LTD, STD

Type of Coverage
Commercial, Individual, Indemnity

Geographic Areas Served
North Dakota and Northwest Minnesota

602　**UnitedHealthcare of North Dakota**

9700 Health Care Lane
Minnetonka, MN 55343
Toll-Free: 800-842-3585
www.uhc.com/contact-us/north-dakota
Subsidiary of: UnitedHealth Group
For Profit Organization: Yes
Year Founded: 1977

Healthplan and Services Defined
PLAN TYPE: HMO/PPO
Model Type: Network
Plan Specialty: Behavioral Health, Dental, Disease
　Management, Lab, PBM, Vision, Radiology
Benefits Offered: Behavioral Health, Dental, Disease
　Management, Home Care, Long-Term Care, Physical
　Therapy, Prescription, Psychiatric, Vision, Wellness,
　AD&D, Life, LTD, STD
Offers Demand Management Patient Information Service:
　Yes

Type of Coverage
Commercial, Individual, Indemnity, Medicare, Supplemental
　Medicare, Medicaid, Catastrophic, Family, Military,
　Veterans, Group,
Catastrophic Illness Benefit: Varies per case

Geographic Areas Served
Statewide. North Dakota is covered by the Minnesota branch

Publishes and Distributes Report Card: Yes

Accreditation Certification
TJC Accreditation, Medicare Approved

Key Personnel
President . . . . David Wichmann
Chief Operating Officer . . . . Dan Schumacher
Chief Strategy Officer . . . . John Cosgriff
Communications Officer . . . . Kirsten Gorsuch
Chief Medical Officer. . . . . Sam Ho
Chief Legal Officer . . . . Thad Johnson
Chief Information Officer . . . . Phil McKoy
Chief Financial Officer. . . . . Jeff Putnam

Specialty Managed Care Partners
Enters into Contracts with Regional Business Coalitions: Yes

HMO/PPO DIRECTORY

OHIO

Health Insurance Coverage Status and Type of Coverage by Age

Category	All Persons		Under 18 years		Under 65 years	
	Number	%	Number	%	Number	%
Total population	11,440	-	2,766	-	9,624	-
Covered by some type of health insurance	10,796 *(17)*	94.4 *(0.2)*	2,662 *(9)*	96.2 *(0.3)*	8,988 *(17)*	93.4 *(0.2)*
Covered by private health insurance	7,953 *(42)*	69.5 *(0.4)*	1,745 *(21)*	63.1 *(0.7)*	6,811 *(39)*	70.8 *(0.4)*
Employer-based	6,777 *(41)*	59.2 *(0.4)*	1,596 *(21)*	57.7 *(0.8)*	6,110 *(39)*	63.5 *(0.4)*
Direct purchase	1,386 *(23)*	12.1 *(0.2)*	150 *(9)*	5.4 *(0.3)*	786 *(19)*	8.2 *(0.2)*
TRICARE	183 *(10)*	1.6 *(0.1)*	37 *(5)*	1.4 *(0.2)*	118 *(8)*	1.2 *(0.1)*
Covered by public health insurance	4,305 *(36)*	37.6 *(0.3)*	1,052 *(20)*	38.0 *(0.7)*	2,545 *(35)*	26.4 *(0.4)*
Medicaid	2,445 *(35)*	21.4 *(0.3)*	1,039 *(21)*	37.6 *(0.8)*	2,269 *(35)*	23.6 *(0.4)*
Medicare	2,088 *(11)*	18.3 *(0.1)*	20 *(3)*	0.7 *(0.1)*	331 *(10)*	3.4 *(0.1)*
VA Care	263 *(7)*	2.3 *(0.1)*	3 *(1)*	0.1 *(Z)*	112 *(5)*	1.2 *(0.1)*
Not covered at any time during the year	644 *(18)*	5.6 *(0.2)*	104 *(7)*	3.8 *(0.3)*	636 *(18)*	6.6 *(0.2)*

Note: Numbers in thousands; Figures cover civilian noninstitutionalized population in 2016; N/A indicates that data was not available; Z represents or rounds to zero; Margin of error appears in parenthesis and is calculated using replicate weights.
Source: U.S. Census Bureau, American Community Survey, Table HIC-4_ACS. Health Insurance Coverage Status and Type of Coverage by State—All People: 2008 to 2016, Table HIC-5_ACS. Health Insurance Coverage Status and Type of Coverage by State—Children Under 18: 2008 to 2016, Table HIC-6_ACS. Health Insurance Coverage Status and Type of Coverage by State—Persons Under 65: 2008 to 2016

Ohio

603 Aetna Health of Ohio

151 Farmington Avenue
Hartford, CT 06156
Toll-Free: 800-872-3862
Phone: 860-273-0123
www.aetna.com
Subsidiary of: Aetna Inc.
For Profit Organization: Yes

Healthplan and Services Defined
PLAN TYPE: HMO/PPO
Other Type: POS
Model Type: Network
Plan Specialty: Behavioral Health, Dental, EPO, Lab, PBM, Vision, Radiology
Benefits Offered: Behavioral Health, Dental, Disease Management, Long-Term Care, Physical Therapy, Podiatry, Prescription, Psychiatric, Vision, Wellness, Life, LTD, STD

Type of Coverage
Commercial, Medicare, Medicaid, Student health

Type of Payment Plans Offered
POS

Geographic Areas Served
Statewide

Subscriber Information
Average Subscriber Co-Payment:
Prescription Drugs: $5.00
Home Health Care Max. Days/Visits Covered: Unlimited

Network Qualifications
Pre-Admission Certification: No

Peer Review Type
Utilization Review: Yes
Second Surgical Opinion: Yes
Case Management: Yes

Publishes and Distributes Report Card: Yes

Accreditation Certification
NCQA
TJC Accreditation, Utilization Review, Pre-Admission Certification, State Licensure, Quality Assurance Program

Key Personnel
CEO . . . . Mark Bertolini

Specialty Managed Care Partners
Enters into Contracts with Regional Business Coalitions: Yes

604 Anthem Blue Cross & Blue Shield of Ohio

4361 Irwin Simpson Road
Mason, OH 45040
Toll-Free: 800-483-2311
www.anthem.com
Subsidiary of: Anthem, Inc.
For Profit Organization: Yes
Year Founded: 1944
Owned by an Integrated Delivery Network (IDN): Yes

Number of Affiliated Hospitals: 568
Number of Primary Care Physicians: 25,000
Number of Referral/Specialty Physicians: 61,728

Healthplan and Services Defined
PLAN TYPE: PPO
Plan Specialty: ASO, Behavioral Health, Chiropractic, Dental, Disease Management, Lab, PBM, Vision, Radiology, Worker's Compensation, UR
Benefits Offered: Behavioral Health, Chiropractic, Dental, Disease Management, Home Care, Inpatient SNF, Physical Therapy, Podiatry, Prescription, Psychiatric, Transplant, Vision, Wellness, Worker's Compensation
Offers Demand Management Patient Information Service: Yes
DMPI Services Offered: Iris Program, Care Wise (24/7 Nurse Line), Dental, Vision

Type of Coverage
Commercial, Individual, Indemnity, Medicare, Catastrophic

Type of Payment Plans Offered
POS, DFFS, Capitated, FFS

Geographic Areas Served
Statewide

Subscriber Information
Average Monthly Fee Per Subscriber
(Employee + Employer Contribution):
Employee Only (Self): Proprietary
Employee & 1 Family Member: Proprietary
Employee & 2 Family Members: Proprierary
Medicare: Proprietary
Average Annual Deductible Per Subscriber:
Employee Only (Self): Proprietary
Employee & 1 Family Member: Proprietary
Employee & 2 Family Members: Proprietary
Medicare: Proprietary

Network Qualifications
Pre-Admission Certification: Yes

Peer Review Type
Utilization Review: Yes
Second Surgical Opinion: Yes
Case Management: Yes

Accreditation Certification
URAC, NCQA
TJC Accreditation, Medicare Approved, Utilization Review, Pre-Admission Certification, State Licensure, Quality Assurance Program

Key Personnel
President & CEO . . . . Scott P. Serota
Chief Financial Officer . . . . Robert Kolodgy
Human Resources . . . . Maureen A. Cahill
Chief Medical Officer. . . . . Trent Haywood
General Counsel. . . . . Scott Nehs

Specialty Managed Care Partners
Anthem Dental, Anthem Prescription Management LLC, Anthem Vision, Anthem Life

605 Aultcare Corporation

2600 Sixth Street SW
Canton, OH 44710
Toll-Free: 800-344-8858
Phone: 330-363-6360
www.aultcare.com
Non-Profit Organization: Yes
Year Founded: 1985
Number of Affiliated Hospitals: 14
Number of Primary Care Physicians: 3,500
Number of Referral/Specialty Physicians: 6,800
Total Enrollment: 500,000
State Enrollment: 5,151

Healthplan and Services Defined
PLAN TYPE: HMO/PPO
Model Type: Network
Benefits Offered: Chiropractic, Dental, Disease Management, Inpatient SNF, Podiatry, Vision, Wellness, Worker's Compensation, STD, Flexible Spending Accounts

Type of Coverage
Commercial, Individual

Geographic Areas Served
Carroll, Holmes, Stark, Summit, Tuscarawas and Wayne counties

Network Qualifications
Pre-Admission Certification: Yes

Peer Review Type
Utilization Review: Yes
Second Surgical Opinion: Yes
Case Management: Yes

Accreditation Certification
NCQA

Key Personnel
CEO/President . . . . Rick Haines

Employer References
Maytag, Timken Company

606 CareSource Ohio

230 N Main Street
Dayton, OH 45402
Toll-Free: 855-475-3163
Phone: 937-224-3300
www.caresource.com
Secondary Address: 5900 Landerbrook Drive, Suite 300, Mayfield Heights, OH 44124, 216-839-1001
Non-Profit Organization: Yes
Total Enrollment: 1,000,000

Healthplan and Services Defined
PLAN TYPE: Medicare
Other Type: Medicaid

Type of Coverage
Medicare, Medicaid

Geographic Areas Served
Statewide

Key Personnel
President & CEO . . . . Pamela Morris
COO . . . . Bobby Jones

607 Delta Dental of Ohio

8044 Montgomery Road
Suite 700
Cincinnati, OH 45236
Toll-Free: 800-524-0149
www.deltadentaloh.com
Non-Profit Organization: Yes
Year Founded: 1960

Healthplan and Services Defined
PLAN TYPE: Dental
Other Type: Dental PPO
Plan Specialty: Dental
Benefits Offered: Dental

Type of Coverage
Commercial

Type of Payment Plans Offered
POS

Geographic Areas Served
Statewide

Peer Review Type
Second Surgical Opinion: Yes
Case Management: No

Publishes and Distributes Report Card: Yes

Accreditation Certification
Utilization Review

Specialty Managed Care Partners
Enters into Contracts with Regional Business Coalitions: Yes

608 EyeMed Vision Care

4000 Luxottica Place
Mason, OH 45040
Toll-Free: 866-939-3633
portal.eyemedvisioncare.com
Subsidiary of: Luxxotica
For Profit Organization: Yes
Year Founded: 1988
Total Enrollment: 43,000,000

Healthplan and Services Defined
PLAN TYPE: Vision
Plan Specialty: Vision
Benefits Offered: Vision

Type of Coverage
Commercial

Key Personnel
President . . . . Lukas Ruecker

609 Humana Health Insurance of Ohio

640 Eden Park Drive
6th Floor
Cincinnati, OH 45202
Toll-Free: 800-941-6172
Phone: 513-826-7207
Fax: 513-442-7668
www.humana.com
Secondary Address: 6050 Oaktree Boulevard, Independence, OH 44131, 216-447-8147
For Profit Organization: Yes
Year Founded: 1979
Owned by an Integrated Delivery Network (IDN): Yes

Healthplan and Services Defined
PLAN TYPE: HMO/PPO
Model Type: Group
Plan Specialty: ASO, Dental, Vision, Radiology, Worker's Compensation
Benefits Offered: Behavioral Health, Chiropractic, Disease Management, Inpatient SNF, Physical Therapy, Podiatry, Prescription, Psychiatric, Transplant, Vision, Wellness
Offers Demand Management Patient Information Service: Yes

Type of Coverage
Commercial, Individual, Medicare, Medicaid

Type of Payment Plans Offered
POS, DFFS, Capitated, FFS, Combination FFS & DFFS

Geographic Areas Served
Statewide

Subscriber Information
Average Subscriber Co-Payment:
Home Health Care: $0
Nursing Home: $0

Peer Review Type
Utilization Review: Yes
Case Management: Yes

Publishes and Distributes Report Card: No

Accreditation Certification
URAC, NCQA, CORE
Utilization Review, Pre-Admission Certification, State Licensure, Quality Assurance Program

Key Personnel
President & CEO . . . . Bruce D. Broussard
Chief Medical Officer. . . . . Roy A. Beveridge
Chief Consumer Officer. . . . . Jody L. Bilney
SVP, Human Resources . . . . Tim Huval
Chief Financial Officer . . . . Brian Kane
Chief Information Officer . . . . Brian LeClaire
SVP, General Counsel . . . . Christopher M. Todoroff

Specialty Managed Care Partners
Enters into Contracts with Regional Business Coalitions: No

610 Medical Mutual

2060 E 9th Street
Cleveland, OH 44115
Toll-Free: 800-382-5729
www.medmutual.com
Year Founded: 1934

Healthplan and Services Defined
PLAN TYPE: HMO
Model Type: Staff
Benefits Offered: Prescription

Type of Coverage
Commercial, Individual, Medicare

Type of Payment Plans Offered
DFFS, Capitated, FFS, Combination FFS & DFFS

Geographic Areas Served
Statewide

Publishes and Distributes Report Card: Yes

Accreditation Certification
NCQA

Key Personnel
Chairman, President & CEO. . . . . Rick Chiricosta
EVP, Chief Health Officer. . . . . Kathy Golovan
EVP, Financial Officer. . . . . Ray Mueller
Chief Information Officer . . . . John Kish
Chief Medical Officer . . . . Tere Koenig
Chief Marketing Officer . . . . Steffany Larkins

Specialty Managed Care Partners
Enters into Contracts with Regional Business Coalitions: Yes

611 Medical Mutual Services

2060 East Ninth Street
Cleveland, OH 44115-1355
Toll-Free: 800-625-2583
Phone: 213-687-6064
Fax: 216-687-7994
www.supermednetwork.com
Subsidiary of: SuperMed Network
Number of Primary Care Physicians: 24,000
Total Enrollment: 144,000

Healthplan and Services Defined
PLAN TYPE: PPO
Benefits Offered: Chiropractic, Physical Therapy, Podiatry, Psychiatric

Type of Coverage
Commercial, Self Funded, Insurance Companies

Geographic Areas Served
South Carolina, Georgia, Ohio

Accreditation Certification
TJC, NCQA

612 MediGold

6150 East Broad Street
Suite EE320
Columbus, OH 43213-1574
Toll-Free: 800-964-4525
Fax: 614-546-3108
www.medigold.com
Subsidiary of: Mount Carmel Health Plan
Non-Profit Organization: Yes
Year Founded: 1997
Federally Qualified: Yes
Number of Affiliated Hospitals: 23
Number of Primary Care Physicians: 1,050
Number of Referral/Specialty Physicians: 1,850
Total Enrollment: 55,000
State Enrollment: 55,000

Healthplan and Services Defined
PLAN TYPE: Medicare
Model Type: Network, Medicare
Benefits Offered: Behavioral Health, Chiropractic, Dental,
   Disease Management, Home Care, Inpatient SNF, Physical
   Therapy, Podiatry, Prescription, Psychiatric, Vision,
   Wellness, Medical, OP Services, Drug Coverage

Type of Coverage
Individual, Medicare
Catastrophic Illness Benefit: Unlimited

Type of Payment Plans Offered
Combination FFS & DFFS

Geographic Areas Served
31 counties in Ohio

Subscriber Information
Average Monthly Fee Per Subscriber
   (Employee + Employer Contribution):
      Employee Only (Self): Varies
      Medicare: Varies
Average Annual Deductible Per Subscriber:
      Employee Only (Self): Varies
      Medicare: Varies
Average Subscriber Co-Payment:
      Primary Care Physician: Varies
      Non-Network Physician: Varies
      Prescription Drugs: Varies
      Hospital ER: Varies
      Home Health Care: Varies
      Home Health Care Max. Days/Visits Covered: Varies
      Nursing Home: Varies
      Nursing Home Max. Days/Visits Covered: Varies

Network Qualifications
Pre-Admission Certification: Yes

Peer Review Type
Utilization Review: Yes
Case Management: Yes

Publishes and Distributes Report Card: Yes

Accreditation Certification
TJC Accreditation, Medicare Approved, Utilization Review,
   Pre-Admission Certification, State Licensure, Quality
   Assurance Program

Specialty Managed Care Partners
PBM-CAREMARK

Employer References
Timken, Mount Carmel Trinity

613 Molina Healthcare of Ohio

3000 Corporate Exchange Drive
Columbus, OH 43231
Toll-Free: 800-642-4168
www.molinahealthcare.com
Subsidiary of: Molina Healthcare, Inc.
For Profit Organization: Yes
Year Founded: 1980
Physician Owned Organization: Yes

Healthplan and Services Defined
PLAN TYPE: Medicare
Model Type: Network
Plan Specialty: Integrated Medicare/Medicaid (Duals)
Benefits Offered: Chiropractic, Dental, Home Care, Inpatient
   SNF, Long-Term Care, Podiatry, Vision

Type of Coverage
Commercial, Medicare, Supplemental Medicare, Medicaid

Accreditation Certification
URAC, NCQA

Key Personnel
Chief Executive Officer . . . . Joseph W. White
Chief Operating Officer . . . . Terry Bayer
General Counsel. . . . . Jeff D. Barlow
SVP, Relations/Marketing . . . . Juan Jos, Orellana
Chief Information Officer . . . . Rick Hopfer

614 Ohio Health Choice

P.O. Box 2090
Akron, OH 44309-2090
Toll-Free: 800-554-0027
www.ohiohealthchoice.com
Mailing Address: P.O. Box 3619, Akron, OH 44309-2090
For Profit Organization: Yes
Year Founded: 1982
Number of Affiliated Hospitals: 199
Number of Primary Care Physicians: 28,000
Total Enrollment: 370,000
State Enrollment: 370,000

Healthplan and Services Defined
PLAN TYPE: PPO
Model Type: Network
Plan Specialty: Chiropractic, Disease Management, EPO, UR
Benefits Offered: Behavioral Health, Chiropractic, Disease
   Management, Home Care, Inpatient SNF, Long-Term Care,
   Physical Therapy, Podiatry, Psychiatric, Transplant,
   Wellness, Audiology, durable medical equipment, sleep
   disorder services, speech therapy

Type of Coverage
Commercial, Individual, Indemnity, Medicare

Type of Payment Plans Offered
POS, FFS

Geographic Areas Served
Throughout Ohio as well as the contiguous counties of Boone, Boyd, Campbell, Grant and Kenton in Kentucky; Dearborn in Indiana; Mercer and Erie in Pennsylvania; and Wood, Hancock and Ohio in West Virginia

Peer Review Type
Utilization Review: Yes
Second Surgical Opinion: Yes
Case Management: Yes

---

615 Ohio State University Health Plan Inc.
700 Ackerman Road
Suite 440
Columbus, OH 43202
Toll-Free: 800-678-6269
Phone: 614-292-4700
osuhealthplancs@osumc.edu
www.osuhealthplan.com
Non-Profit Organization: Yes
Year Founded: 1991
Number of Affiliated Hospitals: 95
Number of Primary Care Physicians: 3,250
Number of Referral/Specialty Physicians: 7,950
Total Enrollment: 52,000
State Enrollment: 52,000

Healthplan and Services Defined
PLAN TYPE: Multiple
Model Type: IPA
Plan Specialty: ASO, Behavioral Health, Disease Management, EPO
Benefits Offered: Behavioral Health, Chiropractic, Complementary Medicine, Dental, Disease Management, Home Care, Inpatient SNF, Physical Therapy, Podiatry, Prescription, Psychiatric, Transplant, Vision, Wellness
Offers Demand Management Patient Information Service: Yes
DMPI Services Offered: Faculty and Staff Assistance Program, University Health Connection

Type of Payment Plans Offered
DFFS, Capitated, Combination FFS & DFFS

Geographic Areas Served
Ohio State University employees and their dependents

Subscriber Information
Average Annual Deductible Per Subscriber:
    Employee Only (Self): $0
    Employee & 1 Family Member: $0
    Employee & 2 Family Members: $0
    Medicare: $0
Average Subscriber Co-Payment:
    Primary Care Physician: $15.00
    Non-Network Physician: 30%
    Prescription Drugs: 20% (generic)
    Hospital ER: $75.00
    Home Health Care: 20%
    Home Health Care Max. Days/Visits Covered: Unlimited
    Nursing Home: $0
    Nursing Home Max. Days/Visits Covered: 60 days

Network Qualifications
Pre-Admission Certification: Yes

Peer Review Type
Utilization Review: Yes
Second Surgical Opinion: No
Case Management: Yes

Publishes and Distributes Report Card: No

Accreditation Certification
NCQA
TJC Accreditation, Medicare Approved, Utilization Review, Pre-Admission Certification, State Licensure, Quality Assurance Program

Key Personnel
CFO & CAO . . . . Kelly Hamilton
Medical Director . . . . Rob Cooper, MD
Dir, Pharmacy Benefits . . . . Greg Wilson
Chief Information Officer . . . . Tom Gessells
Dir, Mkting/Communication . . . . Susan Meyer

Specialty Managed Care Partners
Enters into Contracts with Regional Business Coalitions: No

Employer References
Ohio State University

---

616 OhioHealth Group
155 East Broad Street
Suite 1700
Columbus, OH 43215
Toll-Free: 800-455-4460
Phone: 614-566-0056
www.ohiohealthgroup.com
For Profit Organization: Yes
Year Founded: 1985
Physician Owned Organization: Yes
Number of Affiliated Hospitals: 75
Number of Primary Care Physicians: 6,900
Total Enrollment: 100,000
State Enrollment: 100,000

Healthplan and Services Defined
PLAN TYPE: PPO
Model Type: TPA
Benefits Offered: Disease Management, Prescription, Wellness

Type of Coverage
Commercial, Individual

Geographic Areas Served
Statewide

Peer Review Type
Utilization Review: Yes
Case Management: Yes

617 Paramount Elite Medicare Plan

1901 Indian Wood Circle
Maumee, OH 43537
Toll-Free: 800-462-3589
Phone: 419-887-2525
Fax: 419-887-2039
paramount.memberservices@promedica.org
www.paramounthealthcare.com
Mailing Address: P.O. Box 928, Toledo, OH 43697-0928
Year Founded: 1988
Number of Affiliated Hospitals: 34
Number of Primary Care Physicians: 1,900
Total Enrollment: 187,000

Healthplan and Services Defined
PLAN TYPE: Medicare
Other Type: HMO
Benefits Offered: Chiropractic, Dental, Disease Management,
Home Care, Inpatient SNF, Physical Therapy, Podiatry,
Prescription, Psychiatric, Vision

Type of Coverage
Individual, Medicare

Geographic Areas Served
Ohio: Lucas and Wood counties; Michigan: Monroe County

Subscriber Information
Average Monthly Fee Per Subscriber
(Employee + Employer Contribution):
Employee Only (Self): Varies
Medicare: Varies
Average Annual Deductible Per Subscriber:
Employee Only (Self): Varies
Medicare: Varies
Average Subscriber Co-Payment:
Primary Care Physician: Varies
Non-Network Physician: Varies
Prescription Drugs: Varies
Hospital ER: Varies
Home Health Care: Varies
Home Health Care Max. Days/Visits Covered: Varies
Nursing Home: Varies
Nursing Home Max. Days/Visits Covered: Varies

Key Personnel
President. . . . . John C Randolph
VP, Financial Officer . . . . Stacey Bock
Dir., Care Management. . . . . Deb Woody
VP, Medical Services. . . . . John Meier

618 Paramount Health Care

1901 Indian Wood Circle
Maumee, OH 43537
Toll-Free: 800-462-3589
Phone: 419-887-2500
Fax: 419-887-2017
paramount.marketing@promedica.org
www.paramounthealthcare.com
Secondary Address: 106 Park Place, Dundee, MI 48131,
734-529-7800
Subsidiary of: ProMedica Health System

For Profit Organization: Yes
Year Founded: 1988
Number of Affiliated Hospitals: 34
Number of Primary Care Physicians: 1,900
Number of Referral/Specialty Physicians: 900
Total Enrollment: 187,000

Healthplan and Services Defined
PLAN TYPE: HMO/PPO
Model Type: Network
Benefits Offered: Prescription

Geographic Areas Served
Northwest Ohio and Southeast Michigan

Subscriber Information
Average Monthly Fee Per Subscriber
(Employee + Employer Contribution):
Employee Only (Self): Varies by plan
Average Annual Deductible Per Subscriber:
Employee Only (Self): Varies
Employee & 1 Family Member: Varies
Employee & 2 Family Members: Varies
Average Subscriber Co-Payment:
Primary Care Physician: Varies
Prescription Drugs: Varies
Hospital ER: $25.00
Home Health Care: $0
Home Health Care Max. Days/Visits Covered: Unlimited
Nursing Home: $0
Nursing Home Max. Days/Visits Covered: 100 days

Network Qualifications
Pre-Admission Certification: Yes

Peer Review Type
Second Surgical Opinion: Yes

Publishes and Distributes Report Card: Yes

Accreditation Certification
URAC, NCQA

Key Personnel
President. . . . . John C Randolph
VP, Financial Officer . . . . Stacey Bock
Dir., Care Management. . . . . Deb Woody
VP, Medical Services. . . . . John Meier

619 Prime Time Health Medicare Plan

214 Dartmouth Avenue SW
Canton, OH 44710
Toll-Free: 800-577-5084
Phone: 330-363-7407
www.primetimehealthplan.com
Mailing Address: P.O. Box 6905, Canton, OH 44706
Subsidiary of: Aultcare
Year Founded: 1997
Total Enrollment: 20,000
State Enrollment: 20,000

Healthplan and Services Defined
PLAN TYPE: Medicare

Benefits Offered: Chiropractic, Dental, Disease Management, Home Care, Inpatient SNF, Physical Therapy, Podiatry, Prescription, Psychiatric, Vision, Wellness

Type of Coverage
Individual, Medicare, Medicaid

Geographic Areas Served
Portage, Medina, Summit, Stark, Carroll, Columbiana, Holmes, Harrison, Trumbull, Mahoning, Tuscarawas and Wayne counties

Subscriber Information
Average Monthly Fee Per Subscriber
  (Employee + Employer Contribution):
    Employee Only (Self): Varies
    Medicare: Varies
Average Annual Deductible Per Subscriber:
    Employee Only (Self): Varies
    Medicare: Varies
Average Subscriber Co-Payment:
    Primary Care Physician: Varies
    Non-Network Physician: Varies
    Prescription Drugs: Varies
    Hospital ER: Varies
    Home Health Care: Varies
    Home Health Care Max. Days/Visits Covered: Varies
    Nursing Home: Varies
    Nursing Home Max. Days/Visits Covered: Varies

Key Personnel
President/CEO . . . . Rick Haines

---

620 S&S HealthCare Strategies

1385 Kemper Meadow Drive
Cincinnati, OH 45240
Toll-Free: 800-717-2872
Fax: 513-772-9174
servicedesk@ss-healthcare.com
www.ss-healthcare.com
Subsidiary of: International Managed Care Strategies
Year Founded: 1994

Healthplan and Services Defined
  PLAN TYPE: Other
  Plan Specialty: Third Party Administrator
  Benefits Offered: Dental, Prescription, Vision

Type of Payment Plans Offered
POS, DFFS, FFS

Peer Review Type
Second Surgical Opinion: No
Case Management: No

Publishes and Distributes Report Card: Yes

Specialty Managed Care Partners
Enters into Contracts with Regional Business Coalitions: Yes

---

621 SummaCare Medicare Advantage Plan

10 North Main Street
Akron, OH 44308
Toll-Free: 800-996-8411
www.summacare.com

Subsidiary of: Summa Health System
For Profit Organization: Yes
Year Founded: 1993
Physician Owned Organization: Yes
Number of Affiliated Hospitals: 60
Number of Primary Care Physicians: 10,000
Total Enrollment: 26,000
State Enrollment: 73,724

Healthplan and Services Defined
  PLAN TYPE: Medicare
  Model Type: IPA, PPO, POS
  Benefits Offered: Behavioral Health, Chiropractic, Complementary Medicine, Dental, Disease Management, Home Care, Inpatient SNF, Physical Therapy, Podiatry, Prescription, Psychiatric, Transplant, Vision, Wellness, AD&D, Life
  Offers Demand Management Patient Information Service: Yes
  DMPI Services Offered: Nurses Line

Type of Coverage
Medicare
Catastrophic Illness Benefit: Covered

Type of Payment Plans Offered
POS, DFFS, FFS

Geographic Areas Served
Northeast Ohio: Cuyahoga, Geauga, Medina, Portage, Stark, Summit, Wayne, Tuscarawas, Ashtabula, Caroll, Mahoning, Trumbull & Lorain counties

Subscriber Information
Average Monthly Fee Per Subscriber
  (Employee + Employer Contribution):
    Employee Only (Self): Proprietary
Average Annual Deductible Per Subscriber:
    Employee Only (Self): $0
    Employee & 1 Family Member: $0
    Employee & 2 Family Members: $0
    Medicare: $45.00
Average Subscriber Co-Payment:
    Primary Care Physician: $5.00/10.00
    Prescription Drugs: $5.00/10.00
    Hospital ER: $50.00
    Home Health Care: $0 if in-network
    Home Health Care Max. Days/Visits Covered: 30 days
    Nursing Home: $0 if in-network
    Nursing Home Max. Days/Visits Covered: 100 days

Network Qualifications
Pre-Admission Certification: Yes

Peer Review Type
Utilization Review: Yes
Second Surgical Opinion: Yes
Case Management: Yes

Accreditation Certification
NCQA
TJC Accreditation, Medicare Approved, Utilization Review, Pre-Admission Certification, State Licensure, Quality Assurance Program

Key Personnel
President . . . . Claude Vincenti

Specialty Managed Care Partners
Enters into Contracts with Regional Business Coalitions: Yes
Akron Regional Development Board, Canton Regional
Chamber of Commerce, Home Builders Association

Employer References
Goodyear, Summa Health System, Cuyahoga County,
University of Akron, Akron Public Schools

622 Superior Dental Care
6683 Centerville Business Parkway
Centerville, OH 45459
Toll-Free: 800-762-3159
Phone: 937-438-0283
www.superiordental.com
Year Founded: 1986
Physician Owned Organization: Yes

Healthplan and Services Defined
PLAN TYPE: Dental
Model Type: Network, POS
Plan Specialty: Dental
Benefits Offered: Dental, Vision

Type of Payment Plans Offered
FFS

Geographic Areas Served
Ohio, Kentucky and Indiana

Publishes and Distributes Report Card: Yes

Key Personnel
Chairman . . . . Richard W. Portune
President . . . . L. Don Shumaker

623 The Dental Care Plus Group
100 Crowne Point Place
Cincinnati, OH 45241
Toll-Free: 800-367-9466
Phone: 513-554-1100
Fax: 513-554-3187
www.dentalcareplus.com
For Profit Organization: Yes
Year Founded: 1986
Physician Owned Organization: Yes
Number of Primary Care Physicians: 246,000
Total Enrollment: 300,000

Healthplan and Services Defined
PLAN TYPE: Multiple
Model Type: IPA
Plan Specialty: Dental, Vision
Benefits Offered: Dental, Vision

Type of Payment Plans Offered
POS

Geographic Areas Served
Ohio, Kentucky and Indiana

Peer Review Type
Utilization Review: Yes

Key Personnel
President and CEO . . . . Anthony A. Cook

VP, Financial Officer . . . . Robert C. Hodgkins, Jr.
Chief Operating Officer . . . . Jodi Fronczek
Chief Information Officer. . . . . Tom Koch
Dir., Provider Relations . . . . Sherri Bode
Director of Sales . . . . Jodi Duncan

624 The Health Plan of the Ohio Valley/Mountaineer Region
52160 National Road E
St Clairsville, OH 43950
Phone: 800-624-6961
mtharp@healthplan.org
www.healthplan.org
Non-Profit Organization: Yes
Year Founded: 1979
Federally Qualified: Yes
Number of Affiliated Hospitals: 63
Number of Primary Care Physicians: 4,000
Number of Referral/Specialty Physicians: 1,000
Total Enrollment: 380,000
State Enrollment: 380,000

Healthplan and Services Defined
PLAN TYPE: HMO/PPO
Other Type: POS
Model Type: IPA
Plan Specialty: ASO, Disease Management, Worker's
Compensation, UR, TPA
Benefits Offered: Behavioral Health, Chiropractic, Disease
Management, Home Care, Inpatient SNF, Physical Therapy,
Podiatry, Prescription, Psychiatric, Transplant, Vision,
Worker's Compensation, AD&D, Life, LTD, STD
Offers Demand Management Patient Information Service: No

Type of Coverage
Individual, Medicare, Medicaid
Catastrophic Illness Benefit: Unlimited

Type of Payment Plans Offered
POS, DFFS

Geographic Areas Served
Ohio & Central West Virginia

Subscriber Information
Average Monthly Fee Per Subscriber
(Employee + Employer Contribution):
Employee Only (Self): Varies
Medicare: Varies
Average Annual Deductible Per Subscriber:
Employee Only (Self): Varies
Medicare: Varies
Average Subscriber Co-Payment:
Primary Care Physician: Varies
Non-Network Physician: Varies
Prescription Drugs: Varies
Hospital ER: Varies
Home Health Care: Varies
Home Health Care Max. Days/Visits Covered: Varies
Nursing Home: Varies
Nursing Home Max. Days/Visits Covered: Varies

Network Qualifications
Pre-Admission Certification: Yes

Peer Review Type
Utilization Review: Yes
Second Surgical Opinion: Yes
Case Management: Yes

Publishes and Distributes Report Card: Yes

Accreditation Certification
NCQA
TJC Accreditation, Medicare Approved, Utilization Review,
Pre-Admission Certification, State Licensure, Quality
Assurance Program

Key Personnel
President & CEO . . . . James M. Pennington
Chief Financial Officer . . . . Jeffrey M. Knight
VP of Operations . . . . Patricia Fast
VP of Clinical Services . . . . John Fischer
Chief Information Officer . . . . Bob Roset
Human Resources . . . . Carla Bell

625   Trinity Health of Ohio

Mount Carmel Health System
6001 E Broad Street
Columbus, OH 43213
Phone: 614-234-6000
www.trinity-health.org
Subsidiary of: Trinity Health
Non-Profit Organization: Yes
Year Founded: 2013
Total Enrollment: 30,000,000

Healthplan and Services Defined
PLAN TYPE: Other
Benefits Offered: Disease Management, Home Care,
Long-Term Care, Psychiatric, Hospice programs, PACE
(Program of All Inclusive Care for the Elderly)

Geographic Areas Served
Greater Central Ohio

Key Personnel
Chief Executive Officer . . . . Richard J. Gilfillan
Chief Financial Officer . . . . Benjamin R. Carter
General Counsel . . . . Paul G. Neumann
Chief Clinical Officer . . . . Daniel J. Roth
Chief Operating Officer . . . . Michael A. Slubowski

626   UnitedHealthcare of Ohio

North Point Tower, 1001 Lakeside Avenue
Suite 1000
Cleveland, OH 44114
Toll-Free: 800-468-5001
Phone: 216-694-4080
www.uhc.com/contact-us/ohio
Subsidiary of: UnitedHealth Group
For Profit Organization: Yes
Year Founded: 1980

Healthplan and Services Defined
PLAN TYPE: HMO/PPO

Model Type: Network
Plan Specialty: Behavioral Health, Dental, Disease
Management, PBM, Vision
Benefits Offered: Behavioral Health, Dental, Disease
Management, Long-Term Care, Prescription, Vision,
Wellness, Life, LTD, STD

Type of Coverage
Individual, Medicare, Supplemental Medicare, Medicaid,
Catastrophic, Family, Military, Veterans, Group,

Geographic Areas Served
Statewide

Subscriber Information
Average Subscriber Co-Payment:
Primary Care Physician: $15.00
Prescription Drugs: $15.00

Accreditation Certification
NCQA

Key Personnel
President . . . . David Wichmann
Chief Operating Officer . . . . Dan Schumacher
Chief Strategy Officer . . . . John Cosgriff
Communications Officer . . . . Kirsten Gorsuch
Chief Medical Officer . . . . Sam Ho
Chief Legal Officer . . . . Thad Johnson
Chief Information Officer . . . . Phil McKoy
Chief Financial Officer . . . . Jeff Putnam

Health Insurance Coverage Status and Type of Coverage by Age

Category	All Persons		Under 18 years		Under 65 years	
	Number	%	Number	%	Number	%
Total population	3,846	-	1,018	-	3,277	-
Covered by some type of health insurance	3,316 (13)	86.2 (0.3)	939 (6)	92.3 (0.5)	2,750 (12)	83.9 (0.4)
Covered by private health insurance	2,461 (18)	64.0 (0.5)	530 (10)	52.1 (1.0)	2,106 (18)	64.3 (0.5)
Employer-based	1,915 (18)	49.8 (0.5)	436 (10)	42.9 (1.0)	1,741 (18)	53.1 (0.5)
Direct purchase	538 (10)	14.0 (0.3)	77 (4)	7.6 (0.4)	347 (9)	10.6 (0.3)
TRICARE	150 (8)	3.9 (0.2)	33 (4)	3.3 (0.4)	101 (7)	3.1 (0.2)
Covered by public health insurance	1,329 (14)	34.6 (0.4)	456 (9)	44.8 (0.9)	776 (13)	23.7 (0.4)
Medicaid	698 (14)	18.2 (0.4)	436 (10)	42.9 (1.0)	634 (14)	19.3 (0.4)
Medicare	686 (5)	17.8 (0.1)	23 (3)	2.2 (0.3)	133 (5)	4.1 (0.1)
VA Care	129 (5)	3.3 (0.1)	2 (1)	0.2 (0.1)	61 (3)	1.9 (0.1)
Not covered at any time during the year	530 (13)	13.8 (0.3)	79 (5)	7.7 (0.5)	526 (13)	16.1 (0.4)

Note: Numbers in thousands; Figures cover civilian noninstitutionalized population in 2016; N/A indicates that data was not available; Z represents or rounds to zero; Margin of error appears in parenthesis and is calculated using replicate weights.
Source: U.S. Census Bureau, American Community Survey, Table HIC-4_ACS. Health Insurance Coverage Status and Type of Coverage by State—All People: 2008 to 2016, Table HIC-5_ACS. Health Insurance Coverage Status and Type of Coverage by State—Children Under 18: 2008 to 2016, Table HIC-6_ACS. Health Insurance Coverage Status and Type of Coverage by State—Persons Under 65: 2008 to 2016

Oklahoma

627 Aetna Health of Oklahoma

151 Farmington Avenue
Hartford, CT 06156
Toll-Free: 800-872-3862
Phone: 860-273-0123
www.aetna.com
Subsidiary of: Aetna Inc.
For Profit Organization: Yes

Healthplan and Services Defined
PLAN TYPE: HMO/PPO
Other Type: POS
Model Type: Network
Plan Specialty: Behavioral Health, EPO, Lab, PBM,
Radiology
Benefits Offered: Behavioral Health, Dental, Disease
Management, Long-Term Care, Physical Therapy,
Podiatry, Prescription, Psychiatric, Vision, Wellness, Life,
LTD, STD

Type of Coverage
Commercial, Student health

Geographic Areas Served
Statewide

628 Ascension At Home

Jane Phillips Regional Home Care
219 N Virginia
Bartlesville, OK 74003
Phone: 918-907-3010
Fax: 844-721-8184
ascensionathome.com
Subsidiary of: Ascension
Non-Profit Organization: Yes

Healthplan and Services Defined
PLAN TYPE: Other
Plan Specialty: Disease Management
Benefits Offered: Dental, Disease Management, Home Care,
Wellness, Ambulance & Transportation; Nursing Service;
Short-and-long-term care management planning; Hospice

Geographic Areas Served
Texas, Alabama, Indiana, Kansas, Michigan, Mississippi,
Oklahoma, Wisconsin

Key Personnel
President. . . . . Kirk Allen
Dir., Home Health Service. . . . . Darcy Burthay

629 Blue Cross & Blue Shield of Oklahoma

1400 S Boston
Tulsa, OK 74119
Toll-Free: 800-942-5837
Phone: 918-551-3500
www.bcbsok.com
Mailing Address: P.O. Box 3283, Tulsa, OK 74102-3283
Non-Profit Organization: Yes
Year Founded: 1940

Number of Affiliated Hospitals: 88
Number of Primary Care Physicians: 1,551
Number of Referral/Specialty Physicians: 6,000
Total Enrollment: 600,000
State Enrollment: 600,000

Healthplan and Services Defined
PLAN TYPE: HMO/PPO
Model Type: IPA
Plan Specialty: ASO, Behavioral Health, Chiropractic, Dental,
Disease Management, Lab, MSO, PBM, Vision, Radiology,
UR
Benefits Offered: Behavioral Health, Chiropractic, Dental,
Disease Management, Home Care, Inpatient SNF,
Long-Term Care, Physical Therapy, Podiatry, Prescription,
Psychiatric, Transplant, Vision, Worker's Compensation,
Life, LTD, STD

Type of Coverage
Commercial, Individual, Indemnity, Medicare, Supplemental
Medicare, Student health, Short-term

Type of Payment Plans Offered
POS, FFS

Geographic Areas Served
Statewide

Subscriber Information
Average Annual Deductible Per Subscriber:
Employee Only (Self): $500.00
Average Subscriber Co-Payment:
Primary Care Physician: $10.00
Prescription Drugs: 10/20/30%

Network Qualifications
Pre-Admission Certification: Yes

Peer Review Type
Utilization Review: Yes
Second Surgical Opinion: Yes
Case Management: Yes

Accreditation Certification
URAC

Key Personnel
President. . . . . Ted Haynes
VP of Sales & Marketing. . . . . Stephania Grober
Media Contact . . . . Lauren Cusick
918-551-2002
lauren_cusick@bcbsok.com

Specialty Managed Care Partners
Enters into Contracts with Regional Business Coalitions: Yes

Employer References
Federal Employee Program, The Williams Companies,
OneOK, Helmerich & Payne, Bank of Oklahoma

630 Cigna HealthCare of Oklahoma

900 Cottage Grove Road
Bloomfield, CT 06002
Toll-Free: 800-997-1654
www.cigna.com
For Profit Organization: Yes

Healthplan and Services Defined
  PLAN TYPE: HMO/PPO
  Plan Specialty: Behavioral Health, Dental, Vision
  Benefits Offered: Behavioral Health, Dental, Disease
    Management, Prescription, Vision, AD&D, Life, LTD,
    STD

Type of Coverage
  Commercial, Individual

Type of Payment Plans Offered
  POS

Accreditation Certification
  URAC, NCQA

Key Personnel
  President/CEO . . . . David M. Cordani

631 Cigna HealthCare of Tennessee

900 Cottage Grove Road
Bloomfield, CT 06002
Toll-Free: 800-997-1654
www.cigna.com
For Profit Organization: Yes

Healthplan and Services Defined
  PLAN TYPE: HMO/PPO
  Plan Specialty: Behavioral Health, Dental, Vision
  Benefits Offered: Behavioral Health, Dental, Disease
    Management, Prescription, Vision, AD&D, Life, LTD,
    STD

Type of Coverage
  Commercial, Individual

Type of Payment Plans Offered
  POS

Key Personnel
  President & CEO . . . . David M. Cordina

632 CommunityCare

218 W 6th Street
Tulsa, OK 74119
Toll-Free: 800-278-7563
Phone: 918-594-5200
ccare@ccok.com
www.ccok.com
For Profit Organization: Yes
Total Enrollment: 500,000

Healthplan and Services Defined
  PLAN TYPE: Multiple
  Benefits Offered: Disease Management, Prescription, Vision,
    Wellness

Type of Coverage
  Commercial, Medicare, Supplemental Medicare

Type of Payment Plans Offered
  POS

Geographic Areas Served
  Oklahoma

633 Delta Dental of Oklahoma

16 NW 63rd Street
Oklahoma City, OK 73116
Toll-Free: 800-522-0188
Phone: 405-607-2100
customerservice@deltadentalok.org
www.deltadentalok.org
Secondary Address: Customer Service Department, P.O. Box
  54709, Oklahoma City, OK 73154-1709
Non-Profit Organization: Yes
Year Founded: 1973
Number of Primary Care Physicians: 1,500
Total Enrollment: 1,000,000

Healthplan and Services Defined
  PLAN TYPE: Dental
  Other Type: Dental PPO
  Model Type: Network
  Plan Specialty: ASO, Dental
  Benefits Offered: Dental

Type of Coverage
  Commercial, Individual, Group
  Catastrophic Illness Benefit: None

Geographic Areas Served
  Statewide

Subscriber Information
  Average Subscriber Co-Payment:
    Prescription Drugs: $0
    Home Health Care: $0
    Nursing Home: $0

Key Personnel
  President & CEO . . . . John Gladden
  Chief Financial Officer . . . . Frank Turbeville
  Chief Operating Officer . . . . Tania Graham
  Chief Information Officer . . . . David Jones
  Vice President of Sales . . . . Lan Miller

634 HCSC Insurance Services Company

1400 S Boston Avenue
Tulsa, OK 74119
Phone: 918-560-3500
hcsc.com
Subsidiary of: Blue Cross Blue Shield Association
Non-Profit Organization: Yes
Year Founded: 1936
Number of Primary Care Physicians: 15,600

Healthplan and Services Defined
  PLAN TYPE: HMO
  Benefits Offered: Behavioral Health, Dental, Disease
    Management, Psychiatric, Wellness

Geographic Areas Served
  Statewide

Key Personnel
  President & CEO . . . . Paula Steiner
  EVP, Plan Operations . . . . Colleen Reitan
  SVP, Clinical Officer . . . . Opella Ernest, MD
  SVP, Financial Officer . . . . Eric Feldstein

SVP, Compliance Officer . . . . Thomas Lubben
SVP, Human Resources . . . . Nazneen Razi
SVP, Chief Legal Officer . . . . Blair Todt
Media Contact . . . . Kristen Cunningham
 312-653-1686
 kristen_cunningham@hcsc.net
Media Contact . . . . Greg Thompson
 312-653-7583
 greg_thompson@hcsc.net

635 Humana Health Insurance of Oklahoma

7104 S Sheridan
Suite 10A
Tulsa, OK 74133
Toll-Free: 800-681-0637
Phone: 918-477-9357
Fax: 918-499-2297
www.humana.com
Subsidiary of: Humana
For Profit Organization: Yes

Healthplan and Services Defined
 PLAN TYPE: HMO/PPO
 Model Type: Network
 Plan Specialty: Dental, Vision
 Benefits Offered: Dental, Vision, Life, LTD, STD

Type of Coverage
 Commercial, Individual

Geographic Areas Served
 Statewide

Accreditation Certification
 URAC, NCQA, CORE

Key Personnel
 President & CEO . . . . Bruce Broussard
 Chief Medical Officer . . . . Roy A. Beveridge
 Chief Consumer Officer . . . . Jody L. Bilney
 Human Resources . . . . Tim Huval
 Chief Financial Officer . . . . Brian Kane
 Chief Information Officer . . . . Brian LeClaire
 General Counsel . . . . Christopher M. Todoroff
 Chief Accounting Officer . . . . Cynthia H. Zipperie

636 Mercy Clinic Oklahoma

500 N Clarence Nash Boulevard
Watonga, OK 73772
Phone: 580-623-7211
mercy.net
Subsidiary of: IBM Watson Health
Non-Profit Organization: Yes
Number of Affiliated Hospitals: 44
Number of Primary Care Physicians: 700
Number of Referral/Specialty Physicians: 2,000

Healthplan and Services Defined
 PLAN TYPE: HMO
 Benefits Offered: Behavioral Health, Disease Management,
 Home Care, Inpatient SNF, Physical Therapy, Podiatry,
 Vision, Wellness, Non-Surgical Weight Loss; Urgent Care;

Dermatology; Rehabilitation; Breast Cancer; Orthopedics;
 Ostoclerosis; Pediatrics

Geographic Areas Served
 Arkansas, Kansas, Missouri, and Oklahoma

Key Personnel
 General Manager . . . . Deborah DiSanzo

637 UnitedHealthcare of Oklahoma

5800 Granite Parkway
Suite 700
Plano, TX 75024
Toll-Free: 800-842-2481
www.uhc.com/contact-us/oklahoma
Subsidiary of: UnitedHealth Group
For Profit Organization: Yes
Year Founded: 1986

Healthplan and Services Defined
 PLAN TYPE: HMO/PPO
 Model Type: Network
 Plan Specialty: Behavioral Health, Dental, Disease
 Management, PBM, Vision
 Benefits Offered: Behavioral Health, Dental, Disease
 Management, Long-Term Care, Prescription, Vision,
 Wellness, AD&D, Life, LTD, STD

Type of Coverage
 Commercial, Individual, Medicare, Supplemental Medicare,
 Medicaid, Catastrophic, Family, Military, Veterans, Group,

Geographic Areas Served
 Statewide. Oklahoma is covered by the Texas branch

Network Qualifications
 Pre-Admission Certification: Yes

Publishes and Distributes Report Card: Yes

Accreditation Certification
 AAPI, NCQA

Key Personnel
 Chief Executive Officer . . . . David Wichmann
 Chief Operating Officer . . . . Dan Schumacher
 Chief Strategy Officer . . . . John Cosgriff
 Communications Officer . . . . Kirsten Gorsuch
 Chief Medical Officer . . . . Sam Ho
 Chief Legal Officer . . . . Thad Johnson
 Chief Information Officer . . . . Phil McKoy
 Chief Financial Officer . . . . Jeff Putnam

Specialty Managed Care Partners
 Enters into Contracts with Regional Business Coalitions: Yes

Health Insurance Coverage Status and Type of Coverage by Age

Category	All Persons		Under 18 years		Under 65 years	
	Number	%	Number	%	Number	%
Total population	4,054	-	920	-	3,376	-
Covered by some type of health insurance	3,802 *(10)*	93.8 *(0.2)*	889 *(5)*	96.6 *(0.5)*	3,128 *(10)*	92.7 *(0.3)*
Covered by private health insurance	2,768 *(22)*	68.3 *(0.5)*	566 *(11)*	61.5 *(1.2)*	2,338 *(21)*	69.3 *(0.6)*
Employer-based	2,168 *(25)*	53.5 *(0.6)*	491 *(12)*	53.3 *(1.3)*	1,979 *(25)*	58.6 *(0.7)*
Direct purchase	660 *(14)*	16.3 *(0.3)*	82 *(6)*	8.9 *(0.6)*	396 *(13)*	11.7 *(0.4)*
TRICARE	81 *(6)*	2.0 *(0.1)*	10 *(3)*	1.1 *(0.3)*	40 *(4)*	1.2 *(0.1)*
Covered by public health insurance	1,614 *(21)*	39.8 *(0.5)*	373 *(12)*	40.6 *(1.2)*	958 *(22)*	28.4 *(0.6)*
Medicaid	947 *(23)*	23.3 *(0.6)*	371 *(12)*	40.3 *(1.2)*	867 *(22)*	25.7 *(0.7)*
Medicare	753 *(6)*	18.6 *(0.2)*	3 *(1)*	0.3 *(0.1)*	99 *(6)*	2.9 *(0.2)*
VA Care	131 *(5)*	3.2 *(0.1)*	3 *(1)*	0.3 *(0.1)*	59 *(4)*	1.7 *(0.1)*
Not covered at any time during the year	253 *(10)*	6.2 *(0.2)*	31 *(4)*	3.4 *(0.5)*	248 *(10)*	7.3 *(0.3)*

Note: Numbers in thousands; Figures cover civilian noninstitutionalized population in 2016; N/A indicates that data was not available; Z represents or rounds to zero; Margin of error appears in parenthesis and is calculated using replicate weights.
Source: U.S. Census Bureau, American Community Survey, Table HIC-4_ACS. Health Insurance Coverage Status and Type of Coverage by State—All People: 2008 to 2016, Table HIC-5_ACS. Health Insurance Coverage Status and Type of Coverage by State—Children Under 18: 2008 to 2016, Table HIC-6_ACS. Health Insurance Coverage Status and Type of Coverage by State—Persons Under 65: 2008 to 2016

Oregon

638 Aetna Health of Oregon

151 Farmington Avenue
Hartford, CT 06156
Toll-Free: 800-872-3862
Phone: 860-273-0123
www.aetna.com
Subsidiary of: Aetna Inc.
For Profit Organization: Yes

Healthplan and Services Defined
PLAN TYPE: PPO
Other Type: POS
Model Type: Network
Plan Specialty: Behavioral Health, EPO, Lab, PBM,
    Radiology
Benefits Offered: Behavioral Health, Disease Management,
    Long-Term Care, Physical Therapy, Podiatry, Prescription,
    Psychiatric, Wellness, Life, LTD, STD

Type of Coverage
Commercial, Student health

Type of Payment Plans Offered
POS, FFS

Geographic Areas Served
Statewide

Key Personnel
CEO . . . . Mark Bertolini

639 AllCare Health

1701 NE 7th Street
Grants Pass, OR 97526
Toll-Free: 888-460-0185
Phone: 541-471-4106
Fax: 541-471-1524
info@allcarehealth.com
www.allcarehealth.com
Secondary Address: 3629 Aviation Way, Medford, OR 97504
Year Founded: 1995
Number of Primary Care Physicians: 1,500
Total Enrollment: 54,000
State Enrollment: 54,000

Healthplan and Services Defined
PLAN TYPE: Medicare
Plan Specialty: Medicaid
Benefits Offered: Chiropractic, Dental, Disease Management,
    Home Care, Inpatient SNF, Physical Therapy, Podiatry,
    Prescription, Psychiatric, Vision, Wellness

Type of Coverage
Individual, Medicare, Medicaid

Geographic Areas Served
Southern Oregon (Josephine, Jackson, Curry counties and
    Glendale and Azalea in Douglas County)

Subscriber Information
Average Monthly Fee Per Subscriber
    (Employee + Employer Contribution):
    Employee Only (Self): Varies

Medicare: Varies
Average Annual Deductible Per Subscriber:
    Employee Only (Self): Varies
    Medicare: Varies
Average Subscriber Co-Payment:
    Primary Care Physician: Varies
    Non-Network Physician: Varies
    Prescription Drugs: Varies
    Hospital ER: Varies
    Home Health Care: Varies
    Home Health Care Max. Days/Visits Covered: Varies
    Nursing Home: Varies
    Nursing Home Max. Days/Visits Covered: Varies

Key Personnel
Chair . . . . Richard Williams
Secretary/Treasurer . . . . Susan Seereiter

640 Atrio Health Plans

2270 NW Aviation Drive
Suite 3
Roseburg, OR 97470
Toll-Free: 877-672-8620
Fax: 541-672-8670
www.atriohp.com
Secondary Address: 3025 Ryan Drive SE, Salem, OR 97701

Healthplan and Services Defined
PLAN TYPE: Medicare
Other Type: HMO, PPO
Benefits Offered: Chiropractic, Dental, Disease Management,
    Home Care, Inpatient SNF, Physical Therapy, Podiatry,
    Prescription, Psychiatric, Vision, Wellness

Type of Coverage
Individual, Medicare

Geographic Areas Served
Douglas, Klamath, Josephine, Jackson, Marion, Polk, and
    Deschutes counties

Subscriber Information
Average Monthly Fee Per Subscriber
    (Employee + Employer Contribution):
    Employee Only (Self): Varies
    Medicare: Varies
Average Annual Deductible Per Subscriber:
    Employee Only (Self): Varies
    Medicare: Varies
Average Subscriber Co-Payment:
    Primary Care Physician: Varies
    Non-Network Physician: Varies
    Prescription Drugs: Varies
    Hospital ER: Varies
    Home Health Care: Varies
    Home Health Care Max. Days/Visits Covered: Varies
    Nursing Home: Varies
    Nursing Home Max. Days/Visits Covered: Varies

Accreditation Certification
URAC

641   CareOregon Health Plan

315 SW Fifth Avenue
Portland, OR 97204
Toll-Free: 800-224-4840
Phone: 503-416-4100
www.careoregon.org
Non-Profit Organization: Yes
Year Founded: 1993
Number of Affiliated Hospitals: 33
Number of Primary Care Physicians: 950
Number of Referral/Specialty Physicians: 3,000
Total Enrollment: 250,000
State Enrollment: 250,000

Healthplan and Services Defined
  PLAN TYPE: Medicare
  Plan Specialty: Dental
  Benefits Offered: Dental, Prescription, Vision, Wellness,
    Maternity and Family Planning

Type of Coverage
Medicare

Geographic Areas Served
20 counties in Oregon. careOregon Advantage is available
for residents of Clackamas, Clatsop, Columbia, Jackson,
Josephine, Marion, Multnomah, Polk and Washington
counties

Key Personnel
President & CEO . . . . Eric C Hunter
Chief Network Officer . . . . Greg Morgan
Chief Operating Officer . . . . Katherine Ellis
Chief Medical Officer . . . . Amit Shah, MD
Director, Human Resources . . . . Chantay Reid
Communications Manager . . . . Jeanie Lunsford
  503-416-3626
  lunsfordj@careoregon.org

642   Dental Health Services of Oregon

205 SE Spokane Street
Suite 334
Portland, OR 97202
Toll-Free: 800-637-6453
Phone: 503-281-1771
Fax: 503-968-0187
www.dentalhealthservices.com
Secondary Address: 100 West Harrison Street, Suite S-440,
South Tower, Seattle, WA 98119, 206-633-2300
For Profit Organization: Yes
Year Founded: 1974

Healthplan and Services Defined
  PLAN TYPE: Dental
  Plan Specialty: Dental
  Benefits Offered: Dental

Geographic Areas Served
California, Oregon, and Washington State

Accreditation Certification
URAC, NCQA

Key Personnel
Founder & Chairman . . . . Godfrey Pernell

643   First Choice Health

11000 SW Stratus Street
Suite 325
Beaverton, OR 97008-7104
Phone: 877-287-2922
Fax: 503-652-8087
contact@fchn.com
www.fchn.com
For Profit Organization: Yes
Year Founded: 1996
Number of Affiliated Hospitals: 94
Number of Primary Care Physicians: 980
Number of Referral/Specialty Physicians: 1,793

Healthplan and Services Defined
  PLAN TYPE: PPO
  Benefits Offered: Wellness

Type of Coverage
Commercial, Individual, Private & Public Plans, Geo-specifi

Geographic Areas Served
Washington, Oregon, Alaska, Idaho, Montana, Wyoming, and
select areas of North Dakota and South Dakota

Key Personnel
Chief Executive Officer . . . . Robert L. Hunter

644   Humana Health Insurance of Oregon

1498 SE Tech Center Pl
Suite 300
Vancouver, WA 98683
Toll-Free: 800-781-4203
Phone: 360-253-7523
Fax: 360-253-7524
www.humana.com
Subsidiary of: Humana
For Profit Organization: Yes

Healthplan and Services Defined
  PLAN TYPE: HMO/PPO
  Model Type: Network
  Plan Specialty: Dental, Vision
  Benefits Offered: Dental, Disease Management, Prescription,
    Vision, Wellness, Life, LTD, STD

Type of Coverage
Commercial

Accreditation Certification
URAC, NCQA, CORE

Key Personnel
President & CEO . . . . Bruce Broussard
Chief Medical Officer . . . . Roy A. Beveridge
Chief Consumer Officer . . . . Jody L. Bilney
Human Resources . . . . Tim Huval
Chief Financial Officer . . . . Brian Kane
Chief Information Officer . . . . Brian LeClaire
General Counsel . . . . Christopher M. Todoroff
Chief Accounting Officer . . . . Cynthia H. Zipperie

645 Kaiser Permanente Northwest

500 NE Multnomah Street
Suite 100
Portland, OR 97232
thrive.kaiserpermanente.org/care-near-oregon-washington
Subsidiary of: Kaiser Permanente
Non-Profit Organization: Yes
Year Founded: 1977
Number of Primary Care Physicians: 880
State Enrollment: 523,967

Healthplan and Services Defined
PLAN TYPE: HMO
Model Type: Network
Plan Specialty: Dental, Lab, Radiology
Benefits Offered: Behavioral Health, Dental, Disease
    Management, Prescription, Vision, Wellness, Worker's
    Compensation

Type of Coverage
Individual, Medicare, Supplemental Medicare, Medicaid

Geographic Areas Served
Oregon & Washington

Accreditation Certification
NCQA

Key Personnel
President & CEO . . . . Imelda Dacones
Interim President . . . . Janet O'Hollaren
Dental Director & CEO . . . . John Snyder
Executive Vice President. . . . . Gregory A. Adams

646 LifeMap

P.O. Box 1271, MS E8L
Portland, OR 97207-1271
Toll-Free: 800-794-5390
Fax: 855-854-4570
lifemapco.com
Subsidiary of: Cambia Health Solutions
Year Founded: 1984

Healthplan and Services Defined
PLAN TYPE: Other
Plan Specialty: Short-term Medical
Benefits Offered: Dental, Vision, AD&D, Life

Geographic Areas Served
Alaska, Idaho, Montana, Oregon, Utah, Washington, and
Wyoming

Key Personnel
President & CEO. . . . . Chris Blanton
Director of Finance. Randy Lowell
VP, Sales & Marketing. . . . . Peter Mueller
Operations & Technology . . . . Scott Wilkinson
VP, Rick Management . . . . Jim Clark

647 Managed HealthCare Northwest

422 East Burnside Street, Suite 215
P.O. Box 4629
Portland, OR 97208-4629
Phone: 503-413-5800
Fax: 503-413-5801
www.mhninc.com
Subsidiary of: Legacy Health & Adventist Medical Center
For Profit Organization: Yes
Year Founded: 1988
Number of Affiliated Hospitals: 21
Number of Primary Care Physicians: 1,228
Number of Referral/Specialty Physicians: 4,757
Total Enrollment: 125,000

Healthplan and Services Defined
PLAN TYPE: PPO
Model Type: Network
Plan Specialty: Worker's Compensation, MCO,
    Precertification, Utilization Review
Benefits Offered: Disease Management, Wellness, Worker's
    Compensation, MCO, Precertification, Utilization Review,
    Case Management

Type of Coverage
Commercial, Individual

Geographic Areas Served
Oregon: Clackamas, Clatsop, Columbia, Coos, Hood River,
Lane, Marion, Multnomah, Polk, Wasco, Washington &
Yamhill; Washington: Clark, Cowlitz, Klickitat & Skamania
counties

Peer Review Type
Utilization Review: Yes
Second Surgical Opinion: Yes
Case Management: Yes

Publishes and Distributes Report Card: No

Key Personnel
President and CEO . . . . Dolores Russell
Director, Inf. & Finance. David Pyle
Provider Relations . . . . Jennifer Harvey
Claims Coordinator . . . . Robyn Fischer

Specialty Managed Care Partners
Enters into Contracts with Regional Business Coalitions: Yes

648 Moda Health Oregon

601 SW Second Avenue
Portland, OR 97204
Phone: 855-718-1767
individualplans@modahealth.com
modahealth.com
Mailing Address: P.O. Box 40384, Portland, OR 97240-0384
Year Founded: 1955

Healthplan and Services Defined
PLAN TYPE: Multiple
Plan Specialty: Dental, Disease Management, Health Coaches
Benefits Offered: Dental, Disease Management, Prescription,
    Wellness

Geographic Areas Served
Statewide, Alaska, and Washington

Key Personnel
Chief Executive Officer . . . . Robert Gootee
President. . . . . William Johnson, MD
Executive Vice President . . . . Steve Wynne
Strategic Communications . . . . Jonathan Nicholas
    503-219-3673
    jonathan.nicholas@modahealth.com

649 PacificSource Health Plans
110 International Way
Springfield, OR 97477
Toll-Free: 800-624-6052
Phone: 541-686-1242
www.pacificsource.com
Mailing Address: P.O. Box 7068, Springfield, OR 97475-0068
Non-Profit Organization: Yes
Year Founded: 1933
Number of Referral/Specialty Physicians: 46,300
Total Enrollment: 275,000

Healthplan and Services Defined
  PLAN TYPE: Multiple
  Plan Specialty: Dental, PBM, Vision
  Benefits Offered: Dental, Disease Management, Prescription,
    Vision, Wellness

Type of Coverage
Commercial, Individual, Medicare

Type of Payment Plans Offered
POS, Combination FFS & DFFS

Geographic Areas Served
Oregon, Montana & Idaho

Key Personnel
President & CEO . . . . Ken Provencher
EVP, Operating Officer . . . . Erick Doolen
EVP, Financial Officer . . . . Peter Davidson
EVP, Medical Officer. . . . . Dan Roth, MD

650 PacificSource Health Plans
110 International Way
Springfield, OR 97477
Toll-Free: 800-624-6052
Phone: 541-686-1242
www.pacificsource.com
Mailing Address: P.O. Box 7068, Springfield, OR 97475-0068
Non-Profit Organization: Yes
Year Founded: 1933
Number of Referral/Specialty Physicians: 46,300
Total Enrollment: 275,000

Healthplan and Services Defined
  PLAN TYPE: HMO/PPO
  Benefits Offered: Dental, Disease Management, Prescription,
    Vision, Wellness

Type of Coverage
Commercial, Individual

Type of Payment Plans Offered
POS, Combination FFS & DFFS

Geographic Areas Served
Oregon, Idaho & Montana

Key Personnel
President & CEO . . . . Ken Provencher
EVP, Financial Officer . . . . Peter Davidson
EVP, Operating Officer . . . . Erick Doolen
EVP, Medical Officer. . . . . Daniel Roth, MD

651 Providence Health Plan
P.O. Box 4327
Portland, OR 97208-4327
Toll-Free: 800-878-4445
Phone: 503-574-7500
healthplans.providence.org
Non-Profit Organization: Yes
Year Founded: 1985

Healthplan and Services Defined
  PLAN TYPE: Multiple
  Model Type: IPA, Group, PHO
  Plan Specialty: Disease Management, EPO, Vision, UR
  Benefits Offered: Behavioral Health, Chiropractic,
    Complementary Medicine, Disease Management, Home
    Care, Inpatient SNF, Physical Therapy, Podiatry,
    Prescription, Psychiatric, Transplant, Vision, Wellness

Type of Coverage
Commercial, Individual, Medicare, Medicaid

Type of Payment Plans Offered
POS, FFS

Geographic Areas Served
Oregon: Clackamas, Clark, Columbia, Crook, Deschutes,
  Hood River, Jefferson, Lane, Marion, Multnomah,
  Washington, Wheeler; Washington: Clark

Peer Review Type
Utilization Review: Yes
Second Surgical Opinion: Yes
Case Management: Yes

Publishes and Distributes Report Card: Yes

Accreditation Certification
NCQA
Medicare Approved, Utilization Review, Pre-Admission
  Certification, State Licensure, Quality Assurance Program

Key Personnel
Chief Executive Officer . . . . Michael Cotton
Chief Financial Officer . . . . Michael White
Chief Medical Officer . . . . Robert Gluckman
Adminstrative Officer. . . . . Alison Schrupp
Chief Compliance Officer. . . . . Carrie Smith
Chief Marketing Officer . . . . Brad Garrigues

Average Claim Compensation
Physician's Fees Charged: 55%
Hospital's Fees Charged: 48%

Specialty Managed Care Partners

PBH Behavioral Health, ARGUS (PBM), Complementary Health Care, Well Partner

Enters into Contracts with Regional Business Coalitions: No

Employer References

Providence Health System, PeaceHealth, Portland Public School District, Oregon PERS, Tektonix

652 Regence BlueCross BlueShield of Oregon

PO Box 1071
Portland, OR 97207
Toll-Free: 888-232-5763
www.regence.com
Subsidiary of: Regence
Non-Profit Organization: Yes
Total Enrollment: 2,400,000
State Enrollment: 730,000

Healthplan and Services Defined
PLAN TYPE: Multiple
Model Type: Network
Benefits Offered: Dental, Prescription, Vision, Wellness, Life, Preventive Care

Type of Coverage
Commercial, Individual, Supplemental Medicare

Key Personnel
President . . . . Angela Dowling
Chief Marketing Officer. . . . . Carol Kruse
Chief Medical Officer . . . . Richard Popiel

653 Samaritan Health Plan Operations

2300 NW Walnut Boulevard
Corvallis, OR 97330
Toll-Free: 800-832-4580
Phone: 541-768-4550
www.samhealthplans.org
Subsidiary of: Samaritan Health Services
Year Founded: 1993

Healthplan and Services Defined
PLAN TYPE: Multiple
Benefits Offered: Chiropractic, Dental, Disease Management, Home Care, Inpatient SNF, Physical Therapy, Podiatry, Prescription, Psychiatric, Vision, Wellness

Type of Coverage
Individual, Medicare

Geographic Areas Served
Statewide

Key Personnel
Chief Executive Officer . . . . Kelley C. Kaiser
Chief Operating Officer . . . . Kim R. Whitley
Chief Medical Officer . . . . Kevin Ewanchyna, MD
Chief Financial Officer . . . . Daniel B. Smith

654 Trillium Community Health Plan

UO Riverfront Research Park
1800 Milrace Drive
Eugene, OR 97403
Toll-Free: 877-600-5472
Phone: 541-485-2155
Fax: 866-703-0958
trilliumchp.com
Mailing Address: P.O. Box 11740, Eugene, OR 97440-3940

Healthplan and Services Defined
PLAN TYPE: Multiple
Benefits Offered: Chiropractic, Dental, Disease Management, Home Care, Inpatient SNF, Physical Therapy, Podiatry, Prescription, Psychiatric, Vision, Wellness, Durable Medical Equipment; Hearing Aids

Type of Coverage
Individual, Medicare

Geographic Areas Served
Serving Eugene, Springfield and the following counties: Benton, Clackamas, Clatsop, Deschutes, Douglas, Hood River, Jackson, Josephine, Klamath, Lane, Lincoln, Linn, Malheur, Marion, Polk, Umatilla, Wasco, Washington and Yamhill

Accreditation Certification
NCQA

Key Personnel
Chief Executive Officer . . . . Chris Ellertson
Vice President, Finance . . . . Justin Lyman
Chief Operating Officer . . . . Amy Williams
Chief Medical Officer. . . . . Thomas K. Wuest, MD

655 United Concordia of Oregon

121 SW Salmon Street
Portland, OR 97024
Phone: 503-471-1449
www.unitedconcordia.com
For Profit Organization: Yes
Year Founded: 1971
Total Enrollment: 7,800,000

Healthplan and Services Defined
PLAN TYPE: Dental
Plan Specialty: Dental
Benefits Offered: Dental

Type of Coverage
Commercial, Individual, Military personnel & families

Geographic Areas Served
Nationwide

Accreditation Certification
URAC

Key Personnel
President & COO . . . . Timothy J. Constantine
Contact. . . . . Beth Rutherford
717-260-7659
beth.rutherford@ucci.com

656 UnitedHealthcare of Oregon

5 Centerpointe Drive
Suite 600
Lake Oswego, OR 97035
Toll-Free: 800-922-1444
www.uhc.com/contact-us/oregon
Subsidiary of: UnitedHealth Group
For Profit Organization: Yes

Healthplan and Services Defined
PLAN TYPE: HMO/PPO
Model Type: Network
Plan Specialty: Behavioral Health, Dental, Disease
   Management, PBM, Vision
Benefits Offered: Behavioral Health, Dental, Disease
   Management, Long-Term Care, Prescription, Vision,
   Wellness, Life, LTD, STD

Type of Coverage
Individual, Medicare, Supplemental Medicare, Medicaid,
   Catastrophic, Family, Military, Veterans, Group,

Geographic Areas Served
Statewide

Key Personnel
President . . . . David Wichmann
Chief Operating Officer . . . . Dan Schumacher
Chief Strategy Officer . . . . John Cosgriff
Communications Officer . . . . Kirsten Gorsuch
Chief Medical Officer. . . . . Sam Ho
Chief Legal Officer . . . . Thad Johnson
Chief Information Officer . . . . Phil McKoy
Chief Financial Officer. . . . . Jeff Putnam

657 Willamette Dental Group

6950 NE Campus Way
Hillsboro, OR 97124
Toll-Free: 855-433-6825
Fax: 503-952-2200
info@willamettedental.com
www.willamettedental.com
For Profit Organization: Yes
Year Founded: 1970

Healthplan and Services Defined
PLAN TYPE: Dental
Model Type: Staff
Plan Specialty: Dental
Benefits Offered: Dental

Type of Payment Plans Offered
POS, FFS

Geographic Areas Served
Oregon, Washington and Idaho

Peer Review Type
Case Management: Yes

Publishes and Distributes Report Card: No

Key Personnel
President & CEO . . . . Dr. Eugene Skourtes, DMD

Specialty Managed Care Partners
Enters into Contracts with Regional Business Coalitions: No

Health Insurance Coverage Status and Type of Coverage by Age

Category	All Persons		Under 18 years		Under 65 years	
	Number	%	Number	%	Number	%
Total population	12,579	-	2,853	-	10,439	-
Covered by some type of health insurance	11,871 *(21)*	94.4 *(0.2)*	2,727 *(8)*	95.6 *(0.3)*	9,741 *(22)*	93.3 *(0.2)*
Covered by private health insurance	9,165 *(42)*	72.9 *(0.3)*	1,831 *(21)*	64.2 *(0.7)*	7,705 *(39)*	73.8 *(0.4)*
Employer-based	7,390 *(46)*	58.7 *(0.4)*	1,635 *(21)*	57.3 *(0.7)*	6,687 *(44)*	64.1 *(0.4)*
Direct purchase	2,041 *(28)*	16.2 *(0.2)*	213 *(9)*	7.5 *(0.3)*	1,152 *(23)*	11.0 *(0.2)*
TRICARE	184 *(8)*	1.5 *(0.1)*	30 *(3)*	1.0 *(0.1)*	109 *(6)*	1.0 *(0.1)*
Covered by public health insurance	4,580 *(31)*	36.4 *(0.3)*	1,057 *(18)*	37.1 *(0.7)*	2,503 *(32)*	24.0 *(0.3)*
Medicaid	2,506 *(34)*	19.9 *(0.3)*	1,051 *(18)*	36.8 *(0.7)*	2,246 *(31)*	21.5 *(0.3)*
Medicare	2,420 *(10)*	19.2 *(0.1)*	14 *(2)*	0.5 *(0.1)*	346 *(10)*	3.3 *(0.1)*
VA Care	277 *(7)*	2.2 *(0.1)*	3 *(1)*	0.1 *(Z)*	103 *(6)*	1.0 *(0.1)*
Not covered at any time during the year	708 *(21)*	5.6 *(0.2)*	126 *(8)*	4.4 *(0.3)*	698 *(21)*	6.7 *(0.2)*

Note: Numbers in thousands; Figures cover civilian noninstitutionalized population in 2016; N/A indicates that data was not available; Z represents or rounds to zero; Margin of error appears in parenthesis and is calculated using replicate weights.
Source: U.S. Census Bureau, American Community Survey, Table HIC-4_ACS. Health Insurance Coverage Status and Type of Coverage by State—All People: 2008 to 2016, Table HIC-5_ACS. Health Insurance Coverage Status and Type of Coverage by State—Children Under 18: 2008 to 2016, Table HIC-6_ACS. Health Insurance Coverage Status and Type of Coverage by State—Persons Under 65: 2008 to 2016

Pennsylvania

658 Aetna Health of Pennsylvania
151 Farmington Avenue
Hartford, CT 06156
Toll-Free: 800-872-3862
Phone: 860-273-0123
www.aetna.com
Subsidiary of: Aetna Inc.
For Profit Organization: Yes

Healthplan and Services Defined
  PLAN TYPE: HMO/PPO
  Other Type: POS
  Model Type: Network
  Plan Specialty: Behavioral Health, EPO, Lab, PBM,
    Radiology
  Benefits Offered: Behavioral Health, Dental, Disease
    Management, Long-Term Care, Physical Therapy,
    Podiatry, Prescription, Psychiatric, Vision, Wellness, Life,
    LTD, STD

Type of Coverage
  Commercial, Medicaid, Student health

Geographic Areas Served
  Statewide

Key Personnel
  CEO . . . . Mark Bertolini

659 American HealthCare Group
1910 Cochran Road
Manor Oak One, Suite 405
Pittsburgh, PA 15220
Phone: 412-563-8800
Fax: 412-563-8319
american-healthcare.net
For Profit Organization: Yes
Year Founded: 1996

Healthplan and Services Defined
  PLAN TYPE: Other
  Model Type: Network
  Plan Specialty: ASO, Chiropractic, Dental, MSO, Worker's
    Compensation
  Benefits Offered: Behavioral Health, Chiropractic,
    Complementary
Medicine, Dental, Disease Management, Home Care,
Inpatient SNF, Long-Term Care, Physical Therapy,
Podiatry, Prescription, Psychiatric, Transplant,
Vision, Wellness, Worker's Compensation, School
wellness programs, on-site immunizations, support
services for public housing

Type of Payment Plans Offered
  FFS

Geographic Areas Served
  Pennsylvania, Eastern Ohio, Northwestern Virginia

Peer Review Type
  Utilization Review: Yes
  Second Surgical Opinion: Yes

Case Management: Yes

Accreditation Certification
  State Licensure

Key Personnel
  President & CEO . . . . Robert E. Hagan, Jr.
    412-563-7804
    bhagan@american-healthcare.net
  Accounts Recievable . . . . Lynn Hagan
    412-563-7805
    lhagan@american-healthcare.net
  Dir., Health Benefits . . . . Erin Hart
    412-563-7807
    ehart@american-healthcare.net
  Dir., Wellness Services . . . . Liz Hagan Kanche
    412-563-7854
    lhkanche@american-healthcare.net
  Marketing Manager . . . . Sarah Kelly
    skelly@american-healthcare.net

660 AmeriHealth Pennsylvania
1901 Market Street
Philadelphia, PA 19103
Toll-Free: 866-681-7373
www.amerihealth.com
Year Founded: 1995
Total Enrollment: 265,000

Healthplan and Services Defined
  PLAN TYPE: HMO/PPO
  Benefits Offered: Dental, Disease Management, Prescription,
    Vision, Wellness

Type of Coverage
  Commercial, Individual

Geographic Areas Served
  Pennsylvania

Key Personnel
  Chief Executive Officer . . . . Judith L. Roman

661 Berkshire Health Partners
P.O. Box 14744
Reading, PA 19612-4744
Toll-Free: 866-257-0445
Phone: 610-372-8044
wickmant@dhp.org
bhp.org
Non-Profit Organization: Yes
Year Founded: 1986
Physician Owned Organization: Yes

Healthplan and Services Defined
  PLAN TYPE: PPO

Type of Coverage
  Commercial, Individual, Indemnity, Catastrophic
  Catastrophic Illness Benefit: Varies per case

Geographic Areas Served
  Berks, Upper Bucks, Carbon, Northern Lancaster, Lehigh,
  Montgomery, Northampton and Schuylkill counties

Peer Review Type
Utilization Review: Yes
Second Surgical Opinion: Yes
Case Management: Yes

Accreditation Certification
URAC, NCQA

---

662 Capital BlueCross

P.O. Box 779519
Harrisburg, PA 17177-9519
Toll-Free: 800-451-1181
Fax: 717-541-6915
www.capbluecross.com
Non-Profit Organization: Yes
Year Founded: 1938

Healthplan and Services Defined
PLAN TYPE: HMO/PPO
Plan Specialty: Dental, Vision
Benefits Offered: Dental, Home Care, Inpatient SNF,
Physical Therapy, Prescription, Psychiatric, Transplant,
Vision, Wellness

Type of Coverage
Commercial

Type of Payment Plans Offered
FFS

Geographic Areas Served
21 counties in central Pennsylvania and the Lehigh Valley

Peer Review Type
Second Surgical Opinion: Yes
Case Management: Yes

Accreditation Certification
TJC Accreditation, Medicare Approved, Utilization Review,
Pre-Admission Certification, State Licensure, Quality
Assurance Program

Key Personnel
President & CEO.................... Gary D. St. Hilaire
SVP, Financial Officer .... Harvey Littman
SVP, Medical Officer .... Jennifer A. Chambers
Chief Information Officer.................. Scott Frank
SVP, Human Resources .... Steven J. Krupinski

---

663 Delta Dental of Pennsylvania

One Delta Drive
Mechanicsburg, PA 17055-6999
Toll-Free: 800-932-0783
www.deltadentalins.com
Non-Profit Organization: Yes

Healthplan and Services Defined
PLAN TYPE: Dental
Other Type: Dental PPO
Plan Specialty: Dental
Benefits Offered: Dental

Type of Coverage
Commercial, Individual

Geographic Areas Served
Statewide

Key Personnel
President & CEO......................... Tony Barth
Chief Financial Officer .... Michael Castro
Chief Legal Officer .... Michael Hankinson
EVP, Sales & Marketing .... Belinda Martinez
Chief Operating Officer .... Nilesh Patel

---

664 Devon Health Services

1100 First Avenue
King of Prussia, PA 19406
Toll-Free: 800-431-2273
Fax: 800-221-0002
customerservice@devonhealth.com
www.devonhealth.com
For Profit Organization: Yes
Year Founded: 1991
Physician Owned Organization: Yes

Healthplan and Services Defined
PLAN TYPE: PPO
Model Type: Network
Plan Specialty: Chiropractic, Dental, Lab, Vision, Radiology,
Worker's Compensation, Group Health & Pharmacy Plans;
Acupuncture
Benefits Offered: Chiropractic, Dental, Inpatient SNF,
Physical Therapy, Vision, Worker's Compensation, Group
Health & Pharmacy Plans

Type of Coverage
Commercial

Type of Payment Plans Offered
DFFS, FFS, Combination FFS & DFFS

Geographic Areas Served
Pennsylvania, New Jersey, and Delaware

Publishes and Distributes Report Card: No

Key Personnel
President................................ Dean Vaden
Chief Operating Officer .... Marie McDaniel
Regional VP of Sales .... David Williams

Average Claim Compensation
Physician's Fees Charged: 55%
Hospital's Fees Charged: 58%

Specialty Managed Care Partners
Medimpact
Enters into Contracts with Regional Business Coalitions: Yes

Employer References
Mid-Jersey trucking Industry & Local 701 Welfare Fund,
Pennsylvania Public School Health Care Trust, International
Brotherhood of Teamsters

665 Gateway Health

Four Gateway Center
444 Liberty Ave, Suite 2100
Pittsburgh, PA 15222-1222
Toll-Free: 800-392-1147
www.gatewayhealthplan.com
For Profit Organization: Yes
Year Founded: 1992
State Enrollment: 300,000

Healthplan and Services Defined
PLAN TYPE: HMO
Other Type: Medicaid
Model Type: Network
Plan Specialty: Dental, Disease Management, Vision, UR, Prospective Care Managment; Dual Eligibility; Chronic Special Needs
Benefits Offered: Chiropractic, Dental, Disease Management, Home Care, Inpatient SNF, Physical Therapy, Podiatry, Prescription, Transplant, Vision, Wellness

Type of Coverage
Medicare, Medicaid

Type of Payment Plans Offered
DFFS, Capitated, FFS

Geographic Areas Served
Allegheny, Armstrong, Beaver, Berks, Blair, Butler, Cambria, Clarion, Cumberland, Dauphin, Erie, Fayette, Greene, Indiana, Jefferson, Lawrence, Lehigh, Mercer, Montour, Northumberland, Schulkill, Somerset, Washington and Westmoreland counties

Peer Review Type
Utilization Review: Yes
Second Surgical Opinion: Yes
Case Management: Yes

Accreditation Certification
NCQA
Utilization Review, State Licensure, Quality Assurance Program

Key Personnel
President & CEO . . . . Patricia J. Darnley
Chief Financial Officer. . . . . Sharon Kelley
Chief Medical Officer. . . . . Steven Szebenyi, MD

Specialty Managed Care Partners
Clarity Vision, Dental Benefit Providers, National Imaging Association, Merck-Medco

666 Geisinger Health Plan

100 North Academy Avenue
Danville, PA 17822-3040
Toll-Free: 800-275-6401
www.geisinger.org/health-plan
Non-Profit Organization: Yes
Year Founded: 1985
Number of Affiliated Hospitals: 110
Number of Primary Care Physicians: 3,500
Number of Referral/Specialty Physicians: 27,000
Total Enrollment: 540,000

Healthplan and Services Defined
PLAN TYPE: HMO/PPO
Model Type: Network
Benefits Offered: Chiropractic, Dental, Disease Management, Home Care, Inpatient SNF, Physical Therapy, Podiatry, Prescription, Psychiatric, Vision, Wellness

Type of Coverage
Commercial, Individual, Medicare, Supplemental Medicare, CHIP

Geographic Areas Served
42 counties in Pennsylvania

Accreditation Certification
NCQA

Key Personnel
President & CEO. . . . . Steven R. Youso

667 Health Partners Plans

901 Market Street
Suite 500
Philadelphia, PA 19107
Phone: 215-849-9606
contact@hpplans.com
www.healthpartnersplans.com
Non-Profit Organization: Yes
Year Founded: 1984
Physician Owned Organization: Yes
Number of Affiliated Hospitals: 43
Number of Primary Care Physicians: 6,400
Total Enrollment: 263,200

Healthplan and Services Defined
PLAN TYPE: Medicare
Other Type: Medicaid
Benefits Offered: Chiropractic, Dental, Disease Management, Home Care, Inpatient SNF, Physical Therapy, Podiatry, Prescription, Psychiatric, Vision, Wellness

Type of Coverage
Medicare, Medicaid, CHIP

Geographic Areas Served
Bucks, Chester, Delaware, Lancaster, Lehigh, Montgomery, Northampton, and Philadelphia counties

Key Personnel
President & CEO . . . . William S. George
Chief Information Officer . . . . Joe Brand
Chief Financial Officer . . . . John Sehi

668 HealthAmerica

3721 TecPort Drive
P.O. Box 67103
Harrisburg, PA 17106-7103
Toll-Free: 800-788-6445
healthamerica.coventryhealthcare.com
Secondary Address: 11 Stanwix Street, Suite 2300, Pittsburgh, PA 15222, 800-735-4404
Subsidiary of: Coventry Health Care
For Profit Organization: Yes
Year Founded: 1974

Owned by an Integrated Delivery Network (IDN): Yes

Healthplan and Services Defined
PLAN TYPE: Multiple
Model Type: Network
Plan Specialty: ASO, Behavioral Health, Chiropractic,
 Dental, Disease Management, Lab, Vision, Radiology
Benefits Offered: Behavioral Health, Chiropractic,
 Complementary Medicine, Dental, Disease Management,
 Home Care, Inpatient SNF, Physical Therapy, Podiatry,
 Prescription, Psychiatric, Transplant, Vision, Wellness

Type of Coverage
Commercial, Individual, Medicare

Type of Payment Plans Offered
POS, Capitated, FFS

Geographic Areas Served
Statewide

Peer Review Type
Utilization Review: Yes
Case Management: Yes

Accreditation Certification
TJC, NCQA
Medicare Approved, Utilization Review, Pre-Admission
 Certification, State Licensure, Quality Assurance Program

Key Personnel
Chief Executive Officer . . . . Mark T. Bertolini

Specialty Managed Care Partners
ValueOptions, CareMark, Dominion Dental (WPA) Delta
 Dental (EPA), Quest Diagnostics (EPA) LabCorp (WPA),
 National Vision Administrators (NVA)

Employer References
Federal Government, Penn State University, US Airways,
 City of Pittsburgh, General Motors

---

669   Highmark Blue Cross Blue Shield
501 Penn Avenue Place
Pittsburgh, PA 15222
Toll-Free: 800-816-5527
www.highmarkbcbs.com
For Profit Organization: Yes
Year Founded: 1996
Owned by an Integrated Delivery Network (IDN): Yes

Healthplan and Services Defined
PLAN TYPE: HMO/PPO
Model Type: IPA
Benefits Offered: Dental, Disease Management, Prescription,
 Vision, Wellness
Offers Demand Management Patient Information Service:
 Yes

Type of Coverage
Commercial, Individual
Catastrophic Illness Benefit: Unlimited

Type of Payment Plans Offered
POS, DFFS, Capitated, FFS, Combination FFS & DFFS

Geographic Areas Served
Western and Northeastern Pennsylvania

Peer Review Type
Utilization Review: Yes
Second Surgical Opinion: No
Case Management: Yes

Publishes and Distributes Report Card: No

Accreditation Certification
URAC, NCQA
Medicare Approved, Pre-Admission Certification, State
 Licensure

Key Personnel
President . . . . Deborah L. Rice-Johnson

Average Claim Compensation
Physician's Fees Charged: 50%
Hospital's Fees Charged: 61%

Specialty Managed Care Partners
Enters into Contracts with Regional Business Coalitions: No

---

670   Highmark Blue Shield
Camp Hill Service Center
1800 Center Street
Camp Hill, PA 17011
Toll-Free: 800-816-5527
www.highmarkblueshield.com
Non-Profit Organization: Yes
Year Founded: 1932
Total Enrollment: 5,300,000

Healthplan and Services Defined
PLAN TYPE: PPO
Model Type: Network
Benefits Offered: Disease Management, Prescription,
 Wellness

Type of Payment Plans Offered
POS, DFFS, Combination FFS & DFFS

Geographic Areas Served
Central Pennsylvania

Peer Review Type
Second Surgical Opinion: Yes

Publishes and Distributes Report Card: Yes

Accreditation Certification
URAC, NCQA

Key Personnel
President . . . . Deborah L. Rice-Johnson

Specialty Managed Care Partners
Enters into Contracts with Regional Business Coalitions: Yes

---

671   Humana Health Insurance of Pennsylvania
5000 Ritter Road
Suite 101
Mechanicsburg, PA 17055
Toll-Free: 866-355-5861
Phone: 717-766-6040
Fax: 717-795-1951
www.humana.com

Secondary Address: 325 Sentry Parkway, Suite 200, Philadelphia, PA 19422
Subsidiary of: Humana
For Profit Organization: Yes

Healthplan and Services Defined
PLAN TYPE: HMO/PPO
Model Type: Network
Plan Specialty: Dental, Vision
Benefits Offered: Dental, Vision, Life, LTD, STD

Type of Coverage
Commercial

Geographic Areas Served
Statewide

Accreditation Certification
URAC, NCQA, CORE

Key Personnel
President & CEO . . . . Bruce Broussard
Chief Medical Officer . . . . Roy A. Beveridge
Chief Consumer Officer . . . . Jody L. Bilney
Human Resources . . . . Tim Huval
Chief Financial Officer . . . . Brian Kane
Chief Information Officer . . . . Brian LeClaire
General Counsel . . . . Christopher M. Todoroff
Chief Accounting Officer . . . . Cynthia H. Zipperie

672   Independence Blue Cross
1901 Market Street
Philadelphia, PA 19103-1480
Toll-Free: 800-275-2583
www.ibx.com
Non-Profit Organization: Yes
Year Founded: 1938

Healthplan and Services Defined
PLAN TYPE: HMO/PPO
Other Type: POS
Benefits Offered: Dental, Disease Management, Prescription, Vision, Wellness, Life

Type of Coverage
Commercial, Individual, Medicare, Supplemental Medicare

Type of Payment Plans Offered
POS, FFS

Geographic Areas Served
Philadelphia and Southeastern Pennsylvania

Key Personnel
President & CEO . . . . Daniel J. Hilferty
Chief Financial Officer . . . . Gregory E. Deavens
EVP, Operating Officer . . . . Yvette D. Bright

Specialty Managed Care Partners
Caremark Rx

673   Independence Blue Cross
1901 Market Street
2nd Floor
Philadelphia, PA 19103-1480
Toll-Free: 800-275-2583
www.ibx.com
Non-Profit Organization: Yes
Year Founded: 1986
Total Enrollment: 9,500,000
State Enrollment: 2,500,000

Healthplan and Services Defined
PLAN TYPE: HMO/PPO
Benefits Offered: Dental, Prescription, Vision, Worker's Compensation, AD&D, Life, LTD, STD

Type of Coverage
Individual, Indemnity, Medicaid

Type of Payment Plans Offered
DFFS, FFS, Combination FFS & DFFS

Geographic Areas Served
24 states and the District of Columbia

Network Qualifications
Pre-Admission Certification: Yes

Peer Review Type
Utilization Review: Yes
Second Surgical Opinion: No
Case Management: Yes

Publishes and Distributes Report Card: Yes

Accreditation Certification
NCQA
TJC Accreditation, Medicare Approved, Utilization Review, Pre-Admission Certification, State Licensure, Quality Assurance Program

Key Personnel
President & CEO . . . . Daniel Hilferty
Chief Operating Officer . . . . Yvette Bright
Chief Financial Officer . . . . Gregory Deavens

Specialty Managed Care Partners
Magellan Behavioral Health, United Concorida, Medco Health Solutions
Enters into Contracts with Regional Business Coalitions: Yes

674   InterGroup Services
401 Shady Avenue
Suite B108
Pittsburgh, PA 15206
Phone: 412-363-0600
Fax: 412-363-0900
www.igs-ppo.com
Secondary Address: 1 S Bacton Hill Road], 2nd Floor, Malvern, PA 19355, 800-537-9389
For Profit Organization: Yes
Year Founded: 1985

Healthplan and Services Defined
PLAN TYPE: PPO
Model Type: Network

Plan Specialty: ASO, Behavioral Health, Chiropractic, EPO, Lab, MSO, PBM, Vision, Radiology, Worker's Compensation
Benefits Offered: Behavioral Health, Disease Management, Prescription, Wellness, Worker's Compensation

Type of Coverage
Commercial

Geographic Areas Served
Pennsylvania, New Jersey, Delaware and West Virginia

Network Qualifications
Pre-Admission Certification: Yes

Specialty Managed Care Partners
Chiropractic Network

675   Penn Highlands Healthcare

204 Hospital Avenue
DuBois, PA 15801
Phone: 814-371-2200
www.phhealthcare.org
Non-Profit Organization: Yes
Year Founded: 2011
Number of Affiliated Hospitals: 4
Number of Primary Care Physicians: 363

Healthplan and Services Defined
    PLAN TYPE: PPO
    Model Type: IPA
    Plan Specialty: ASO, Behavioral Health, Disease Management, EPO, Lab, MSO, Radiology, Worker's Compensation, UR
    Benefits Offered: Behavioral Health, Chiropractic, Disease Management, Home Care, Inpatient SNF, Long-Term Care, Physical Therapy, Podiatry, Psychiatric, Transplant, Wellness, Worker's Compensation
    Offers Demand Management Patient Information Service: Yes

Type of Coverage
Commercial

Type of Payment Plans Offered
POS, DFFS, Combination FFS & DFFS

Geographic Areas Served
Cameron, Centre, Clarion, Clearfield, Elk, Forest, Jefferson and McKean counties

Network Qualifications
Pre-Admission Certification: Yes

Peer Review Type
Utilization Review: Yes
Second Surgical Opinion: No
Case Management: Yes

Publishes and Distributes Report Card: Yes

Accreditation Certification
AAAHC, URAC
TJC Accreditation, Medicare Approved, Pre-Admission Certification, State Licensure

Key Personnel
Chief Executive Officer . . . . Steven M. Fontaine

Average Claim Compensation
Physician's Fees Charged: 1%
Hospital's Fees Charged: 1%

Specialty Managed Care Partners
Enters into Contracts with Regional Business Coalitions: No

676   Preferred Health Care

Urban Place
480 New Holland Ave, Suite 7203
Lancaster, PA 17602
Phone: 717-560-9290
Fax: 717-560-2312
info@phcunity.com
www.phcunity.com
Non-Profit Organization: Yes
Year Founded: 1984
Number of Affiliated Hospitals: 19
Number of Primary Care Physicians: 1,900

Healthplan and Services Defined
    PLAN TYPE: PPO
    Model Type: Network
    Offers Demand Management Patient Information Service: Yes

Type of Payment Plans Offered
FFS

Geographic Areas Served
Statewide

Peer Review Type
Utilization Review: Yes
Case Management: Yes

Accreditation Certification
TJC Accreditation, Medicare Approved, Utilization Review, Pre-Admission Certification, State Licensure, Quality Assurance Program

Key Personnel
President & CEO. . . . . Eric E. Buck
VP, Operations. Sherry Wolgemuth
Financial Services . . . . Kathy Roth
Provider Relations . . . . Lynne Ostrowski

677   Preferred Healthcare System

P.O. Box 1015
Duncansville, PA 16635
Toll-Free: 800-238-9900
Phone: 814-317-5063
Fax: 814-317-5139
www.phsppo.com
For Profit Organization: Yes
Year Founded: 1985
Physician Owned Organization: Yes

Healthplan and Services Defined
    PLAN TYPE: PPO
    Model Type: Network
    Plan Specialty: ASO, Behavioral Health, Chiropractic, Dental, Disease Management, EPO, PBM, Vision, Worker's Compensation, Health

Benefits Offered: Behavioral Health, Chiropractic,
Complementary Medicine, Dental, Disease Management,
Home Care, Inpatient SNF, Long-Term Care, Physical
Therapy, Podiatry, Prescription, Psychiatric, Transplant,
Vision, Wellness, AD&D, Life, STD, Durable Medical
Equipment

Type of Coverage
Commercial, Individual, Indemnity
Catastrophic Illness Benefit: Maximum $1M

Type of Payment Plans Offered
Combination FFS & DFFS

Geographic Areas Served
South Central Pennsylvania

Peer Review Type
Utilization Review: Yes
Second Surgical Opinion: Yes

Publishes and Distributes Report Card: No

Accreditation Certification
TJC Accreditation, Utilization Review, Pre-Admission
Certification, State Licensure, Quality Assurance Program

Key Personnel
President . . . . Maureen Frucella
Chief Executive Officer . . . . Brian Brumbaugh

Average Claim Compensation
Physician's Fees Charged: 70%
Hospital's Fees Charged: 70%

Specialty Managed Care Partners
Enters into Contracts with Regional Business Coalitions: Yes

---

678   South Central Preferred Health Network
3421 Concord Road
York, PA 17402
Toll-Free: 800-842-1768
Phone: 717-851-6800
www.scp-ppo.com
Non-Profit Organization: Yes
Year Founded: 1992
Number of Affiliated Hospitals: 16
Number of Primary Care Physicians: 6,150
Number of Referral/Specialty Physicians: 1,275
Total Enrollment: 33,000
State Enrollment: 33,000

Healthplan and Services Defined
PLAN TYPE: PPO
Model Type: PHO
Plan Specialty: Behavioral Health, Chiropractic, Radiology
Benefits Offered: Behavioral Health, Chiropractic, Home
Care, Inpatient SNF, Long-Term Care, Physical Therapy,
Podiatry, Psychiatric, Transplant

Type of Coverage
Catastrophic Illness Benefit: None

Type of Payment Plans Offered
Capitated

Geographic Areas Served
Cumberland, Dauphin, Lebanon, Perry and Northern York
counties

Subscriber Information
Average Monthly Fee Per Subscriber
(Employee + Employer Contribution):
Employee Only (Self): $6.75 per employee

Network Qualifications
Pre-Admission Certification: No

Peer Review Type
Utilization Review: Yes

Average Claim Compensation
Physician's Fees Charged: 64%
Hospital's Fees Charged: 70%

---

679   Trinity Health of Pennsylvania
Mercy Health System
One W Elm St, Suite 100
Conshohocken, PA 19428
Phone: 610-567-6000
www.trinity-health.org
Secondary Address: St Mary Medical Center, 1201
Langhorne-Newtown Road, Langhorne, PA 19047,
215-710-2000
Subsidiary of: Trinity Health
Non-Profit Organization: Yes
Year Founded: 2013
Total Enrollment: 30,000,000

Healthplan and Services Defined
PLAN TYPE: Other
Benefits Offered: Disease Management, Home Care,
Long-Term Care, Psychiatric, Hospice programs, PACE
(Program of All Inclusive Care for the Elderly)

Geographic Areas Served
Statewide

Key Personnel
Chief Executive Officer . . . . Richard J. Gilfillan
Chief Financial Officer. . . . . Benjamin R. Carter
Human Resources. . . . . Edmund F. Hodge
General Counsel . . . . Paul G. Neumann
Chief Clinical Officer. . . . . Daniel J. Roth
Chief Operating Officer. . . . . Michael A. Slubowski

---

680   United Concordia Dental
4401 Deer Path Road
Harrisburg, PA 17110
Toll-Free: 800-332-0366
www.unitedconcordia.com
Secondary Address: Claims Submission, PO Box 69421,
Harrisburg, PA 17106-9421
Subsidiary of: Highmark, Inc.
For Profit Organization: Yes
Year Founded: 1971
Total Enrollment: 7,800,000

Healthplan and Services Defined
PLAN TYPE: Dental

Plan Specialty: Dental
Benefits Offered: Dental

Type of Coverage
Commercial, Individual

Geographic Areas Served
Nationwide

Accreditation Certification
URAC

Key Personnel
President & COO . . . . Timothy J. Constantine
Contact. . . . . Beth Rutherford
   717-260-7659
   beth.rutherford@ucci.com

681   United Concordia of Pennsylvania

4401 Deer Path Road
Harrisburg, PA 17110
Phone: 717-260-6800
www.unitedconcordia.com
For Profit Organization: Yes
Year Founded: 1971
Total Enrollment: 7,800,000

Healthplan and Services Defined
PLAN TYPE: Dental
Plan Specialty: Dental
Benefits Offered: Dental

Type of Coverage
Commercial, Individual, Military personnel & families

Geographic Areas Served
Nationwide

Accreditation Certification
URAC

Key Personnel
President & COO . . . . Timothy J. Constantine
Contact. . . . . Beth Rutherford
   717-260-7659
   beth.rutherford@ucci.com

682   UnitedHealthcare of Pennsylvania

6095 Marshalee Drive
Suite 200
Elkridge, MD 21075
Toll-Free: 800-307-7820
www.uhc.com/contact-us/pennsylvania
Subsidiary of: UnitedHealth Group
For Profit Organization: Yes

Healthplan and Services Defined
PLAN TYPE: HMO/PPO
Model Type: Network
Plan Specialty: Behavioral Health, Dental, Disease
   Management, PBM, Vision
Benefits Offered: Behavioral Health, Dental, Disease
   Management, Long-Term Care, Prescription, Vision,
   Wellness, Life, LTD, STD

Type of Coverage
Individual, Medicare, Supplemental Medicare, Medicaid,
   Catastrophic, Family, Military, Veterans, Group,

Type of Payment Plans Offered
DFFS

Geographic Areas Served
Statewide. Pennsylvania is covered by the Maryland branch

Publishes and Distributes Report Card: Yes

Accreditation Certification
AAPI, NCQA

Key Personnel
President . . . . David Wichmann
Chief Operating Officer. . . . . Dan Schummacher
Chief Strategy Officer . . . . John Cosgriff
Communications Officer . . . . Kirsten Gorsuch
Chief Medical Officer. . . . . Sam Ho
Chief Legal Officer . . . . Thad Johnson
Chief Information Officer . . . . Phil McKoy
Chief Financial Officer. . . . . Jeff Putnam

683   UPMC Health Plan

5580 Goods Lane
Altoona, PA 16602
Toll-Free: 866-406-8762
www.upmchealthplan.com
Secondary Address: U.S. Steel Tower, 600 Grant Street,
   Pittsburgh, PA 15219
Subsidiary of: University of Pittsburgh Medical Center
For Profit Organization: Yes
Year Founded: 1996
Physician Owned Organization: Yes
Number of Affiliated Hospitals: 125
Number of Primary Care Physicians: 11,500
Total Enrollment: 101,000
State Enrollment: 209,211

Healthplan and Services Defined
PLAN TYPE: Multiple
Benefits Offered: Behavioral Health, Chiropractic,
   Complementary Medicine, Dental, Disease Management,
   Home Care, Inpatient SNF, Physical Therapy, Podiatry,
   Prescription, Psychiatric, Transplant, Vision, Wellness

Type of Coverage
Commercial, Individual, Medicare, Medicaid

Type of Payment Plans Offered
POS

Geographic Areas Served
26 counties in western Pennsylvania

Subscriber Information
Average Monthly Fee Per Subscriber
   (Employee + Employer Contribution):
      Employee Only (Self): Varies
      Employee & 1 Family Member: Varies
      Employee & 2 Family Members: Varies
      Medicare: Varies
Average Annual Deductible Per Subscriber:
      Employee Only (Self): Varies

Employee & 1 Family Member: Varies
Employee & 2 Family Members: Varies
Medicare: Varies
Average Subscriber Co-Payment:
Primary Care Physician: Varies
Non-Network Physician: Varies
Prescription Drugs: Varies
Hospital ER: Varies
Home Health Care: Varies
Home Health Care Max. Days/Visits Covered: Varies
Nursing Home: Varies
Nursing Home Max. Days/Visits Covered: Varies

Accreditation Certification
NCQA

Key Personnel
Executive VP and CEO . . . . Diane Holder
CFO. . . . . Scott Lammie
Senior VP and COF . . . . Mary Beth Jenkins
VP, Medicare . . . . Cathy Batteer
VP, Network Management. . . . . Sandra McAnallen
VP, Marketing & Comm . . . . Sheri Manning
VP, Business Development . . . . Kim Jacobs
VP, Human Resources . . . . Sharon Czyzewski
Chief Medical Officer . . . . William Shrank, MD
President . . . . David Weir

684   UPMC Susquehanna
700 High Street
Williamsport, PA 17701
Phone: 570-321-1000
www.susquehannahealth.org
For Profit Organization: Yes
Year Founded: 1994
Physician Owned Organization: Yes
Number of Affiliated Hospitals: 24
Number of Primary Care Physicians: 1,090

Healthplan and Services Defined
PLAN TYPE: PPO
Model Type: Network
Plan Specialty: Disease Management, Lab, Cancer,
orthopedics, heart & vascular, maternaty care
Benefits Offered: Disease Management, Home Care,
Long-Term Care, Prescription, Wellness

Type of Coverage
Catastrophic Illness Benefit: Maximum $2M

Geographic Areas Served
Central & Northeastern Pennsylvania

Subscriber Information
Average Monthly Fee Per Subscriber
(Employee + Employer Contribution):
Employee Only (Self): $140
Employee & 1 Family Member: $275
Employee & 2 Family Members: $410
Average Annual Deductible Per Subscriber:
Employee Only (Self): $500
Average Subscriber Co-Payment:
Primary Care Physician: $30.00

Non-Network Physician: $52.00
Hospital ER: $75.00
Home Health Care: 15%
Home Health Care Max. Days/Visits Covered: 100 days
Nursing Home Max. Days/Visits Covered:
30/confinement

Network Qualifications
Pre-Admission Certification: Yes

Peer Review Type
Utilization Review: Yes
Second Surgical Opinion: Yes

Publishes and Distributes Report Card: No

Accreditation Certification
Medicare Approved, Utilization Review, Pre-Admission
Certification, State Licensure, Quality Assurance Program

Key Personnel
President/CEO . . . . Steven P. Johnson, Jr

Specialty Managed Care Partners
Enters into Contracts with Regional Business Coalitions: Yes

685   Vale-U-Health
800 Plaza Dr
Suite 230
Belle Vernon, PA 15012
Phone: 724-379-4011
Fax: 724-379-4354
www.valeuhealth.com
Non-Profit Organization: Yes
Year Founded: 1995
Number of Affiliated Hospitals: 1
Number of Primary Care Physicians: 156
Total Enrollment: 2,375

Healthplan and Services Defined
PLAN TYPE: PPO
Model Type: PHO
Plan Specialty: Radiology
Benefits Offered: Disease Management, Podiatry, Psychiatric,
Wellness, 40 specialties including allergy & immunology,
cardiology, dermatology & geriatrics.

Type of Coverage
Commercial, Individual
Catastrophic Illness Benefit: Covered

Geographic Areas Served
Monongahela Valley

Subscriber Information
Average Annual Deductible Per Subscriber:
Employee Only (Self): $200.00
Employee & 1 Family Member: $400.00
Employee & 2 Family Members: $400.00

Peer Review Type
Case Management: Yes

Accreditation Certification
TJC, CARF, COA and AOA

Key Personnel

Chief Executive Officer . . . . Susan Flynn
smf@vuhealth.com
Director of Operations . . . . Jois J. Weaver
ljw@vuhealth.com
Care & Quality Management . . . . Trina L. Curcio
tlc@vuhealth.com
Claims Adjudicator . . . . Hillary Rodenz
hrodenz@vuhealth.com

686   Valley Preferred

1605 N Cedar Crest Blvd.
Suite 411
Allentown, PA 18104-2351
Toll-Free: 800-955-6620
Phone: 610-969-0485
Fax: 610-969-0439
info@valleypreferred.com
www.valleypreferred.com
Non-Profit Organization: Yes
Year Founded: 1994
Physician Owned Organization: Yes
Federally Qualified: Yes
Number of Affiliated Hospitals: 18
Number of Primary Care Physicians: 778
Number of Referral/Specialty Physicians: 2,977
Total Enrollment: 174,309
State Enrollment: 174,209

Healthplan and Services Defined
 PLAN TYPE: Multiple
 Model Type: PHO

Geographic Areas Served
 Lehigh, Northampton, Berks, Bucks, Montgomery, Dauphin, Schuylkill, Columbia, Luzerne, Carbon and Lackawanna counties

Accreditation Certification
 TJC, NCQA

Key Personnel
 Chair. . . . . Gregory Kile
 Executive Director . . . . Mark Wendling
 General Manager . . . . Laura J. Mertz
 Finance Manager . . . . Tracy Hujsa
 Medical Director. . . . . Jonathan Burke

Specialty Managed Care Partners
 Enters into Contracts with Regional Business Coalitions: No
 NPRHCC

687   Value Behavioral Health of Pennsylvania

520 Pleasant Valley Road
Trafford, PA 15085
Toll-Free: 877-615-8503
vbhpawebmaster@valueoptions.com
www.vbh-pa.com
Subsidiary of: A Beacon Health Options Company
For Profit Organization: Yes
Year Founded: 1999
Physician Owned Organization: Yes

Number of Referral/Specialty Physicians: 6,000
Total Enrollment: 22,000,000

Healthplan and Services Defined
 PLAN TYPE: PPO
 Model Type: Network
 Plan Specialty: ASO, Behavioral Health, UR
 Benefits Offered: Behavioral Health, Psychiatric, EAP

Type of Coverage
 Commercial, Indemnity, Medicaid

Type of Payment Plans Offered
 POS, DFFS, Combination FFS & DFFS

Geographic Areas Served
 Armstrong, Beaver, Butler, Crawford, Fayette, Greene, Indiana, Lawrence, Mercer, Venango, Washington and Westmoreland counties

Peer Review Type
 Case Management: Yes

Publishes and Distributes Report Card: Yes

Accreditation Certification
 TJC, URAC, NCQA, CARF, COA and AOA

Key Personnel
 CEO . . . . Mark Fuller
 CFO . . . . Diane Werksman

Health Insurance Coverage Status and Type of Coverage by Age

Category	All Persons		Under 18 years		Under 65 years	
	Number	%	Number	%	Number	%
Total population	N/A	-	N/A	-	N/A	-
Covered by some type of health insurance	N/A	N/A	N/A	N/A	N/A	N/A
Covered by private health insurance	N/A	N/A	N/A	N/A	N/A	N/A
Employer-based	N/A	N/A	N/A	N/A	N/A	N/A
Direct purchase	N/A	N/A	N/A	N/A	N/A	N/A
TRICARE	N/A	N/A	N/A	N/A	N/A	N/A
Covered by public health insurance	N/A	N/A	N/A	N/A	N/A	N/A
Medicaid	N/A	N/A	N/A	N/A	N/A	N/A
Medicare	N/A	N/A	N/A	N/A	N/A	N/A
VA Care	N/A	N/A	N/A	N/A	N/A	N/A
Not covered at any time during the year	N/A	N/A	N/A	N/A	N/A	N/A

Note: Figures cover civilian noninstitutionalized population in 2016; N/A indicates that data was not available.
Source: U.S. Census Bureau, American Community Survey, Table HIC-4_ACS. Health Insurance Coverage Status and Type of Coverage by State—All People: 2008 to 2016, Table HIC-5_ACS. Health Insurance Coverage Status and Type of Coverage by State—Children Under 18: 2008 to 2016, Table HIC-6_ACS. Health Insurance Coverage Status and Type of Coverage by State—Persons Under 65: 2008 to 2016

Puerto Rico

688 BlueCross BlueShield of Puerto Rico

P.O. Box 363628
San Juan, PR 00936-3628
Toll-Free: 800-981-4860
Phone: 787-277-6544
Fax: 855-887-8275
Year Founded: 1959

Healthplan and Services Defined
PLAN TYPE: Multiple

Benefits Offered: Chiropractic, Dental, Disease Management, Home Care, Inpatient SNF, Physical Therapy, Podiatry, Prescription, Psychiatric, Vision, Wellness

Type of Coverage
Individual, Medicare, Supplemental Medicare

Geographic Areas Served
Puerto Rico

Accreditation Certification
TJC, URAC, NCQA

689 First Medical Health Plan

Lote #510 00966, Frontage Road
Guaynabo, PR 00966
Toll-Free: 888-318-0274
Phone: 787-474-3999
www.firstmedicalpr.com
For Profit Organization: Yes
Year Founded: 1977
Number of Affiliated Hospitals: 12
Total Enrollment: 180,000
State Enrollment: 180,000

Healthplan and Services Defined
PLAN TYPE: Multiple
Plan Specialty: Dental
Benefits Offered: Dental, Disease Management, Wellness

Key Personnel
President . . . . Francisco Javier Artau Feliciano

690 Humana Health Insurance of Puerto Rico

383 Franklin Delano Roosevelt Avenue
San Juan, PR 00918
Toll-Free: 866-250-0000
Fax: 888-899-6762
www.humana.com
Subsidiary of: Humana
For Profit Organization: Yes

Healthplan and Services Defined
PLAN TYPE: HMO/PPO
Model Type: Network
Plan Specialty: Dental, Vision
Benefits Offered: Dental, Vision, Life, LTD, STD

Type of Coverage
Commercial

Accreditation Certification
URAC, NCQA, CORE

Key Personnel
President & CEO. Bruce Broussard
Chief Medical Officer. . . . . Roy A. Beveridge
Chief Consumer Officer. . . . . Jody L. Bilney
Human Resources. . . . . Tim Huval
Chief Financial Officer . . . . Brian Kane
Chief Information Officer . . . . Brian LeClaire
General Counsel . . . . Christopher M. Todoroff
Chief Accounting Officer . . . . Cynthia H. Zipperie

691 InnovaCare Health

173 Bridge Plaza N
Fort Lee, NJ 07024
Phone: 201-969-2300
info@innovacarehealth.com
innovacarehealth.com

Healthplan and Services Defined
PLAN TYPE: Medicare

Type of Coverage
Medicare

Geographic Areas Served
Puerto Rico

Key Personnel
President & CEO . . . . Richard Shinto
Chief Financial Officer . . . . Douglas Malton
General Counsel . . . . Christopher Joyce
Administrative Officer. . . . . Penelope Kokkinides
Chief Accounting Officer. . . . . Michael J. Sortino
Chief Actuary Officer . . . . Jonathan A. Meyers
Chief Information Officer . . . . S Bhasker

692 Medical Card System (MCS)

San Juan, PR 00917
Toll-Free: 888-758-1616
Phone: 787-281-2800
www.mcs.com.pr
For Profit Organization: Yes
Year Founded: 1983
Number of Affiliated Hospitals: 57
Number of Primary Care Physicians: 11
Total Enrollment: 300,000

Healthplan and Services Defined
PLAN TYPE: Multiple
Model Type: Group, Network
Plan Specialty: ASO, Behavioral Health, Chiropractic, Dental, Disease Management, EPO, Lab, MSO, PBM, Vision, Radiology
Benefits Offered: Behavioral Health, Chiropractic, Complementary Medicine, Dental, Disease Management, Home Care, Inpatient SNF, Physical Therapy, Podiatry, Prescription, Psychiatric, Transplant, Vision, Wellness, Life, LTD

Type of Coverage
Commercial, Individual, Indemnity, Medicare, Supplemental Medicare, Medicaid, Catastrophic

Type of Payment Plans Offered
POS, Capitated

Geographic Areas Served
Statewide

Subscriber Information
Average Monthly Fee Per Subscriber
(Employee + Employer Contribution):
Employee Only (Self): Varies
Employee & 1 Family Member: Varies
Employee & 2 Family Members: Varies
Medicare: Varies
Average Annual Deductible Per Subscriber:
Employee Only (Self): Varies
Employee & 1 Family Member: Varies
Employee & 2 Family Members: Varies
Medicare: Varies
Average Subscriber Co-Payment:
Primary Care Physician: Varies
Non-Network Physician: Varies
Prescription Drugs: Varies
Hospital ER: Varies
Home Health Care: Varies
Home Health Care Max. Days/Visits Covered: Varies
Nursing Home: Varies
Nursing Home Max. Days/Visits Covered: Varies

Network Qualifications
Pre-Admission Certification: Yes

Peer Review Type
Utilization Review: Yes
Second Surgical Opinion: Yes
Case Management: Yes

Accreditation Certification
Medicare Approved, Pre-Admission Certification, State Licensure

Key Personnel
President . . . . Roberto Pando
Chief Financial Officer . . . . Jos, Aponte Amador
Chief Executive Officer . . . . Jim O 'Drobinak
Chief Compliance Officer . . . . Maite Morales Martinez
VP of Clinical Operations . . . . Ixel Rivera
Membership Senior VP . . . . Richard Luna
VP Marketing & Comm. . . . . Ricardo Martinez
Human Resources Senior VP. . . . . Gretchen Muniz
Chief Medical Officer. . . . . Ines Hernandez, MD

Employer References
Sensormatic, El Nuevo Dia, Pan Pepin, Nypro Puerto Rico, Cardinal Health

693 MMM Holdings
P.O. Box 71114
San Juan, PR 00936-8014
Toll-Free: 866-333-5470
Phone: 787-620-2397
www.mmm-pr.com

Subsidiary of: InnovaCare, Inc.
For Profit Organization: Yes
Year Founded: 2001
Total Enrollment: 126,000

Healthplan and Services Defined
PLAN TYPE: Multiple

Type of Coverage
Individual, Medicare, Medicaid

Geographic Areas Served
Puerto Rico

Accreditation Certification
NCQA

Key Personnel
President . . . . Orlando Gonzalez
CEO. . . . . Richard Shinto
Chief Operating Officer . . . . Manuel Sanchez
Chief Financial Officer. . . . . Carlos Vivaldi
Chief Medical Officer . . . . Diego Rosso Flores

694 PMC Medicare Choice
350 Chardon Avenue
Suite 500, Torre Chardon
San Juan, PR 00926-2709
Toll-Free: 866-516-7700
Phone: 787-625-2126
www.pmcpr.org
Mailing Address: P.O. Box 366292, San Juan, PR 00936-6292
Subsidiary of: MMM Holdings, Inc.
For Profit Organization: Yes
Year Founded: 2000
Number of Primary Care Physicians: 7
Total Enrollment: 53,000

Healthplan and Services Defined
PLAN TYPE: Medicare
Model Type: Network
Benefits Offered: Behavioral Health, Chiropractic, Home Care, Inpatient SNF, Podiatry, Prescription, Vision, Wellness

Type of Coverage
Medicare

Geographic Areas Served
Puerto Rico

Accreditation Certification
NCQA

Key Personnel
President . . . . Orlando Gonzalez, Esq.
Chief Executive Officer. . . . . Richard Shinto, MD

695 UnitedHealthcare of Puerto Rico
9700 Health Care Lane
Minnetonka, MN 55343
Toll-Free: 800-842-3585
www.uhc.com/contact-us/puerto-rico
Subsidiary of: UnitedHealth Group
Year Founded: 1977

Healthplan and Services Defined
PLAN TYPE: HMO/PPO
Model Type: Network
Plan Specialty: Behavioral Health, Dental, Disease
    Management, Lab, PBM, Vision, Radiology
Benefits Offered: Behavioral Health, Chiropractic, Dental,
    Disease Management, Long-Term Care, Physical Therapy,
    Prescription, Vision, Wellness, AD&D, Life, LTD, STD

Type of Coverage
Commercial, Individual, Indemnity, Medicare, Supplemental
    Medicare, Medicaid, Catastrophic, Family, Military,
    Veterans, Group,

Geographic Areas Served
Statewide. Puerto Rico is covered by the Minnesota branch

Network Qualifications
Pre-Admission Certification: Yes

Peer Review Type
Utilization Review: Yes
Second Surgical Opinion: Yes
Case Management: Yes

Publishes and Distributes Report Card: Yes

Accreditation Certification
TJC, NCQA

Key Personnel
President . . . . David Wichmann
Chief Operating Officer . . . . Dan Schumacher
Chief Strategy Officer . . . . John Cosgriff
Communications Officer . . . . Kirsten Gorsuch
Chief Medical Officer. . . . . Sam Ho
Chief Legal Officer . . . . Thad Johnson
Chief Information Officer . . . . Phil McKoy
Chief Financial Officer. . . . . Jeff Putnam

Specialty Managed Care Partners
Enters into Contracts with Regional Business Coalitions: Yes

Health Insurance Coverage Status and Type of Coverage by Age

Category	All Persons		Under 18 years		Under 65 years	
	Number	%	Number	%	Number	%
Total population	1,040	-	225	-	874	-
Covered by some type of health insurance	995 *(5)*	95.7 *(0.5)*	220 *(2)*	97.8 *(0.6)*	829 *(5)*	94.9 *(0.5)*
Covered by private health insurance	746 *(11)*	71.7 *(1.1)*	152 *(5)*	67.6 *(2.3)*	643 *(11)*	73.6 *(1.2)*
Employer-based	598 *(14)*	57.5 *(1.3)*	135 *(6)*	60.2 *(2.4)*	551 *(13)*	63.1 *(1.5)*
Direct purchase	170 *(8)*	16.4 *(0.8)*	18 *(3)*	8.0 *(1.3)*	106 *(7)*	12.1 *(0.8)*
TRICARE	18 *(3)*	1.7 *(0.3)*	3 *(1)*	1.3 *(0.5)*	12 *(2)*	1.3 *(0.3)*
Covered by public health insurance	389 *(10)*	37.4 *(1.0)*	83 *(5)*	36.7 *(2.1)*	227 *(10)*	26.0 *(1.2)*
Medicaid	230 *(11)*	22.1 *(1.1)*	81 *(5)*	36.2 *(2.1)*	204 *(10)*	23.4 *(1.2)*
Medicare	197 *(4)*	19.0 *(0.3)*	2 *(1)*	0.9 *(0.4)*	36 *(3)*	4.1 *(0.4)*
VA Care	23 *(2)*	2.2 *(0.2)*	Z *(Z)*	Z *(Z)*	9 *(2)*	1.1 *(0.2)*
Not covered at any time during the year	45 *(5)*	4.3 *(0.5)*	5 *(1)*	2.2 *(0.6)*	45 *(5)*	5.1 *(0.5)*

Note: Numbers in thousands; Figures cover civilian noninstitutionalized population in 2016; N/A indicates that data was not available; Z represents or rounds to zero; Margin of error appears in parenthesis and is calculated using replicate weights.
Source: U.S. Census Bureau, American Community Survey, Table HIC-4_ACS. Health Insurance Coverage Status and Type of Coverage by State—All People: 2008 to 2016, Table HIC-5_ACS. Health Insurance Coverage Status and Type of Coverage by State—Children Under 18: 2008 to 2016, Table HIC-6_ACS. Health Insurance Coverage Status and Type of Coverage by State—Persons Under 65: 2008 to 2016

Rhode Island

696 Aetna Health of Rhode Island

151 Farmington Avenue
Hartford, CT 06156
Toll-Free: 800-872-3862
Phone: 860-273-0123
www.aetna.com
Subsidiary of: Aetna Inc.
For Profit Organization: Yes

Healthplan and Services Defined
PLAN TYPE: PPO
Other Type: POS
Model Type: Network
Plan Specialty: Behavioral Health, EPO, Lab, PBM,
   Radiology
Benefits Offered: Behavioral Health, Disease Management,
   Long-Term Care, Physical Therapy, Podiatry, Prescription,
   Psychiatric, Wellness, Life, LTD, STD

Type of Coverage
Commercial, Student health

Type of Payment Plans Offered
POS, FFS

Geographic Areas Served
Statewide

Key Personnel
CEO . . . . Mark Bertolini

697 Blue Cross & Blue Shield of Rhode Island

500 Exchange Street
Providence, RI 02903
Toll-Free: 800-637-3718
Phone: 401-459-1000
www.bcbsri.com
Subsidiary of: Health and Wellness Institute
Non-Profit Organization: Yes
Year Founded: 1939
Number of Primary Care Physicians: 100,000
Total Enrollment: 600,000

Healthplan and Services Defined
PLAN TYPE: HMO
Model Type: Staff
Plan Specialty: Dental, Vision
Benefits Offered: Dental, Disease Management, Home Care,
   Inpatient SNF, Prescription, Vision, Wellness

Type of Coverage
Commercial, Individual, Medicare

Type of Payment Plans Offered
DFFS

Geographic Areas Served
Statewide

Subscriber Information
Average Monthly Fee Per Subscriber
   (Employee + Employer Contribution):
      Employee Only (Self): Varies
      Employee & 1 Family Member: Varies
      Employee & 2 Family Members: Varies
      Medicare: Varies
Average Annual Deductible Per Subscriber:
      Employee Only (Self): Varies
      Employee & 1 Family Member: Varies
      Employee & 2 Family Members: Varies

Peer Review Type
Case Management: Yes

Publishes and Distributes Report Card: Yes

Accreditation Certification
URAC, NCQA

Key Personnel
President & CEO . . . . Kim A. Keck
Chief Financial Officer . . . . Mark Stewart
EVP, General Counsel . . . . Michele Lederberg
SVP, Care Integration . . . . Mark Waggoner
SVP/Chief Medical Officer . . . . Gus Manocchia, MD
Chief Customer Officer. . . . . Melissa Cummings

698 Coventry Health Care of Rhode Island

6720-B Rockledge Drive
Suite 700
Bethesda, MD 20817
Phone: 301-581-0600
www.coventryhealthcare.com
Subsidiary of: Aetna Inc.
For Profit Organization: Yes

Healthplan and Services Defined
PLAN TYPE: HMO/PPO
Model Type: Network
Plan Specialty: Behavioral Health, Dental, Worker's
   Compensation
Benefits Offered: Behavioral Health, Dental, Prescription,
   Wellness, Worker's Compensation

Type of Coverage
Commercial, Medicare, Medicaid

Geographic Areas Served
Statewide

Key Personnel
Chief Executive Officer. . . . . Mark T. Bertolini
President . . . . Karen S. Lynch
Chief Financial Officer . . . . Shawn M. Guertin
Operations & Technology . . . . Meg McCarthy
Chief Medical Officer . . . . Harold L. Paz
General Counsel . . . . Thomas Sabatino Jr.
Government Services . . . . Fran S. Soistman

699 CVS CareMark

P.O. Box 6590
Lee's Summit, MO 64064-6590
Toll-Free: 800-552-8159
cvshealth.com/
Secondary Address: One CVS Drive, Woonsocket, RI 02895,
   800-746-7287
For Profit Organization: Yes

Year Founded: 1963
Owned by an Integrated Delivery Network (IDN): Yes
Number of Affiliated Hospitals: 650
Number of Primary Care Physicians: 60,000
Total Enrollment: 70,000,000

Healthplan and Services Defined
PLAN TYPE: Other
Other Type: PBM
Model Type: Staff
Plan Specialty: Disease Management, PBM
Benefits Offered: Disease Management, Prescription

Type of Payment Plans Offered
POS, DFFS, FFS

Geographic Areas Served
Nationwide

Peer Review Type
Second Surgical Opinion: Yes
Case Management: Yes

Publishes and Distributes Report Card: Yes

Accreditation Certification
TJC, URAC

Key Personnel
President & CEO . . . . Larry J Merlo
EVP/COO . . . . Jonathan C. Roberts
EVP, Chief Financial Offc . . . . David M Denton
Executive Vice President. . . . . Thomas M Moriarty
Executive Vice President. . . . . Helena B Foulkes
EVP & Chief Medical Off. . . . . Troyen A. Brennan, MD
SVP, Chief Human Resource . . . . Lisa Bisaccia
SVP, Chief Info Officer . . . . Stephen J Gold
Executive Vice President . . . . J David Joyner

Specialty Managed Care Partners
Enters into Contracts with Regional Business Coalitions: Yes

700 Humana Health Insurance of Rhode Island

1 International Boulevard
Suite 904
Mahwah, NJ 07495
Toll-Free: 800-967-2370
www.humana.com
Subsidiary of: Humana
For Profit Organization: Yes

Healthplan and Services Defined
PLAN TYPE: HMO/PPO
Model Type: Network
Plan Specialty: Dental, Vision
Benefits Offered: Dental, Vision, Life, LTD, STD

Type of Coverage
Commercial

Geographic Areas Served
Rhode Island is covered by the New Jersey branch

Accreditation Certification
URAC, NCQA, CORE

Key Personnel
President & CEO. Bruce Broussard

Chief Medical Officer. . . . . Roy A. Beveridge
Chief Consumer Officer. . . . . Jody L. Bilney
Human Resources. . . . . Tim Huval
Chief Financial Officer . . . . Brian Kane
Chief Information Officer . . . . Brian LeClaire
General Counsel . . . . Christopher M. Todoroff

701 Neighborhood Health Plan of Rhode Island

910 Douglas Pike
Smithfield, RI 02917
Toll-Free: 800-963-1001
Phone: 401-459-6000
Fax: 401-459-6175
www.nhpri.org
Non-Profit Organization: Yes
Year Founded: 1994
Number of Primary Care Physicians: 900
Number of Referral/Specialty Physicians: 2,700
Total Enrollment: 190,000
State Enrollment: 190,000

Healthplan and Services Defined
PLAN TYPE: HMO
Model Type: Network
Benefits Offered: Behavioral Health, Disease Management,
Inpatient SNF, Prescription, Wellness

Type of Coverage
Commercial, Individual, Medicare, Medicaid

Peer Review Type
Case Management: Yes

Publishes and Distributes Report Card: Yes

Accreditation Certification
NCQA

Key Personnel
President/CEO. . . . . Peter M. Marino
Chief Financial Officer. . . . . Frank Meaney
Chief of Staff. . . . . David Burnett
Chief Marketing Officer . . . . Brenda Whittle
Chief Medical Officer . . . . Francisco Trilla, MD
Chief Information Officer . . . . Jeffrey Meyer

702 Tufts Health Plan: Rhode Island

1 W Exchange Street
Providence, RI 02903
Toll-Free: 866-738-4116
Phone: 401-272-3499
www.tuftshealthplan.com
Secondary Address: 705 Mt Auburn Street, Watertown, MA
02742, 617-972-9400
Non-Profit Organization: Yes
Year Founded: 1979
Number of Affiliated Hospitals: 90
Number of Primary Care Physicians: 25,000
Number of Referral/Specialty Physicians: 12,500
Total Enrollment: 1,018,589

Healthplan and Services Defined
PLAN TYPE: Multiple

Model Type: IPA

Plan Specialty: ASO, Behavioral Health, Chiropractic, Disease Management, EPO, Lab, PBM, Vision, Radiology, UR, Pharmacy

Benefits Offered: Behavioral Health, Chiropractic, Complementary Medicine, Disease Management, Home Care, Inpatient SNF, Physical Therapy, Podiatry, Prescription, Psychiatric, Transplant, Vision, Wellness

Type of Coverage

Commercial, Individual, Medicare, Supplemental Medicare, Medicaid

Type of Payment Plans Offered

POS, DFFS, FFS, Combination FFS & DFFS

Geographic Areas Served

Massachusetts, New Hampshire and Rhode Island

Subscriber Information

Average Monthly Fee Per Subscriber
(Employee + Employer Contribution):
Employee Only (Self): $190.00-220.00
Employee & 2 Family Members: $800.00-950.00
Medicare: $150.00
Average Annual Deductible Per Subscriber:
Employee Only (Self): $1000.00
Employee & 1 Family Member: $500.00
Employee & 2 Family Members: $3000.00
Average Subscriber Co-Payment:
Primary Care Physician: $10.00
Non-Network Physician: 20%
Prescription Drugs: $10/20/35
Hospital ER: $50.00
Home Health Care: $0
Home Health Care Max. Days/Visits Covered: 120 days
Nursing Home: $0
Nursing Home Max. Days/Visits Covered: 120 days

Network Qualifications

Pre-Admission Certification: No

Peer Review Type

Utilization Review: Yes
Case Management: Yes

Publishes and Distributes Report Card: Yes

Accreditation Certification

TJC, AAPI, NCQA

Average Claim Compensation

Physician's Fees Charged: 75%
Hospital's Fees Charged: 70%

Specialty Managed Care Partners

Advance PCS, Private Healthe Care Systems

Employer References

Commonwealth of Massachuestts, Fleet Boston, Roman Catholic Archdiocese of Boston, City of Boston, State Street Corporation

703　UnitedHealthcare of Rhode Island

475 Kilvert Street
Warwick, RI 02886
Toll-Free: 800-447-1245
Phone: 401-737-6900
www.uhc.com/contact-us/rhode-island
Subsidiary of: UnitedHealth Group
For Profit Organization: Yes
Year Founded: 1983
Owned by an Integrated Delivery Network (IDN): Yes

Healthplan and Services Defined

PLAN TYPE: HMO/PPO

Model Type: Network

Plan Specialty: Behavioral Health, Chiropractic, Dental, Disease Management, Lab, PBM, Vision, Radiology

Benefits Offered: Behavioral Health, Dental, Disease Management, Long-Term Care, Prescription, Vision, Wellness, Life, LTD, STD

Type of Coverage

Commercial, Individual, Medicare, Supplemental Medicare, Medicaid, Catastrophic, Family, Military, Veterans, Group,

Type of Payment Plans Offered

Combination FFS & DFFS

Geographic Areas Served

Rhode Island, Massachusetts, Maine, New Hampshire, Vermont

Publishes and Distributes Report Card: Yes

Accreditation Certification

AAPI, NCQA

Key Personnel

President . . . . David Wichmann
Chief Operating Officer . . . . Dan Schumacher
Chief Strategy Officer . . . . John Cosgriff
Communications Officer . . . . Kirsten Gorsuch
Chief Medical Officer. . . . . Sam Ho
Chief Legal Officer . . . . Thad Johnson
Chief Information Officer . . . . Phil McKoy
Chief Financial Officer. . . . . Jeff Putnam

Specialty Managed Care Partners

G Tec, State of RI

Health Insurance Coverage Status and Type of Coverage by Age

Category	All Persons		Under 18 years		Under 65 years	
	Number	%	Number	%	Number	%
Total population	4,861	-	1,168	-	4,049	-
Covered by some type of health insurance	4,375 *(14)*	90.0 *(0.3)*	1,118 *(6)*	95.7 *(0.4)*	3,566 *(14)*	88.1 *(0.3)*
Covered by private health insurance	3,242 *(24)*	66.7 *(0.5)*	653 *(13)*	55.9 *(1.1)*	2,735 *(23)*	67.5 *(0.6)*
Employer-based	2,509 *(28)*	51.6 *(0.6)*	545 *(14)*	46.7 *(1.1)*	2,251 *(26)*	55.6 *(0.6)*
Direct purchase	718 *(16)*	14.8 *(0.3)*	74 *(5)*	6.3 *(0.5)*	448 *(14)*	11.1 *(0.3)*
TRICARE	256 *(12)*	5.3 *(0.3)*	58 *(6)*	5.0 *(0.5)*	166 *(11)*	4.1 *(0.3)*
Covered by public health insurance	1,811 *(21)*	37.2 *(0.4)*	515 *(12)*	44.1 *(1.1)*	1,016 *(21)*	25.1 *(0.5)*
Medicaid	966 *(21)*	19.9 *(0.4)*	510 *(12)*	43.7 *(1.1)*	861 *(20)*	21.3 *(0.5)*
Medicare	955 *(8)*	19.6 *(0.2)*	5 *(1)*	0.4 *(0.1)*	161 *(7)*	4.0 *(0.2)*
VA Care	159 *(7)*	3.3 *(0.1)*	2 *(1)*	0.2 *(0.1)*	77 *(5)*	1.9 *(0.1)*
Not covered at any time during the year	486 *(14)*	10.0 *(0.3)*	50 *(5)*	4.3 *(0.4)*	483 *(14)*	11.9 *(0.3)*

Note: Numbers in thousands; Figures cover civilian noninstitutionalized population in 2016; N/A indicates that data was not available; Z represents or rounds to zero; Margin of error appears in parenthesis and is calculated using replicate weights.
Source: U.S. Census Bureau, American Community Survey, Table HIC-4_ACS. Health Insurance Coverage Status and Type of Coverage by State—All People: 2008 to 2016, Table HIC-5_ACS. Health Insurance Coverage Status and Type of Coverage by State—Children Under 18: 2008 to 2016, Table HIC-6_ACS. Health Insurance Coverage Status and Type of Coverage by State—Persons Under 65: 2008 to 2016

South Carolina

704   Aetna Health of South Carolina

151 Farmington Avenue
Hartford, CT 06156
Toll-Free: 800-872-3862
Phone: 860-273-0123
www.aetna.com
Secondary Address: 6730-B Rockledge Drive, Suite 700,
    Bethesda, MD 20817, 301-581-0600
Subsidiary of: Aetna Inc.
For Profit Organization: Yes

Healthplan and Services Defined
PLAN TYPE: PPO
Other Type: POS
Model Type: Network
Plan Specialty: Behavioral Health, EPO, Lab, PBM,
    Radiology
Benefits Offered: Behavioral Health, Dental, Disease
    Management, Long-Term Care, Physical Therapy,
    Podiatry, Prescription, Psychiatric, Vision, Wellness, Life,
    LTD, STD

Type of Coverage
Commercial, Supplemental Medicare, Student health

Geographic Areas Served
29 counties

Key Personnel
CEO . . . . Mark Bertolini

705   Blue Cross & Blue Shield of South Carolina

51 Clemson Road
Columbia, SC 29229
Toll-Free: 800-868-2520
Phone: 736-1576
www.southcarolinablues.com
For Profit Organization: Yes
Year Founded: 1946
Number of Affiliated Hospitals: 64
Number of Primary Care Physicians: 3,434
Number of Referral/Specialty Physicians: 5,473
Total Enrollment: 950,000
State Enrollment: 950,000

Healthplan and Services Defined
PLAN TYPE: HMO/PPO
Model Type: Network
Plan Specialty: ASO, Behavioral Health, Chiropractic,
    Dental, Disease Management, EPO, Lab, PBM, Vision,
    Radiology, UR
Benefits Offered: Behavioral Health, Chiropractic,
    Complementary Medicine, Dental, Disease Management,
    Physical Therapy, Podiatry, Prescription, Psychiatric,
    Transplant, Vision, Wellness
Offers Demand Management Patient Information Service:
    Yes

Type of Coverage
Commercial, Individual, Medicare

Type of Payment Plans Offered
POS, DFFS, Capitated, FFS, Combination FFS & DFFS

Geographic Areas Served
Statewide

Network Qualifications
Pre-Admission Certification: Yes

Peer Review Type
Utilization Review: Yes
Second Surgical Opinion: Yes

Publishes and Distributes Report Card: Yes

Accreditation Certification
URAC, NCQA
TJC Accreditation, Utilization Review, Pre-Admission
    Certification, State Licensure, Quality Assurance Program

Key Personnel
President . . . . Scott Graves

Specialty Managed Care Partners
Enters into Contracts with Regional Business Coalitions: Yes

706   BlueChoice Health Plan of South Carolina

2501 Faraway Drive
Columbia, SC 29223
Phone: 803-788-0222
www.bluechoicesc.com
For Profit Organization: Yes
Year Founded: 1984
Owned by an Integrated Delivery Network (IDN): Yes
Federally Qualified: Yes
Number of Affiliated Hospitals: 68
Number of Primary Care Physicians: 7,700
Number of Referral/Specialty Physicians: 4,199
Total Enrollment: 205,000
State Enrollment: 205,000

Healthplan and Services Defined
PLAN TYPE: Multiple
Model Type: IPA
Plan Specialty: ASO, Disease Management, EPO, PBM,
    Vision, UR
Benefits Offered: Behavioral Health, Chiropractic,
    Complementary Medicine, Dental, Disease Management,
    Home Care, Inpatient SNF, Physical Therapy, Podiatry,
    Prescription, Psychiatric, Transplant, Vision, Wellness,
    AD&D, Life, LTD, STD, EAP
Offers Demand Management Patient Information Service: Yes

Type of Coverage
Commercial, Individual, Medicare, Medicaid, Medicare
    Advantage
Catastrophic Illness Benefit: Maximum $2M

Type of Payment Plans Offered
POS, DFFS, Combination FFS & DFFS

Geographic Areas Served
Statewide

Subscriber Information
Average Annual Deductible Per Subscriber:
    Employee Only (Self): $0

Employee & 1 Family Member: $0
Employee & 2 Family Members: $0
Average Subscriber Co-Payment:
    Primary Care Physician: $15.00
    Non-Network Physician: $25.00
    Prescription Drugs: $3 tier
    Hospital ER: 10%
    Home Health Care: 10%
    Home Health Care Max. Days/Visits Covered: Unlimited
    Nursing Home Max. Days/Visits Covered: 120 days

Network Qualifications
Pre-Admission Certification: Yes

Peer Review Type
Utilization Review: Yes
Second Surgical Opinion: Yes
Case Management: Yes

Publishes and Distributes Report Card: Yes

Accreditation Certification
NCQA
Quality Assurance Program

Key Personnel
President . . . . Scott Graves

Average Claim Compensation
Physician's Fees Charged: 65%
Hospital's Fees Charged: 65%

Specialty Managed Care Partners
Companion Benefit Alternatives (CBA)

Employer References
Alltel Corporation, Bank of America, Kimberley Clark,
BellSouth, United Parcel Service

707   Delta Dental of South Carolina

1320 Main Street
Suite 650
Columbia, SC 29201
Toll-Free: 800-529-3268
Phone: 803-731-2495
service@deltadentalmo.com
www.deltadentalsc.com
Mailing Address: P.O. Box 8690, St. Louis, MO 63126-0690
Non-Profit Organization: Yes
Year Founded: 1969

Healthplan and Services Defined
  PLAN TYPE: Dental
  Other Type: Dental PPO
  Model Type: Network
  Plan Specialty: ASO, Dental
  Benefits Offered: Dental

Type of Coverage
Commercial, Individual
Catastrophic Illness Benefit: None

Geographic Areas Served
South Carolina and Missouri

708   Humana Health Insurance of South Carolina

240 Harbison Boulevard
Suite H
Columbia, SC 29212
Toll-Free: 877-486-2622
Phone: 803-865-7663
Fax: 803-865-1760
www.humana.com
Secondary Address: 1025 Woodruff Roadf, Suite J108,
  Greenville, SC 29607, 864-968-2307
Subsidiary of: Humana
For Profit Organization: Yes

Healthplan and Services Defined
  PLAN TYPE: HMO/PPO
  Model Type: Network
  Plan Specialty: Dental, Vision
  Benefits Offered: Dental, Vision, Life, LTD, STD

Type of Coverage
Commercial

Geographic Areas Served
Statewide

Accreditation Certification
URAC, NCQA, CORE

Key Personnel
President & CEO. Bruce Broussard
Chief Medical Officer. . . . . Roy A. Beveridge
Chief Consumer Officer . . . . Jody L. Bilner
Human Resources. . . . . Tim Huval
Chief Financial Officer . . . . Brian Kane
Chief Information Officer . . . . Brian LeClaire
General Counsel . . . . Christopher M. Todoroff
Chief Accounting Officer . . . . Cynthia H. Zipperie

709   InStil Health

P.O. Box 100294
Mail Code AG-795
Columbia, SC 29202-3294
Toll-Free: 800-444-5445
Phone: 803-763-6620
Fax: 803-666-3705
sandy.collins@myinstil.com
www.myinstil.com
Total Enrollment: 30,000

Healthplan and Services Defined
  PLAN TYPE: Medicare
  Plan Specialty: ASO
  Benefits Offered: Behavioral Health, Disease Management,
    Home Care, Physical Therapy, Psychiatric, Wellness

Type of Coverage
Medicare, Supplemental Medicare

Accreditation Certification
URAC

Key Personnel
Network Manager . . . . Sandy Collins
Provider Relations . . . . Carlotta Rose
  carlotta.rose@myinstil.com

Service Consultant . . . . Julie Drews

---

710   Molina Healthcare of South Carolina

4105 Faber Place Drive
Suite 120
North Charleston, SC 29405
Toll-Free: 855-882-3901
www.molinahealthcare.com
Subsidiary of: Molina Healthcare, Inc.
For Profit Organization: Yes

Healthplan and Services Defined
PLAN TYPE: Medicare
Model Type: Network
Plan Specialty: Dental, PBM, Vision, Integrated
   Medicare/Medicaid (Duals)
Benefits Offered: Dental, Prescription, Vision, Wellness, Life

Type of Coverage
Individual, Medicare, Supplemental Medicare, Medicaid

Geographic Areas Served
Statewide

Key Personnel
Chief Executive Officer . . . . Joseph W. White
Chief Operating Officer . . . . Terry Bayer
General Counsel. . . . . Jeff D. Barlow
SVP, Relations/Marketing . . . . Juan Jos, Orellana
Chief Information Officer . . . . Rick Hopfer

---

711   Select Health of South Carolina

P.O. Box 40849
Charleston, SC 29423
Toll-Free: 800-741-6605
Phone: 843-569-1759
Fax: 843-569-0702
www.selecthealthofsc.com
Subsidiary of: AmeriHealth Mercy
For Profit Organization: Yes
Total Enrollment: 330,000
State Enrollment: 330,000

Healthplan and Services Defined
PLAN TYPE: HMO
Model Type: Medicaid
Plan Specialty: Medicaid
Benefits Offered: Chiropractic, Disease Management, Home
   Care, Inpatient SNF, Physical Therapy, Prescription,
   Psychiatric, Transplant, Vision, Wellness, Transportation;
   Hearing; Durable Medical Equipment; Family Planning;
   Labs & X-rays; Speech Therapy

Type of Coverage
Medicaid

Geographic Areas Served
Statewide

Peer Review Type
Case Management: Yes

Publishes and Distributes Report Card: Yes

Accreditation Certification
TJC, URAC, NCQA

Key Personnel
Founder/Regional Pres. . . . . J. Michael Jernigan
Chief Medical Officer. . . . . Fred Hill, MD
Director, Finance. . . . . Sean Popson
Plan Operations & Admin. . . . . Courtnay Thompson
Director, Member Services . . . . Kevin Vaughan
Provider Services. Phillip Fairchild
Director, Communications. . . . . Tricia Crimminger

---

712   UnitedHealthcare of South Carolina

107 Westpark Boulevard
Suite 110
Columbia, SC 29210
Toll-Free: 800-660-5378
Phone: 803-551-1170
www.uhc.com/contact-us/south-carolina
Subsidiary of: UnitedHealth Group
For Profit Organization: Yes

Healthplan and Services Defined
PLAN TYPE: HMO/PPO
Model Type: Network
Plan Specialty: Behavioral Health, Dental, Disease
   Management, PBM, Vision
Benefits Offered: Behavioral Health, Dental, Disease
   Management, Long-Term Care, Prescription, Vision,
   Wellness, Life, LTD, STD

Type of Coverage
Individual, Medicare, Supplemental Medicare, Medicaid,
   Catastrophic, Family, Military, Veterans, Group,

Geographic Areas Served
Statewide

Accreditation Certification
AAPI, NCQA

Key Personnel
President . . . . David Wichmann
Chief Operating Officer . . . . Dan Schumacher
Chief Strategy Officer . . . . John Cosgriff
Communications Officer . . . . Kirsten Gorsuch
Chief Medical Officer. . . . . Sam Ho
Chief Legal Officer . . . . Thad Johnson
Chief Information Officer . . . . Phil McKoy
Chief Financial Officer. . . . . Jeff Putnam

Health Insurance Coverage Status and Type of Coverage by Age

Category	All Persons		Under 18 years		Under 65 years	
	Number	%	Number	%	Number	%
Total population	849	-	225	-	718	-
Covered by some type of health insurance	775 (4)	91.3 (0.5)	215 (2)	95.3 (0.8)	644 (5)	89.7 (0.6)
Covered by private health insurance	623 (8)	73.5 (0.9)	148 (5)	65.8 (2.0)	539 (8)	75.1 (1.1)
Employer-based	462 (11)	54.4 (1.2)	122 (5)	54.1 (2.3)	438 (10)	60.9 (1.4)
Direct purchase	166 (8)	19.6 (0.9)	26 (3)	11.7 (1.4)	105 (7)	14.6 (1.0)
TRICARE	35 (4)	4.2 (0.4)	10 (2)	4.2 (0.8)	28 (3)	3.8 (0.5)
Covered by public health insurance	263 (7)	31.0 (0.8)	75 (5)	33.5 (2.0)	135 (7)	18.8 (1.0)
Medicaid	125 (7)	14.8 (0.8)	74 (5)	33.0 (2.0)	112 (7)	15.6 (0.9)
Medicare	147 (3)	17.3 (0.4)	1 (1)	0.5 (0.3)	19 (3)	2.7 (0.4)
VA Care	32 (2)	3.8 (0.3)	Z (Z)	0.2 (0.2)	15 (2)	2.1 (0.2)
Not covered at any time during the year	74 (4)	8.7 (0.5)	11 (2)	4.7 (0.8)	74 (4)	10.3 (0.6)

Note: Numbers in thousands; Figures cover civilian noninstitutionalized population in 2016; N/A indicates that data was not available; Z represents or rounds to zero; Margin of error appears in parenthesis and is calculated using replicate weights.
Source: U.S. Census Bureau, American Community Survey, Table HIC-4_ACS. Health Insurance Coverage Status and Type of Coverage by State—All People: 2008 to 2016, Table HIC-5_ACS. Health Insurance Coverage Status and Type of Coverage by State—Children Under 18: 2008 to 2016, Table HIC-6_ACS. Health Insurance Coverage Status and Type of Coverage by State—Persons Under 65: 2008 to 2016

South Dakota

713 Avera Health Plans

3816 S Elmwood Avenue
Sioux Falls, SD 57105-6583
Toll-Free: 855-692-8372
Phone: 605-322-4500
sales@averahealthplans.com
www.averahealthplans.com
Total Enrollment: 63,000
State Enrollment: 63,000

Healthplan and Services Defined
PLAN TYPE: HMO
Benefits Offered: Disease Management, Prescription,
Wellness, Health Education, EAP

Type of Coverage
Commercial, Individual

Type of Payment Plans Offered
POS

Geographic Areas Served
Statewide

Accreditation Certification
URAC

Key Personnel
President . . . . Gary Gaspar
SVP, Financial Services . . . . Jim Breckenridge
Chief Operations Officer . . . . Fred Slunecka
Chief Executive Officer . . . . Debra Muller
Physician . . . . Thomas Dean
Physician . . . . Clark Likness

714 DakotaCare

2600 W 49th Street
P.O. Box 7406
Sioux Falls, SD 57117-7406
Toll-Free: 800-325-5598
Phone: 605-334-4000
customer-service@dakotacare.com
www.dakotacare.com
Subsidiary of: Avera Health
For Profit Organization: Yes
Year Founded: 1986
Physician Owned Organization: Yes
Number of Affiliated Hospitals: 74
Number of Primary Care Physicians: 825
Number of Referral/Specialty Physicians: 950
Total Enrollment: 118,600
State Enrollment: 24,310

Healthplan and Services Defined
PLAN TYPE: HMO
Model Type: IPA
Plan Specialty: ASO, Behavioral Health, Chiropractic,
Dental, Disease Management, Lab, PBM, Vision,
Radiology, UR
Benefits Offered: Behavioral Health, Chiropractic,
Complementary Medicine, Dental, Disease Management,

Home Care, Inpatient SNF, Physical Therapy, Podiatry,
Prescription, Psychiatric, Transplant, Vision, Wellness,
AD&D, Life, LTD, STD
Offers Demand Management Patient Information Service: No

Type of Payment Plans Offered
POS, FFS

Geographic Areas Served
HMO: all counties in South Dakota; TPA: Nationwide

Subscriber Information
Average Monthly Fee Per Subscriber
(Employee + Employer Contribution):
Employee Only (Self): Varies by plan
Average Annual Deductible Per Subscriber:
Employee & 1 Family Member: $1500
Average Subscriber Co-Payment:
Primary Care Physician: $25.00
Non-Network Physician: $25.00
Hospital ER: $150.00

Network Qualifications
Pre-Admission Certification: Yes

Peer Review Type
Utilization Review: Yes
Case Management: Yes

Publishes and Distributes Report Card: No

Accreditation Certification
URAC
Utilization Review, Pre-Admission Certification, State
Licensure, Quality Assurance Program

Key Personnel
Chief Operating Officer . . . . Rhonda K. Mack
dkrogman@dakotacare.com
VP, Medical Management . . . . Rich Jones

Specialty Managed Care Partners
Prescription benefits - CVS Caremark, Chiropractic - CASD,
Transplant - Optum, Dental Benefits - Companion Life, Life
Insurance Benefits - Companion Life, Sun Life Standard,
STD/LTD - Companion Life
Enters into Contracts with Regional Business Coalitions: No

715 Delta Dental of South Dakota

P.O. Box 1157
Pierre, SD 57501
Toll-Free: 877-841-1478
Fax: 605-494-2566
benefit@deltadentalsd.com
www.deltadentalsd.com
Non-Profit Organization: Yes
Year Founded: 1963
Total Enrollment: 60,000,000
State Enrollment: 340,000

Healthplan and Services Defined
PLAN TYPE: Dental
Other Type: Dental PPO
Model Type: Network
Plan Specialty: ASO, Dental
Benefits Offered: Dental

Type of Coverage
Commercial, Individual
Catastrophic Illness Benefit: None

Geographic Areas Served
Statewide

Key Personnel
President & CEO........................ Scott Jones
VP, Operations..................... Mick Heckenlaible
VP, Finance............................. Kirby Scott
VP, Underwriting .... Jeff Miller
VP, Information Tech.................... Gene Tetzlaff

716   First Choice of the Midwest
100 S Spring Avenue
Suite 220
Sioux Falls, SD 57104-3660
Toll-Free: 888-246-9949
Phone: 605-332-5955
Fax: 605-332-5953
info@1choicem.com
www.1choicem.com
Mailing Address: PO Box 5078, Sioux Falls, SD 57117-5078
For Profit Organization: Yes
Year Founded: 1997
Owned by an Integrated Delivery Network (IDN): Yes
Number of Referral/Specialty Physicians: 6,924
Total Enrollment: 87,000
State Enrollment: 25,000

Healthplan and Services Defined
PLAN TYPE: PPO
Model Type: Network, Open Staff
Plan Specialty: ASO, Behavioral Health, Chiropractic,
   Disease Management, EPO, Lab, Radiology, Worker's
   Compensation
Benefits Offered: Behavioral Health, Chiropractic,
   Complementary Medicine, Home Care, Inpatient SNF,
   Long-Term Care, Physical Therapy, Podiatry, Prescription,
   Psychiatric, Transplant, Vision, Wellness, Worker's
   Compensation, Durable Medical Equipment

Type of Payment Plans Offered
DFFS

Geographic Areas Served
Colorado, Idaho, Iowa, Minnesota, Montana, Nebraska,
North Dakota, South Dakota, Utah, and Wyoming

Network Qualifications
Pre-Admission Certification: No

Accreditation Certification
TJC, NCQA

Average Claim Compensation
Physician's Fees Charged: 85%
Hospital's Fees Charged: 90%

Specialty Managed Care Partners
Enters into Contracts with Regional Business Coalitions: Yes

717   Humana Health Insurance of South Dakota
1415 Kimberly Road
Bettendorf, SD 52722
Toll-Free: 800-653-7275
Phone: 563-344-1242
Fax: 563-355-0730
www.humana.com
Subsidiary of: Humana
For Profit Organization: Yes

Healthplan and Services Defined
PLAN TYPE: HMO/PPO
Model Type: Network
Plan Specialty: Dental, Vision
Benefits Offered: Dental, Vision, Life, LTD, STD

Type of Coverage
Commercial, Medicare

Geographic Areas Served
Statewide

Accreditation Certification
URAC, NCQA, CORE

Key Personnel
President & CEO..................... Bruce Broussard
Chief Medical Officer................. Roy A. Beveridge
Chief Consumer Officer.................. Jody L. Bilney
Human Resources........................ Tim Huval
Chief Financial Officer .... Brian Kane
Chief Information Officer .... Brian LeClaire
General Counsel............... Christopher M. Todoroff
Chief Accounting Officer .... Cynthia H. Zipperie

718   UnitedHealthcare of South Dakota
9700 Health Care Lane
Minnetonka, MN 55343
Toll-Free: 800-842-3585
www.uhc.com/contact-us/south-dakota
Subsidiary of: UnitedHealth Group
Year Founded: 1977

Healthplan and Services Defined
PLAN TYPE: HMO/PPO
Model Type: Network
Plan Specialty: Behavioral Health, Dental, Disease
   Management, Lab, PBM, Vision, Radiology
Benefits Offered: Behavioral Health, Chiropractic, Dental,
   Disease Management, Long-Term Care, Physical Therapy,
   Prescription, Vision, Wellness, AD&D, Life, LTD, STD

Type of Coverage
Commercial, Individual, Indemnity, Medicare, Supplemental
   Medicare, Medicaid, Catastrophic, Family, Military,
   Veterans, Group,

Geographic Areas Served
Statewide. South Dakota is covered by the Minnesota branch

Network Qualifications
Pre-Admission Certification: Yes

Peer Review Type
Utilization Review: Yes
Second Surgical Opinion: Yes

Case Management: Yes

Publishes and Distributes Report Card: Yes

Accreditation Certification
TJC, NCQA

Key Personnel

President . . . . David Wichmann
Chief Operating Officer . . . . Dan Schumacher
Chief Strategy Officer . . . . Jeff Cosgriff
Communications Officer . . . . Kirsten Gorsuch
Chief Medical Officer. . . . . Sam Ho
Chief Legal Officer . . . . Thad Johnson
Chief Information Officer . . . . Phil McKoy
Chief Financial Officer. . . . . Jeff Putnam

Specialty Managed Care Partners
Enters into Contracts with Regional Business Coalitions: Yes

719　Wellmark Blue Cross & Blue Shield of South Dakota

1601 W Madison Street
Sioux Falls, SD 57104
Toll-Free: 800-524-9242
Phone: 605-373-7200
www.wellmark.com
For Profit Organization: Yes
Owned by an Integrated Delivery Network (IDN): Yes
Number of Affiliated Hospitals: 6,000
Number of Primary Care Physicians: 600,000
Total Enrollment: 1,800,000
State Enrollment: 300,000

Healthplan and Services Defined
PLAN TYPE: Multiple
Model Type: Network
Plan Specialty: ASO, Behavioral Health, Chiropractic,
Dental, Disease Management, EPO, Lab, PBM, Vision,
Radiology, UR
Benefits Offered: Behavioral Health, Chiropractic,
Complementary Medicine, Dental, Disease Management,
Home Care, Inpatient SNF, Physical Therapy, Podiatry,
Prescription, Psychiatric, Transplant, Vision, Wellness,
AD&D, Life, LTD, STD

Type of Coverage
Commercial, Individual, Indemnity, Medicare, Supplemental
Medicare, Medicaid, Catastrophic
Catastrophic Illness Benefit: Maximum $1M

Geographic Areas Served
South Dakota and Iowa

Publishes and Distributes Report Card: Yes

Accreditation Certification
AAAHC, TJC, URAC, NCQA

Key Personnel

Chairman/CEO . . . . John D Forsyth
Chief Financial Officer . . . . David Brown
Chief Information Officer . . . . Paul Eddy
Administrative & Legal . . . . Cory R. Harris
Business Development . . . . Laura Jackson
Executive VP, Operations . . . . Vicki Signor

Specialty Managed Care Partners
American Health Ways

Health Insurance Coverage Status and Type of Coverage by Age

Category	All Persons		Under 18 years		Under 65 years	
	Number	%	Number	%	Number	%
Total population	6,547	-	1,589	-	5,530	-
Covered by some type of health insurance	5,955 *(16)*	91.0 *(0.2)*	1,530 *(8)*	96.3 *(0.4)*	4,943 *(16)*	89.4 *(0.3)*
Covered by private health insurance	4,339 *(30)*	66.3 *(0.5)*	917 *(16)*	57.7 *(1.0)*	3,739 *(29)*	67.6 *(0.5)*
Employer-based	3,420 *(29)*	52.2 *(0.4)*	776 *(14)*	48.9 *(0.9)*	3,137 *(26)*	56.7 *(0.5)*
Direct purchase	955 *(19)*	14.6 *(0.3)*	122 *(9)*	7.7 *(0.5)*	603 *(17)*	10.9 *(0.3)*
TRICARE	219 *(10)*	3.4 *(0.1)*	47 *(4)*	2.9 *(0.3)*	145 *(9)*	2.6 *(0.2)*
Covered by public health insurance	2,442 *(25)*	37.3 *(0.4)*	686 *(15)*	43.2 *(0.9)*	1,452 *(25)*	26.3 *(0.5)*
Medicaid	1,411 *(25)*	21.6 *(0.4)*	681 *(15)*	42.9 *(0.9)*	1,277 *(24)*	23.1 *(0.4)*
Medicare	1,202 *(9)*	18.4 *(0.1)*	8 *(2)*	0.5 *(0.1)*	214 *(8)*	3.9 *(0.1)*
VA Care	173 *(6)*	2.6 *(0.1)*	2 *(1)*	0.1 *(0.1)*	84 *(5)*	1.5 *(0.1)*
Not covered at any time during the year	592 *(16)*	9.0 *(0.2)*	58 *(7)*	3.7 *(0.4)*	588 *(15)*	10.6 *(0.3)*

Note: Numbers in thousands; Figures cover civilian noninstitutionalized population in 2016; N/A indicates that data was not available; Z represents or rounds to zero; Margin of error appears in parenthesis and is calculated using replicate weights.
Source: U.S. Census Bureau, American Community Survey, Table HIC-4_ACS. Health Insurance Coverage Status and Type of Coverage by State—All People: 2008 to 2016, Table HIC-5_ACS. Health Insurance Coverage Status and Type of Coverage by State—Children Under 18: 2008 to 2016, Table HIC-6_ACS. Health Insurance Coverage Status and Type of Coverage by State—Persons Under 65: 2008 to 2016

Tennessee

720 Aetna Health of Tennessee

151 Farmington Avenue
Hartford, CT 06156
Toll-Free: 800-872-3862
Phone: 860-273-0123
www.aetna.com
Subsidiary of: Aetna Inc.
For Profit Organization: Yes

Healthplan and Services Defined
PLAN TYPE: HMO/PPO
Other Type: POS
Model Type: Network
Plan Specialty: Behavioral Health, EPO, Lab, PBM,
Radiology
Benefits Offered: Behavioral Health, Dental, Disease
Management, Long-Term Care, Physical Therapy,
Podiatry, Prescription, Psychiatric, Vision, Wellness, Life,
LTD, STD

Type of Coverage
Commercial, Student health

Geographic Areas Served
Statewide

Key Personnel
CEO . . . . Mark Bertolini

721 Amerigroup Tennessee

22 Century Boulevard
Suite 310
Nashville, TN 37214
Toll-Free: 800-600-4441
Phone: 615-316-2400
www.myamerigroup.com/tn
Subsidiary of: Anthem, Inc.
For Profit Organization: Yes
Year Founded: 2007

Healthplan and Services Defined
PLAN TYPE: HMO

Type of Coverage
Taking Care of Baby and Me

Geographic Areas Served
Statewide

Accreditation Certification
NCQA

Key Personnel
EVP/Pres., Gov. Business . . . . Peter D. Haytaian

722 Baptist Health Services Group

350 N Humphreys Boulevard
4th Floor
Memphis, TN 38120
Toll-Free: 800-522-2474
Phone: 901-227-2474
bhsginfo@bmhcc.org

www.bhsgonline.org
Subsidiary of: Baptist Memorial Health Care Corporation
Non-Profit Organization: Yes
Year Founded: 1984
Number of Affiliated Hospitals: 52
Number of Primary Care Physicians: 4,000
Number of Referral/Specialty Physicians: 2,073
Total Enrollment: 423,244

Healthplan and Services Defined
PLAN TYPE: Other
Model Type: Network, Provider Spons. Network
Plan Specialty: Disease Management, Lab, Worker's
Compensation
Benefits Offered: Disease Management, Home Care,
Long-Term Care, Physical Therapy, Podiatry, Transplant,
Wellness, Orthopedics; Diabeties; Dialysis; Durable
Medical Equipment; Occupational Therapy; Prosthetics
Offers Demand Management Patient Information Service: No

Geographic Areas Served
E Arkansas, SW Kentucky, N Mississipi, SE Missouri, and W
Tennessee

Subscriber Information
Average Monthly Fee Per Subscriber
(Employee + Employer Contribution):
Employee Only (Self): n/a
Average Annual Deductible Per Subscriber:
Employee Only (Self): n/a
Average Subscriber Co-Payment:
Primary Care Physician: n/a

Publishes and Distributes Report Card: No

Key Personnel
President/CEO . . . . Jason Little
Chief Operating Officer . . . . Paul DePriest
Chief Financial Officer . . . . Bill Griffin
Chief Legal Officer . . . . Gregory M. Duckett
CEO, Health Service Group . . . . David Elliott

Average Claim Compensation
Physician's Fees Charged: 1%
Hospital's Fees Charged: 1%

Specialty Managed Care Partners
Enters into Contracts with Regional Business Coalitions: Yes

723 Blue Cross & Blue Shield of Tennessee

1 Cameron Hill Circle
Chattanooga, TN 37402
Toll-Free: 800-565-9140
Phone: 423-535-3040
www.bcbst.com
Secondary Address: 85 North Danny Thomas Boulevard,
Memphis, TN 38103-2398
Non-Profit Organization: Yes
Year Founded: 1945
Number of Affiliated Hospitals: 130
Number of Primary Care Physicians: 2,490
Number of Referral/Specialty Physicians: 15,000
Total Enrollment: 3,000,000
State Enrollment: 3,000,000

Healthplan and Services Defined
PLAN TYPE: Multiple

Plan Specialty: Dental, Disease Management, Vision

Benefits Offered: Dental, Disease Management, Prescription, Vision, Wellness

Type of Coverage
Medicaid

Key Personnel
President & CEO .... JD Hickey
EVP, CFO .... John Giblin
EVP, COO .... Scott Pierce
SVP, Human Resources .... Karen Ward
SVP, Marketing Officer................... Henry Smith
VP, General Manager....................... Todd Ray
Chief Medical Officer................. Andrea D. Willis
SVP, General Counsel .... Anne Hance
Communications Officer .... Roy Vaughn
Government Relations................. Dakasha Winton

Specialty Managed Care Partners
Magellen Health Services

Employer References
State, local and government employees

---

724 Cigna-HealthSpring
P.O. Box 20002
Nashville, TN 37202
Toll-Free: 800-668-3813
www.cigna.com/medicare/cigna-healthspring
Subsidiary of: Cigna Corporation
For Profit Organization: Yes
Year Founded: 2000

Healthplan and Services Defined
PLAN TYPE: Medicare

Type of Coverage
Medicare, Supplemental Medicare, Medicaid

Geographic Areas Served
Certain counties in Alabama, Arizona, Delaware, Florida, Georgia, Illinois, Indiana, Maryland, Mississippi, North Carolina, Pennsylvania, South Carolina, Tennessee, Texas and Washington, DC

Accreditation Certification
URAC, NCQA

---

725 Cigna-HealthSpring
500 Great Circle Road
Nashville, TN 37228
Toll-Free: 888-705-2933
info@myhealthspring.com
www.healthspring.com
For Profit Organization: Yes
Year Founded: 1995
Number of Affiliated Hospitals: 42
Number of Primary Care Physicians: 4,300
Total Enrollment: 345,000
State Enrollment: 17,844

Healthplan and Services Defined
PLAN TYPE: Medicare

Model Type: Network

Plan Specialty: ASO, EPO

Benefits Offered: Behavioral Health, Chiropractic, Disease Management, Home Care, Inpatient SNF, Physical Therapy, Podiatry, Prescription, Psychiatric, Transplant, Vision

Type of Coverage
Commercial, Medicare, Supplemental Medicare, Catastrophic, Medicare PPO

Catastrophic Illness Benefit: Covered

Type of Payment Plans Offered
POS, DFFS, Capitated, Combination FFS & DFFS

Geographic Areas Served
Tennessee, Northern Mississippi, Northern Georgia

Subscriber Information
Average Monthly Fee Per Subscriber
(Employee + Employer Contribution):
Employee Only (Self): Varies by plan
Medicare: $0
Average Subscriber Co-Payment:
Primary Care Physician: Varies by plan

Network Qualifications
Minimum Years of Practice: 3
Pre-Admission Certification: Yes

Peer Review Type
Utilization Review: Yes
Case Management: Yes

Accreditation Certification
AAAHC, URAC

Average Claim Compensation
Physician's Fees Charged: 65%
Hospital's Fees Charged: 80%

Specialty Managed Care Partners
Magellaw, Black Vision, MedImpact

Employer References
Lifeway, Ingram Industries, AmSouth Banks

---

726 Coventry Health & Life Ins. Co. of Tennessee
5350 Poplar Avenue
Suite 390
Memphis, TN 38119
Phone: 901-462-2380
www.coventryhealthcare.com
Subsidiary of: Aetna Inc.
For Profit Organization: Yes

Healthplan and Services Defined
PLAN TYPE: HMO/PPO

Model Type: Network

Plan Specialty: Behavioral Health, Dental, Worker's Compensation

Benefits Offered: Behavioral Health, Dental, Prescription, Wellness, Worker's Compensation, Life

Type of Coverage
Commercial, Individual, Medicare, Medicaid

Geographic Areas Served
Tennessee, Mississippi and Arkansas

Key Personnel
Chief Executive Officer . . . . Mark T. Bertolini
President . . . . Karen S. Lynch
Chief Financial Officer . . . . Shawn M. Guertin
Operations & Technology . . . . Meg McCarthy
Chief Medical Officer . . . . Harold L. Paz
General Counsel . . . . Thomas Sabatino Jr.
Government Services . . . . Fran S. Soistman

727 Delta Dental of Tennessee

240 Venture Circle
Nashville, TN 37228
Toll-Free: 800-223-3104
www.deltadentaltn.com
Non-Profit Organization: Yes
Year Founded: 1965
State Enrollment: 1,500,000

Healthplan and Services Defined
PLAN TYPE: Dental
Other Type: Dental PPO
Model Type: Network
Plan Specialty: ASO, Dental
Benefits Offered: Dental

Type of Coverage
Commercial, Individual
Catastrophic Illness Benefit: None

Geographic Areas Served
Statewide

Key Personnel
President & CEO. . . . . Philip A. Wenk
Senior VP, Operations . . . . Kaye Martin
Chief Financial Officer . . . . Jeff Ballard

728 Health Choice LLC

1661 International Place
Suite 150
Memphis, TN 38120
Phone: 901-821-6700
Fax: 901-821-4900
contactus@myhealthchoice.com
www.myhealthchoice.com
Year Founded: 1985
Number of Affiliated Hospitals: 24
Number of Primary Care Physicians: 1,400
Total Enrollment: 518,000
State Enrollment: 518,000

Healthplan and Services Defined
PLAN TYPE: PPO
Model Type: PHO
Plan Specialty: ASO, Behavioral Health, Chiropractic,
Disease Management, EPO, Lab, MSO, PBM, Radiology,
Worker's Compensation, UR

Type of Payment Plans Offered
DFFS, FFS, Combination FFS & DFFS

Geographic Areas Served
Tennessee: Shelby, Tipton, Fayette; Arkansas: Crittenden,
Cross; Mississippi: Tunica, Desoto; Missouri: Pemiscott

Network Qualifications
Pre-Admission Certification: Yes

Peer Review Type
Utilization Review: Yes
Second Surgical Opinion: Yes
Case Management: Yes

Accreditation Certification
AAAHC
TJC Accreditation, Medicare Approved, Utilization Review,
Pre-Admission Certification, State Licensure, Quality
Assurance Program

Key Personnel
President/CEO . . . . Mitch Graves

Specialty Managed Care Partners
Lakeside Behavioral Health, Med Impact PEM
Memphis Business Group On Health

Employer References
City of Memphis Employees, Shelby County Government,
Memphis Light Gas and Water, Methodist HealthCare
Associates, St. Jude Children's Hospital

729 HealthPartners

620 Skyline Drive
Jackson, TN 38301
Phone: 731-541-5000
Fax: 731-424-4109
info@wth.org
www.wth.org
Subsidiary of: West Tennessee Healthcare
Non-Profit Organization: Yes
Number of Affiliated Hospitals: 14
Total Enrollment: 48,477
State Enrollment: 48,477

Healthplan and Services Defined
PLAN TYPE: PPO
Other Type: TPA
Plan Specialty: Disease Management, Lab, Radiology,
Worker's Compensation, Anesthesia; Cancer; Pediatric;
Inpatient Rehabilitation; Orthopedics; Outpatient Therapy;
Sleep Disorders
Benefits Offered: Dental, Disease Management, Home Care,
Prescription, Wellness
Offers Demand Management Patient Information Service: Yes
DMPI Services Offered: Classes and Events

Type of Coverage
Commercial, Individual

Geographic Areas Served
West Tennessee

Peer Review Type
Utilization Review: Yes
Case Management: Yes

Key Personnel
President/CEO. . . . . James Ross

Chairwoman............................ Vicki Burch
Secretary............................ Curtis Mansfield
Vice Chairman .... Danny Wheeler
Board Member .... Phil Bryant
Board Member........................ Greg Milam

Specialty Managed Care Partners
Express Scripts

730 Humana Health Insurance of Tennessee
6515 Poplar Avenue
Suite 108
Memphis, TN 38119
Toll-Free: 866-254-1218
Fax: 901-685-0194
www.humana.com
Secondary Address: 320 Seven Springs Way, Suite 200, Brentwood, TN 37027, 877-365-1197
For Profit Organization: Yes

Healthplan and Services Defined
PLAN TYPE: HMO/PPO
Plan Specialty: ASO
Benefits Offered: Disease Management, Prescription, Wellness

Type of Coverage
Commercial, Individual

Geographic Areas Served
Statewide

Accreditation Certification
URAC, NCQA, CORE

Key Personnel
President & CEO .... Bruce D. Broussard
Chief Medical Officer................ Roy A. Beveridge
Chief Consumer Officer................. Jody L. Bilney
SVP, Human Resources .... Tim Huval
Chief Financial Officer .... Brian Kane
Chief Information Officer .... Brian LeClaire
SVP, General Counsel .... Christopher M. Todoroff

Specialty Managed Care Partners
Caremark Rx

Employer References
Tricare

731 Initial Group
6556 Jocelyn Hollow Road
Nashville, TN 37205
Toll-Free: 866-295-6586
Phone: 865-546-1893
Fax: 615-352-8782
www.initialgroup.com
Mailing Address: P.O. Box 58735, Nashville, TN 37205-8735
Subsidiary of: Baptist Health System of East Tennessee
For Profit Organization: Yes
Year Founded: 1994
Number of Affiliated Hospitals: 190
Number of Primary Care Physicians: 12,000
Number of Referral/Specialty Physicians: 4,000

Total Enrollment: 200,000
State Enrollment: 106,364

Healthplan and Services Defined
PLAN TYPE: PPO
Model Type: Network
Plan Specialty: Behavioral Health, Lab, Radiology, Worker's Compensation
Benefits Offered: Behavioral Health, Home Care, Inpatient SNF, Physical Therapy, Podiatry, Psychiatric, Transplant, Wellness, Worker's Compensation, Life, LTD

Type of Coverage
Commercial, Medicare
Catastrophic Illness Benefit: Covered

Type of Payment Plans Offered
POS

Geographic Areas Served
East Tennessee region (i.e., KY, NC, VA, TN, GA and AL)

Subscriber Information
Average Monthly Fee Per Subscriber
(Employee + Employer Contribution):
Employee Only (Self): Varies by plan
Average Annual Deductible Per Subscriber:
Employee Only (Self): $250.00
Employee & 2 Family Members: $500.00
Average Subscriber Co-Payment:
Primary Care Physician: $15.00
Prescription Drugs: $5.00/10.00
Hospital ER: $30.00
Home Health Care: $30.00

Network Qualifications
Pre-Admission Certification: Yes

Peer Review Type
Utilization Review: Yes
Second Surgical Opinion: Yes
Case Management: Yes

Accreditation Certification
URAC
TJC Accreditation, Medicare Approved, Utilization Review, Pre-Admission Certification, State Licensure, Quality Assurance Program

Key Personnel
President/CEO .... Lisa J Wear

Specialty Managed Care Partners
Health System

732 UnitedHealthcare of Tennessee
10 Cadillac Drive
Suite 200
Brentwood, TN 37027
Toll-Free: 800-695-1273
www.uhc.com/contact-us/tennessee
Secondary Address: 3175 Lenox Park Boulevard, Memphis, TN 38115, 866-314-9794
Subsidiary of: UnitedHealth Group
For Profit Organization: Yes
Year Founded: 1992

Healthplan and Services Defined
PLAN TYPE: HMO/PPO
Model Type: Network
Plan Specialty: ASO, Behavioral Health, Chiropractic,
   Dental, Disease Management, EPO, Lab, MSO, PBM,
   Vision, Radiology, UR
Benefits Offered: Behavioral Health, Dental, Disease
   Management, Long-Term Care, Prescription, Vision,
   Wellness, AD&D, Life, LTD, STD

Type of Coverage
Commercial, Individual, Indemnity, Medicare, Supplemental
   Medicare, Medicaid, Catastrophic, Family, Military,
   Veterans, Group,
Catastrophic Illness Benefit: Covered

Geographic Areas Served
Statewide

Network Qualifications
Pre-Admission Certification: Yes

Accreditation Certification
AAPI, NCQA

Key Personnel
President & CEO . . . . David Wichmann
Chief Operating Officer . . . . Dan Schumacher
Chief Strategy Officer . . . . John Cosgriff
Communications Officer . . . . Kirsten Gorsuch
Chief Medical Officer. . . . . Sam Ho
Chief Legal Officer . . . . Thad Johnson
Chief Information Officer . . . . Phil McKoy
Chief Financial Officer. Jeff Putnam

Specialty Managed Care Partners
United Health Group, Spectra, United Behavioral Health
Enters into Contracts with Regional Business Coalitions: Yes

Health Insurance Coverage Status and Type of Coverage by Age

Category	All Persons		Under 18 years		Under 65 years	
	Number	%	Number	%	Number	%
Total population	27,386	-	7,696	-	24,126	-
Covered by some type of health insurance	22,841 *(56)*	83.4 *(0.2)*	6,944 *(21)*	90.2 *(0.3)*	19,639 *(55)*	81.4 *(0.2)*
Covered by private health insurance	17,190 *(81)*	62.8 *(0.3)*	4,023 *(42)*	52.3 *(0.6)*	15,406 *(80)*	63.9 *(0.3)*
Employer-based	13,940 *(75)*	50.9 *(0.3)*	3,410 *(39)*	44.3 *(0.5)*	12,949 *(74)*	53.7 *(0.3)*
Direct purchase	3,311 *(42)*	12.1 *(0.2)*	536 *(18)*	7.0 *(0.2)*	2,453 *(41)*	10.2 *(0.2)*
TRICARE	821 *(22)*	3.0 *(0.1)*	189 *(10)*	2.5 *(0.1)*	565 *(20)*	2.3 *(0.1)*
Covered by public health insurance	7,987 *(57)*	29.2 *(0.2)*	3,116 *(41)*	40.5 *(0.5)*	4,893 *(57)*	20.3 *(0.2)*
Medicaid	4,792 *(57)*	17.5 *(0.2)*	3,091 *(41)*	40.2 *(0.5)*	4,328 *(55)*	17.9 *(0.2)*
Medicare	3,620 *(17)*	13.2 *(0.1)*	32 *(3)*	0.4 *(Z)*	532 *(15)*	2.2 *(0.1)*
VA Care	603 *(13)*	2.2 *(Z)*	11 *(2)*	0.1 *(Z)*	318 *(11)*	1.3 *(Z)*
Not covered at any time during the year	4,545 *(55)*	16.6 *(0.2)*	752 *(21)*	9.8 *(0.3)*	4,487 *(55)*	18.6 *(0.2)*

Note: Numbers in thousands; Figures cover civilian noninstitutionalized population in 2016; N/A indicates that data was not available; Z represents or rounds to zero; Margin of error appears in parenthesis and is calculated using replicate weights.
Source: U.S. Census Bureau, American Community Survey, Table HIC-4_ACS. Health Insurance Coverage Status and Type of Coverage by State—All People: 2008 to 2016, Table HIC-5_ACS. Health Insurance Coverage Status and Type of Coverage by State—Children Under 18: 2008 to 2016, Table HIC-6_ACS. Health Insurance Coverage Status and Type of Coverage by State—Persons Under 65: 2008 to 2016

Texas

733 Aetna Health of Texas

151 Farmington Avenue
Hartford, CT 06156
Toll-Free: 800-872-3862
Phone: 860-273-0123
www.aetna.com
Subsidiary of: Aetna Inc.
For Profit Organization: Yes

Healthplan and Services Defined
PLAN TYPE: HMO/PPO
Other Type: POS
Model Type: Network
Plan Specialty: Behavioral Health, EPO, Lab, PBM,
   Radiology
Benefits Offered: Behavioral Health, Dental, Disease
   Management, Long-Term Care, Physical Therapy,
   Podiatry, Prescription, Psychiatric, Vision, Wellness, Life,
   LTD, STD

Type of Coverage
Commercial, Medicaid, Student health

Geographic Areas Served
Statewide

Key Personnel
CEO . . . . Mark Bertolini

734 Alliance Regional Health Network

1501 S. Coulter Street
Amarillo, TX 79106
Phone: 806-354-1000
www.nwtexashealthcare.com
Subsidiary of: Northwest Texas Healthcare System
For Profit Organization: Yes
Year Founded: 1986
Number of Affiliated Hospitals: 25
Number of Primary Care Physicians: 1,000
Number of Referral/Specialty Physicians: 900
Total Enrollment: 80,000
State Enrollment: 79,500

Healthplan and Services Defined
PLAN TYPE: PPO
Model Type: Network
Plan Specialty: Behavioral Health, Radiology, Blood
   Management Program; Diabetes; Sleep Disorders; Surgery
Benefits Offered: Behavioral Health, Disease Management,
   Prescription, Wellness, Worker's Compensation,
   Occupational therapy

Geographic Areas Served
Northwest Texas

Network Qualifications
Pre-Admission Certification: Yes

Accreditation Certification
Medicare Approved, Utilization Review, State Licensure,
   Quality Assurance Program

Key Personnel
Chief Executive Officer . . . . Mark Crawford
Chief Operating Officer. . . . . Randall Castillo
Chief Medical Officer . . . . Brian Weis
Chief Nursing Officer. . . . . Douglas Coffey
Assistant Administrator. . . . . Jason Madsen
Chairman. . . . . Lilia Escajeda

Employer References
City of Amarillo, Affilate Foods, Potter County,
   TPMHMR/State Center, Boys Ranch

735 American National Insurance Company

One Moody Plaza
1 Moody Avenue
Galveston, TX 77550
Toll-Free: 800-899-6503
Phone: 409-763-4661
www.americannational.com
Total Enrollment: 5,000,000

Healthplan and Services Defined
PLAN TYPE: PPO
Benefits Offered: AD&D, Life

Type of Coverage
Supplemental Medicare, Supplemental health, credit disabil

Geographic Areas Served
Nationwide and Puerto Rico

Key Personnel
President & CEO . . . . James Pozzi

736 American PPO

391 East Las Colinas Boulevard
Suite 130
Irving, TX 75039
Phone: 972-533-0081
Fax: 972-871-2005
www.americanppo.com
For Profit Organization: Yes
Year Founded: 2000
Number of Affiliated Hospitals: 305
Number of Primary Care Physicians: 10,000
Number of Referral/Specialty Physicians: 13,000

Healthplan and Services Defined
PLAN TYPE: PPO
Model Type: Network
Benefits Offered: Behavioral Health, Chiropractic, Dental,
   Disease Management, Home Care, Inpatient SNF,
   Long-Term Care, Physical Therapy, Prescription, Vision
Offers Demand Management Patient Information Service: Yes

Type of Coverage
Commercial

Type of Payment Plans Offered
Combination FFS & DFFS

Geographic Areas Served
Arkansas, Louisiana, Mississippi, Missouri, Oklahoma,
   Tennessee and Texas

Specialty Managed Care Partners
Enters into Contracts with Regional Business Coalitions: Yes

737 Amerigroup Texas

2505 N Highway 360 Service Road E
Suite 300
Grand Prairie, TX 75050
Toll-Free: 800-600-4441
www.myamerigroup.com/tx
Subsidiary of: Anthem, Inc.
For Profit Organization: Yes

Healthplan and Services Defined
PLAN TYPE: HMO

Type of Coverage
Medicaid

Accreditation Certification
URAC, NCQA

Key Personnel
EVP/Pres. Gov. Business .... Peter D. Haytaian

738 Ascension At Home

13737 Noel Road
Suite 1400
Dallas, TX 75240
Phone: 314-733-8000
ascensionathome.com
Secondary Address: Providence Home Care, 301 Owen Lane,
Waco, TX 76710, 254-523-6970
Subsidiary of: Ascension

Healthplan and Services Defined
PLAN TYPE: Other
Plan Specialty: Disease Management
Benefits Offered: Dental, Disease Management, Home Care,
Vision, Wellness, Ambulance & Transportation; Nursing
Service; Short-and-long-term care management planning;
Hospice

Geographic Areas Served
Texas, Alabama, Indiana, Kansas, Michigan, Mississippi,
Oklahoma, Wisconsin

Key Personnel
President................................. Kirk Allen
Dir., Home Health Service .... Darcy Burthay

739 Avesis: Texas

8000 W Interstate 10
San Antonio, TX 78230
Phone: 210-366-8071
www.avesis.com
Subsidiary of: Guardian Life Insurance Co.
Year Founded: 1978
Number of Primary Care Physicians: 25,000
Total Enrollment: 3,500,000

Healthplan and Services Defined
PLAN TYPE: PPO
Other Type: Vision, Dental

Model Type: Network
Plan Specialty: Dental, Vision, Hearing
Benefits Offered: Dental, Vision

Type of Coverage
Commercial

Type of Payment Plans Offered
POS, Capitated, Combination FFS & DFFS

Geographic Areas Served
Nationwide and Puerto Rico

Publishes and Distributes Report Card: Yes

Accreditation Certification
AAAHC, NCQA
TJC Accreditation

Key Personnel
Chief Executive Officer .... Chris Swanker
Business Development .... Alan Cohn

740 Blue Cross & Blue Shield of Texas

1001 E Lookout Drive
Richardson, TX 75082
Phone: 972-766-6900
www.bcbstx.com
Year Founded: 1984
Number of Affiliated Hospitals: 451
Number of Primary Care Physicians: 3,800
State Enrollment: 4,700,000

Healthplan and Services Defined
PLAN TYPE: HMO/PPO
Model Type: Network
Plan Specialty: Behavioral Health, Disease Management, Lab
Benefits Offered: Behavioral Health, Disease Management,
Physical Therapy, Prescription, Psychiatric, Wellness

Type of Coverage
Commercial, Individual, Medicare, Supplemental Medicare
Catastrophic Illness Benefit: Unlimited

Type of Payment Plans Offered
POS, DFFS, Capitated, FFS, Combination FFS & DFFS

Geographic Areas Served
Statewide

Subscriber Information
Average Monthly Fee Per Subscriber
(Employee + Employer Contribution):
Employee Only (Self): Varies by plan
Average Subscriber Co-Payment:
Home Health Care Max. Days/Visits Covered: 60 days
Nursing Home Max. Days/Visits Covered: 60 days

Network Qualifications
Pre-Admission Certification: Yes

Peer Review Type
Utilization Review: Yes
Second Surgical Opinion: Yes
Case Management: Yes

Publishes and Distributes Report Card: Yes

Accreditation Certification

NCQA

TJC Accreditation, Medicare Approved, Utilization Review,
Pre-Admission Certification, State Licensure, Quality
Assurance Program

Key Personnel

President . . . . Dan McCoy
Chief Medical Officer . . . . Esteban Lopez
DSVP of Sales & Marketing . . . . Darrell Beckett
VP, Government Relations . . . . Lee Spangler
VP, Business Performance . . . . Erin Barney

Average Claim Compensation

Physician's Fees Charged: 1%
Hospital's Fees Charged: 1%

Specialty Managed Care Partners

Magellen Behavioral Health
Enters into Contracts with Regional Business Coalitions: Yes

Employer References

American Airlines, Halliburton, Texas Instruments, Texas
A&M System, JBS

---

741   Care N' Care

1701 River Run
Suite 402
Fort Worth, TX 76107
Toll-Free: 800-994-1076
cnchealthplan.com
Year Founded: 2008

Healthplan and Services Defined

PLAN TYPE: Medicare

Other Type: HMO & PPO

Benefits Offered: Dental, Home Care, Physical Therapy,
Podiatry, Prescription, Durable Medical Equipment; Labs
& X-rays; Ocupational & Speech Therapy; Outpatient
Surgery; Therapeutic Radiology

Geographic Areas Served

Tarrant, Johnson, Dallas, Collin, Denton, Rockwall and parts
of Parker County

Key Personnel

Chief Executive Officer . . . . Wendy Karsten
Medical Director . . . . S. David Lloyd, MD
SVP, Sales & Operations . . . . Scott Hancock
Compliance Director . . . . Nakia Smith

---

742   Cigna HealthCare of Texas

900 Cottage Grove Road
Bloomfield, CT 06002
Toll-Free: 800-997-1654
www.cigna.com
For Profit Organization: Yes

Healthplan and Services Defined

PLAN TYPE: HMO

Plan Specialty: Behavioral Health, Dental, Vision

Benefits Offered: Behavioral Health, Dental, Disease
Management, Prescription, Vision, AD&D, Life, LTD, STD

Type of Coverage

Commercial, Individual

Type of Payment Plans Offered

POS, DFFS, Capitated, FFS, Combination FFS & DFFS

Peer Review Type

Utilization Review: Yes
Second Surgical Opinion: Yes
Case Management: Yes

Publishes and Distributes Report Card: Yes

Accreditation Certification

URAC, NCQA

Utilization Review, Pre-Admission Certification, State
Licensure, Quality Assurance Program

Average Claim Compensation

Physician's Fees Charged: 1%
Hospital's Fees Charged: 1%

Specialty Managed Care Partners

Quest
Enters into Contracts with Regional Business Coalitions: Yes

---

743   Community First Health Plans

12238 Silicon Drive
Suite 100
San Antonio, TX 78249
Toll-Free: 800-434-2347
Phone: 210-358-3000
www.cfhp.com
Secondary Address: Avenida Guadalupe, 1410 Guadalupe
Street, Suite 222, San Antonio, TX 78207
Subsidiary of: University Health System
Non-Profit Organization: Yes
Year Founded: 1995
Total Enrollment: 110,000
State Enrollment: 110,000

Healthplan and Services Defined

PLAN TYPE: HMO/PPO

Benefits Offered: Disease Management, Wellness

Type of Coverage

Commercial, Medicaid, CHIP

Geographic Areas Served

Bexar and surrounding seven counties

Key Personnel

Chairman. . . . . Rene Escobedo
Vice-Chair. . . . . Paul Nguyen
President/CEO . . . . Greg Gieseman
Chief Financial Officer . . . . Barbara Holmes
Chief Medical Officer. . . . . Priti Mody-Bailey
President of Operations . . . . Brian Wheeler

744 Concentra

5080 Spectrum Drive
Suite 1200W
Addison, TX 75001
Toll-Free: 866-944-6046
www.concentra.com
For Profit Organization: Yes

Healthplan and Services Defined
PLAN TYPE: Other
Plan Specialty: Worker's Compensation, Workers' compensation and occupational health (wellness, ergonomics, drug screening and occupational therapy)
Benefits Offered: Wellness, Worker's Compensation

Type of Coverage
Commercial

Key Personnel
President & CEO . . . . Keith Newton
Chief Financial Officer . . . . Su Zan Nelson
SVP, Human Resources . . . . Dani Kendall
SVP, Medical Officer . . . . John Anderson
EVP, Marketing & Sales . . . . John deLorimier

745 Consumers Direct Insurance Services (CDIS)

14785 Preston Road
Suite 550
Dallas, TX 75254
Toll-Free: 855-788-2583
texasmedicarehealth.com
Subsidiary of: Blue Cross Blue Shield of Texas
Year Founded: 1997

Healthplan and Services Defined
PLAN TYPE: Multiple
Benefits Offered: Dental, Wellness

Type of Coverage
Individual, Medicare, Supplemental Medicare, Medicaid, Short-term Insurance

Geographic Areas Served
Statewide

Key Personnel
President . . . . Scott Loochtan
Executive Vice President . . . . Jenn Hemann

746 Coventry Health Care of Texas

100 E Royal Lane
Irving, TX 75039
Phone: 972-807-4100
www.coventryhealthcare.com
Subsidiary of: Aetna Inc.
For Profit Organization: Yes

Healthplan and Services Defined
PLAN TYPE: HMO/PPO
Model Type: Network
Plan Specialty: Behavioral Health, Dental, Worker's Compensation

Benefits Offered: Behavioral Health, Dental, Prescription, Wellness, Worker's Compensation

Type of Coverage
Commercial, Medicare, Medicaid

Geographic Areas Served
Statewide

Key Personnel
Chief Executive Officer . . . . Mark T. Bertolini
President . . . . Karen S. Lynch
Chief Financial Officer . . . . Shawn M. Guertin
Operations & Technology . . . . Meg McCarthy
Chief Medical Officer . . . . Harold L. Paz
General Counsel . . . . Thomas Sabatino Jr.
Government Services . . . . Fran S. Soistman

747 Dental Source: Dental Health Care Plans

101 Parklane Boulevard
Suite 301
Sugar Land, TX 77478
Toll-Free: 877-493-6282
Phone: 866-481-9473
Fax: 281-313-7155
www.densource.com
For Profit Organization: Yes
Number of Primary Care Physicians: 149
State Enrollment: 1,500

Healthplan and Services Defined
PLAN TYPE: Dental
Model Type: Network
Plan Specialty: Dental
Benefits Offered: Dental

Type of Coverage
Commercial, Individual, Indemnity

Geographic Areas Served
Kansas and Missouri

748 FCL Dental

101 Parklane Boulevard
Suite 301
Sugar Land, TX 77478
Toll-Free: 877-493-6282
Phone: 281-313-7150
www.fcldental.com
For Profit Organization: Yes
Year Founded: 1986

Healthplan and Services Defined
PLAN TYPE: Dental
Other Type: PPO
Plan Specialty: Dental, Vision
Benefits Offered: Dental, Vision

Subscriber Information
Average Annual Deductible Per Subscriber:
Employee Only (Self): $0
Employee & 1 Family Member: $0
Employee & 2 Family Members: $0
Medicare: $0

Average Subscriber Co-Payment:
Primary Care Physician: $9.00

749 Galaxy Health Network

631 106th Street
Arlington, TX 76011
Toll-Free: 800-975-3322
Phone: 817-633-5822
Fax: 817-633-5729
contracting@ghn-mci.com
www.galaxyhealth.net
Mailing Address: PO Box 201425, Arlington, TX 76006
For Profit Organization: Yes
Year Founded: 1993
Number of Affiliated Hospitals: 2,700
Number of Primary Care Physicians: 400,000
Number of Referral/Specialty Physicians: 47,000
Total Enrollment: 3,500,000
State Enrollment: 3,200,000

Healthplan and Services Defined
PLAN TYPE: PPO
Model Type: Network
Benefits Offered: Disease Management, Prescription,
Wellness
Offers Demand Management Patient Information Service:
Yes

Type of Coverage
Catastrophic Illness Benefit: Varies per case

Type of Payment Plans Offered
POS, DFFS, FFS, Combination FFS & DFFS

Geographic Areas Served
Nationwide

Subscriber Information
Average Monthly Fee Per Subscriber
(Employee + Employer Contribution):
Employee Only (Self): Varies by plan
Average Annual Deductible Per Subscriber:
Employee Only (Self): $500.00
Employee & 1 Family Member: $1000.00
Employee & 2 Family Members: $1000.00
Average Subscriber Co-Payment:
Primary Care Physician: $10.00

Network Qualifications
Pre-Admission Certification: Yes

Peer Review Type
Utilization Review: Yes
Second Surgical Opinion: Yes
Case Management: Yes

Publishes and Distributes Report Card: Yes

Accreditation Certification
URAC
Utilization Review, Pre-Admission Certification, State
Licensure, Quality Assurance Program

Key Personnel
President. . . . . P.J. Shane, Jr, Jr
pjshanejr@ghn-mci.com

Executive Vice President. . . . . Dan Shadle
dshadle@ghn-mci.com
Administrative Manager . . . . Venus Warner
vmatthews@ghn-mci.com
Director of Operations . . . . Susdey Sud
susdeys@ghn-mci.com
Chief Technology Offier . . . . Stephen Ferraro
sferraro@ghn-mci.com
Manager, Info Services . . . . Brandie Santillan
bsantillan@ghn-mci.com
Vice President, Sales. . . . . Stacey Hollinger
shollinger@ghn-mci.com

Specialty Managed Care Partners
Enters into Contracts with Regional Business Coalitions: Yes

750 HCSC Insurance Services Company

1001 E Lookout Drive
Richardson, TX 75082
Phone: 912-766-6900
hcsc.com
Subsidiary of: Blue Cross Blue Shield Association
Non-Profit Organization: Yes
Year Founded: 1936
Number of Primary Care Physicians: 111,500

Healthplan and Services Defined
PLAN TYPE: HMO
Benefits Offered: Behavioral Health, Dental, Disease
Management, Psychiatric, Wellness

Geographic Areas Served
Statewide

Key Personnel
President & CEO . . . . Paula Steiner
EVP, Plan Operations. . . . . Colleen Reitan
SVP, Clinical Officer. . . . . Opella Ernest, MD
SVP, Financial Officer. . . . . Eric Feldstein
SVP, Compliance Officer. . . . . Thomas Lubben
SVP, Human Resources. . . . . Nazneen Razi
SVP, Chief Legal Officer. . . . . Blair Todt
Media Contact . . . . Kristen Cunningham
312-653-1686
kristen_cunningham@hcsc.net
Media Contact . . . . Greg Thompson
312-653-7581
greg_thompson@hcsc.net

751 HealthSmart

222 West Las Colinas Boulevard
Suite 600N
Irving, TX 75039
Toll-Free: 800-687-0500
Phone: 214-574-3546
Fax: 214-574-2368
www.healthsmart.com
For Profit Organization: Yes
Year Founded: 1983
Total Enrollment: 1,000,000

Healthplan and Services Defined
PLAN TYPE: PPO
Model Type: Network
Plan Specialty: MSO, PBM
Benefits Offered: Disease Management, Wellness, Business
    intelligence; web-based reporting; employer clinics

Type of Coverage
Catastrophic Illness Benefit: Varies per case

Type of Payment Plans Offered
POS, DFFS, FFS, Combination FFS & DFFS

Subscriber Information
Average Monthly Fee Per Subscriber
    (Employee + Employer Contribution):
        Employee Only (Self): Varies
        Employee & 1 Family Member: Varies
        Employee & 2 Family Members: Varies
        Medicare: Varies
Average Annual Deductible Per Subscriber:
        Employee Only (Self): Varies
        Employee & 1 Family Member: Varies
        Employee & 2 Family Members: Varies
        Medicare: Varies
Average Subscriber Co-Payment:
        Primary Care Physician: Varies
        Non-Network Physician: Varies
        Hospital ER: Varies
        Home Health Care: Varies
        Home Health Care Max. Days/Visits Covered: Varies
        Nursing Home: Varies
        Nursing Home Max. Days/Visits Covered: Varies

Network Qualifications
Minimum Years of Practice: 1
Pre-Admission Certification: Yes

Peer Review Type
Utilization Review: Yes
Second Surgical Opinion: Yes
Case Management: Yes

Publishes and Distributes Report Card: Yes

Accreditation Certification
URAC
Medicare Approved, Utilization Review, Pre-Admission
    Certification, State Licensure, Quality Assurance Program

Key Personnel
Chief Executive Officer . . . . Phil Christianson
Executive Vice President . . . . Bill Wallace
Chief Operating Officer . . . . Loren W. Claypool
VP, Strategic Markets. Marc Zech
Chief Clinical Officer . . . . Pamela Coffey
General Counsel . . . . Sarah Bittner
Chief Financial Officer . . . . Matthew Thompson
Chief Sales Officer. . . . . Tom Mafale
Chief Information Officer. . . . . Donald Couch

Specialty Managed Care Partners
Enters into Contracts with Regional Business Coalitions: Yes

Employer References
Garland ISD, Richardson ISD, Nokia, Tenet Health System,
    Gulf Stream Aerospace

---

752 Horizon Health Corporation
1965 Lakepointe Drive
Suite 100
Lewisville, TX 75057
Toll-Free: 800-727-2407
Phone: 972-420-8300
Fax: 972-420-8383
bhs@horizonhealth.com
www.horizonhealth.com
Subsidiary of: Universal Health Solutions, Inc.
For Profit Organization: Yes
Year Founded: 1981
Number of Affiliated Hospitals: 2,000
Number of Primary Care Physicians: 17,000
Number of Referral/Specialty Physicians: 18,531
Total Enrollment: 120,000

Healthplan and Services Defined
PLAN TYPE: PPO
Model Type: Staff
Plan Specialty: Behavioral Health, UR
Benefits Offered: Behavioral Health, Psychiatric,
    Rehabilitation Services

Type of Coverage
Commercial, Indemnity

Type of Payment Plans Offered
POS, DFFS, Capitated, FFS, Combination FFS & DFFS

Geographic Areas Served
All 50 United States, Canada, Puerto Rico, Mexico, England,
and the Virgin Islands

Subscriber Information
Average Monthly Fee Per Subscriber
    (Employee + Employer Contribution):
        Employee & 2 Family Members: Varies by plan

Network Qualifications
Pre-Admission Certification: Yes

Peer Review Type
Utilization Review: Yes
Case Management: Yes

Publishes and Distributes Report Card: Yes

Accreditation Certification
URAC, NCQA

Key Personnel
President . . . . Jack DeVaney
Chief Financial Officer. . . . . Jack E. Polson
VP/Assistant Secretary . . . . Steven T. Davidson

Specialty Managed Care Partners
Enters into Contracts with Regional Business Coalitions: Yes
Employer Health Coalition

Employer References
American Greetings, Saint Gobain Corporation, Broodwing,
    Jeld-Wen, The Pep Boys

753   Humana Health Insurance of Texas
8119 Datapoint Drive
San Antonio, TX 78229
Toll-Free: 800-611-1456
Phone: 210-615-5100
Fax: 210-617-1251
www.humana.com
Secondary Address: 10710 Research Boulevard, Suite 120,
   Austin, TX 78759, 512-808-2821
For Profit Organization: Yes
Year Founded: 1983

Healthplan and Services Defined
   PLAN TYPE: HMO/PPO
   Model Type: Network
   Benefits Offered: Disease Management, Prescription,
      Wellness
   Offers Demand Management Patient Information Service:
      Yes

Type of Coverage
   Commercial, Individual
   Catastrophic Illness Benefit: Covered

Geographic Areas Served
   Statewide

Peer Review Type
   Utilization Review: Yes
   Second Surgical Opinion: Yes
   Case Management: Yes

Publishes and Distributes Report Card: Yes

Accreditation Certification
   URAC, NCQA, CORE
   TJC Accreditation, Medicare Approved, Utilization Review,
      Pre-Admission Certification, State Licensure, Quality
      Assurance Program

Key Personnel
   President & CEO . . . . Bruce D. Broussard
   Chief Medical Officer. . . . . Roy A. Beveridge
   Chief Consumer Officer. . . . . Jody L. Bilney
   SVP, Human Resources . . . . Tim Huval
   Chief Financial Officer . . . . Brian Kane
   Chief Information Officer . . . . Brian LeClaire
   General Counsel . . . . Christopher M. Todoroff

Average Claim Compensation
   Physician's Fees Charged: 80%
   Hospital's Fees Charged: 80%

Specialty Managed Care Partners
   Enters into Contracts with Regional Business Coalitions: Yes

754   KelseyCare Advantage
11511 Shadow Creek Parkway
Pearland, TX 77584
Toll-Free: 866-302-9336
Phone: 713-442-5646
www.kelseycareadvantage.com

Healthplan and Services Defined
   PLAN TYPE: Multiple
   Other Type: HMO/POS

   Benefits Offered: Behavioral Health, Chiropractic, Dental,
      Disease Management, Home Care, Podiatry, Prescription,
      Vision, Wellness, Hearing; Outpatient Rehabilitation;
      Prosthetic

Type of Coverage
   Medicare, Medicare Advantage

Key Personnel
   President . . . . Marnie Matheny
   VP, Operations . . . . Theresa Devivar
   Medical Director . . . . Dr. Donald Aga

755   Liberty Dental Plan of Texas
P.O. Box 26110
Santa Ana, CA 92799-6110
Toll-Free: 877-558-6489
www.libertydentalplan.com
For Profit Organization: Yes
Year Founded: 2008
Total Enrollment: 3,000,000

Healthplan and Services Defined
   PLAN TYPE: Dental
   Other Type: Dental HMO
   Plan Specialty: Dental
   Benefits Offered: Dental

Type of Coverage
   Commercial, Individual, Medicare, Medicaid, Unions

Geographic Areas Served
   Statewide

Accreditation Certification
   NCQA

Key Personnel
   Senior Vice President . . . . Bill Henderson
      bhenderson@libertydentalplan.com
   Network Manager, Texas . . . . Deborah Kinder
      dkinder@libertydentalplan.com
   Operations Manager, Texas . . . . Margaret Stark
      mstark@libertydentalplan.com
   Chief Dental Officer . . . . Rick Goren
      rgoren@libertydentalplan.com

756   MHNet Behavioral Health
9606 N. Mopac Expressway
Stonebridge Plaza 1, Suite 600
Austin, TX 78759
Toll-Free: 888-646-6889
Fax: 724-741-4552
www.mhnet.com
Mailing Address: PO Box 209010, Austin, TX 78720-9010
For Profit Organization: Yes
Year Founded: 1985
Number of Affiliated Hospitals: 134
Number of Referral/Specialty Physicians: 2,000
Total Enrollment: 2,000,000

Healthplan and Services Defined
   PLAN TYPE: Multiple
   Model Type: IPA

Plan Specialty: Behavioral Health, Employee Assistance
Programs and Managed Behavioral Health Care
Benefits Offered: Behavioral Health, Psychiatric
Offers Demand Management Patient Information Service:
Yes
DMPI Services Offered: Psychiatric Illness

Type of Payment Plans Offered
POS, DFFS, Capitated, FFS, Combination FFS & DFFS

Geographic Areas Served
Nationwide

Network Qualifications
Minimum Years of Practice: 1
Pre-Admission Certification: Yes

Peer Review Type
Utilization Review: Yes
Second Surgical Opinion: Yes
Case Management: Yes

Publishes and Distributes Report Card: Yes

Accreditation Certification
URAC, NCQA

Key Personnel
Chairman & CEO . . . . Mark T. Bertolini
President . . . . Karen S. Lynch
Chief Financial Officer . . . . Shawn M. Guertin
Corporate Affairs . . . . Steven B. Kelmar
President of Operations . . . . Meg McCarthy
Chief Medical Officer . . . . Harold L. Paz

Average Claim Compensation
Physician's Fees Charged: 30%
Hospital's Fees Charged: 30%

Specialty Managed Care Partners
Enters into Contracts with Regional Business Coalitions: Yes

757   Molina Healthcare of Texas

5605 N MacArthur Boulevard
Suite 400
Irving, TX 75038
Toll-Free: 877-665-4622
www.molinahealthcare.com
Subsidiary of: Molina Healthcare, Inc.
For Profit Organization: Yes
Year Founded: 1980
Physician Owned Organization: Yes

Healthplan and Services Defined
PLAN TYPE: Medicare
Model Type: Network
Plan Specialty: Integrated Medicare/Medicaid (Duals)
Benefits Offered: Chiropractic, Dental, Home Care, Inpatient
SNF, Long-Term Care, Podiatry, Vision

Type of Coverage
Commercial, Medicare, Supplemental Medicare, Medicaid

Accreditation Certification
URAC, NCQA

Key Personnel
Chief Executive Officer . . . . Joseph W. White

Chief Operating Officer . . . . Terry Bayer
General Counsel . . . . Jeff D. Barlow
SVP, Relations/Marketing . . . . Juan Jos, Orellana
Chief Information Officer . . . . Rick Hopfer

758   Ora Quest Dental Plans

101 Parklane Boulevard
Suite 301
Sugar Land, TX 77478
Toll-Free: 800-660-6064
Phone: 281-313-7170
Fax: 281-313-7155
info@oraquest.com
www.oraquest.com
For Profit Organization: Yes

Healthplan and Services Defined
PLAN TYPE: Dental
Other Type: Dental HMO
Model Type: Network
Plan Specialty: Dental
Benefits Offered: Dental

Type of Coverage
Commercial, Individual, Medicare, Medicaid

Subscriber Information
Average Annual Deductible Per Subscriber:
Employee Only (Self): $0

759   Parkland Community Health Plan

P.O. Box 569005
Dallas, TX 75356-9005
Toll-Free: 888-672-2277
www.parklandhmo.com
Non-Profit Organization: Yes
Year Founded: 1999
Number of Affiliated Hospitals: 25
Number of Primary Care Physicians: 3,000

Healthplan and Services Defined
PLAN TYPE: HMO
Model Type: Network
Benefits Offered: Behavioral Health, Chiropractic, Home
Care, Inpatient SNF, Physical Therapy, Podiatry,
Prescription, Psychiatric, Transplant, Vision

Type of Coverage
Medicaid, Medicaid STAR, CHIP

Type of Payment Plans Offered
POS, FFS

Geographic Areas Served
Dallas, Collin, Ellis, Hunt, Kaufman, Navarro and Rockwall
counties

Network Qualifications
Pre-Admission Certification: Yes

Peer Review Type
Utilization Review: Yes
Second Surgical Opinion: Yes
Case Management: Yes

Accreditation Certification
Utilization Review, Pre-Admission Certification, State Licensure, Quality Assurance Program

Key Personnel
President & CEO. . . . . Frederick P. Cerise, MD
EVP, Financial Officer . . . . Richard Humphrey
Chief Operating Officer . . . . David Lopez
EVP, Medical Officer . . . . Roberto de la Cruz, MD

Specialty Managed Care Partners
Comprehensive Behavioral Care, Block Vision

---

760 Scott & White Health Plan
1206 West Campus Drive
Temple, TX 76502
Toll-Free: 800-321-7947
Fax: 254-298-3385
www.swhp.org
Secondary Address: 204 S IH 35, Suite 100, Georgetown, TX 78628
Non-Profit Organization: Yes
Year Founded: 1982
Owned by an Integrated Delivery Network (IDN): Yes
Number of Affiliated Hospitals: 18
Number of Primary Care Physicians: 1,000
Total Enrollment: 200,000
State Enrollment: 200,000

Healthplan and Services Defined
PLAN TYPE: Multiple
Other Type: POS, CDHP
Model Type: Group
Benefits Offered: Behavioral Health, Dental, Disease Management, Home Care, Inpatient SNF, Long-Term Care, Physical Therapy, Podiatry, Prescription, Psychiatric, Transplant, Vision, Life
Offers Demand Management Patient Information Service: Yes
DMPI Services Offered: Secondary prevention of Coronary Artery Disease, Pediatric Asthma, Diabetes Mellitius, Congestive Heart Failure, Hypertension

Type of Coverage
Commercial, Individual, Medicare, Medicare cost
Catastrophic Illness Benefit: Covered

Type of Payment Plans Offered
DFFS, Capitated

Geographic Areas Served
77 counties in the Central, East, North, and West Texas regions

Subscriber Information
Average Monthly Fee Per Subscriber
(Employee + Employer Contribution):
Employee Only (Self): Varies by plan
Average Annual Deductible Per Subscriber:
Employee Only (Self): $0.00
Employee & 1 Family Member: $0.00
Employee & 2 Family Members: $0.00
Average Subscriber Co-Payment:
Primary Care Physician: $10.00

Prescription Drugs: $5.00/20.00/50.00
Hospital ER: $75.00
Home Health Care: $10.00
Nursing Home: $0

Network Qualifications
Pre-Admission Certification: No

Peer Review Type
Utilization Review: Yes
Second Surgical Opinion: No
Case Management: Yes

Publishes and Distributes Report Card: Yes

Accreditation Certification
NCQA
TJC Accreditation, Medicare Approved, Utilization Review, State Licensure, Quality Assurance Program

Key Personnel
Chief Executive Officer . . . . Jeff Ingrum
Chief Financial Officer . . . . Stephen Bush
Chief Sales Officer . . . . Linza Jones
Vp, Government Programs . . . . Stephanie Rogersl

Average Claim Compensation
Physician's Fees Charged: 57%
Hospital's Fees Charged: 43%

Employer References
Texas A&M, ERS, Wiliamson County

---

761 Script Care, Ltd.
6380 Folsom Drive
Beaumont, TX 77706
Toll-Free: 800-880-9988
customerservice@scriptcare.com
www.scriptcare.com
Year Founded: 1989
Number of Primary Care Physicians: 60,000

Healthplan and Services Defined
PLAN TYPE: PPO
Other Type: PBM
Plan Specialty: PBM
Benefits Offered: Prescription

Type of Payment Plans Offered
Capitated, FFS

Geographic Areas Served
Nationwide

Subscriber Information
Average Subscriber Co-Payment:
Prescription Drugs: Variable

Peer Review Type
Case Management: Yes

Key Personnel
President. . . . . Jim Brown
VP Sales/Marketing . . . . Tab Bryan

762   Seton Healthcare Family

4515 Seton Center Pkwy, Suite 310
Austin, TX 78759
Toll-Free: 1-800-749-7624
Phone: 512-324-3350
www.setonhealthplan.com
Subsidiary of: Ascension
Non-Profit Organization: Yes
Year Founded: 1902
Number of Affiliated Hospitals: 100
Total Enrollment: 15,000

Healthplan and Services Defined
  PLAN TYPE: HMO
  Benefits Offered: Behavioral Health, Disease Management,
    Long-Term Care, Physical Therapy, Podiatry, Prescription,
    Wellness, Cancer; Cardiac; Orthopedic; Plastic &
    Reconstructive Surgery; Pediatric;Dermatology; Trauma &
    Emergency

Type of Coverage
  Commercial

Geographic Areas Served
  Central Texas

Key Personnel
  President & CEO . . . . Jesus Garza
  Chief Operating Officer. . . . . Michelle L. Robertson
  VP, Human Resources . . . . Joe Canales
  Marketing & Comm . . . . Mike Dollen

763   Sterling Insurance

P.O. Box 26580
Austin, TX 78755-0580
Toll-Free: 800-688-0010
www.cigna.com/sterlinginsurance/products
Subsidiary of: CIGNA/Sterling Life Insurance
Total Enrollment: 44,000
State Enrollment: 44,000

Healthplan and Services Defined
  PLAN TYPE: Medicare
  Benefits Offered: Prescription, Life

Type of Coverage
  Individual, Medicare, Supplemental Medicare

Geographic Areas Served
  39 States

764   TexanPlus Medicare Advantage HMO

P.O. Box 18400
Austin, TX 78760-8400
Toll-Free: 866-249-8668
www.universal-american-medicare.com/texanplus-hmo
For Profit Organization: Yes
Total Enrollment: 42,000

Healthplan and Services Defined
  PLAN TYPE: Multiple
  Benefits Offered: Chiropractic, Dental, Disease Management,
    Home Care, Inpatient SNF, Physical Therapy, Podiatry,
    Prescription, Psychiatric, Vision, Wellness

Type of Coverage
  Individual, Medicare

Geographic Areas Served
  Statewide

Subscriber Information
  Average Monthly Fee Per Subscriber
    (Employee + Employer Contribution):
      Employee Only (Self): Varies
      Medicare: Varies
  Average Annual Deductible Per Subscriber:
      Employee Only (Self): Varies
      Medicare: Varies
  Average Subscriber Co-Payment:
      Primary Care Physician: Varies
      Non-Network Physician: Varies
      Prescription Drugs: Varies
      Hospital ER: Varies
      Home Health Care: Varies
      Home Health Care Max. Days/Visits Covered: Varies
      Nursing Home: Varies
      Nursing Home Max. Days/Visits Covered: Varies

Key Personnel
  Chairman & CEO . . . . Richard A Barasch
  Chief Financial Officer . . . . Adam C. Thackery
  Administrative Officer. . . . . Steven H. Black
  President of Medicare . . . . Erin Page
  General Counsel/Secretary . . . . Anthony L. Wolk
  Executive Vice President. . . . . Theodore Carpenter

765   Texas HealthSpring

2900 North Loop West, Suite 1300
Houston, TX 77092
Phone: 832-553-3300
www.cigna.com/medicare/cigna-healthspring
Subsidiary of: Cigna Corporation
For Profit Organization: Yes
Year Founded: 2000

Healthplan and Services Defined
  PLAN TYPE: Medicare

Type of Coverage
  Medicare, Medicaid

Geographic Areas Served
  Houston, Golden Triangle & Valley, North Texas & Lubbock

Key Personnel
  President & CEO . . . . David Cordani
  VP, Marketing Officer . . . . Lisa Bacus
  Chief Information Officer . . . . Mark Boxer
  General Counsel . . . . Nicole Jones
  Human Resources. John Murabito

766   UniCare Texas

3820 American Drive
Plano, TX 75075
Toll-Free: 800-333-2203
Phone: 972-599-3888
www.unicare.com

Secondary Address: 106 East Sixth Street, Suite 333, Austin, TX 78701

Subsidiary of: Anthem, Inc.

For Profit Organization: Yes

Year Founded: 1995

Healthplan and Services Defined
PLAN TYPE: HMO/PPO
Model Type: Network
Plan Specialty: Dental, EPO, Lab, Radiology
Benefits Offered: Dental, Inpatient SNF, Long-Term Care, Prescription, Transplant, Wellness, AD&D, Life, LTD, STD, EAP

Type of Coverage
Individual, Indemnity, Medicare, Supplemental Medicare

Geographic Areas Served
Statewide

Network Qualifications
Pre-Admission Certification: Yes

Peer Review Type
Utilization Review: Yes
Second Surgical Opinion: Yes
Case Management: Yes

Publishes and Distributes Report Card: No

Accreditation Certification
URAC, NCQA
TJC Accreditation, Utilization Review, Pre-Admission Certification, State Licensure, Quality Assurance Program

Specialty Managed Care Partners
Wellpoint Pharmacy Management, Wellpoint Dental Services, Wellpoint Behavioral Health
Enters into Contracts with Regional Business Coalitions: No

767 United Concordia of Texas

8214 Westchester Drive
Suite 600
Dallas, TX 75225
Phone: 214-378-6410
www.unitedconcordia.com
For Profit Organization: Yes
Year Founded: 1971
Total Enrollment: 7,800,000

Healthplan and Services Defined
PLAN TYPE: Dental
Plan Specialty: Dental
Benefits Offered: Dental

Type of Coverage
Commercial, Individual, Military personnel & families

Geographic Areas Served
Nationwide

Accreditation Certification
URAC

Key Personnel
President & COO . . . . Timothy J. Constantine

Contact. . . . . Beth Rutherford
717-260-7659
beth.rutherford@ucci.com

768 UnitedHealthcare of Texas

1250 Capital of Texas Highway
Building 1, Suite 360
Austin, TX 78746
Toll-Free: 877-294-1429
www.uhc.com/contact-us/texas
Secondary Address: 1311 W President George Bush Highway, Richardson, TX 75080, 800-458-5653
Subsidiary of: UnitedHealth Group
For Profit Organization: Yes
Year Founded: 1986

Healthplan and Services Defined
PLAN TYPE: HMO/PPO
Model Type: Network
Plan Specialty: Behavioral Health, Dental, Disease Management, PBM, Vision
Benefits Offered: Behavioral Health, Dental, Disease Management, Long-Term Care, Prescription, Vision, Wellness, AD&D, Life, LTD, STD

Type of Coverage
Commercial, Individual, Medicare, Supplemental Medicare, Medicaid, Catastrophic, Family, Military, Veterans, Group,

Geographic Areas Served
Texas and Oklahoma

Network Qualifications
Pre-Admission Certification: Yes

Publishes and Distributes Report Card: Yes

Accreditation Certification
AAPI, NCQA

Key Personnel
Chief Executive Officer. . . . . David Wichmann
Chief Operating Officer . . . . Dan Schumacher
Chief Strategy Officer . . . . John Cosgriff
Communications Officer . . . . Kirsten Gorsuch
Chief Medical Officer. . . . . Sam Ho
Chief Legal Officer . . . . Thad Johnson
Chief Information Officer . . . . Phil McKoy
Chief Financial Officer. . . . . Jeff Putnam

Specialty Managed Care Partners
Enters into Contracts with Regional Business Coalitions: Yes

769 USA Managed Care Organization

1250 S Capital of Texas Highway
Bldg 3, Suite 500
Austin, TX 78746
Toll-Free: 800-872-0020
info@usamco.com
www.usamco.com
Secondary Address: 7301 North 16th Street, Suite 201, Phoenix, AZ 85020
For Profit Organization: Yes
Year Founded: 1984

Number of Affiliated Hospitals: 5,000
Number of Primary Care Physicians: 430,000
Total Enrollment: 5,427,579
State Enrollment: 1,118,582

Healthplan and Services Defined
PLAN TYPE: PPO
Model Type: Group
Plan Specialty: Behavioral Health, Chiropractic, Dental, Disease Management, EPO, Lab, PBM, Vision, Radiology, Worker's Compensation, UR
Benefits Offered: Behavioral Health, Chiropractic, Dental, Disease Management, Physical Therapy, Prescription, Vision, Wellness, Worker's Compensation

Type of Coverage
Commercial, Medicare

Type of Payment Plans Offered
POS, DFFS, FFS, Combination FFS & DFFS

Network Qualifications
Pre-Admission Certification: Yes

Peer Review Type
Utilization Review: Yes
Second Surgical Opinion: Yes
Case Management: Yes

Publishes and Distributes Report Card: No

Accreditation Certification
TJC Accreditation, Pre-Admission Certification, State Licensure, Quality Assurance Program

Key Personnel
President and CEO . . . . Michael Bogle
CFO . . . . Joseph Dulin

Average Claim Compensation
Physician's Fees Charged: 34%
Hospital's Fees Charged: 32%

---

770 UTMB HealthCare Systems

301 University Boulevard
Galveston, TX 77555-0915
Toll-Free: 855-256-7876
Phone: 409-766-4064
www.utmbhcs.org
Subsidiary of: The University of Texas Medical Branch
Non-Profit Organization: Yes
Year Founded: 1998
Total Enrollment: 1,000

Healthplan and Services Defined
PLAN TYPE: HMO
Benefits Offered: Disease Management

Type of Coverage
Commercial, Medicare, CHIP

Geographic Areas Served
Statewide

Key Personnel
Chief Executive Officer . . . . Donna Sollenberger
President . . . . David L. Callender
Vice President . . . . Danny O. Jacobs

Sr. VP & General Counsel . . . . Carolee King

771 Valley Baptist Health Plan

2101 Pease Street
Harlingen, TX 78550
Toll-Free: 855-720-7448
Phone: 956-389-1100
www.valleybaptist.net
Subsidiary of: Valley Baptist Insurance Company
Non-Profit Organization: Yes
Total Enrollment: 22,000
State Enrollment: 12,004

Healthplan and Services Defined
PLAN TYPE: HMO
Plan Specialty: Lab, Surgical and Medical Weight Loss Program
Benefits Offered: Behavioral Health, Chiropractic, Dental, Disease Management, Home Care, Inpatient SNF, Physical Therapy, Podiatry, Prescription, Psychiatric, Transplant, Vision, Wellness, Durable Medical Equipment; Orthopedics; Rehabilitation

Type of Coverage
Commercial

Type of Payment Plans Offered
POS

Geographic Areas Served
Statewide

Subscriber Information
Average Monthly Fee Per Subscriber
(Employee + Employer Contribution):
Employee Only (Self): Varies
Employee & 1 Family Member: Varies
Employee & 2 Family Members: Varies
Medicare: Varies
Average Annual Deductible Per Subscriber:
Employee Only (Self): Varies
Employee & 1 Family Member: Varies
Employee & 2 Family Members: Varies
Medicare: Varies
Average Subscriber Co-Payment:
Primary Care Physician: Varies
Non-Network Physician: Varies
Prescription Drugs: Varies
Hospital ER: Varies
Home Health Care: Varies
Home Health Care Max. Days/Visits Covered: Varies
Nursing Home: Varies
Nursing Home Max. Days/Visits Covered: Varies

Key Personnel
Chief Executive Officer . . . . Manny Vela
Chief Financial Officer . . . . Patrick Clune
Business Devevelopment . . . . Megan Drake
Chief Operating Officer . . . . Daniel Listi
Chief Medical Officer . . . . Jose Ayala

Specialty Managed Care Partners
Express Scripts

Health Insurance Coverage Status and Type of Coverage by Age

Category	All Persons		Under 18 years		Under 65 years	
	Number	%	Number	%	Number	%
Total population	3,025	-	973	-	2,709	-
Covered by some type of health insurance	2,760 *(12)*	91.2 *(0.4)*	914 *(7)*	94.0 *(0.6)*	2,446 *(12)*	90.3 *(0.4)*
Covered by private health insurance	2,379 *(17)*	78.7 *(0.6)*	755 *(10)*	77.6 *(1.0)*	2,180 *(16)*	80.5 *(0.6)*
Employer-based	1,967 *(20)*	65.0 *(0.7)*	648 *(11)*	66.6 *(1.1)*	1,854 *(19)*	68.5 *(0.7)*
Direct purchase	438 *(16)*	14.5 *(0.5)*	106 *(7)*	10.9 *(0.8)*	341 *(14)*	12.6 *(0.5)*
TRICARE	72 *(6)*	2.4 *(0.2)*	19 *(3)*	2.0 *(0.3)*	49 *(6)*	1.8 *(0.2)*
Covered by public health insurance	651 *(12)*	21.5 *(0.4)*	191 *(9)*	19.6 *(0.9)*	348 *(12)*	12.9 *(0.5)*
Medicaid	342 *(13)*	11.3 *(0.4)*	189 *(8)*	19.5 *(0.9)*	310 *(12)*	11.4 *(0.4)*
Medicare	345 *(4)*	11.4 *(0.1)*	2 *(1)*	0.2 *(0.1)*	43 *(3)*	1.6 *(0.1)*
VA Care	46 *(3)*	1.5 *(0.1)*	Z *(Z)*	Z *(Z)*	19 *(2)*	0.7 *(0.1)*
Not covered at any time during the year	265 *(12)*	8.8 *(0.4)*	59 *(6)*	6.0 *(0.6)*	262 *(12)*	9.7 *(0.4)*

Note: Numbers in thousands; Figures cover civilian noninstitutionalized population in 2016; N/A indicates that data was not available; Z represents or rounds to zero; Margin of error appears in parenthesis and is calculated using replicate weights.
Source: U.S. Census Bureau, American Community Survey, Table HIC-4_ACS. Health Insurance Coverage Status and Type of Coverage by State—All People: 2008 to 2016, Table HIC-5_ACS. Health Insurance Coverage Status and Type of Coverage by State—Children Under 18: 2008 to 2016, Table HIC-6_ACS. Health Insurance Coverage Status and Type of Coverage by State—Persons Under 65: 2008 to 2016

Utah

772 Aetna Health of Utah

151 Farmington Avenue
Hartford, CT 06156
Toll-Free: 800-872-3862
Phone: 860-273-0123
www.aetna.com
Secondary Address: 6730-B Rockledge Drive, Suite 700,
    Bethesda, MD 20817, 301-581-0600
Subsidiary of: Aetna Inc.
For Profit Organization: Yes

Healthplan and Services Defined
PLAN TYPE: PPO
Other Type: POS
Model Type: Network
Plan Specialty: Behavioral Health, Dental, EPO, Lab, PBM,
    Vision, Radiology
Benefits Offered: Behavioral Health, Dental, Disease
    Management, Long-Term Care, Physical Therapy,
    Podiatry, Prescription, Psychiatric, Wellness, Life, LTD,
    STD

Type of Coverage
Commercial, Student health

Type of Payment Plans Offered
POS, FFS

Geographic Areas Served
Statewide

Key Personnel
CEO. . . . . Mark Bertolini

773 Altius Health Plans

10150 S Centennial Parkway
Suite 450
Sandy, UT 84070
Toll-Free: 800-377-4161
www.altiushealthplans.com
Subsidiary of: Coventry Health Care
For Profit Organization: Yes
Year Founded: 1998
Number of Affiliated Hospitals: 46
Number of Primary Care Physicians: 3,800
Number of Referral/Specialty Physicians: 1,850
Total Enrollment: 148,000
State Enrollment: 84,000

Healthplan and Services Defined
PLAN TYPE: Multiple
Model Type: Group, POS
Plan Specialty: Behavioral Health, Chiropractic, Disease
    Management, Lab, PBM, Vision, Radiology, UR
Benefits Offered: Behavioral Health, Chiropractic, Dental,
    Disease Management, Home Care, Inpatient SNF, Physical
    Therapy, Podiatry, Prescription, Psychiatric, Transplant,
    Vision, Wellness
Offers Demand Management Patient Information Service:
    Yes

Type of Coverage
Commercial, Catastrophic
Catastrophic Illness Benefit: Unlimited

Type of Payment Plans Offered
POS, DFFS

Geographic Areas Served
Utah, Idaho, Wyoming, and Nevada

Subscriber Information
Average Monthly Fee Per Subscriber
    (Employee + Employer Contribution):
        Employee Only (Self): Varies
        Employee & 1 Family Member: Varies
        Employee & 2 Family Members: Varies
        Medicare: Varies
Average Annual Deductible Per Subscriber:
        Employee Only (Self): Varies
        Employee & 1 Family Member: Varies
        Employee & 2 Family Members: Varies
        Medicare: Varies
Average Subscriber Co-Payment:
        Primary Care Physician: $15.00
        Non-Network Physician: 70%
        Prescription Drugs: Varies
        Hospital ER: Varies
        Home Health Care: Varies
        Home Health Care Max. Days/Visits Covered: 60 visits
        Nursing Home: Varies
        Nursing Home Max. Days/Visits Covered: 60 visits

Network Qualifications
Pre-Admission Certification: Yes

Peer Review Type
Utilization Review: Yes
Second Surgical Opinion: Yes
Case Management: Yes

Publishes and Distributes Report Card: Yes

Accreditation Certification
URAC
TJC Accreditation, Medicare Approved, Utilization Review,
    Pre-Admission Certification, State Licensure, Quality
    Assurance Program

Key Personnel
Chief Executive Officer. . . . . Mark T. Bertolini

Specialty Managed Care Partners
Horizon Behavioral Health, ESI

Employer References
Federal Government, State of Utah, Davis County School
    District, Wells Fargo, DMBA

774 Altius Health Plans of Utah

10150 S Centennial Parkway
Suite 450
Sandy, UT 84070
Toll-Free: 800-377-4161
Phone: 800-346-4128
altius.coventryhealthcare.com
Subsidiary of: Coventry Health Care, Inc.

For Profit Organization: Yes
Year Founded: 1976

Healthplan and Services Defined
PLAN TYPE: HMO/PPO
Model Type: Network
Plan Specialty: Behavioral Health, Dental, Worker's
  Compensation
Benefits Offered: Behavioral Health, Dental, Prescription,
  Wellness, Worker's Compensation

Type of Coverage
Commercial, Individual, Medicare, Medicaid

Geographic Areas Served
Utah, Wyoming, Idaho, and Nevada

Accreditation Certification
NCQA

Key Personnel
Chairman & CEO . . . . Mark T. Bertolini
President . . . . Karen S. Lynch
Chief Financial Officer . . . . Shawn M. Guertin
Operations & Technology . . . . Meg McCarthy
Chief Medical Officer . . . . Harold L. Paz
General Counsel . . . . Thomas Sabatino
Government Services . . . . Fran S. Soistman

775 BridgeSpan Health
2890 E Cottonwood Parkway
Salt Like City, UT 84121
Toll-Free: 855-857-9943
www.bridgespanhealth.com
Subsidiary of: Cambia Health Solutions
Non-Profit Organization: Yes
Year Founded: 2012

Healthplan and Services Defined
PLAN TYPE: HMO
Benefits Offered: Behavioral Health, Physical Therapy,
  Prescription, Wellness, Abulance Care; Hospice; Labs &
  Imaging; Maternity; Substance Abuse; Rehabilitation;
  Pediatrics

Geographic Areas Served
Idaho, Oregon, Utah, and Washington

Key Personnel
President . . . . Chris Blanton

776 Emi Health
852 E Arrowhead Lane
Murray, UT 84107-5298
Toll-Free: 800-662-5851
Phone: 801-262-7475
Fax: 801-269-9734
cs@emihealth.com
www.emihealth.com
Subsidiary of: Educators Mutual
Non-Profit Organization: Yes
Year Founded: 1935
Physician Owned Organization: Yes
Federally Qualified: Yes

Number of Affiliated Hospitals: 25
Number of Primary Care Physicians: 3,500
Total Enrollment: 6,000
State Enrollment: 65,000

Healthplan and Services Defined
PLAN TYPE: HMO/PPO
Model Type: Network
Plan Specialty: Behavioral Health, Chiropractic, Disease
  Management, Radiology, UR
Benefits Offered: Behavioral Health, Chiropractic,
  Complementary Medicine, Dental, Disease Management,
  Home Care, Inpatient SNF, Physical Therapy, Podiatry,
  Prescription, Psychiatric, Transplant, Vision, Wellness,
  AD&D, Life, LTD, STD
Offers Demand Management Patient Information Service: Yes
DMPI Services Offered: Wellness Web

Type of Coverage
Commercial, Individual

Type of Payment Plans Offered
POS

Geographic Areas Served
counties: Box Elder; Cache; Davis; Salt Lake; Weber

Subscriber Information
Average Monthly Fee Per Subscriber
  (Employee + Employer Contribution):
  Employee Only (Self): Varies by plan
Average Annual Deductible Per Subscriber:
  Employee Only (Self): $0
  Employee & 1 Family Member: $0
  Employee & 2 Family Members: $0
  Medicare: $0
Average Subscriber Co-Payment:
  Primary Care Physician: $5.00
  Prescription Drugs: 30%
  Hospital ER: $25.00
  Home Health Care: $0
  Nursing Home: $0

Network Qualifications
Pre-Admission Certification: Yes

Peer Review Type
Utilization Review: Yes
Second Surgical Opinion: No
Case Management: Yes

Publishes and Distributes Report Card: Yes

Accreditation Certification
TJC Accreditation, Utilization Review, Pre-Admission
  Certification, State Licensure, Quality Assurance Program

Key Personnel
President/CEO . . . . Steven C. Morrison
EVP/CFO/Treasurer . . . . Mike Greenhalgh
EVP/COO/Secretary . . . . Ryan Lowther
Compliance Officer . . . . Brandon L. Smart
Chief Actuary . . . . David Wood
Information Technology VP . . . . Joe Campbell
Corporate Communications . . . . Christie Hawkes
Sales & Marketing . . . . Cindy Dunnavant

Specialty Managed Care Partners
Enters into Contracts with Regional Business Coalitions: No

Chief Strategy Officer . . . . Greg Poulsen
Chief Financial Officer . . . . Bert Zimmerli

777 Humana Health Insurance of Utah

9815 South Monroe Street
Suite 300
Sandy, UT 84070
Toll-Free: 800-884-8328
Phone: 801-256-6200
Fax: 801-256-0782
www.humana.com
Subsidiary of: Humana
For Profit Organization: Yes

Healthplan and Services Defined
PLAN TYPE: HMO/PPO
Model Type: Network
Plan Specialty: Dental, Vision
Benefits Offered: Dental, Vision, Life, LTD, STD

Type of Coverage
Commercial, Individual

Accreditation Certification
URAC, NCQA, CORE

Key Personnel
President & CEO. Bruce Broussard
Chief Medical Officer. . . . . Roy A. Beveridge
Chief Consumer Officer. . . . . Jody L. Bilney
Human Resources. . . . . Tim Huval
Chief Financial Officer . . . . Brain Kane
Chief Information Officer . . . . Brian LeClaire
General Counsel . . . . Christopher M. Todoroff
Chief Accounting Officer . . . . Cynthia H. Zipperie

778 Intermountain Healthcare

36 S State Street
Salt Lake City, UT 84111
Phone: 801-442-2000
www.intermountainhealthcare.org
Non-Profit Organization: Yes
Year Founded: 1975
Total Enrollment: 750,000

Healthplan and Services Defined
PLAN TYPE: HMO
Benefits Offered: Chiropractic, Complementary Medicine,
Dental, Home Care, Inpatient SNF, Long-Term Care,
Podiatry, Prescription, Psychiatric, Transplant, Vision,
Wellness, Worker's Compensation

Type of Coverage
Commercial, Individual, Medicare, Medicaid

Geographic Areas Served
Utah and SE Idaho

Accreditation Certification
NCQA

Key Personnel
President & CEO. A. Marc Harrison
Chief Operating Officer. . . . . Robert W. Allen
Chief Physician Executive . . . . Mark Briesacher

779 Molina Healthcare of Utah

7050 Union Park Center
Suite 200
Midvale, UT 84047
Toll-Free: 866-449-6817
Phone: 801-858-0400
www.molinahealthcare.com
Subsidiary of: Molina Healthcare, Inc.
For Profit Organization: Yes
Year Founded: 1980
Physician Owned Organization: Yes

Healthplan and Services Defined
PLAN TYPE: Medicare
Model Type: Network
Plan Specialty: Integrated Medicare/Medicaid (Duals)
Benefits Offered: Chiropractic, Dental, Home Care, Inpatient
SNF, Long-Term Care, Podiatry, Vision

Type of Coverage
Commercial, Medicare, Supplemental Medicare, Medicaid

Accreditation Certification
URAC, NCQA

Key Personnel
Chief Executive Officer . . . . Joseph W. White
Chief Operating Officer . . . . Terry Bayer
General Counsel. . . . . Jeff D. Barlow
SVP, Relations/Marketing . . . . Juan Jos, Orellana
Chief Information Officer . . . . Rick Hopfer

780 Opticare of Utah

1901 W Parkway Boulevard
Salt Lake City, UT 84119
Toll-Free: 800-363-0950
Phone: 801-869-2020
service@opticareofutah.com
www.opticareofutah.com
For Profit Organization: Yes
Year Founded: 1985
Number of Referral/Specialty Physicians: 40
Total Enrollment: 150,000
State Enrollment: 150,000

Healthplan and Services Defined
PLAN TYPE: Vision
Other Type: Optical
Model Type: Network
Plan Specialty: Vision
Benefits Offered: Vision

Type of Payment Plans Offered
POS, Capitated, FFS

Geographic Areas Served
Statewide

Subscriber Information
Average Subscriber Co-Payment:
Primary Care Physician: Varies

Network Qualifications
Pre-Admission Certification: Yes

Peer Review Type
Utilization Review: Yes
Second Surgical Opinion: Yes
Case Management: Yes

Key Personnel
CEO/ABO . . . . Aaron Schubach
  800-363-0950
  aaron@standardoptical.net
President . . . . Stephen Schubach
  stephen@standardoptical.net
Account Manager . . . . Madeline Draper
  801-910-3978
  madeline@opticareofutah.com
Sales Director . . . . Jennine Ashley
  801-869-2019
  jennine@opticareofutah.com
Office Manager . . . . Carliedane Livingston
  801-869-2021

Specialty Managed Care Partners
Enters into Contracts with Regional Business Coalitions: Yes

Employer References
State of Utah Employees

---

781 Premier Access Insurance/Access Dental
P.O. Box 659010
Sacramento, CA 95865-9010
Toll-Free: 888-634-6074
Phone: 916-920-2500
Fax: 916-563-9000
info@premierlife.com
www.premierppo.com
Subsidiary of: Guardian Life Insurance Co.
For Profit Organization: Yes
Year Founded: 1989
Number of Primary Care Physicians: 1,000

Healthplan and Services Defined
PLAN TYPE: PPO
Other Type: Dental
Plan Specialty: Dental
Benefits Offered: Dental

Key Personnel
President & CEO . . . . Deanna M. Mulligan

---

782 Public Employees Health Program
560 East 200 South
Salt Lake City, UT 84102-2099
Toll-Free: 800-765-7347
Phone: 801-366-7555
www.pehp.org
Subsidiary of: Utah Retirement Systems
Non-Profit Organization: Yes
Year Founded: 1977
Number of Affiliated Hospitals: 49
Number of Primary Care Physicians: 12,000
Number of Referral/Specialty Physicians: 2,900

Total Enrollment: 177,854
State Enrollment: 177,854

Healthplan and Services Defined
PLAN TYPE: PPO
Model Type: Network
Plan Specialty: Dental, Disease Management, Lab, PBM, Radiology, UR
Benefits Offered: Dental, Disease Management, Home Care, Prescription, Transplant, Wellness, AD&D, Life, LTD

Type of Coverage
Supplemental Medicare, Children's Health Insurance Program
Catastrophic Illness Benefit: None

Type of Payment Plans Offered
FFS

Subscriber Information
Average Monthly Fee Per Subscriber
  (Employee + Employer Contribution):
    Employee Only (Self): Varies by plan
    Employee & 1 Family Member: $583.00
Average Annual Deductible Per Subscriber:
    Employee Only (Self): $0
    Employee & 1 Family Member: $0
    Employee & 2 Family Members: $0
    Medicare: $0
Average Subscriber Co-Payment:
    Primary Care Physician: $15.00
    Non-Network Physician: 15.00 + 30%
    Prescription Drugs: 20%
    Hospital ER: $80.00
    Home Health Care Max. Days/Visits Covered: Unlimited

Network Qualifications
Pre-Admission Certification: No

Peer Review Type
Utilization Review: Yes
Second Surgical Opinion: Yes
Case Management: Yes

Publishes and Distributes Report Card: Yes

Accreditation Certification
TJC Accreditation, Medicare Approved, State Licensure

Key Personnel
Director . . . . R. Chet Loftis
Provider Relations . . . . Cortney Larson
Operations Director . . . . G. Steven Baker
Marketing Director . . . . Joel Sheppard
Chief Actuary . . . . John Borer

Average Claim Compensation
Physician's Fees Charged: 70%
Hospital's Fees Charged: 80%

Specialty Managed Care Partners
Managed Mental Healthcare, Chiropratic Health Plan, IHC Auesst
Enters into Contracts with Regional Business Coalitions: Yes

Employer References
State of Utah, Jordon School District, Salt Lake County, Salt Lake City, Utah School Boards Association

783 Regence BlueCross BlueShield of Utah
PO Box 1071
Portland, OR 97207
Toll-Free: 888-232-5763
www.regence.com
Subsidiary of: Regence
Non-Profit Organization: Yes
Total Enrollment: 2,400,000
State Enrollment: 330,000

Healthplan and Services Defined
  PLAN TYPE: Multiple
  Model Type: Network
  Benefits Offered: Dental, Prescription, Vision, Wellness,
    Life, Preventive Care

Type of Coverage
  Commercial, Individual, Supplemental Medicare

Key Personnel
  President................................ Jim Swayze
  Chief Marketing Officer.................... Carol Kruse
  Chief Medical Officer .... Richard Popiel

784 SelectHealth
5381 S Green Street
Murray, UT 84123
Toll-Free: 800-538-5038
selecthealth.org
Non-Profit Organization: Yes

Healthplan and Services Defined
  PLAN TYPE: HMO

Type of Coverage
  Commercial, Individual

Geographic Areas Served
  Utah and Idaho

Accreditation Certification
  NCQA

785 Total Dental Administrators
6985 Union Park Center
Suite 675
Cottonwood Heights, UT 84047
Toll-Free: 800-880-3536
Phone: 801-268-9840
Fax: 801-268-9873
www.tdadental.com
Secondary Address: 2111 E. Highland Avenue, Suite 250,
  Phoenix, AZ 85016-4735, 602-266-1995
Subsidiary of: Companion Life Insurance Co.

Healthplan and Services Defined
  PLAN TYPE: Dental

Key Personnel
  President & CEO .... Jeremy Spencer

786 UnitedHealthcare of Utah
2525 Lake Park Boulevard
Salt Lake City, UT 84120
Toll-Free: 800-624-2942
www.uhc.com/contact-us/utah
Subsidiary of: UnitedHealth Group
For Profit Organization: Yes

Healthplan and Services Defined
  PLAN TYPE: HMO/PPO
  Model Type: Network
  Plan Specialty: Behavioral Health, Dental, Disease
    Management, PBM, Vision
  Benefits Offered: Behavioral Health, Dental, Disease
    Management, Long-Term Care, Prescription, Vision,
    Wellness, Life, LTD, STD

Type of Coverage
  Individual, Medicare, Supplemental Medicare, Medicaid,
    Catastrophic, Family, Military, Veterans, Group,

Geographic Areas Served
  Statewide

Key Personnel
  Chief Executive Officer................ David Wichmann
  Chief Operating Officer .... Dan Schumacher
  Chief Strategy Officer .... John Cosgriff
  Communications Officer .... Kirsten Gorsuch
  Chief Medical Officer....................... Sam Ho
  Chief Legal Officer .... Thad Johnson
  Chief Information Officer .... Phil McKoy
  Chief Financial Officer.................... Jeff Putnam

787 University Health Plans
6053 Fashion Square Drive
Suite 110
Murray, UT 84107
Toll-Free: 888-271-5870
Phone: 801-587-6480
Fax: 801-281-6121
uuhp@hsc.utah.edu
uhealthplan.utah.edu
Mailing Address: P.O. Box 45180, Salt Lake City, UT
  84145-0180
Non-Profit Organization: Yes
Number of Affiliated Hospitals: 28
Number of Primary Care Physicians: 1,750
Total Enrollment: 86,000
State Enrollment: 50,000

Healthplan and Services Defined
  PLAN TYPE: HMO/PPO
  Benefits Offered: Disease Management, Wellness

Type of Coverage
  Commercial, Medicare, Medicaid

Geographic Areas Served
  Statewide

Health Insurance Coverage Status and Type of Coverage by Age

Category	All Persons		Under 18 years		Under 65 years	
	Number	%	Number	%	Number	%
Total population	619	-	128	-	508	-
Covered by some type of health insurance	596 (2)	96.3 (0.4)	126 (2)	98.5 (0.4)	485 (2)	95.5 (0.5)
Covered by private health insurance	422 (9)	68.2 (1.4)	74 (4)	57.8 (2.9)	349 (8)	68.8 (1.6)
Employer-based	337 (8)	54.4 (1.4)	66 (4)	51.7 (2.9)	300 (7)	59.2 (1.5)
Direct purchase	96 (5)	15.5 (0.8)	8 (1)	6.0 (1.1)	55 (4)	10.8 (0.8)
TRICARE	11 (2)	1.8 (0.3)	2 (1)	1.6 (0.6)	7 (2)	1.4 (0.3)
Covered by public health insurance	264 (7)	42.7 (1.2)	59 (4)	45.8 (2.9)	157 (7)	30.9 (1.5)
Medicaid	162 (8)	26.2 (1.2)	58 (4)	45.7 (2.9)	146 (8)	28.7 (1.5)
Medicare	127 (2)	20.5 (0.4)	Z (Z)	0.3 (0.2)	19 (2)	3.8 (0.4)
VA Care	15 (1)	2.4 (0.2)	Z (Z)	0.1 (0.1)	6 (1)	1.2 (0.2)
Not covered at any time during the year	23 (2)	3.7 (0.4)	2 (1)	1.5 (0.4)	23 (2)	4.5 (0.5)

Note: Numbers in thousands; Figures cover civilian noninstitutionalized population in 2016; N/A indicates that data was not available; Z represents or rounds to zero; Margin of error appears in parenthesis and is calculated using replicate weights.
Source: U.S. Census Bureau, American Community Survey, Table HIC-4_ACS. Health Insurance Coverage Status and Type of Coverage by State—All People: 2008 to 2016, Table HIC-5_ACS. Health Insurance Coverage Status and Type of Coverage by State—Children Under 18: 2008 to 2016, Table HIC-6_ACS. Health Insurance Coverage Status and Type of Coverage by State—Persons Under 65: 2008 to 2016

Vermont

788   Aetna Health of Vermont

151 Farmington Avenue
Hartford, CT 06156
Toll-Free: 800-872-3862
Phone: 860-273-0123
www.aetna.com
Subsidiary of: Aetna Inc.
For Profit Organization: Yes

Healthplan and Services Defined
  PLAN TYPE: PPO
  Other Type: POS
  Model Type: Network
  Plan Specialty: Behavioral Health, EPO, Lab, PBM,
    Radiology
  Benefits Offered: Behavioral Health, Disease Management,
    Long-Term Care, Physical Therapy, Podiatry, Prescription,
    Psychiatric, Wellness, Life, LTD, STD

Type of Coverage
  Commercial, Student health

Type of Payment Plans Offered
  POS, FFS

Geographic Areas Served
  Statewide

Key Personnel
  CEO . . . . Mark Bertolini

789   Blue Cross & Blue Shield of Vermont

445 Industrial Lane
Berlin, VT 05602
Toll-Free: 800-247-2583
Phone: 802-223-6131
www.bcbsvt.com
Mailing Address: P.O. Box 186, Montpelier, VT 05601-0186
Subsidiary of: Blue Cross Blue Shield Association
Non-Profit Organization: Yes
Year Founded: 1944
Total Enrollment: 180,000
State Enrollment: 54,023

Healthplan and Services Defined
  PLAN TYPE: PPO
  Model Type: Network
  Plan Specialty: Behavioral Health, Chiropractic, Disease
    Management, PBM, Vision, UR
  Benefits Offered: Behavioral Health, Chiropractic, Physical
    Therapy, Prescription, Psychiatric, Vision, AD&D, Life,
    LTD, STD, Alternative Healthcare discounts, Vermont
    Medigap Blue

Type of Coverage
  Commercial, Individual, Indemnity, Medicare, Supplemental
    Medicare, Catastrophic
  Catastrophic Illness Benefit: Maximum $1M

Type of Payment Plans Offered
  Capitated

Geographic Areas Served
  Statewide

Subscriber Information
  Average Monthly Fee Per Subscriber
    (Employee + Employer Contribution):
      Employee Only (Self): Varies by plan
  Average Annual Deductible Per Subscriber:
      Employee Only (Self): $400.00
      Employee & 1 Family Member: $400.00
      Employee & 2 Family Members: $200.00
  Average Subscriber Co-Payment:
      Primary Care Physician: $10.00
      Prescription Drugs: $10.00/20.00/35.00
      Hospital ER: $50.00
      Home Health Care: $40.00

Network Qualifications
  Pre-Admission Certification: Yes

Peer Review Type
  Utilization Review: Yes
  Second Surgical Opinion: No
  Case Management: Yes

Publishes and Distributes Report Card: No

Accreditation Certification
  Utilization Review, State Licensure, Quality Assurance
    Program

Key Personnel
  President and CEO . . . . Don George
  VP, External Affairs . . . . Kevin Goddard
  VP, Con Svcs & Planning . . . . Catherine Hamilton, PhD
  VP/ General Counsel/ CAO . . . . Christopher R Gannon
  Chief Marketing Executive . . . . Ellen Yakubik
  VP/CFO . . . . Ruth K Greene
  VP/Chief Medical Officer. . . . . Robert R Wheeler
  VP/CIO . . . . Daniel Galdenzi
  VP/External Affairs. . . . . Andrew Garland

Average Claim Compensation
  Physician's Fees Charged: 85%
  Hospital's Fees Charged: 92%

Specialty Managed Care Partners
  Magellan, Restat
  Enters into Contracts with Regional Business Coalitions: Yes

790   Coventry Health Care of Vermont

6720-B Rockledge Drive
Suite 700
Bethesda, MD 20817
Phone: 301-581-0600
www.coventryhealthcare.com
Subsidiary of: Aetna Inc.
For Profit Organization: Yes

Healthplan and Services Defined
  PLAN TYPE: HMO/PPO
  Model Type: Network
  Plan Specialty: Behavioral Health, Dental, Worker's
    Compensation

Benefits Offered: Behavioral Health, Dental, Prescription, Wellness, Worker's Compensation

Type of Coverage
Commercial, Medicare, Medicaid

Geographic Areas Served
Statewide

Key Personnel
Chief Executive Officer . . . . Mark T. Bertolini
President . . . . Karen S. Lynch
Chief Financial Officer . . . . Shawn M. Guertin
Operations & Technology . . . . Meg McCarthy
Chief Medical Officer . . . . Harold L. Paz
General Counsel . . . . Thomas Sabatino Jr.
Government Services . . . . Fran S. Soistman

791   UnitedHealthcare of Vermont

475 Kilvert Street
Warwick, RI 02886
Toll-Free: 888-735-5842
www.uhc.com/contact-us/vermont
Subsidiary of: UnitedHealth Group
For Profit Organization: Yes
Year Founded: 1986

Healthplan and Services Defined
PLAN TYPE: HMO/PPO
Model Type: Network
Plan Specialty: Behavioral Health, Dental, Disease Management, MSO, PBM, Vision
Benefits Offered: Behavioral Health, Chiropractic, Complementary Medicine, Dental, Disease Management, Home Care, Inpatient SNF, Long-Term Care, Physical Therapy, Podiatry, Prescription, Psychiatric, Transplant, Vision, Wellness, AD&D, Life, LTD, STD

Type of Coverage
Commercial, Individual, Medicare, Supplemental Medicare, Medicaid, Catastrophic, Family, Military, Veterans, Group,

Type of Payment Plans Offered
DFFS, FFS, Combination FFS & DFFS

Geographic Areas Served
Statewide. Vermont is covered by the Rhode Island branch

Subscriber Information
Average Monthly Fee Per Subscriber
    (Employee + Employer Contribution):
        Employee Only (Self): Varies
Average Subscriber Co-Payment:
    Primary Care Physician: $10
    Prescription Drugs: $10/15/30
    Hospital ER: $50

Network Qualifications
Pre-Admission Certification: Yes

Peer Review Type
Case Management: Yes

Publishes and Distributes Report Card: Yes

Accreditation Certification
URAC, NCQA

State Licensure, Quality Assurance Program

Key Personnel
President . . . . David Wichmann
Chief Operating Officer . . . . Dan Schumacher
Chief Strategy Officer . . . . John Cosgriff
Communications Officer . . . . Kirsten Gorsuch
Chief Medical Officer . . . . Sam Ho
Chief Legal Officer . . . . Thad Johnson
Chief Information Officer . . . . Phil McKoy
Chief Financial Officer . . . . Jeff Putnam

Average Claim Compensation
Physician's Fees Charged: 70%
Hospital's Fees Charged: 55%

Specialty Managed Care Partners
United Behavioral Health
Enters into Contracts with Regional Business Coalitions: No

Health Insurance Coverage Status and Type of Coverage by Age

Category	All Persons		Under 18 years		Under 65 years	
	Number	%	Number	%	Number	%
Total population	8,200	-	1,989	-	6,999	-
Covered by some type of health insurance	7,485 (22)	91.3 (0.3)	1,890 (10)	95.0 (0.4)	6,294 (21)	89.9 (0.3)
Covered by private health insurance	6,282 (32)	76.6 (0.4)	1,414 (15)	71.1 (0.7)	5,446 (30)	77.8 (0.4)
Employer-based	4,892 (39)	59.7 (0.5)	1,141 (17)	57.3 (0.8)	4,436 (36)	63.4 (0.5)
Direct purchase	1,285 (21)	15.7 (0.3)	180 (8)	9.0 (0.4)	872·(19)	12.5 (0.3)
TRICARE	643 (18)	7.8 (0.2)	169 (8)	8.5 (0.4)	488 (16)	7.0 (0.2)
Covered by public health insurance	2,252 (22)	27.5 (0.3)	532 (14)	26.8 (0.7)	1,101 (21)	15.7 (0.3)
Medicaid	951 (22)	11.6 (0.3)	515 (14)	25.9 (0.7)	848 (21)	12.1 (0.3)
Medicare	1,338 (10)	16.3 (0.1)	14 (3)	0.7 (0.2)	189 (8)	2.7 (0.1)
VA Care	240 (8)	2.9 (0.1)	9 (2)	0.5 (0.1)	147 (7)	2.1 (0.1)
Not covered at any time during the year	715 (21)	8.7 (0.3)	99 (8)	5.0 (0.4)	705 (21)	10.1 (0.3)

Note: Numbers in thousands; Figures cover civilian noninstitutionalized population in 2016; N/A indicates that data was not available; Z represents or rounds to zero; Margin of error appears in parenthesis and is calculated using replicate weights.
Source: U.S. Census Bureau, American Community Survey, Table HIC-4_ACS. Health Insurance Coverage Status and Type of Coverage by State—All People: 2008 to 2016, Table HIC-5_ACS. Health Insurance Coverage Status and Type of Coverage by State—Children Under 18: 2008 to 2016, Table HIC-6_ACS. Health Insurance Coverage Status and Type of Coverage by State—Persons Under 65: 2008 to 2016

Virginia

792   Aetna Health of Virginia

151 Farmington Avenue
Hartford, CT 06156
Toll-Free: 800-872-3862
Phone: 860-273-0123
www.aetna.com
Subsidiary of: Aetna Inc.
For Profit Organization: Yes
Year Founded: 1984

Healthplan and Services Defined
PLAN TYPE: HMO/PPO
Other Type: POS
Model Type: Network
Plan Specialty: Behavioral Health, Dental, EPO, Lab, PBM, Vision, Radiology
Benefits Offered: Behavioral Health, Dental, Disease Management, Long-Term Care, Physical Therapy, Podiatry, Prescription, Psychiatric, Vision, Wellness, Life, LTD, STD

Type of Coverage
Commercial, Medicaid, Catastrophic, Student health

Type of Payment Plans Offered
POS, DFFS

Geographic Areas Served
Alexandria City, Arlington, Fairfax, Fairfax City, Falls Church City, Loudoun, Stafford, Spotsylvania, Fredericksburg City, Prince William County, Manassas City, Manassas Park City, Winchester City, Frederick County, Clarke County, Shenandoah County, Warren County and Page County

Subscriber Information
Average Annual Deductible Per Subscriber:
    Employee Only (Self): Varies
    Employee & 1 Family Member: Varies
    Employee & 2 Family Members: Varies
    Medicare: Varies

Network Qualifications
Pre-Admission Certification: Yes

Peer Review Type
Utilization Review: No
Second Surgical Opinion: Yes
Case Management: Yes

Publishes and Distributes Report Card: Yes

Accreditation Certification
NCQA
TJC Accreditation, Utilization Review, Pre-Admission Certification, State Licensure, Quality Assurance Program

Key Personnel
CEO . . . . Mark Bertolini

Specialty Managed Care Partners
Enters into Contracts with Regional Business Coalitions: Yes

793   Anthem Blue Cross & Blue Shield of Virginia

2015 Staples Mill Road
Richmond, VA 23230
Toll-Free: 866-755-2680
www.anthem.com
For Profit Organization: Yes
Year Founded: 1980
Total Enrollment: 2,800,000
State Enrollment: 2,800,000

Healthplan and Services Defined
PLAN TYPE: HMO
Model Type: Network
Plan Specialty: ASO, Behavioral Health, Chiropractic, Dental, Disease Management, Lab, PBM, Vision, Radiology, Worker's Compensation, UR
Benefits Offered: Behavioral Health, Chiropractic, Dental, Disease Management, Home Care, Inpatient SNF, Physical Therapy, Podiatry, Prescription, Psychiatric, Transplant, Vision, Wellness, Worker's Compensation, Life

Type of Coverage
Commercial, Individual, Medicare, Catastrophic
Catastrophic Illness Benefit: Unlimited

Type of Payment Plans Offered
Capitated

Geographic Areas Served
All of Virginia except for the City of Fairfax, the Town of Vienna and the area east of State Route 123

Subscriber Information
Average Subscriber Co-Payment:
    Primary Care Physician: $5.00/10.00
    Prescription Drugs: $5.00/10.00
    Hospital ER: $25.00
    Home Health Care Max. Days/Visits Covered: 100 days

Peer Review Type
Case Management: Yes

Publishes and Distributes Report Card: Yes

Accreditation Certification
URAC, NCQA
TJC Accreditation, Medicare Approved, Utilization Review, Pre-Admission Certification, State Licensure, Quality Assurance Program

Key Personnel
President & CEO . . . . Joseph Swedish
Corperate Communications . . . . Scott Golden
    804-354-5252
    scott.golden@anthem.com

Specialty Managed Care Partners
Enters into Contracts with Regional Business Coalitions: Yes

Employer References
Commonwealth of Virginia, GE

794 CareFirst Blue Cross & Blue Shield of Virginia

10455 Mill Run Circle
Owings Mills, MD 21117
Toll-Free: 800-544-8703
www.carefirst.com
Non-Profit Organization: Yes
Year Founded: 1985
Number of Affiliated Hospitals: 165
Number of Primary Care Physicians: 4,500
Number of Referral/Specialty Physicians: 15,068
Total Enrollment: 3,400,000

Healthplan and Services Defined
PLAN TYPE: HMO/PPO
Model Type: IPA
Plan Specialty: ASO, Behavioral Health, Dental, Vision
Benefits Offered: Behavioral Health, Chiropractic, Dental,
Disease Management, Home Care, Physical Therapy,
Podiatry, Prescription, Psychiatric, Transplant, Vision,
Wellness

Type of Coverage
Commercial, Individual

Type of Payment Plans Offered
POS

Geographic Areas Served
Arlington County and portions of Fairfax and Prince William
counties east of State Route 123

Accreditation Certification
NCQA

Key Personnel
Chief Actuary . . . . Peter Berry
EVO, Medical Affairs . . . . Jon Blum
EVP & General Counsel . . . . Meryl Burgin
Chief Financial Officer . . . . G. Mark Chaney
Chief Medical Officer . . . . Rahul Rajkumar
Human Resources . . . . Michelle Wright

795 Delta Dental of Virginia

4818 Starkey Road
Roanoke, VA 24018
Toll-Free: 800-237-6060
Phone: 540-989-8000
www.deltadentalva.com
Secondary Address: 4860 Cox Road, Suite 130, Glen Allen,
VA 23060
Non-Profit Organization: Yes
Year Founded: 1964
Total Enrollment: 68,000,000
State Enrollment: 2,000,000

Healthplan and Services Defined
PLAN TYPE: Dental
Other Type: Dental PPO/POS
Plan Specialty: Dental
Benefits Offered: Dental

Type of Coverage
Commercial, Individual

Type of Payment Plans Offered
FFS

Geographic Areas Served
Statewide

Accreditation Certification
TJC

796 Dominion Dental Services

251 18th Street South
Suite 900
Arlington, VA 22314
Toll-Free: 888-518-5338
www.dominionnational.com
Mailing Address: P.O. Box 1126, Claims/Utilization, Elk Grove
Village, IL 60009
For Profit Organization: Yes
Year Founded: 1996
Physician Owned Organization: Yes
Total Enrollment: 24,000,000
State Enrollment: 490,000

Healthplan and Services Defined
PLAN TYPE: Dental
Plan Specialty: Dental
Benefits Offered: Dental

Type of Coverage
Commercial, Individual

Type of Payment Plans Offered
DFFS, Capitated, Combination FFS & DFFS

Geographic Areas Served
Maryland; Delaware; Pennsylvania; District of Columbia;
Virginia and New Jersey

Network Qualifications
Pre-Admission Certification: Yes

Peer Review Type
Utilization Review: Yes
Case Management: Yes

Publishes and Distributes Report Card: No

Accreditation Certification
NCQA

Key Personnel
President and COO . . . . Mike Davis
VP of Business Management . . . . Jay Rausch
VP of Operations . . . . Ann Quinlan
VP of Accounting . . . . Dee Dee Brooks
Dental Director . . . . Wayne Silverman, DDS
Director of Marketing . . . . Jeff Schwab
Member Services . . . . Pete Harris
Media Contact . . . . Jeff Schwab

Specialty Managed Care Partners
Enters into Contracts with Regional Business Coalitions: Yes

797   EPIC Pharmacy Network

8703 Studley Road
Suite B
Mechanicsville, VA 23116-2016
Toll-Free: 800-876-3742
Phone: 804-559-4597
Fax: 804-559-2038
www.epicrx.com
Subsidiary of: EPIC Pharmacies, Inc.
For Profit Organization: Yes
Year Founded: 1992
Number of Primary Care Physicians: 1,400

Healthplan and Services Defined
PLAN TYPE: Multiple
Plan Specialty: PBM
Benefits Offered: Prescription

Geographic Areas Served
Mid-Atlantic states

Key Personnel
Chief Executive Officer . . . . Jay Romero
VP of Contracts . . . . Thomas E. Scono
Executive Vice President. . . . . Mark P Barwig

798   Humana Health Insurance of Virginia

4191 Innslake Drive
Suite 100
Glen Allen, VA 23060
Toll-Free: 800-350-7213
Phone: 804-253-0060
Fax: 804-217-6514
www.humana.com
Secondary Address: 3800 Electric Road, Suite 406, Roanoke,
    VA 24018, 540-772-5762
Subsidiary of: Humana
For Profit Organization: Yes

Healthplan and Services Defined
PLAN TYPE: HMO/PPO
Model Type: Network
Plan Specialty: Dental, Vision
Benefits Offered: Dental, Vision, Life, LTD, STD

Type of Coverage
Commercial, Individual

Geographic Areas Served
Statewide

Accreditation Certification
URAC, NCQA, CORE

Key Personnel
President & CEO. . . . . Bruce Broussard
Chief Medical Officer. . . . . Roy A. Beveridge
Chief Consumer Officer. . . . . Jody L. Bilney
Human Resources. . . . . Tim Huval
Chief Financial Officer . . . . Brian Kane
Chief Information Officer . . . . Brian LeClaire
General Counsel. . . . . Christopher M. Todoroff
Chief Accounting Officer . . . . Cynthia H. Zipperie

799   Molina Healthcare of Virgina

4050 Innslake Drive
Suite 202
Glen Allen, VA 23060
Phone: 844-509-7583
molinahealthcare.com
Subsidiary of: Monlina Healthcare, Inc.
For Profit Organization: Yes
Year Founded: 1980

Healthplan and Services Defined
PLAN TYPE: Medicare
Plan Specialty: Dental, PBM, Vision, intergrated
    Medicare/Medicaid (Duals)
Benefits Offered: Dental, Prescription, Vision, Wellness, Life

Geographic Areas Served
Statewide

Key Personnel
Chief Executive Officer . . . . Joseph W. White
Chief Operating Officer . . . . Terry Bayer
SVP, General Counsel . . . . Jeff D. Barlow
SVP, Marketing. . . . . Juan Jos, Orellana

800   Optima Health Plan

4417 Corporation Lane
Virginia Beach, VA 23462-3162
Toll-Free: 877-828-1140
Phone: 757-552-7401
www.optimahealth.com
Secondary Address: 1604 Santa Rosa Road, Suite 100,
    Richmond, VA 23229
Subsidiary of: Sentara Health Plans
Non-Profit Organization: Yes
Year Founded: 1984
Federally Qualified: Yes
Number of Affiliated Hospitals: 12
Number of Primary Care Physicians: 15,000
Number of Referral/Specialty Physicians: 3,870
Total Enrollment: 430,000
State Enrollment: 430,000

Healthplan and Services Defined
PLAN TYPE: HMO/PPO
Other Type: POS
Model Type: Network
Plan Specialty: ASO, Behavioral Health, Chiropractic, Dental,
    PBM, Vision
Benefits Offered: Behavioral Health, Chiropractic,
    Complementary Medicine, Dental, Disease Management,
    Home Care, Inpatient SNF, Long-Term Care, Physical
    Therapy, Podiatry, Prescription, Psychiatric, Transplant,
    Vision, Wellness
Offers Demand Management Patient Information Service: Yes
DMPI Services Offered: After hours nurse triage

Type of Coverage
Commercial, Individual, Medicare, Medicaid
Catastrophic Illness Benefit: Covered

Type of Payment Plans Offered
FFS

Geographic Areas Served
Selected counties in Virginia

Subscriber Information
Average Monthly Fee Per Subscriber
(Employee + Employer Contribution):
Employee Only (Self): Varies by plan
Medicare: Varies
Average Annual Deductible Per Subscriber:
Employee Only (Self): $0
Employee & 1 Family Member: $0
Employee & 2 Family Members: $0
Medicare: Varies
Average Subscriber Co-Payment:
Primary Care Physician: $15.00
Non-Network Physician: 70 %
Prescription Drugs: 50/20%
Hospital ER: 80%
Home Health Care: 80%

Network Qualifications
Pre-Admission Certification: Yes

Peer Review Type
Utilization Review: Yes
Second Surgical Opinion: No
Case Management: Yes

Accreditation Certification
URAC, NCQA

Key Personnel
President & CEO. . . . . Michael M Dudley
SVP/Chief Financial Offc. . . . . Andy Hilbert
SVP, Sales & Marketing . . . . John DeGruttola
VP, Medical Director . . . . Thomas Lundquist

Specialty Managed Care Partners
Cole Vision, American Specialty Health, Doral Dental,
Sentara Mental Health
Enters into Contracts with Regional Business Coalitions: Yes

Employer References
City of Virginia Beach, City of Norfolk, Bank of America,
Nexcom, CHKD

801   **Piedmont Community Health Plan**
2316 Atherholt Road
Lynchburg, VA 24501
Toll-Free: 800-400-7247
Phone: 434-947-4463
Fax: 434-947-3670
www.pchp.net
Subsidiary of: Centra Health System
For Profit Organization: Yes
Year Founded: 1995
Physician Owned Organization: Yes
Total Enrollment: 30,000
State Enrollment: 30,000

Healthplan and Services Defined
PLAN TYPE: Multiple
Other Type: POS
Benefits Offered: Disease Management, Prescription,
Wellness

Type of Payment Plans Offered
POS

Geographic Areas Served
Cities of Lynchburg and Bedford and the counties of
Albemarle, Amherst, Appomattox, Bedford, Buchkingham,
Campbell, Cumberland, Lunenburg, Nottoway and Price
Edward

Key Personnel
Marketing Executive . . . . Lori Carter
434-947-4463

Specialty Managed Care Partners
Caremark Rx

802   **United Concordia of Virginia**
4860 Cox Road
Suite 200
Glen Allen, VA 23060
Phone: 804-217-8336
www.unitedconcordia.com
For Profit Organization: Yes
Year Founded: 1971
Total Enrollment: 7,800,000

Healthplan and Services Defined
PLAN TYPE: Dental
Plan Specialty: Dental
Benefits Offered: Dental

Type of Coverage
Commercial, Individual, Military personnel & families

Geographic Areas Served
Nationwide

Accreditation Certification
URAC

Key Personnel
President & COO . . . . Timothy J. Constantine
Contact. . . . . Beth Rutherford
717-260-7659
beth.rutherford@ucci.com

803   **UnitedHealthcare of Virginia**
9020 Stony Point Parkway
Suite 400
Richmond, VA 23235
Toll-Free: 877-842-3210
Phone: 800-357-0978
www.uhc.com/contact-us/virginia
Subsidiary of: UnitedHealth Group
For Profit Organization: Yes

Healthplan and Services Defined
PLAN TYPE: HMO/PPO
Model Type: Network
Plan Specialty: Behavioral Health, Dental, Disease
Management, PBM, Vision
Benefits Offered: Behavioral Health, Dental, Disease
Management, Long-Term Care, Prescription, Vision,
Wellness, Life, LTD, STD

Type of Coverage
Individual, Medicare, Supplemental Medicare, Medicaid, Catastrophic, Family, Military, Veterans, Group,

Geographic Areas Served
Statewide, and West Virgnia

Accreditation Certification
TJC

Key Personnel
Chief Executive Officer . . . . David Wichmann
Cheif Operating Officer . . . . Dan Schumacher
Chief Strategy Officer . . . . John Cosgriff
Communications Officer . . . . Kirsten Gorsuch
Chief Medical Officer. . . . . Sam Ho
Chief Legal Officer . . . . Thad Johnson
Chief Information Officer . . . . Phil McKoy
Chief Financial Officer. . . . . Jeff Putnam

804 Virginia Health Network

812 Moorefield Park Drive
Suite 204
Richmond, VA 23236
Phone: 804-320-3837
Fax: 804-320-5984
jhoover@vhn.com
www.vhn.com
For Profit Organization: Yes
Year Founded: 1988
Physician Owned Organization: No
Federally Qualified: No
Number of Primary Care Physicians: 75,000
Total Enrollment: 88,366
State Enrollment: 88,366

Healthplan and Services Defined
PLAN TYPE: PPO
Model Type: Network
Plan Specialty: Worker's Compensation, Medical PPO
Offers Demand Management Patient Information Service: No

Type of Coverage
Commercial

Geographic Areas Served
Virginia, North and South Carolina

Network Qualifications
Pre-Admission Certification: Yes

Publishes and Distributes Report Card: No

Accreditation Certification
Medicare; State License
TJC Accreditation, Medicare Approved, Utilization Review, State Licensure

Key Personnel
President . . . . Jim Brittain
jbrittain@vhn.com
Provider Relations . . . . Betty Walters
bwalters@vhn.com
Administrative Assistant . . . . Sandra Newby
snewby@vhn.comÿ

Average Claim Compensation
Physician's Fees Charged: 79%
Hospital's Fees Charged: 67%

Specialty Managed Care Partners
Enters into Contracts with Regional Business Coalitions: Yes

Health Insurance Coverage Status and Type of Coverage by Age

Category	All Persons		Under 18 years		Under 65 years	
	Number	%	Number	%	Number	%
Total population	7,184	-	1,723	-	6,125	-
Covered by some type of health insurance	6,756 *(15)*	94.0 *(0.2)*	1,677 *(7)*	97.3 *(0.3)*	5,703 *(16)*	93.1 *(0.2)*
Covered by private health insurance	5,130 *(27)*	71.4 *(0.4)*	1,089 *(16)*	63.2 *(0.9)*	4,434 *(27)*	72.4 *(0.4)*
Employer-based	4,110 *(30)*	57.2 *(0.4)*	916 *(16)*	53.2 *(0.9)*	3,751 *(28)*	61.2 *(0.5)*
Direct purchase	1,010 *(18)*	14.1 *(0.2)*	131 *(8)*	7.6 *(0.5)*	636 *(16)*	10.4 *(0.3)*
TRICARE	318 *(13)*	4.4 *(0.2)*	80 *(7)*	4.6 *(0.4)*	231 *(12)*	3.8 *(0.2)*
Covered by public health insurance	2,568 *(24)*	35.8 *(0.3)*	678 *(15)*	39.3 *(0.9)*	1,550 *(25)*	25.3 *(0.4)*
Medicaid	1,519 *(26)*	21.1 *(0.4)*	671 *(16)*	39.0 *(0.9)*	1,390 *(25)*	22.7 *(0.4)*
Medicare	1,177 *(11)*	16.4 *(0.1)*	8 *(3)*	0.4 *(0.2)*	161 *(9)*	2.6 *(0.1)*
VA Care	193 *(9)*	2.7 *(0.1)*	3 *(1)*	0.2 *(0.1)*	103 *(7)*	1.7 *(0.1)*
Not covered at any time during the year	428 *(15)*	6.0 *(0.2)*	46 *(5)*	2.7 *(0.3)*	421 *(15)*	6.9 *(0.2)*

Note: Numbers in thousands; Figures cover civilian noninstitutionalized population in 2016; N/A indicates that data was not available; Z represents or rounds to zero; Margin of error appears in parenthesis and is calculated using replicate weights.
Source: U.S. Census Bureau, American Community Survey, Table HIC-4_ACS. Health Insurance Coverage Status and Type of Coverage by State—All People: 2008 to 2016, Table HIC-5_ACS. Health Insurance Coverage Status and Type of Coverage by State—Children Under 18: 2008 to 2016, Table HIC-6_ACS. Health Insurance Coverage Status and Type of Coverage by State—Persons Under 65: 2008 to 2016

Washington

805 Aetna Health of Washington

151 Farmington Avenue
Hartford, CT 06156
Toll-Free: 800-872-3862
Phone: 860-273-0123
www.aetna.com
Subsidiary of: Aetna Inc.
For Profit Organization: Yes

Healthplan and Services Defined
PLAN TYPE: PPO
Other Type: POS
Model Type: Network
Plan Specialty: Behavioral Health, EPO, Lab, PBM,
   Radiology
Benefits Offered: Chiropractic, Dental, Disease Management,
   Home Care, Long-Term Care, Physical Therapy, Podiatry,
   Prescription, Vision

Type of Coverage
Commercial, Student Health

Type of Payment Plans Offered
Capitated

Geographic Areas Served
Statewide

Publishes and Distributes Report Card: Yes

Accreditation Certification
AAAHC

Key Personnel
CEO . . . . Mark Bertolini

806 Amerigroup Washington

705 5th Avenue S
Suite 300
Seattle, WA 98104
Toll-Free: 800-600-4441
Phone: 206-695-7081
www.myamerigroup.com/wa
Subsidiary of: Anthem, Inc.
For Profit Organization: Yes

Healthplan and Services Defined
PLAN TYPE: Other
Model Type: Network
Plan Specialty: Disease Management, Managed health care
   for people in public programs.
Benefits Offered: Disease Management, Prescription

Type of Coverage
Medicaid

Geographic Areas Served
Statewide

Key Personnel
EVP/Pres., Gov. Business . . . . Peter D. Haytaian

807 Asuris Northwest Health

Toll-Free: 888-367-2109
asurisnwealth@gmail.com
www.asuris.com
Subsidiary of: Cambia Health Solutions
Non-Profit Organization: Yes
Year Founded: 1998
Total Enrollment: 71,000

Healthplan and Services Defined
PLAN TYPE: Multiple
Model Type: Network, TPA
Plan Specialty: ASO, Behavioral Health, Chiropractic,
   Disease Management, Lab, Vision, Radiology
Benefits Offered: Chiropractic, Dental, Disease Management,
   Home Care, Inpatient SNF, Physical Therapy, Podiatry,
   Prescription, Psychiatric, Vision, Wellness, AD&D, Life,
   LTD, STD

Type of Coverage
Individual, Medicare, Supplemental Medicare, Medicaid

Geographic Areas Served
Eastern Washington

Peer Review Type
Utilization Review: Yes
Second Surgical Opinion: Yes

Accreditation Certification
URAC
TJC Accreditation, Medicare Approved, State Licensure

Key Personnel
President . . . . Brady Cass

Average Claim Compensation
Physician's Fees Charged: 80%
Hospital's Fees Charged: 80%

808 Community Health Plan of Washington

1111 3rd Avenue
Suite 400
Seattle, WA 98101
Toll-Free: 800-440-1561
Phone: 206-652-7213
Fax: 206-521-8834
customercare@chpw.org
www.chpw.org
Non-Profit Organization: Yes
Year Founded: 1992
Number of Affiliated Hospitals: 100
Number of Primary Care Physicians: 2,500
Number of Referral/Specialty Physicians: 14,000
Total Enrollment: 300,000
State Enrollment: 300,000

Healthplan and Services Defined
PLAN TYPE: Multiple
Benefits Offered: Disease Management, Prescription,
   Wellness

Type of Coverage
Commercial, Individual, Medicare, Medicaid

Geographic Areas Served
38 counties in Washington State

Subscriber Information
Average Monthly Fee Per Subscriber
(Employee + Employer Contribution):
Employee Only (Self): Varies
Employee & 1 Family Member: Varies
Employee & 2 Family Members: Varies
Medicare: Varies
Average Annual Deductible Per Subscriber:
Employee Only (Self): Varies
Employee & 1 Family Member: Varies
Employee & 2 Family Members: Varies
Medicare: Varies
Average Subscriber Co-Payment:
Primary Care Physician: Varies
Non-Network Physician: Varies
Prescription Drugs: Varies
Hospital ER: Varies
Home Health Care: Varies
Home Health Care Max. Days/Visits Covered: Varies
Nursing Home: Varies
Nursing Home Max. Days/Visits Covered: Varies

Key Personnel
Chief Executive Officer. . . . . Leanne Berge
Administrative Officer . . . . Alan Lederman
Chief Financial Officer . . . . Stacy Kessel
Chief Operating Officer. . . . . Marilee McGuire
Media. . . . . Jackie Micucci
jackie.mcucci@chpw.org

Specialty Managed Care Partners
Express Scripts

---

809 Coventry Health Care of Washington
6720-B Rockledge Drive
Suite 700
Bethesda, MD 20817
Phone: 301-581-0600
www.coventryhealthcare.com
Subsidiary of: Aetna Inc.
For Profit Organization: Yes

Healthplan and Services Defined
PLAN TYPE: HMO/PPO
Model Type: Network
Plan Specialty: Behavioral Health, Dental, Worker's
Compensation
Benefits Offered: Behavioral Health, Dental, Prescription,
Wellness, Worker's Compensation

Type of Coverage
Commercial, Medicare, Medicaid

Geographic Areas Served
Statewide

Key Personnel
Chief Executive Officer. . . . . Mark T. Bertolini
President. . . . . Karen S. Lynch
Chief Financial Officer . . . . Shawn M. Guertin
Operations & Technology . . . . Meg McCarthy

Chief Medical Officer . . . . Harold L. Paz
General Counsel . . . . Thomas Sabatino Jr.
Government Services . . . . Fran S. Soistman

---

810 Delta Dental of Washington
P.O. Box 75688
Seattle, WA 98175
Toll-Free: 800-554-1907
www.deltadentalwa.com
Non-Profit Organization: Yes
Year Founded: 1954

Healthplan and Services Defined
PLAN TYPE: Dental
Other Type: Dental PPO
Model Type: Network
Plan Specialty: ASO, Dental
Benefits Offered: Dental

Type of Coverage
Commercial, Individual
Catastrophic Illness Benefit: None

Geographic Areas Served
Statewide

Key Personnel
President & CEO . . . . Jim Dwyer
COO & CFO . . . . Brad Berg
Human Resources . . . . Karen Aliabadi
VP, Underwriting. . . . . Eric Lo
Marketing & Sales Officer. . . . . Kristin Merlo
Prodiver Relations . . . . Cindy Snyder

---

811 First Choice Health
600 Univeristy Street
Suite 1400
Seattle, WA 98101-3129
Toll-Free: 800-467-5281
Fax: 206-667-8062
contact@fchn.com
www.fchn.com
Secondary Address: 120 W Cataldo Avenue, Suite 200,
Spokane, WA 99201, 509-227-5700
For Profit Organization: Yes
Year Founded: 1996
Number of Affiliated Hospitals: 94
Number of Primary Care Physicians: 980
Number of Referral/Specialty Physicians: 1,793

Healthplan and Services Defined
PLAN TYPE: PPO
Benefits Offered: Wellness

Type of Coverage
Commercial, Individual, Private & Public Plans, Geo-specifi

Geographic Areas Served
Washington, Oregon, Alaska, Idaho, Montana, Wyoming, and
select areas of North Dakota and South Dakota

Key Personnel
Chief Executive Officer . . . . Robert L. Hunter

812 Humana Health Insurance of Washington

1498 SE Tech Center Place
Suite 300
Vancouver, WA 98683
Toll-Free: 800-781-4203
Phone: 360-253-7523
Fax: 360-253-7524
www.humana.com
Subsidiary of: Humana
For Profit Organization: Yes

Healthplan and Services Defined
PLAN TYPE: HMO/PPO
Model Type: Network
Plan Specialty: Dental, Vision
Benefits Offered: Dental, Disease Management, Prescription,
  Vision, Wellness, Life, LTD, STD

Type of Coverage
Commercial, Medicare

Accreditation Certification
URAC, NCQA, CORE

Key Personnel
President & CEO. Bruce Broussard
Chief Medical Officer. . . . . Roy A. Beveridge
Chief Consumer Officer. . . . . Jody L. Bilney
Human Resources. . . . . Tim Huval
Chief Financial Officer . . . . Brian Kane
Chief Information Officer . . . . Brian LeClaire
General Counsel. . . . . Christopher M. Todoroff
Chief Accounting Officer . . . . Cynthia H. Zipperie

813 LifeWise

7001 220th Street SW
Building 1
Mountlake Terrace, WA 98043
Toll-Free: 800-592-6804
www.lifewisewa.com
Secondary Address: 3900 E Sprague Avenue, Spokane, WA
  99220
For Profit Organization: Yes
Year Founded: 1986
Number of Primary Care Physicians: 9,000
Total Enrollment: 1,900,000

Healthplan and Services Defined
PLAN TYPE: PPO
Benefits Offered: Acupuncture, Naturopathy

Geographic Areas Served
Washington and Alaska

Accreditation Certification
NCQA

Key Personnel
President & CEO . . . . Jim Havens

814 Molina Healthcare of Washington

21540 30th Drive SE
Suite 400
Bothell, WA 98021
Toll-Free: 800-869-7175
www.molinahealthcare.com
Mailing Address: P.O. Box 4004, Bothell, WA 98041-4004
Subsidiary of: Molina Healthcare, Inc.
For Profit Organization: Yes

Healthplan and Services Defined
PLAN TYPE: Medicare
Model Type: Network
Plan Specialty: Dental, PBM, Vision, Integrated
  Medicare/Medicaid (Duals)
Benefits Offered: Dental, Prescription, Vision, Wellness, Life

Type of Coverage
Individual, Medicare, Supplemental Medicare, Medicaid

Geographic Areas Served
Statewide

Key Personnel
Chief Executive Officer . . . . Joseph W. White
Chief Operating Officer . . . . Terry Bayer
General Counsel. . . . . Jeff D. Barlow
SVP, Relations/Marketing . . . . Juan Jos, Orellana
Chief Information Officer . . . . Rick Hopfer

815 Soundpath Health

33820 Weyerhaeuser Way S
Suite 200
Federal Way, WA 98001
Toll-Free: 866-789-7747
Fax: 844-612-4062
www.soundpathhealth.com
Mailing Address: P.O. Box 27510, Federal Way, WA 98093
Subsidiary of: Catholic Health Initiatives
Year Founded: 2007
Number of Affiliated Hospitals: 76
Total Enrollment: 17,000
State Enrollment: 17,000

Healthplan and Services Defined
PLAN TYPE: Medicare

Type of Coverage
Medicare

Accreditation Certification
TJC, URAC

816 United Concordia of Washington

2200 6th Ave
Seattle, WA 98121
Phone: 206-441-3853
www.unitedconcordia.com
For Profit Organization: Yes
Year Founded: 1971
Total Enrollment: 7,800,000

Healthplan and Services Defined
PLAN TYPE: Dental

Plan Specialty: Dental
Benefits Offered: Dental

Type of Coverage
Commercial, Individual, Military personnel & families

Geographic Areas Served
Nationwide

Accreditation Certification
URAC

Key Personnel
President & COO . . . . Timothy J. Constantine
Contact. . . . . Beth Rutherford
   717-260-7659
   beth.rutherford@ucci.com

817   UnitedHealthcare of Washington

1111 Third Avenue
Suite 1100
Seattle, WA 98101
Phone: 206-926-0251
www.uhc.com/contact-us/washington
Subsidiary of: UnitedHealth Group
For Profit Organization: Yes

Healthplan and Services Defined
PLAN TYPE: HMO/PPO
Model Type: Network
Plan Specialty: Behavioral Health, Dental, Disease
   Management, PBM, Vision
Benefits Offered: Behavioral Health, Dental, Disease
   Management, Long-Term Care, Prescription, Vision,
   Wellness, Life, LTD, STD

Type of Coverage
Individual, Medicare, Supplemental Medicare, Medicaid,
   Catastrophic, Family, Military, Veterans, Group,

Geographic Areas Served
Washington and Montana

Accreditation Certification
URAC

Key Personnel
Chief Executive Officer. . . . . David Wichmann
Chief Operating Officer . . . . Dan Schumacher
Chief Strategy Officer . . . . John Cosgriff
Communications Officer . . . . Kirsten Gorsuch
Chief Medical Officer. . . . . Sam Ho
Chief Legal Officer . . . . Thad Johnson
Chief Information Officer . . . . Phil McKoy
Chief Financial Officer. Jeff Putnam

Health Insurance Coverage Status and Type of Coverage by Age

Category	All Persons		Under 18 years		Under 65 years	
	Number	%	Number	%	Number	%
Total population	1,803	-	400	-	1,467	-
Covered by some type of health insurance	1,707 (6)	94.7 (0.3)	391 (3)	97.7 (0.5)	1,372 (6)	93.5 (0.4)
Covered by private health insurance	1,123 (16)	62.3 (0.9)	213 (8)	53.4 (1.9)	909 (15)	62.0 (1.0)
Employer-based	949 (15)	52.7 (0.8)	196 (7)	48.9 (1.8)	818 (14)	55.8 (0.9)
Direct purchase	197 (9)	10.9 (0.5)	19 (3)	4.7 (0.7)	102 (7)	6.9 (0.5)
TRICARE	41 (4)	2.3 (0.2)	6 (2)	1.4 (0.4)	23 (3)	1.6 (0.2)
Covered by public health insurance	872 (13)	48.4 (0.7)	200 (8)	50.0 (2.0)	543 (14)	37.0 (0.9)
Medicaid	520 (15)	28.8 (0.8)	198 (8)	49.6 (2.0)	479 (14)	32.6 (0.9)
Medicare	413 (6)	22.9 (0.3)	3 (1)	0.6 (0.3)	85 (5)	5.8 (0.4)
VA Care	66 (4)	3.6 (0.2)	Z (Z)	0.1 (0.1)	27 (3)	1.9 (0.2)
Not covered at any time during the year	96 (6)	5.3 (0.3)	9 (2)	2.3 (0.5)	95 (6)	6.5 (0.4)

Note: Numbers in thousands; Figures cover civilian noninstitutionalized population in 2016; N/A indicates that data was not available; Z represents or rounds to zero; Margin of error appears in parenthesis and is calculated using replicate weights.
Source: U.S. Census Bureau, American Community Survey, Table HIC-4_ACS. Health Insurance Coverage Status and Type of Coverage by State—All People: 2008 to 2016, Table HIC-5_ACS. Health Insurance Coverage Status and Type of Coverage by State—Children Under 18: 2008 to 2016, Table HIC-6_ACS. Health Insurance Coverage Status and Type of Coverage by State—Persons Under 65: 2008 to 2016

West Virginia

818   Aetna Better Health of West Virginia
500 Virginia Street East
Suite 400
Charleston, WV 25301
Toll-Free: 888-348-2922
abh-wv-memberservices@aetna.com
www.aetnabetterhealth.com/westvirginia
Mailing Address: P.O. Box 67450, Phoenix, AZ 85082-7450
For Profit Organization: Yes
Year Founded: 1995

Healthplan and Services Defined
PLAN TYPE: HMO/PPO
Benefits Offered: Behavioral Health, Disease Management,
Prescription, Vision, Wellness

Type of Coverage
Commercial, Medicare, Medicaid

Geographic Areas Served
Statewide

Peer Review Type
Case Management: Yes

Publishes and Distributes Report Card: Yes

Accreditation Certification
URAC

Key Personnel
Chief Executive Officer. . . . . Mark T. Bertolini
President. . . . . Karen S. Lynch
Chief Financial Officer . . . . Shawn M. Guertin
Chief Operating Officer . . . . Meg McCarthy
Chief Medical Officer . . . . Harold L. Paz
General Counsel . . . . Thomas Sabatino Jr.
Government Services . . . . Fran Soistman

819   Aetna Health of West Virginia
151 Farmington Avenue
Hartford, CT 06156
Toll-Free: 800-872-3862
Phone: 860-273-0123
www.aetna.com
Subsidiary of: Aetna Inc.
For Profit Organization: Yes

Healthplan and Services Defined
PLAN TYPE: PPO
Other Type: POS
Model Type: Network
Plan Specialty: Behavioral Health, EPO, Lab, PBM,
Radiology
Benefits Offered: Behavioral Health, Dental, Disease
Management, Long-Term Care, Physical Therapy,
Podiatry, Prescription, Psychiatric, Vision, Wellness, Life,
LTD, STD

Type of Coverage
Commercial, Student health

Geographic Areas Served
Statewide

Key Personnel
CEO. . . . . Mark Bertolini

820   CareSource West Virginia
230 N Main Street
Dayton, OH 45402
Phone: 937-224-3300
www.caresource.com
Non-Profit Organization: Yes
Total Enrollment: 1,000,000

Healthplan and Services Defined
PLAN TYPE: Medicare

Type of Coverage
Medicare, Medicaid

Geographic Areas Served
West Virginia counties: Barbour, Boone, Calhoun, Clay,
Doddridge, Fayette, Gilmer, Harrison, Jackson, Logan,
Marion, Monongalia, Pleasants, Preston, Raleigh, Ritchie,
Roane, Taylor, Tyler, Wetzel, Wirt and Wood

Key Personnel
President & CEO . . . . Pamela Morris
EVP, COO & CFO . . . . L. Tarlton Thomas III
EVP, General Counsel . . . . Mark Chilson
Administrative Officer . . . . Dan McCabe
Chief Information Officer . . . . Paul Stoddard
President, Ohio Market . . . . Steve Ringel

821   Delta Dental of West Virginia
One Delta Drive
Mechanicsburg, PA 17055-6999
Toll-Free: 800-932-0783
www.deltadentalins.com
Non-Profit Organization: Yes

Healthplan and Services Defined
PLAN TYPE: Dental
Other Type: Dental PPO
Plan Specialty: Dental
Benefits Offered: Dental

Type of Coverage
Commercial, Individual

Geographic Areas Served
Statewide

822   Highmark BCBS West Virginia
300 Wharton Circle
Suite 150
Triadelphia, WV 26059
Toll-Free: 800-876-7639
Phone: 412-544-0100
www.highmarkbcbswv.com
Subsidiary of: Highmark, Inc.
For Profit Organization: Yes
Year Founded: 1932

Number of Affiliated Hospitals: 65
Number of Primary Care Physicians: 1,400
Number of Referral/Specialty Physicians: 3,200
Total Enrollment: 5,300,000
State Enrollment: 500,000

Healthplan and Services Defined
PLAN TYPE: PPO
Model Type: Network, PPO, POS, TPA
Plan Specialty: ASO, Behavioral Health, Chiropractic, EPO, Lab, Radiology, UR, Case Management
Benefits Offered: Behavioral Health, Chiropractic, Home Care, Inpatient SNF, Long-Term Care, Physical Therapy, Podiatry, Prescription, Psychiatric, Transplant

Type of Coverage
Commercial, Individual, Supplemental Medicare

Type of Payment Plans Offered
POS, DFFS

Geographic Areas Served
West Virginia and Washington County, Ohio

Network Qualifications
Pre-Admission Certification: Yes

Peer Review Type
Utilization Review: Yes
Second Surgical Opinion: Yes
Case Management: Yes

Publishes and Distributes Report Card: No

Accreditation Certification
URAC

Key Personnel
President . . . . Deborah L. Rice-Johnson
Chief Medical Officer . . . . Charles Deshazer
Chief Executive Officer . . . . David L. Holmberg

Specialty Managed Care Partners
WV University, Charleston Area Medical Center (CAMC)
Enters into Contracts with Regional Business Coalitions: No

---

823   Humana Health Insurance of West Virginia

4202A MacCorkle Avenue
SE Charleston, WV 25304
Toll-Free: 800-951-0130
Phone: 304-925-0972
Fax: 304-925-0976
www.humana.com
Subsidiary of: Humana
For Profit Organization: Yes

Healthplan and Services Defined
PLAN TYPE: HMO/PPO
Model Type: Network
Plan Specialty: Dental, Vision
Benefits Offered: Dental, Vision, Life, LTD, STD

Type of Coverage
Commercial

Accreditation Certification
URAC, NCQA

Key Personnel
President/CEO . . . . Bruce D. Broussard
Chief Medical Officer . . . . Roy A. Beveridge
Chief Consumer Officer . . . . Jody L. Bilney
Human Resources . . . . Tim Huval
Chief Financial Officer . . . . Brian Kane
Chief Information Officer . . . . Brian LeClaire
General Counsel . . . . Christopher M. Todoroff
Accounting Officer . . . . Cynthia H. Zipperie

---

824   Molina Medicaid Solutions

1600 Pennsylvania Avenue
Charleston, WV 25302
Phone: 304-348-3200
molinahealthcare.com
Subsidiary of: Molina Healthcare, Inc.
For Profit Organization: Yes
Year Founded: 1980

Healthplan and Services Defined
PLAN TYPE: Medicare
Plan Specialty: Dental, PBM, Vision, Intergrated Medicaid/Medicare (Duals)
Benefits Offered: Dental, Prescription, Vision, Wellness, Life

Geographic Areas Served
Statewide

Key Personnel
Chief Executive Officer . . . . Joseph W. White
Chief Operating Officer . . . . Terry Bayer
SVP, General Counsel . . . . Jeff D. Barlow
SVP, Marketing . . . . Juan Jos, Orellana

---

825   Mountain Health Trust/Physician Assured Access System

231 Capitol Street
Suite 310
Charleston, WV 25301
Toll-Free: 800-449-8466
Fax: 304-345-1581
www.mountainhealthtrust.com
Year Founded: 1996

Healthplan and Services Defined
PLAN TYPE: HMO
Benefits Offered: Dental, Disease Management, Home Care, Inpatient SNF, Prescription, Vision, Wellness, Hearing; Durable Medical Equipment; Midwife Services

Type of Coverage
Medicaid

Geographic Areas Served
Statewide

---

826   UniCare West Virginia

200 Association Drive
Suite 200
Charleston, WV 25311
Toll-Free: 888-611-9958
www.unicare.com

Subsidiary of: Anthem, Inc.
For Profit Organization: Yes
Year Founded: 1985
Number of Affiliated Hospitals: 102
Number of Primary Care Physicians: 3,500
Number of Referral/Specialty Physicians: 8,000
Total Enrollment: 80,000

Healthplan and Services Defined
  PLAN TYPE: Multiple
  Model Type: Network
  Plan Specialty: Dental, Vision
  Benefits Offered: Chiropractic, Dental, Physical Therapy,
    Prescription, Vision, Life

Type of Coverage
  Medicare, Supplemental Medicare, Medicaid

Geographic Areas Served
  Statewide

Subscriber Information
  Average Monthly Fee Per Subscriber
    (Employee + Employer Contribution):
      Employee Only (Self): Varies
      Employee & 1 Family Member: Varies
      Employee & 2 Family Members: Varies
      Medicare: Varies
  Average Annual Deductible Per Subscriber:
      Employee Only (Self): Varies
      Employee & 1 Family Member: Varies
      Employee & 2 Family Members: Varies
      Medicare: Varies
  Average Subscriber Co-Payment:
      Primary Care Physician: Varies
      Non-Network Physician: Varies
      Prescription Drugs: Varies
      Hospital ER: Varies
      Home Health Care: Varies
      Home Health Care Max. Days/Visits Covered: Varies
      Nursing Home: Varies
      Nursing Home Max. Days/Visits Covered: Varies

Network Qualifications
  Pre-Admission Certification: Yes

Peer Review Type
  Utilization Review: Yes
  Second Surgical Opinion: Yes
  Case Management: Yes

Publishes and Distributes Report Card: No

Accreditation Certification
  URAC
  TJC Accreditation, Medicare Approved, Utilization Review,
    Pre-Admission Certification, State Licensure, Quality
    Assurance Program

---

827 UnitedHealthcare of West Virginia
9020 Stony Point Parkway
Suite 400
Richmond, VA 23235
Toll-Free: 877-842-3210
www.uhc.com/contact-us/west-virginia

Subsidiary of: UnitedHealth Group
Year Founded: 1977

Healthplan and Services Defined
  PLAN TYPE: HMO/PPO
  Model Type: Network
  Plan Specialty: Behavioral Health, Dental, Disease
    Management, Lab, PBM, Vision, Radiology
  Benefits Offered: Behavioral Health, Chiropractic, Dental,
    Disease Management, Long-Term Care, Physical Therapy,
    Prescription, Vision, Wellness, AD&D, Life, LTD, STD

Type of Coverage
  Commercial, Individual, Indemnity, Medicare, Supplemental
    Medicare, Medicaid, Catastrophic, Family, Military,
    Veterans, Group,

Geographic Areas Served
  Statewide. West Virginia is covered by the Virginia branch

Network Qualifications
  Pre-Admission Certification: Yes

Peer Review Type
  Utilization Review: Yes
  Second Surgical Opinion: Yes
  Case Management: Yes

Publishes and Distributes Report Card: Yes

Accreditation Certification
  TJC, NCQA

Key Personnel
  Chief Executive Officer . . . . David Wichmann
  Chief Operating Officer . . . . Dan Schumacher
  Chief Strategy Officer . . . . John Cosgriff
  Communications Officer . . . . Kirsten Gorsuch
  Chief Medical Officer. . . . . Sam Ho
  Chief Legal Officer . . . . Thad Johnson
  Chief Information Officer . . . . Phil McKoy
  Chief Financial Officer. . . . . Jeff Putnam

Specialty Managed Care Partners
  Enters into Contracts with Regional Business Coalitions: Yes

Health Insurance Coverage Status and Type of Coverage by Age

Category	All Persons		Under 18 years		Under 65 years	
	Number	%	Number	%	Number	%
Total population	5,707	-	1,365	-	4,806	-
Covered by some type of health insurance	5,406 *(10)*	94.7 *(0.2)*	1,315 *(6)*	96.3 *(0.3)*	4,508 *(11)*	93.8 *(0.2)*
Covered by private health insurance	4,294 *(20)*	75.2 *(0.4)*	943 *(11)*	69.1 *(0.8)*	3,708 *(20)*	77.1 *(0.4)*
Employer-based	3,521 *(22)*	61.7 *(0.4)*	867 *(12)*	63.5 *(0.9)*	3,276 *(22)*	68.2 *(0.5)*
Direct purchase	867 *(15)*	15.2 *(0.3)*	77 *(5)*	5.7 *(0.4)*	481 *(13)*	10.0 *(0.3)*
TRICARE	88 *(5)*	1.5 *(0.1)*	17 *(3)*	1.3 *(0.2)*	54 *(5)*	1.1 *(0.1)*
Covered by public health insurance	1,883 *(19)*	33.0 *(0.3)*	448 *(12)*	32.8 *(0.9)*	1,003 *(19)*	20.9 *(0.4)*
Medicaid	1,014 *(20)*	17.8 *(0.3)*	444 *(12)*	32.6 *(0.9)*	901 *(19)*	18.8 *(0.4)*
Medicare	1,013 *(6)*	17.8 *(0.1)*	6 *(1)*	0.4 *(0.1)*	133 *(6)*	2.8 *(0.1)*
VA Care	138 *(4)*	2.4 *(0.1)*	3 *(1)*	0.2 *(0.1)*	55 *(3)*	1.2 *(0.1)*
Not covered at any time during the year	300 *(10)*	5.3 *(0.2)*	50 *(4)*	3.7 *(0.3)*	298 *(10)*	6.2 *(0.2)*

Note: Numbers in thousands; Figures cover civilian noninstitutionalized population in 2016; N/A indicates that data was not available; Z represents or rounds to zero; Margin of error appears in parenthesis and is calculated using replicate weights.
Source: U.S. Census Bureau, American Community Survey, Table HIC-4_ACS. Health Insurance Coverage Status and Type of Coverage by State—All People: 2008 to 2016, Table HIC-5_ACS. Health Insurance Coverage Status and Type of Coverage by State—Children Under 18: 2008 to 2016, Table HIC-6_ACS. Health Insurance Coverage Status and Type of Coverage by State—Persons Under 65: 2008 to 2016

Wisconsin

828 Aetna Health of Wisconsin

151 Farmington Avenue
Hartford, CT 06156
Toll-Free: 800-872-3862
Phone: 860-273-0123
www.aetna.com
Subsidiary of: Aetna Inc.
For Profit Organization: Yes

Healthplan and Services Defined
  PLAN TYPE: PPO
  Other Type: POS
  Plan Specialty: Behavioral Health, EPO, Lab, PBM,
    Radiology
  Benefits Offered: Behavioral Health, Dental, Disease
    Management, Long-Term Care, Physical Therapy,
    Podiatry, Prescription, Psychiatric, Wellness, Life, LTD,
    STD

Type of Coverage
  Commercial, Student health

Type of Payment Plans Offered
  POS, FFS

Geographic Areas Served
  Statewide

Key Personnel
  CEO . . . . Mark Bertolini

829 American Family Insurance

6000 Madison Parkway
Madison, WI 53783
Toll-Free: 800-692-6326
www.amfam.com

Healthplan and Services Defined
  PLAN TYPE: Multiple
  Benefits Offered: Life

Type of Coverage
  Commercial, Individual, Supplemental Medicare, Short-term

Geographic Areas Served
  Arizona, Colorado, Georgia, Idaho, Illinois, Indiana, Iowa,
  Kansas, Minnesota, Missouri, Nebraska, Nevada, North
  Dakota, Ohio, Oregon, South Dakota, Utah, Washington,
  Wisconsin

Key Personnel
  Chairman, President & CEO . . . . Jack Salzwedel

830 Anthem Blue Cross & Blue Shield of Wisconsin

6775 W Washington Street
Milwaukee, WI 53214
Phone: 414-459-5057
www.anthem.com
Subsidiary of: Anthem, Inc.
For Profit Organization: Yes

Healthplan and Services Defined
  PLAN TYPE: HMO/PPO
  Model Type: Network
  Plan Specialty: ASO, Behavioral Health, Chiropractic, Dental,
    Disease Management, Lab, PBM, Vision, Radiology,
    Worker's Compensation, UR
  Benefits Offered: Behavioral Health, Chiropractic, Dental,
    Disease Management, Home Care, Inpatient SNF, Physical
    Therapy, Podiatry, Prescription, Psychiatric, Transplant,
    Vision, Wellness, Worker's Compensation, Life

Type of Coverage
  Commercial, Individual, Medicare, Supplemental Medicare,
  Medicaid, Catastrophic

Geographic Areas Served
  Statewide

Accreditation Certification
  URAC, NCQA

Key Personnel
  President & CEO . . . . Scott P. Serota
  Chief Financial Officer . . . . Robert Kolodgy
  Human Resources . . . . Maureen A. Cahill
  Chief Medical Officer. . . . . Trent Haywood
  General Counsel. . . . . Scott Nehs

831 Ascension At Home

Affinity Home Care Plus
2074 American Drive, Suite A
Neenah, WI 54956
Phone: 920-735-8100
Fax: 920-735-8101
ascensionathome.com
Subsidiary of: Ascension
Non-Profit Organization: Yes

Healthplan and Services Defined
  PLAN TYPE: Other
  Plan Specialty: Disease Management
  Benefits Offered: Dental, Disease Management, Home Care,
    Wellness, Ambulance & Transportation; Nursing Service;
    Short-and-long-term care management planning; Hospice

Geographic Areas Served
  Texas, Alabama, Indiana, Kansas, Michigan, Mississippi,
  Oklahoma, wisconsin

Key Personnel
  President. . . . . Kirk Allen
  Dir., Home Health Service . . . . Darcy Burthay

832 Assurant Employee Benefits Wisconsin

125 N Executive Drive
Brookfield, WI 53005
Phone: 262-798-0280
www.assurantemployeebenefits.com
Subsidiary of: Sun Life Financial, US
For Profit Organization: Yes

Healthplan and Services Defined
  PLAN TYPE: Multiple
  Plan Specialty: Dental, Vision

Benefits Offered: Dental, Disease Management, Vision, Wellness, AD&D, Life, LTD, STD

Type of Coverage
Commercial, Individual

Geographic Areas Served
Statewide

Subscriber Information
Average Monthly Fee Per Subscriber
(Employee + Employer Contribution):
Employee Only (Self): Varies by plan

Accreditation Certification
URAC, NCQA

Key Personnel
President . . . . Dan Fishbein
Senior Vice President . . . . Kevin Krzeminski
Human Resources . . . . Kathy deCastro
Marketing . . . . Ed Milano
Chairman . . . . William Anderson

---

833 Care Plus Dental Plans

1135 S Cesar Chavez Drive
Milwaukee, WI 53204
Toll-Free: 800-318-7007
www.careplusdentalplans.com
Subsidiary of: Dental Associates Ltd
Non-Profit Organization: Yes
Year Founded: 1983
Physician Owned Organization: Yes
Total Enrollment: 200,000

Healthplan and Services Defined
PLAN TYPE: Dental
Model Type: Staff
Plan Specialty: Dental
Benefits Offered: Dental, Prescription

Type of Coverage
Commercial, Individual

Type of Payment Plans Offered
Capitated

Geographic Areas Served
Appleton, Fond Du Lac, Green Bay, Greenville, Kenosha, Milwaukee & Waukesha

Peer Review Type
Utilization Review: Yes

Accreditation Certification
AAAHC

Key Personnel
Vice President . . . . Kati Gruneberg
Sales Manager . . . . James Schmitz
Senior Client Service Mgn . . . . Brenda Boyd

---

834 ChiroCare of Wisconsin

250 Bishops Way
Suite 101
Brookfield, WI 53005
Toll-Free: 800-397-1541
Phone: 414-476-4733
www.chirocare.com
Subsidiary of: Fulcrum Health, Inc.
Non-Profit Organization: Yes
Year Founded: 1986
Total Enrollment: 150,000

Healthplan and Services Defined
PLAN TYPE: PPO
Model Type: IPA, Network
Plan Specialty: Chiropractic, Complimentary Medicine Networks
Benefits Offered: Chiropractic

Type of Coverage
Commercial, Indemnity, Medicare, Supplemental Medicare, Medicaid

Type of Payment Plans Offered
POS, DFFS, Capitated, FFS, Combination FFS & DFFS

Geographic Areas Served
Statewide

Network Qualifications
Pre-Admission Certification: Yes

Peer Review Type
Utilization Review: Yes
Second Surgical Opinion: Yes
Case Management: Yes

Accreditation Certification
URAC, NCQA
Quality Assurance Program

Key Personnel
CEO . . . . Patricia Dennis

---

835 Coventry Health Care of Wisconsin

1238 Market Place
Waukesha, WI 53189
Phone: 262-650-9221
www.coventryhealthcare.com
Subsidiary of: Aetna Inc.
For Profit Organization: Yes

Healthplan and Services Defined
PLAN TYPE: HMO/PPO
Model Type: Network
Plan Specialty: Behavioral Health, Dental, Worker's Compensation
Benefits Offered: Behavioral Health, Dental, Prescription, Wellness, Worker's Compensation

Type of Coverage
Commercial, Medicare, Medicaid

Geographic Areas Served
Statewide

Key Personnel

Chief Executive Officer . . . . Mark T. Bertolini

President . . . . Karen S. Lynch

Chief Financial Officer . . . . Shawn M. Guertin

Operations & Technology . . . . Meg McCarthy

Chief Medical Officer . . . . Harold L. Paz

General Counsel . . . . Thomas Sabatino Jr.

Government Services . . . . Fran S. Soistman

836 Dean Health Plan

1277 Deming Way

Madison, WI 53717

Toll-Free: 800-279-1301

Phone: 608-827-4420

Fax: 608-827-4212

www.deancare.com

For Profit Organization: Yes

Year Founded: 1983

Physician Owned Organization: Yes

Federally Qualified: Yes

Number of Affiliated Hospitals: 26

Number of Primary Care Physicians: 1,500

Total Enrollment: 247,881

Healthplan and Services Defined

PLAN TYPE: Multiple

Model Type: Network

Benefits Offered: Behavioral Health, Chiropractic, Dental, Disease Management, Home Care, Inpatient SNF, Physical Therapy, Podiatry, Prescription, Psychiatric, Transplant, Vision, Wellness

Offers Demand Management Patient Information Service: Yes

DMPI Services Offered: On Call Nurse Line

Type of Coverage

Commercial, Individual, Indemnity, Medicare, Supplemental Medicare, Medicaid

Type of Payment Plans Offered

Capitated

Geographic Areas Served

20 counties in Southern Wisconsin

Subscriber Information

Average Monthly Fee Per Subscriber

(Employee + Employer Contribution):

Employee Only (Self): Varies

Employee & 1 Family Member: Varies

Employee & 2 Family Members: Varies

Medicare: Varies

Average Annual Deductible Per Subscriber:

Employee Only (Self): Varies

Employee & 1 Family Member: Varies

Employee & 2 Family Members: Varies

Medicare: Varies

Average Subscriber Co-Payment:

Primary Care Physician: Varies

Non-Network Physician: Varies

Prescription Drugs: Varies

Hospital ER: Varies

Home Health Care: Varies

Home Health Care Max. Days/Visits Covered: Varies

Nursing Home: Varies

Nursing Home Max. Days/Visits Covered: Varies

Network Qualifications

Pre-Admission Certification: Yes

Peer Review Type

Utilization Review: Yes

Publishes and Distributes Report Card: Yes

Accreditation Certification

NCQA

Key Personnel

President & CEO . . . . Frank L. Lucia

Executive Director . . . . David Docherty

Director of Compliance . . . . Stephanie Cook

VP of Operations . . . . Marcus Julian

Chief Medical Offier . . . . Ron Parton

Chief Financial Officer . . . . Randy Ruplinger

Specialty Managed Care Partners

Enters into Contracts with Regional Business Coalitions: No

Employer References

State of Wisconsin Employees

837 Delta Dental of Wisconsin

P.O. Box 828

Stevens Point, WI 54481-0828

Toll-Free: 800-236-3712

www.deltadentalwi.com

Non-Profit Organization: Yes

Year Founded: 1962

Healthplan and Services Defined

PLAN TYPE: Dental

Other Type: Dental PPO

Model Type: Network

Plan Specialty: Dental, Vision

Benefits Offered: Dental, Vision

Type of Coverage

Commercial, Individual

Type of Payment Plans Offered

POS, FFS

Geographic Areas Served

Statewide

Peer Review Type

Case Management: Yes

Publishes and Distributes Report Card: No

Accreditation Certification

TJC

Key Personnel

President & CEO . . . . Dennis Peterson

Specialty Managed Care Partners

Enters into Contracts with Regional Business Coalitions: No

838 Dental Protection Plan

7130 W Greenfield Avenue
West Allis, WI 53214-4708
Phone: 414-259-9522
www.bayviewdentalcare.com
Subsidiary of: Bayview Dental Care
Year Founded: 1987

Healthplan and Services Defined
  PLAN TYPE: Dental
  Other Type: Dental HMO
  Plan Specialty: Dental
  Benefits Offered: Dental

Geographic Areas Served
  Nationwide

Subscriber Information
  Average Monthly Fee Per Subscriber
    (Employee + Employer Contribution):
    Employee Only (Self): $35/year

Peer Review Type
  Case Management: Yes

Publishes and Distributes Report Card: Yes

839 Group Health Cooperative of Eau Claire

2503 N Hillcrest Parkway
Altoona, WI 54702
Toll-Free: 888-203-7770
Phone: 715-552-4300
Fax: 715-836-7683
www.group-health.com
Non-Profit Organization: Yes
Year Founded: 1976
Number of Primary Care Physicians: 7,700
Total Enrollment: 75,000

Healthplan and Services Defined
  PLAN TYPE: HMO
  Model Type: Network
  Benefits Offered: Dental, Disease Management, Prescription,
    Wellness, Comprehensive Health
  Offers Demand Management Patient Information Service:
    Yes
  DMPI Services Offered: FirstCare Nurseline

Type of Coverage
  Commercial, Medicaid, SSI
  Catastrophic Illness Benefit: Varies per case

Geographic Areas Served
  Barron, Buffalo, Chippewa, Clark, Dunn, Eau Claire,
  Jackson, Pepin, Rusk, Sawyer, Taylor, Trempealeau,
  Washburn, Ashland, Bayfield, Douglas, Burnett, Polk, St.
  Croix, Pierce, LaCrosse, Monroe, Juneau, Veronn, Crawford,
  Richland, Sauk, Columbia, Grant, Iowa, Lafayette, Green
  counties

Peer Review Type
  Utilization Review: Yes
  Second Surgical Opinion: Yes
  Case Management: Yes

Publishes and Distributes Report Card: Yes

Accreditation Certification
  AAAHC
  TJC Accreditation, Medicare Approved, Utilization Review,
    State Licensure, Quality Assurance Program

Key Personnel
  General Manager & CEO . . . . Peter Farrow
  Chief Medical Officer . . . . Michele Bauer, MD
  Chief Operating Officer . . . . Darin McFadden
  Chief Financial Officer . . . . Bob Tanner

Specialty Managed Care Partners
  CMS, OMNE
  Enters into Contracts with Regional Business Coalitions: Yes

840 Group Health Cooperative of South Central Wisconsin

1265 John Q Hammons Drive
Madison, WI 53717-1962
Toll-Free: 800-605-4327
Phone: 608-828-4853
member_services@ghcscw.com
www.ghcscw.com
Non-Profit Organization: Yes
Year Founded: 1976
Owned by an Integrated Delivery Network (IDN): Yes
Federally Qualified: Yes
Total Enrollment: 80,000

Healthplan and Services Defined
  PLAN TYPE: HMO
  Model Type: Staff
  Plan Specialty: Dental, Lab, Vision, Radiology
  Benefits Offered: Chiropractic, Disease Management,
    Physical Therapy, Prescription, Vision, Wellness,
    Acupuncture
  Offers Demand Management Patient Information Service: Yes

Type of Coverage
  Commercial, Medicare, Medicaid

Type of Payment Plans Offered
  DFFS, Capitated

Geographic Areas Served
  Dane County

Publishes and Distributes Report Card: Yes

Accreditation Certification
  AAAHC, NCQA
  Medicare Approved, Utilization Review, Pre-Admission
    Certification, State Licensure, Quality Assurance Program

Key Personnel
  President . . . . Ann Hoyt

Specialty Managed Care Partners
  UW Hospitals
  Enters into Contracts with Regional Business Coalitions: Yes

841   Gundersen Lutheran Health Plan

3190 Gundersen Drive
Onalaska, WI 54650
Toll-Free: 800-897-1923
Phone: 608-881-8271
Fax: 608-775-8091
customerservice@quartzbenefits.com
www.gundersenhealthplan.org
Secondary Address: Mail: 1836 South Avenue, NCA2-01,
   LaCrosse, WI 54601
Subsidiary of: Quartz Health Solutions, Inc
Non-Profit Organization: Yes
Year Founded: 1995
Physician Owned Organization: Yes
Federally Qualified: Yes
Number of Affiliated Hospitals: 14
Number of Primary Care Physicians: 850
Number of Referral/Specialty Physicians: 200
Total Enrollment: 90,000
State Enrollment: 90,000

Healthplan and Services Defined
   PLAN TYPE: HMO
   Other Type: POS
   Model Type: Network
   Plan Specialty: ASO, Behavioral Health, Chiropractic,
      Disease Management, Lab, PBM, Radiology, UR
   Benefits Offered: Behavioral Health, Chiropractic, Disease
      Management, Home Care, Inpatient SNF, Physical
      Therapy, Podiatry, Prescription, Psychiatric, Transplant,
      Vision, Wellness, AD&D
   Offers Demand Management Patient Information Service:
      Yes
   DMPI Services Offered: Nurse Advisor Line

Type of Coverage
   Commercial, Individual, Medicare

Geographic Areas Served
   Western Wisconsin

Subscriber Information
   Average Monthly Fee Per Subscriber
      (Employee + Employer Contribution):
         Employee Only (Self): Varies
   Average Annual Deductible Per Subscriber:
      Employee & 2 Family Members: Varies

Accreditation Certification
   TJC, URAC, NCQA
   Pre-Admission Certification

842   Health Tradition

1808 East Main Street
Onalaska, WI 54650
Toll-Free: 888-459-3020
Phone: 608-781-9692
www.healthtradition.com
For Profit Organization: Yes
Year Founded: 1986
Number of Affiliated Hospitals: 17
Number of Primary Care Physicians: 800

Number of Referral/Specialty Physicians: 100
Total Enrollment: 34,000
State Enrollment: 40,000

Healthplan and Services Defined
   PLAN TYPE: HMO
   Model Type: Group
   Benefits Offered: Disease Management, Prescription,
      Wellness
   Offers Demand Management Patient Information Service: Yes
   DMPI Services Offered: 24 hour nurse line

Type of Coverage
   Medicare, Medicaid
   Catastrophic Illness Benefit: Maximum $2M

Type of Payment Plans Offered
   POS, Combination FFS & DFFS

Geographic Areas Served
   Iowa: Allamakee; Minnesota: Houston; Buffalo, Crawford,
   Fillmore, Jackson, La Crosse, Monroe, Trempealeau, Vernon,
   Winneshiek, Winona counties

Subscriber Information
   Average Monthly Fee Per Subscriber
      (Employee + Employer Contribution):
         Employee Only (Self): Varies by plan
   Average Annual Deductible Per Subscriber:
      Employee Only (Self): $50.00
      Employee & 1 Family Member: $100.00
      Employee & 2 Family Members: $150.00
   Average Subscriber Co-Payment:
      Primary Care Physician: $0
      Prescription Drugs: $11.00
      Hospital ER: $25.00-50.00
      Home Health Care: $0
      Home Health Care Max. Days/Visits Covered: 345 days
      Nursing Home: $0
      Nursing Home Max. Days/Visits Covered: 60 days

Network Qualifications
   Pre-Admission Certification: Yes

Peer Review Type
   Utilization Review: Yes
   Second Surgical Opinion: Yes
   Case Management: Yes

Publishes and Distributes Report Card: No

Accreditation Certification
   TJC Accreditation, Medicare Approved, Utilization Review,
      Pre-Admission Certification, State Licensure, Quality
      Assurance Program

Key Personnel
   Director/Sales & Market . . . . Michael Eckstein

Average Claim Compensation
   Physician's Fees Charged: 85%
   Hospital's Fees Charged: 85%

Specialty Managed Care Partners
   Franciscon Scam Health Care
   Enters into Contracts with Regional Business Coalitions: No

843   Humana Health Insurance of Wisconsin

N19W24133 Riverwood Drive
Suite 110
Waukesha, WI 53188
Toll-Free: 800-289-0260
Phone: 262-408-4300
Fax: 920-632-9508
www.humana.com
For Profit Organization: Yes
Year Founded: 1985
Physician Owned Organization: Yes

Healthplan and Services Defined
  PLAN TYPE: HMO/PPO
  Model Type: IPA, Network
  Plan Specialty: UR
  Benefits Offered: Behavioral Health, Chiropractic, Dental,
    Disease Management, Home Care, Inpatient SNF, Physical
    Therapy, Podiatry, Prescription, Psychiatric, Transplant,
    Vision, Wellness, Worker's Compensation, AD&D, Life,
    LTD
  Offers Demand Management Patient Information Service:
    Yes

Type of Coverage
  Commercial, Individual

Type of Payment Plans Offered
  POS, DFFS, Capitated, FFS, Combination FFS & DFFS

Geographic Areas Served
  Dodge, Jefferson, Kenosha, Milwaukee, Ozaukee, Racine,
  Sheboygan, Walworth, Washington, Fond du Luc, Green,
  Montowoe, Rock & Waukesha counties

Peer Review Type
  Utilization Review: Yes
  Second Surgical Opinion: Yes
  Case Management: Yes

Accreditation Certification
  AAAHC, URAC, NCQA, CORE

Key Personnel
  President & CEO . . . . Bruce D. Broussard
  Chief Medical Officer . . . . Roy A. Beverridge
  Chief Consumer Officer. . . . . Jody L. Bilney
  SVP, Human Resources . . . . Tim Huval
  Chief Financial Officer . . . . Brian Kane
  Chief Information Officer . . . . Brian LeClaire
  SVP, General Counsel . . . . Christopher M. Todoroff

Specialty Managed Care Partners
  Aurora Behavioral, Chirotech, Accordant, Health Service

844   Managed Health Services

10700 W Research Drive
Wauwatosa, WI 53226
Toll-Free: 888-713-6180
www.mhswi.com
For Profit Organization: Yes
Year Founded: 1984
Number of Affiliated Hospitals: 57
Number of Primary Care Physicians: 5,500

Number of Referral/Specialty Physicians: 1,255
Total Enrollment: 130,000
State Enrollment: 164,700

Healthplan and Services Defined
  PLAN TYPE: HMO
  Model Type: IPA, Network
  Benefits Offered: Disease Management, Prescription,
    Wellness
  Offers Demand Management Patient Information Service: Yes

Type of Coverage
  Medicare, Medicaid
  Catastrophic Illness Benefit: Varies per case

Type of Payment Plans Offered
  POS, FFS

Geographic Areas Served
  22 counties in Wisconsin, Northern Indiana, and Illinois,
  Racine, Kenosha; Indiana: Indianapolis; Illinois: Chicago

Subscriber Information
  Average Monthly Fee Per Subscriber
    (Employee + Employer Contribution):
      Employee Only (Self): Varies
      Employee & 1 Family Member: Varies
      Employee & 2 Family Members: Varies
      Medicare: Varies
  Average Annual Deductible Per Subscriber:
      Employee Only (Self): Varies
      Employee & 1 Family Member: Varies
      Employee & 2 Family Members: Varies
      Medicare: Varies
  Average Subscriber Co-Payment:
      Primary Care Physician: $10.00/15.00
      Non-Network Physician: 100%
      Prescription Drugs: $5.00/10.00
      Hospital ER: $25.00
      Home Health Care: $0

Network Qualifications
  Pre-Admission Certification: Yes

Peer Review Type
  Utilization Review: Yes

Publishes and Distributes Report Card: Yes

Accreditation Certification
  NCQA
  TJC Accreditation, Medicare Approved, Utilization Review,
    Pre-Admission Certification, State Licensure, Quality
    Assurance Program

Key Personnel
  Chairman . . . . John Finerty, Jr.
  President & CEO . . . . Sherry Husa
  Executive Director. . . . . Tony Perez

Specialty Managed Care Partners
  Enters into Contracts with Regional Business Coalitions: Yes

845 MercyHealth System

1000 Mineral Point Avenue
Janesville, WI 53547
Toll-Free: 888-396-3729
Phone: 815-971-5000
mercyhealthsystem.org
Non-Profit Organization: Yes
Year Founded: 1889
Number of Affiliated Hospitals: 5
Number of Primary Care Physicians: 650

Healthplan and Services Defined
PLAN TYPE: HMO
Benefits Offered: Disease Management, Orthopedic surgery; neurosurgery; cancer care; plastic/reconstructive sergery; trauma centers

Geographic Areas Served
Southern Wisconsin and Northern Illinois counties

Key Personnel
President & CEO . . . . Javon R. Bea

846 Molina Healthcare of Wisconsin

11200 W Parkland Avenue
Milwaukee, WI 53224
Toll-Free: 888-999-2404
www.molinahealthcare.com
Subsidiary of: Molina Healthcare, Inc.
For Profit Organization: Yes

Healthplan and Services Defined
PLAN TYPE: Medicare
Model Type: Network
Plan Specialty: Dental, PBM, Vision, Integrated Medicare/Medicaid (Duals)
Benefits Offered: Dental, Prescription, Vision, Wellness, Life

Type of Coverage
Individual, Medicare, Supplemental Medicare, Medicaid

Geographic Areas Served
Statewide

Key Personnel
Chief Executive Officer . . . . Joseph W. White
Chief Operating Officer . . . . Terry Bayer
General Counsel. . . . . Jeff D. Barlow
SVP, Relations/Marketing . . . . Juan Jos, Orellana
Chief Information Officer . . . . Rick Hopfer

847 Network Health Plan of Wisconsin

1570 Midway Place
Menasha, WI 54952
Toll-Free: 800-826-0940
Phone: 920-720-1300
www.networkhealth.com
Subsidiary of: Affinity Health System
For Profit Organization: Yes
Year Founded: 1982
Total Enrollment: 118,000
State Enrollment: 67,812

Healthplan and Services Defined
PLAN TYPE: HMO
Model Type: Group, Network
Plan Specialty: Behavioral Health, Chiropractic, Disease Management, Lab
Benefits Offered: Chiropractic, Disease Management, Prescription, Wellness, Maternity care

Type of Coverage
Commercial, Medicare, Medicaid

Type of Payment Plans Offered
POS, Combination FFS & DFFS

Geographic Areas Served
Brown, Calumet, Dodge, Door, Fond du Lac, Green Lake, Kewaunee, Manitowoc, Marquette, Outagamie, Portage, Shawano, Sheboygan, Waupaca, Waushara, Winnebago counties

Subscriber Information
Average Monthly Fee Per Subscriber
(Employee + Employer Contribution):
Employee Only (Self): Varies
Employee & 1 Family Member: Varies
Employee & 2 Family Members: Varies
Medicare: Varies
Average Annual Deductible Per Subscriber:
Employee Only (Self): Varies
Employee & 1 Family Member: Varies
Employee & 2 Family Members: Varies
Medicare: Varies
Average Subscriber Co-Payment:
Primary Care Physician: $10.00
Prescription Drugs: $5.00-7.00
Home Health Care: $0

Network Qualifications
Pre-Admission Certification: Yes

Peer Review Type
Utilization Review: Yes
Second Surgical Opinion: No
Case Management: Yes

Publishes and Distributes Report Card: Yes

Accreditation Certification
NCQA
TJC Accreditation, Medicare Approved, Utilization Review, Pre-Admission Certification, State Licensure, Quality Assurance Program

Key Personnel
President. . . . . Sheila Jenkins
Dir, Health Promotions . . . . Deborah Anderson
Chief Administrative Offi . . . . Penny Ransom
VP/General Manager . . . . Marcia Broeren
VP/Network Development. . . . . Donald Schumann
Medical Director . . . . Edward Scanlan, MD
President & CEO . . . . Coreen Dicus-Johnson
Administrative Officer. . . . . Penny Ransom
Chief Financial Officer . . . . Brian Ollech
Chief Actuary . . . . Kevin Borchert
General Counsel. . . . . Kathryn Finerty
Chief Medical Officer . . . . Gregory Buran

Public Relations & Events . . . . Hannah Zillmer
262-788-9525
hzillmer@networkhealth.org
Marketing Manager . . . . Lisa Endl
920-720-1789
lendl@networkhealth.org

Specialty Managed Care Partners
Enters into Contracts with Regional Business Coalitions: Yes

848   Physicians Plus Insurance Corporation

2650 Novation Parkway
Madison, WI 53713
Toll-Free: 800-545-5015
Phone: 608-282-8900
ppicinfo@pplusic.com
www.pplusic.com
Mailing Address: PO Box 2078, Madison, WI 53701-2078
Subsidiary of: Meriter Health Services
For Profit Organization: Yes
Year Founded: 1986
Physician Owned Organization: Yes
Number of Primary Care Physicians: 4,900
Total Enrollment: 112,000
State Enrollment: 112,000

Healthplan and Services Defined
PLAN TYPE: HMO/PPO
Other Type: POS
Model Type: Network
Plan Specialty: Behavioral Health, Chiropractic, Dental,
Disease Management, Lab, X-Ray
Benefits Offered: Behavioral Health, Chiropractic, Dental,
Disease Management, Home Care, Inpatient SNF, Physical
Therapy, Podiatry, Prescription, Transplant, Vision,
Wellness, Durable Medical Equipment

Type of Coverage
Individual, Supplemental Medicare, Commercial Small
Group, Large Group
Catastrophic Illness Benefit: Covered

Type of Payment Plans Offered
Capitated, FFS, Combination FFS & DFFS

Geographic Areas Served
South Central Wisconsin

Subscriber Information
Average Monthly Fee Per Subscriber
(Employee + Employer Contribution):
Employee Only (Self): Varies by plan
Average Annual Deductible Per Subscriber:
Employee Only (Self): Varies by plan
Employee & 1 Family Member: $0
Employee & 2 Family Members: $0
Medicare: $0
Average Subscriber Co-Payment:
Primary Care Physician: Varies by plan
Hospital ER: $100.00
Home Health Care Max. Days/Visits Covered: 100 visits
Nursing Home Max. Days/Visits Covered: 100 days

Network Qualifications
Pre-Admission Certification: Yes

Peer Review Type
Utilization Review: Yes
Second Surgical Opinion: Yes
Case Management: Yes

Publishes and Distributes Report Card: Yes

Accreditation Certification
NCQA
State Licensure, Quality Assurance Program

Key Personnel
Chief Operating Officer . . . . Jim Thomson
Sales & Marketing . . . . Tom Luddyÿ
Chief Medical Officer. . . . . Jason Yelk
Chief Finance Officer. . . . . Michael Lorhan

Average Claim Compensation
Physician's Fees Charged: 70%
Hospital's Fees Charged: 75%

Specialty Managed Care Partners
Enters into Contracts with Regional Business Coalitions: No

849   Prevea Health Network

P.O. Box 19070
Green Bay, WI 54307
Toll-Free: 888-277-3832
Phone: 920-496-4700
Fax: 920-272-1120
www.prevea.com
For Profit Organization: Yes
Year Founded: 1996
Number of Affiliated Hospitals: 14
Number of Primary Care Physicians: 1,602
Total Enrollment: 119,712
State Enrollment: 15,706

Healthplan and Services Defined
PLAN TYPE: PPO
Model Type: Group
Plan Specialty: UR
Benefits Offered: Behavioral Health, Chiropractic, Disease
Management, Home Care, Prescription, Transplant,
Wellness, Allergy; Asthma; Cancer Rehab; Cardiac;
Dermatology; Lab & Pathology; Pediatric; Reconstructive
Plastic Surgery

Type of Coverage
Commercial, Supplemental Medicare

Geographic Areas Served
Northeast Wisconsin and Western Wisconsin's Chippewa
Valley region

Subscriber Information
Average Annual Deductible Per Subscriber:
Employee Only (Self): $0
Employee & 1 Family Member: $0
Employee & 2 Family Members: $0
Medicare: $0
Average Subscriber Co-Payment:
Primary Care Physician: $0

Accreditation Certification
  TJC
  Pre-Admission Certification

Key Personnel
  President,CEO . . . . Ashok Rai, MD
  SVP/Chief Medical Officer . . . . Karla Roth, MD
  SVP/Chief Financial Offic . . . . Lorrie Jacobetti
  SVP/Chief Operating Offic . . . . Brian Charlier
  SVP/Human Resources . . . . Deb Mauthe
  SVP/General Counsel . . . . Larry Gille
  Health Promotions Coord . . . . Candy Blaney
  Client Support Coord . . . . Deb Rhode
  Client Services . . . . Cherie Heath
  Provider Network Coord . . . . Trisha Paulson

Specialty Managed Care Partners
  Express Scripts

---

850 Security Health Plan of Wisconsin

1515 Saint Joseph Avenue
P.O. Box 8000
Marshfield, WI 54449-8000
Toll-Free: 800-472-2363
Phone: 715-221-9555
Fax: 715-221-9500
shpwebmaster@securityhealth.org
www.securityhealth.org
Non-Profit Organization: Yes
Year Founded: 1986
Physician Owned Organization: Yes
Total Enrollment: 187,000
State Enrollment: 187,000

Healthplan and Services Defined
  PLAN TYPE: Multiple
  Model Type: Network
  Plan Specialty: Behavioral Health, Chiropractic, Disease
    Management, EPO, Lab, PBM, Vision, Radiology,
    Worker's Compensation, UR
  Benefits Offered: Behavioral Health, Chiropractic,
    Complementary Medicine, Dental, Disease Management,
    Home Care, Inpatient SNF, Long-Term Care, Podiatry,
    Prescription, Psychiatric, Transplant, Vision, Wellness,
    Worker's Compensation, AD&D, Durable Medical
    Equipment
  Offers Demand Management Patient Information Service:
    Yes
  DMPI Services Offered: Nurse Line, Health Information Line

Type of Coverage
  Commercial, Individual, Indemnity, Medicare, Supplemental
    Medicare, Medicaid, TPA
  Catastrophic Illness Benefit: Covered

Type of Payment Plans Offered
  Capitated, FFS

Geographic Areas Served
  Northern, Western and Central Wisconsin

Subscriber Information
  Average Monthly Fee Per Subscriber
    (Employee + Employer Contribution):

  Employee Only (Self): Varies by plan
  Average Annual Deductible Per Subscriber:
    Employee Only (Self): $200.00
    Employee & 2 Family Members: $100.00
    Medicare: $0
  Average Subscriber Co-Payment:
    Primary Care Physician: $20.00
    Non-Network Physician: $20.00
    Prescription Drugs: $3.00
    Hospital ER: $50.00
    Home Health Care: $0
    Home Health Care Max. Days/Visits Covered: 40 days
    Nursing Home: $0
    Nursing Home Max. Days/Visits Covered: 30 days

Network Qualifications
  Pre-Admission Certification: No

Peer Review Type
  Utilization Review: Yes

Publishes and Distributes Report Card: Yes

Accreditation Certification
  NCQA
  Medicare Approved, Pre-Admission Certification

Key Personnel
  Chief Medical Officer . . . . Eric Quivers

Specialty Managed Care Partners
  Enters into Contracts with Regional Business Coalitions: Yes

---

851 Trilogy Health Insurance

18000 West Sarah Lane
Suite 310
Brookfield, WI 53045
Toll-Free: 866-429-3241
Phone: 262-432-9140
www.trilogycares.com
For Profit Organization: Yes
Number of Affiliated Hospitals: 75
Number of Primary Care Physicians: 3,300
Total Enrollment: 5,000

Healthplan and Services Defined
  PLAN TYPE: PPO
  Other Type: HSA
  Benefits Offered: Disease Management, Prescription,
    Wellness
  Offers Demand Management Patient Information Service: Yes
  DMPI Services Offered: 24-Hour Nurse Line

Type of Coverage
  Commercial

Accreditation Certification
  URAC

---

852 UnitedHealthcare of Wisconsin

10701 W. Research Drive
Milwaukee, WI 53226
Toll-Free: 800-879-0071
Phone: 414-443-4000
www.uhc.com

Subsidiary of: UnitedHealth Group
For Profit Organization: Yes

Healthplan and Services Defined
PLAN TYPE: HMO/PPO
Model Type: Network
Plan Specialty: Behavioral Health, Dental, Disease
Management, PBM, Vision
Benefits Offered: Behavioral Health, Dental, Disease
Management, Long-Term Care, Prescription, Vision,
Wellness, Life, LTD, STD

Type of Coverage
Commercial, Individual, Medicare, Supplemental Medicare,
Medicaid, Catastrophic, Family, Military, Veterans, Group,

Geographic Areas Served
Statewide

Key Personnel
CEO . . . . David S. Wichmann
President & CFO . . . . Dan Schumacher
Chief Strategy Officer . . . . John Cosgriff
Communications Officer . . . . Kirsten Gorsuch
Chief Medical Officer . . . . Sam Ho
Chief Legal Officer . . . . Thad Johnson
Chief Information Officer . . . . Phil McKoy
Chief Financial Officer . . . . Jeff Putnam

853   Unity Health Insurance
840 Carolina Street
Sauk City, WI 53583
Toll-Free: 800-362-3310
Phone: 608-644-3430
www.unityhealth.com
Subsidiary of: University Health Care Inc
For Profit Organization: Yes
Year Founded: 1994
Number of Affiliated Hospitals: 44
Number of Primary Care Physicians: 908
Number of Referral/Specialty Physicians: 3,227
Total Enrollment: 90,000
State Enrollment: 75,000

Healthplan and Services Defined
PLAN TYPE: Multiple
Model Type: Network
Benefits Offered: Behavioral Health, Chiropractic, Dental,
Disease Management, Home Care, Inpatient SNF, Physical
Therapy, Podiatry, Prescription, Psychiatric, Transplant,
Vision, Wellness

Type of Coverage
Commercial, Individual, Medicare, Medicaid

Type of Payment Plans Offered
POS, DFFS, FFS, Combination FFS & DFFS

Geographic Areas Served
20 counties in Southwestern and South Central Wisconsin

Network Qualifications
Pre-Admission Certification: Yes

Peer Review Type
Utilization Review: Yes

Second Surgical Opinion: Yes
Case Management: Yes

Publishes and Distributes Report Card: Yes

Accreditation Certification
NCQA
Medicare Approved, Utilization Review, Pre-Admission
Certification, State Licensure, Quality Assurance Program

Key Personnel
CEO/President . . . . Terry Bolz
Chief Operating Office . . . . Gail Midlikowski
Chief Medical Officer . . . . Gary Lenth
VP/CFO/Treasurer . . . . Jim Hiveley

Specialty Managed Care Partners
Behavioral Health Consultation System, UW Hospital and
Clinics, APS Healthcare
Enters into Contracts with Regional Business Coalitions: No

Employer References
University of Wisconsin Medical Foundation, Middleton
Cross Plains School District, Rockwell Automation,
Brakebush Brothers, Epic Systemss Corporation

854   Wisconsin Physician's Service
1717 West Broadway
P.O. Box 8190
Madison, WI 53708-8190
Toll-Free: 800-223-6048
Phone: 608-977-5000
member@wpsic.com
www.wpsic.com
Non-Profit Organization: Yes
Year Founded: 1946
Owned by an Integrated Delivery Network (IDN): Yes
Number of Affiliated Hospitals: 129
Number of Primary Care Physicians: 14,500
Total Enrollment: 175,000
State Enrollment: 223,000

Healthplan and Services Defined
PLAN TYPE: Multiple
Model Type: Network
Plan Specialty: ASO, Behavioral Health, Chiropractic, Dental,
Disease Management, EPO, Lab, PBM, Vision, Radiology,
Worker's Compensation, UR, Rational Med
Benefits Offered: Behavioral Health, Chiropractic, Dental,
Disease Management, Home Care, Inpatient SNF, Physical
Therapy, Podiatry, Prescription, Psychiatric, Transplant,
Vision, Wellness, AD&D, Life, LTD, STD
Offers Demand Management Patient Information Service: Yes

Type of Coverage
Commercial, Individual, Indemnity, Medicare, Supplemental
Medicare, Catastrophic
Catastrophic Illness Benefit: Varies per case

Type of Payment Plans Offered
POS, DFFS

Subscriber Information
Average Annual Deductible Per Subscriber:
Employee Only (Self): $0

Employee & 1 Family Member: $0
Employee & 2 Family Members: $0
Medicare: $0

Peer Review Type
Case Management: Yes

Publishes and Distributes Report Card: Yes

Accreditation Certification
AAAHC, URAC
Medicare Approved, Utilization Review, State Licensure,
   Quality Assurance Program

Key Personnel
President and CEO . . . . Mike Hamerlik
Chief Operating Officer . . . . Jay Mertinson
Chief Financial Officer . . . . Vicki Bernards
Administrative Officer . . . . Craig Campbell
VP, Government Relations . . . . Rob Palmer

Specialty Managed Care Partners
Delta Dental
Enters into Contracts with Regional Business Coalitions: Yes

Employer References
US Department of Defense

Health Insurance Coverage Status and Type of Coverage by Age

Category	All Persons		Under 18 years		Under 65 years	
	Number	%	Number	%	Number	%
Total population	576	-	150	-	491	-
Covered by some type of health insurance	510 (6)	88.5 (1.0)	136 (3)	91.2 (1.9)	425 (6)	86.6 (1.2)
Covered by private health insurance	427 (8)	74.1 (1.4)	106 (5)	70.9 (3.2)	370 (8)	75.4 (1.6)
Employer-based	337 (9)	58.5 (1.5)	90 (5)	60.4 (3.3)	311 (9)	63.4 (1.9)
Direct purchase	94 (6)	16.3 (1.0)	14 (3)	9.5 (2.0)	59 (6)	12.0 (1.2)
TRICARE	19 (3)	3.3 (0.5)	5 (1)	3.2 (1.0)	14 (2)	2.8 (0.5)
Covered by public health insurance	157 (5)	27.3 (0.9)	36 (3)	24.4 (2.3)	74 (5)	15.1 (1.1)
Medicaid	70 (5)	12.1 (0.9)	36 (3)	24.3 (2.3)	61 (5)	12.4 (1.0)
Medicare	94 (2)	16.3 (0.4)	Z (Z)	0.1 (0.1)	11 (2)	2.2 (0.4)
VA Care	22 (2)	3.8 (0.4)	Z (Z)	0.1 (0.1)	10 (2)	2.0 (0.3)
Not covered at any time during the year	67 (6)	11.5 (1.0)	13 (3)	8.8 (1.9)	66 (6)	13.4 (1.2)

Note: Numbers in thousands; Figures cover civilian noninstitutionalized population in 2016; N/A indicates that data was not available; Z represents or rounds to zero; Margin of error appears in parenthesis and is calculated using replicate weights.
Source: U.S. Census Bureau, American Community Survey, Table HIC-4_ACS. Health Insurance Coverage Status and Type of Coverage by State—All People: 2008 to 2016, Table HIC-5_ACS. Health Insurance Coverage Status and Type of Coverage by State—Children Under 18: 2008 to 2016, Table HIC-6_ACS. Health Insurance Coverage Status and Type of Coverage by State—Persons Under 65: 2008 to 2016

Wyoming

855 Aetna Health of Wyoming

151 Farmington Avenue
Hartford, CT 06156
Toll-Free: 800-872-3862
Phone: 860-273-0123
www.aetna.com
Secondary Address: 6730-B Rockledge Drive, Suite 700,
Bethesda, MD 20817, 301-581-0600
Subsidiary of: Aetna Inc.
For Profit Organization: Yes

Healthplan and Services Defined
PLAN TYPE: PPO
Other Type: POS
Model Type: Network
Plan Specialty: Behavioral Health, EPO, Lab, PBM,
Radiology
Benefits Offered: Behavioral Health, Dental, Disease
Management, Long-Term Care, Physical Therapy,
Podiatry, Prescription, Psychiatric, Wellness, Life, LTD,
STD

Type of Coverage
Commercial, Student health

Type of Payment Plans Offered
POS, FFS

Geographic Areas Served
Statewide

Key Personnel
CEO . . . . Mark Bertolini

856 Blue Cross & Blue Shield of Wyoming

4000 House Avenue
Cheyenne, WY 82001
Toll-Free: 800-442-2376
www.bcbswy.com
Non-Profit Organization: Yes
Year Founded: 1976
Total Enrollment: 100,000
State Enrollment: 100,000

Healthplan and Services Defined
PLAN TYPE: HMO
Benefits Offered: Disease Management, Physical Therapy,
Wellness

Type of Coverage
Commercial, Individual, Medicare, Medicaid

Type of Payment Plans Offered
FFS

Geographic Areas Served
Statewide

Key Personnel
President & CEO . . . . Rick Schum

Specialty Managed Care Partners
Prime Therapeutics

Employer References
Tricare

857 Delta Dental of Wyoming

6234 Yellowstone Road
P.O. Box 29
Cheyenne, WY 82009
Toll-Free: 800-735-3379
Phone: 307-632-3313
Fax: 307-632-7309
customerservice@deltadentalwy.org
www.deltadentalwy.org
Non-Profit Organization: Yes

Healthplan and Services Defined
PLAN TYPE: Dental
Other Type: Dental PPO
Model Type: Network
Plan Specialty: ASO, Dental
Benefits Offered: Dental

Type of Coverage
Commercial, Individual
Catastrophic Illness Benefit: None

Geographic Areas Served
Statewide

Accreditation Certification
URAC, NCQA

Key Personnel
President & CEO . . . . Kerry P. Hall

858 Humana Health Insurance of Wyoming

12300 Whitewater Drive
Suite 150
Minnetonka, MT 55343
Toll-Free: 877-368-6990
Fax: 952-938-2787
www.humana.com
Subsidiary of: Humana
For Profit Organization: Yes

Healthplan and Services Defined
PLAN TYPE: HMO/PPO
Model Type: Network
Plan Specialty: Dental, Vision
Benefits Offered: Dental, Vision, Life, LTD, STD

Type of Coverage
Commercial

Geographic Areas Served
Statewide. Wyoming is covered by the Minnesota branch

Accreditation Certification
URAC, NCQA, CORE

Key Personnel
President & CEO. . . . . Bruce Broussard
Chief Medical Officr. . . . . Roy A. Beveridge
Chief Consumer Officer. . . . . Jody L. Bilney
Human Resources. . . . . Tim Huval
Chief Financial Officer . . . . Brian Kane

Chief Information Officer .... Brian LeClaire
General Counsel .... Christopher M. Todoroff

859 UnitedHealthcare of Wyoming

6465 S Greenwood Plaza Boulevard
Suite 300
Centennial, CO 80111
Toll-Free: 866-574-6088
www.uhc.com/contact-us/wyoming
Subsidiary of: UnitedHealth Group

Healthplan and Services Defined
PLAN TYPE: HMO/PPO
Model Type: Network
Plan Specialty: Behavioral Health, Dental, Disease
   Management, MSO, PBM, Vision
Benefits Offered: Behavioral Health, Chiropractic,
   Complementary
Medicine, Dental, Disease Management, Home Care,
Inpatient SNF, Long-Term Care, Physical Therapy,
Podiatry, Prescription, Psychiatric, Transplant,
Vision, Wellness, AD&D, Life, Benefits vary
according to plan

Type of Coverage
Commercial, Individual, Medicare, Medicaid, Family,
   Military, Veterans, Group,

Type of Payment Plans Offered
DFFS, FFS, Combination FFS & DFFS

Geographic Areas Served
Statewide. Wyoming is covered by the Colorado branch

Subscriber Information
Average Monthly Fee Per Subscriber
   (Employee + Employer Contribution):
      Employee Only (Self): Varies

Network Qualifications
Pre-Admission Certification: Yes

Peer Review Type
Case Management: Yes

Publishes and Distributes Report Card: Yes

Accreditation Certification
URAC, NCQA
State Licensure, Quality Assurance Program

Average Claim Compensation
Physician's Fees Charged: 70%
Hospital's Fees Charged: 55%

Specialty Managed Care Partners
United Behavioral Health
Enters into Contracts with Regional Business Coalitions: No

Appendix A: Glossary of Terms

A

Access
A person's ability to obtain healthcare services.

Acute Care
Medical treatment rendered to people whose illnesses or medical problems are short-term or don't require long-term continuing care. Acute care facilities are hospitals that mainly treat people with short-term health problems.

Aggregate Indemnity
The maximum amount of payment provided by an insurer for each covered service for a group of insured people.

Aid to Families with Dependent Children (AFDC)
A state-based federal assistance program that provided cash payments to needy children (and their caretakers), who met certain income requirements. AFDC has now been replaced by a new block grant program, but the requirements, or criteria, can still be used for determining eligibility for Medicaid.

Alliance
Large businesses, small businesses, and individuals who form a group for insurance coverage.

All-payer System
A proposed healthcare system in which, no matter who is paying, prices for health services and payment methods are the same. Federal or state government, a private insurance company, a self-insured employer plan, an individual, or any other payer would pay the same rates. Also called Multiple Payer system.

Ambulatory Care
All health services that are provided on an out-patient basis, that don't require overnight care. Also called out-patient care.

Ancillary Services
Supplemental services, including laboratory, radiology and physical therapy, that are provided along with medical or hospital care.

B

Beneficiary
A person who is eligible for or receiving benefits under an insurance policy or plan.

Benefits
The services that members are entitled to receive based on their health plan.

Blue Cross/Blue Shield
Non-profit, tax-exempt insurance service plans that cover hospital care, physician care and related services. Blue Cross and Blue Shield are separate organizations that have different benefits, premiums and policies. These organizations are in all states, and The Blue Cross and Blue Shield Association of America is their national organization.

Board Certified
Status granted to a medical specialist who completes required training and passes and examination in his/her specialized area. Individuals who have met all requirements, but have not completed the exam are referred to as "board eligible."

Board Eligible
Reference to medical specialists who have completed all required training but have not completed the exam in his/her specialized area.

C

Cafeteria Plan
This benefit plan gives employees a set amount of funds that they can choose to spend on a different benefit options, such as health insurance or retirement savings

Capitation
A fixed prepayment, per patient covered, to a healthcare provider to deliver medical services to a particular group of patients. The payment is the same no matter how many services or what type of services each patient actually gets. Under capitation, the provider is financially responsible.

Care Guidelines
A set of medical treatments for a particular condition or group of patients that has been reviewed and endorsed by a national organization, such as the Agency for Healthcare Policy Research.

Carrier
A private organization, usually an insurance company, that finances healthcare.

Carve-out
Medical services that are separated out and contracted for independently from any other benefits.

Case management
Intended to improve health outcomes or control costs, services and education are tailored to a patient's needs, which are designed to improve health outcomes and/or control costs

Catastrophic Health Insurance
Health insurance that provides coverage for treating severe or lengthy illnesses or disability.

CHAMPUS
(Civilian Health and Medical Program of the Uniformed Services) A health plan that serves the dependents of active duty military personnel and retired military personnel and their dependents.

Chronic Care
Treatment given to people whose health problems are long-term and continuing. Nu nursing homes, mental hospitals and rehabilitation facilities are chronic care facilities.

Chronic Disease
A medical problem that will not improve, that lasts a lifetime, or recurs.

Claims
Bills for services. Doctors, hospitals, labs and other providers send billed claims to health insurance plans, and what the plans pay are called paid claims.

COBRA
(Consolidated Omnibus Budget Reconciliation Act of 1985) Designed to provide health coverage to workers between jobs, this legal act lets workers who leave a company buy health insurance from that company at the employer's group rate rather than an individual rate.

Co-insurance
A cost-sharing requirement under some health insurance policies in which the insured person pays some of the costs of covered services.

Cooperatives/Co-ops
HMOs that are managed by the members of the health plan or insurance purchasing arrangements in which businesses or other groups join together to gain the buying power of large employers or groups.

Co-pay
Flat fees or payments (often $5-10) that a patient pays for each doctor visit or prescription.

Cost Containment
The method of preventing healthcare costs from increasing beyond a set level by controlling or reducing inefficiency and waste in the healthcare system.

Cost Sharing
An insurance policy requires the insured person to pay a portion of the costs of covered services. Deductibles, co-insurance and co-payments are cost sharing.

Cost Shifting
When one group of patients does not pay for services, such as uninsured or Medicare patients, healthcare providers pass on the costs for these health services to other groups of patients.

Coverage
A person's healthcare costs are paid by their insurance or by the government..

Covered services
Treatments or other services for which a health plan pays at least part of the charge.

D

Deductible
The amount of money, or value of certain services (such as one physician visit), a patient or family must pay before costs (or percentages of costs) are covered by the health plan or insurance company, usually per year.

Diagnostic related groups (DRGs)
A system for classifying hospital stays according to the diagnosis of the medical problem being treated, for the purposes of payment.

Direct access
The ability to see a doctor or receive a medical service without a referral from your primary care physician.

Disease management
Programs for people who have chronic illnesses, such as asthma or diabetes, that try to encourage them to have a healthy lifestyle, to take medications as prescribed, and that coordinate care.

Disposable Personal Income
The amount of a person's income that is left over after money has been spent on basic necessities such as rent, food, and clothing.

E

Early and Periodic Screening, Diagnosis, and Treatment Program (EPSDT)
As part of the Medicaid program, the law requires that all states have a program for eligible children under age 21 to receive a medical assessment, medical treatments and other measures to correct any problems and treat chronic conditions.

Elective
A healthcare procedure that is not an emergency and that the patient and doctor plan in advance.

Emergency
A medical condition that starts suddenly and requires immediate care.

Employee Retirement Income Security Act (ERISA)
A Federal act, passed in 1974, that established new standards for employer-funded health benefit and pension programs. Companies that have self-funded health benefit plans operating under ERISA are not subject to state insurance regulations and healthcare legislation.

Employer Contribution
The contribution is the money a company pays for its employees' healthcare. Exclusions
Health conditions that are explicitly not covered in an insurance package and that your insurance will not pay for.

Exclusive Provider Organizations (EPO)/Exclusive Provider Arrangement (EPA)
An indemnity or service plan that provides benefits only if those hospitals or doctors with which it contracts provide the medical services, with some exceptions for emergency and out-of-area services.

F

Federal Employee Health Benefit Program (FEP)
Health insurance program for Federal workers and their dependents, established in 1959 under the Federal Employees Health Benefits Act. Federal employees may choose to participate in one of two or more plans.

Fee-for-Service

Physicians or other providers bill separately for each patient encounter or service they provide. This method of billing means the insurance company pays all or some set percentage of the fees that hospitals and doctors set and charge. Expenditures increase if the increaseThis is still the main system of paying for healthcare services in the United States.

First Dollar Coverage

A system in which the insurer pays for all employee out-of-pocket healthcare costs. Under first dollar coverage, the beneficiary has no deductible and no co-payments.

Flex plan

An account that lets workers set aside pretax dollars to pay for medical benefits, childcare, and other services.

Formulary

A list of medications that a managed care company encourages or requires physicians to prescribe as necessary in order to reduce costs.

G

Gag clause

A contractual agreement between a managed care organization and a provider that restricts what the provider can say about the managed care company

Gatekeeper

The person in a managed care organization, often a primary care provider, who controls a patient's access to healthcare services and whose approval is required for referrals to other services or other specialists.

General Practice

Physicians without specialty training who provide a wide range of primary healthcare services to patients.

Global Budgeting

A way of containing hospital costs in which participating hospitals share a budget, agreeing together to set the maximum amount of money that will be paid for healthcare.

Group Insurance

Health insurance offered through business, union trusts or other groups and associations. The most common system of health insurance in the United States, in which the cost of insurance is based on the age, sex, health status and occupation of the people in the group.

Group model HMO

An HMO that contracts with an independent group practice to provide medical services

Guaranteed Issue

The requirement that an insurance plan accept everyone who applies for coverage and guarantee the renewal of that coverage as long as the covered person pays the policy premium.

H

Healthcare Benefits

The specific services and procedures covered by a health plan or insurer.

Healthcare Financing Administration (HCFA)

The federal government agency within the Department of Health and Human Services that directs the Medicare and Medicaid programs. HCFA also does research to support these programs and oversees more than a quarter of all healthcare costs in the United States.

Health Insurance

Financial protection against the healthcare costs caused by treating disease or accidental injury.

Health Insurance Portability and Accountability Act (HIPAA)

Also known as Kennedy-Kassebaum law, this guarantees that people who lose their group health insurance will have access to individual insurance, regardless of pre-existing medical problems. The law also allows employees to secure health insurance from their new employer when they switch jobs even if they have a pre-existing medical condition.

Health Insurance Purchasing Cooperatives (HIPCs)

Public or private organizations that get health insurance coverage for certain populations of people, combining everyone in a specific geographic region and basing insurance rates on the people in that area.

Health Maintenance Organization (HMO)

A health plan provides comprehensive medical services to its members for a fixed, prepaid premium. Members must use participating providers and are enrolled for a fixed period of time. HMOs can do business either on a for-profit or not-for-profit basis.

Health Plan Employer Data and Information Set (HEDIS)

Performance measures designed by the National Committee for Quality Assurance to give participating managed health plans and employers to information about the value of their healthcare and trends in their health plan performance compared with other health plans.

Home healthcare

Skilled nurses and trained aides who provide nursing services and related care to someone at home.

Hospice Care

Care given to terminally ill patients. Hospital Alliances Groups of hospitals that join together to cut their costs by purchasing services and equipment in volume.

I

Indemnity Insurance

A system of health insurance in which the insurer pays for the costs of covered services after care has been given, and which usually defines the maximum amounts which will be paid for covered services. This is the most common type of insurance in the United States.

Independent Practice Association (IPA)
A group of private physicians who join together in an association to contract with a managed care organization.

Indigent Care
Care provided, at no cost, to people who do not have health insurance or are not covered by Medicare, Medicaid, or other public programs.

In-patient
A person who has been admitted to a hospital or other health facility, for a period of at least 24 hours.

Integrated Delivery System (IDS)
An organization that usually includes a hospital, a large medical group, and an insurer such as an HMO or PPO.

Integrated Provider (IP)
A group of providers that offer comprehensive and coordinated care, and usually provides a range of medical care facilities and service plans including hospitals, group practices, a health plan and other related healthcare services.

J

Joint Commission on the Accreditation of Healthcare Organizations (JCAHO)
A national private, non-profit organization that accredits healthcare organizations and agencies and sets guidelines for operation for these facilities.

L

Limitations
A "cap" or limit on the amount of services that may be provided. It may be the maximum cost or number of days that a service or treatment is covered.

Limited Service Hospital
A hospital, often located in a rural area, that provides a limited set of medical and surgical services.

Long-term Care
Healthcare, personal care and social services provided to people who have a chronic illness or disability and do not have full functional capacity. This care can take place in an institution or at home, on a long-term basis.

M

Malpractice Insurance
Coverage for medical professionals which pays the costs of legal fees and/or any damages assessed by the court in a lawsuit brought against a professional who has been charged with negligence.

Managed care
This term describes many types of health insurance, including HMOs and PPOs. They control the use of health services by their members so that they can contain healthcare costs and/or improve the quality of care.

Mandate
Law requiring that a health plan or insurance carrier must offer a particular procedure or type of coverage.

Means Test
An assessment of a person's or family's income or assets so that it can be determined if they are eligible to receive public support, such as Medicaid.

Medicaid
An insurance program for people with low incomes who are unable to afford healthcare. Although funded by the federal government, Medicaid is administered by each state. Following very broad federal guidelines, states determine specific benefits and amounts of payment for providers.

Medical IRAs
Personal accounts which, like individual retirement plans, allow a person to accumulate funds for future use. The money in these accounts must be used to pay for medical services. The employee decides how much money he or she will spend on healthcare.

Medically Indigent
A person who does not have insurance and is not covered by Medicaid, Medicare or other public programs.

Medicare
A federal program of medical care benefits created in 1965 designed for those over age 65 or permanently disabled. Medicare consists of two separate programs: A and B. Medicare Part A, which is automatic at age 65, covers hospital costs and is financed largely by employer payroll taxes. Medicare Part B covers outpatient care and is financed through taxes and individual payments toward a premium.

Medicare Supplements or Medigap
A privately-purchased health insurance policy available to Medicare beneficiaries to cover costs of care that Medicare does not pay. Some policies cover additional costs, such as preventive care, prescription drugs, or at-home care.

Member
The person enrolled in a health plan.

N

National Committee on Quality Assurance (NCQA)
An independent national organization that reviews and accredits managed care plans and measures the quality of care offered by managed care plans.

Network

A group of affiliated contracted healthcare providers (physicians, hospitals, testing centers, rehabilitation centers etc.), such as an HMO, PPO, or Point of Service plan.

Non-contributory Plan

A group insurance plan that requires no payment from employees for their healthcare coverage.

Non-participating Provider

A healthcare provider who is not part of a health plan. Usually patients must pay their own healthcare costs to see a non-participating provider.

Nurse practitioner

A nurse specialist who provides primary and/or specialty care to patients. In some states nurse practitioners do not have to be supervised by a doctor.

O

Open Enrollment Period

A specified period of time during which people are allowed to change health plans.

Open Panel

A right included in an HMO, which allows the covered person to get non-emergency covered services from a specialist without getting a referral from the primary care physician or gatekeeper.

Out of Pocket costs or expenditures

The amount of money that a person must pay for his or her healthcare, including: deductibles, co-pays, payments for services that are not covered, and/or health insurance premiums that are not paid by his or her employer.

Outcomes

Measures of the effectiveness of particular kinds of medical treatment. This refers to what is quantified to determine if a specific treatment or type of service works.

Out of Pocket Maximum

The maximum amount that a person must pay under a plan or insurance contract.

Outpatient Care

Healthcare services that do not require a patient to receive overnight care in a hospital.

P

Participating Physician or Provider

Healthcare providers who have contracted with a managed care plan to provide eligible healthcare services to members of that plan.

Payer

The organization responsible for the costs of healthcare services. A payer may be private insurance, the government, or an employer's self-funded plan.

Peer Review Organization (PRO or PSRO)

An agency that monitors the quality and appropriateness of medical care delivered to Medicare and Medicaid patients. Healthcare professionals in these agencies review other professionals with similar training and experience. [See Quality Improvement Organizations]

Percent of Poverty

A term that describes the income level a person or family must have to be eligible for Medicaid.

Physician Assistant

A health professional who provides primary and/or specialty care to patients under the supervision of a physician.

Physician Hospital Organizations (PHOs)

An organization that contracts with payers on behalf of one or more hospitals and affiliated physicians. Physicians still own their practices.

Play or Pay

This system would provide coverage for all people by requiring employers either to provide health insurance for their employees and dependents (play) or pay a contribution to a publicly-provided system that covers uninsured or unemployed people without private insurance (pay).

Point of Service (POS)

A type of insurance where each time healthcare services are needed, the patient can choose from different types of provider systems (indemnity plan, PPO or HMO). Usually, members are required to pay more to see PPO or non-participating providers than to see HMO providers.

Portability

A person's ability to keep his or her health coverage during times of change in health status or personal situation (such as change in employment or unemployment, marriage or divorce) or while moving between health plans.

Postnatal Care

Healthcare services received by a woman immediately following the delivery of her child

Pre-authorization

The process where, before a patient can be admitted to the hospital or receive other types of specialty services, the managed care company must approve of the proposed service in order to cover it.

Pre-existing Condition

A medical condition or diagnosis that began before coverage began under a current plan or insurance contract. The insurance company may provide coverage but will specifically exclude treatment for such a condition from that person's coverage for a certain period of time, often six months to a year.

Preferred Provider Organization (PPO)

A type of insurance in which the managed care company pays a higher percentage of the costs when a preferred (in-plan) provider is used. The participating providers have agreed to provide their services at negotiated discount fees.

Premium
The amount paid periodically to buy health insurance coverage. Employers and employees usually share the cost of premiums.

Premium Cap
The maximum amount of money an insurance company can charge for coverage.

Premium Tax
A state tax on insurance premiums.

Prepaid Group Practice
A type of HMO where participating providers receive a fixed payment in advance for providing particular healthcare services.

Preventive Care
Healthcare services that prevent disease or its consequences. It includes primary prevention to keep people from getting sick (such as immunizations), secondary prevention to detect early disease (such as Pap smears) and tertiary prevention to keep ill people or those at high risk of disease from getting sicker (such as helping someone with lung disease to quit smoking).

Primary Care
Basic or general routine office medical care, usually from an internist, obstetrician-gynecologist, family practitioner, or pediatrician.

Primary care provider (PCP)
The health professional who provides basic healthcare services. The PCP may control patients' access to the rest of the healthcare system through referrals.

Private Insurance
Health insurance that is provided by insurance companies such as commercial insurers and Blue Cross plans, self-funded plans sponsored by employers, HMOs or other managed care arrangements.

Provider
An individual or institution who provides medical care, including a physician, hospital, skilled nursing facility, or intensive care facility.

Provider-Sponsored Organization (PSO)
Healthcare providers (physicians and/or hospitals) who form an affiliation to act as insurer for an enrolled population.

Q

Quality Assessment
Measurement of the quality of care.

Quality Assurance and Quality Improvement
A systematic process to improve quality of healthcare by monitoring quality, finding out what is not working, and fixing the problems of healthcare delivery.

Quality Improvement Organization (QIO)
An organization contracting with HCFA to review the medical necessity and quality of care provided to Medicare beneficiaries.

Quality of care
How well health services result in desired health outcomes.

R

Rate Setting
These programs were developed by several states in the 1970's to establish in advance the amount that hospitals would be paid no matter how high or low their costs actually were in any particular year. (Also known as hospital rate setting or prospective reimbursement programs)

Referral system
The process through which a primary care provider authorizes a patient to see a specialist to receive additional care.

Reimbursement
The amount paid to providers for services they provide to patients.

Risk
The responsibility for profiting or losing money based on the cost of healthcare services provided. Traditionally, health insurance companies have carried the risk. Under capitation, healthcare providers bear risk.

S

Self-insured
A type of insurance arrangement where employers, usually large employers, pay for medical claims out of their own funds rather than contracting with an insurance company for coverage. This puts the employer at risk for its employees' medical expenses rather than an insurance company.

Single Payer System
A healthcare reform proposal in which healthcare costs are paid by taxes rather than by the employer and employee. All people would have coverage paid by the government.

Socialized Medicine
A healthcare system in which providers are paid by the government, and healthcare facilities are run by the government.

Staff Model HMO
A type of managed care where physicians are employees of the health plan, usually in the health plan's own health center or facility.

Standard Benefit Package
A defined set of benefits provided to all people covered under a health plan.

T

Third Party Administrator (TPA)
An organization that processes health plan claims but does not carry any insurance risk.

Third Party Payer
An organization other than the patient or healthcare provider involved in the financing of personal health services.

U

Uncompensated Care
Healthcare provided to people who cannot pay for it and who are not covered by any insurance. This includes both charity care which is not billed and the cost of services that were billed but never paid.

Underinsured
People who have some type of health insurance but not enough insurance to cover their the cost of necessary healthcare. This includes people who have very high deductibles of $1000 to $5000 per year, or insurance policies that have specific exclusions for costly services.

Underwriting
This process is the basis of insurance. It analyzes the health status and history, claims experience (cost), age and general health risks of the individual or group who is applying for insurance coverage.

Uninsured
People who do not have health insurance of any type. Over 80 percent of the uninsured are working adults and their family members.

Universal Coverage
This refers to the proposal that all people could get health insurance, regardless of the way that the system is financed.

Utilization Review
A program designed to help reduce unnecessary medical expenses by studying the appropriateness of when certain services are used and by how many patients they are used.

Utilization
How many times people use particular healthcare services during particular periods of time.

V

Vertical Integration
A healthcare system that includes the entire range of healthcare services from out-patient to hospital and long-term care.

W

Waiting Period
The amount of time a person must wait from the date he or she is accepted into a health plan (or from when he or she applies) until the insurance becomes effective and he or she can receive benefits.

Withhold
A percentage of providers' fees that managed care companies hold back from providers which is only given to them if the amount of care they provide (or that the entire plan provides) is under a budgeted amount for each quarter or the whole year.

Worker's Compensation Coverage
States require employers to provide coverage to compensate employees for work-related injuries or disabilities.

Source: Public Broadcasting Service, http://www.pbs.org/ healthcarecrisis/glossary.htm. Reprinted with permission of www.issuestv.com and www.pbs.com.

Appendix B: Industry Websites

Alliance of Community Health Plans (ACHP)

http://www.achp.org

Offers information on health care so that it is safe, effective, patient-centered, timely, efficient and equitable. Members use this web site to collaborate, share strategies and work toward solutions to some of health care's biggest challenges.

America's Health Insurance Plans (AHIP)

http://www.ahip.org

AHIP is a national trade association representing nearly 1,300 member companies providing health insurance coverage to more than 200 million Americans.

American Academy of Medical Administrators (AAMA)

http://www.aameda.org

Supports individuals involved in medical administration at the executive - or middle-management levels. Promotes educational courses for the training of persons in medical administration. Conducts research. Offers placement service.

American Accreditation Healthcare Commission/URAC

http://www.urac.org

URAC (Utilization Review Accreditation Commission) is a 501(c)(3) non-profit charitable organization founded in 1990 to establish standards for the managed care industry. URAC's broad-based membership includes representation from all the constituencies affected by managed care - employers, consumers, regulators, health care providers, and the workers' compensation and managed care industries.

American Association of Healthcare Administrative Management (AAHAM)

http://www.aaham.org

A professional organization in healthcare administrative management that offers information, education and advocacy in the areas of reimbursement, admitting and registration, data management, medical records, patient relations and more. Founded in 1968, AAHAM represents a broad-based constituency of healthcare professionals through a comprehensive program of legislative and regulatory monitoring and its participation in industry groups such as ANSI, DISA and NUBC.

American Association of Integrated Healthcare Delivery Systems (AAIHDS)

http://www.aaihds.org

AAIHDS was founded in 1993 as a non-profit organization dedicated to the educational advancement of provider-based managed care professionals involved in integrated healthcare delivery.

American Association of Preferred Provider Organizations (AAPPO)

http://www.aappo.org

A national association of preferred provider organizations (PPOs) and affiliate organizations, established in 1983 to advance awareness of the benefits - greater access, choice and flexibility - that PPOs bring to American health care.

American College of Health Care Administrators (ACHCA)

http://achca.org

Founded in 1962, ACHCA provides superior educational programming, professional certification, and career development opportunities for its members. It identifies, recognizes, and supports long term care leaders, advocating for their mission and promoting excellence in their profession.

American College of Healthcare Executives (ACHE)

http://www.ache.org

International professional society of more than 30,000 healthcare executives, including credentialing and educational programs and sponsors the Congress on Healthcare Management. ACHE's publishing division, Health Administration Press, is one of the largest publishers of books.

American College of Physician Executives (ACPE)

http://www.acpe.org

Supports physicians whose primary professional responsibility is the management of healthcare organizations. Provides for continuing education and certification of the physician executive. Offers specialized career planning, counseling, recruitment and placement services, and research and information data on physician managers.

American Health Care Association (AHCA)

http://www.ahcancal.org

A non-profit federation of affiliated state health organizations, representing more than 10,000 non-profit and for-profit assisted living, nursing facility, developmentally-disabled, and subacute care providers that care for more than 1.5 million elderly and disabled individuals nationally.

American Health Planning Association (AHPA)

http://www.ahpanet.org

A non-profit public interest organization that brings together individuals and organizations interested in the availability, affordability and equitable distribution of health services. AHPA supports community participation in health policy formulation and in the organization and operation of local health services.

American Health Quality Association (AHQA)

http://www.ahqa.org

The American Health Quality Association represents Quality Improvement Organizations (QIOs) and professionals working to improve the quality of health care in communities across America. QIOs share information about best practices with physicians, hospitals, nursing homes, home health agencies, and others. Working together with health care providers, QIOs identify opportunities and provide assistance for improvement.

American Medical Association (AMA)

http://www.ama-assn.org

Founded more than 150 years ago, the AMA's work includes the development and promotion of standards in medical practice, research, and education. This site offers medical information for physicians, medical students, other health professionals, and patients.

American Medical Directors Association (AMDA)

http://www.amda.com

A professional association of medical directors, attending physicians, and others practicing in the long term care continuum, that provides education, advocacy, information, and professional development to promote the delivery of quality long term care medicine.

American Medical Group Association (AMGA)

http://www.amga.org

Association that supports various medical groups and organized systems of care at the national level.

Association of Family Medicine Residency Directors (AFMRD)

http://www.afmrd.org

Provides representation for residency directors at a national level and provides a political voice for them to appropriate arenas. Promotes cooperation and communication between residency programs and different branches of the family medicine specialty. Dedicated to improving of education of family physicians. Provides a network for mutual assistance among FP, residency directors.

Association of Family Practice Administrators (AFPA)

http://www.uams.edu/afpa/afpa1.htm

Promotes professionalism in family practice administration. Serves as a network for sharing of information and fellowship among members. Provides technical assistance to members and functions as a liaison to related professional organizations.

Association of Healthcare Internal Auditors (AHIA)

http://www.ahia.org

Promotes cost containment and increased productivity in health care institutions through internal auditing. Serves as a forum for the exchange of experience, ideas, and information among members; provides continuing professional education courses and informs members of developments in health care internal auditing. Offers employment clearinghouse services.

Case Management Society of America (CMSA)

http://www.cmsa.org

Information for the case management profession.

Centers for Medicare and Medicaid Services (CMS)

http://cms.hhs.gov

Formerly known as the Health Care Financing Administration (HCFA), this is the federal agency that administers Medicare, Medicaid and the State Children's Health Insurance Program (SCHIP). CMS provides health insurance for over 74 million Americans through these programs.

College of Healthcare Information Management Executives (CHIME)

http://www.cio-chime.org

Serves the professional development needs of healthcare CIOs, and advocating the more effective use of information management within healthcare.

Electronic Healthcare Network Accreditation Commission (EHNAC)

http://www.ehnac.org

A federally-recognized standards development organization and non-profit accrediting body designed to improve transactional quality, operational efficiency and data security in healthcare.

Healthcare Financial Management Association (HFMA)

http://www.hfma.org

HFMA is a membership organization for healthcare financial management executives and leaders. The association brings perspective and clarity to the industry's complex issues for the purpose of preparing members to succeed. Programs, publications and partnerships enhance the capabilities that strengthen not only individuals careers, but also the organizations from which members come.

Healthcare Information and Management Systems Society (HIMSS)

http://www.himss.org

The healthcare industry's membership organization exclusively focused on providing global leadership for the optimal use of healthcare information technology (IT) and management systems. HIMSS represents more than 20,000 individual members and over 300 corporate members leads healthcare public policy and industry practices through its advocacy, educational and professional development initiatives designed to promote information and management systems' contributions to ensuring quality patient care.

Healthfinder.gov

http://www.healthfinder.gov

A comprehensive guide to resources for health information from the federal government and related agencies.

The Joint Commission (JC)

http://www.jointcommission.org

An independent, not-for-profit organization, JC accredits and certifies more than 15,000 health care organizations and programs in the United States which is recognized nationwide as a symbol of quality that reflects an organization's commitment to meeting certain performance standards.

Managed Care Information Center (MCIC)

http://www.managedcaremarketplace.com

An online yellow pages for companies providing services to Managed Care Organizations (MCO), hospitals and physician groups. There are more than three dozen targeted categories, offering information on vendors from claims processing to transportation services to health care compliance.

National Association for Healthcare Quality (NAHQ)

http://www.nahq.org

Provides vital research, education, networking, certification and professional practice resources, designed to empower healthcare quality professionals from every specialty. This leading resource for healthcare quality professionals is an essential connection for leadership, excellence and innovation in healthcare quality.

National Association for Health Care Recruitment (NAHCR)

http://www.nahcr.com

Supports individuals employed directly by hospitals and other health care organizations which are involved in the practice of professional health care recruitment. Promotes sound principles of professional healthcare recruitment. Provides financial assistance to aid members in planning and implementing regional educational programs. Offers technical assistance and consultation services. Compiles statistics.

National Association Medical Staff Services (NAMSS)

http://www.namss.org

Supports individuals involved in the management and administration of health care provider services. Seeks to enhance the knowledge and experience of medical staff services professionals and promote the certification of those involved in the profession.

National Association of Dental Plans (NADP)

http://www.nadp.org

Promotes and advances the dental benefits industry to improve consumer access to affordable, quality dental care.

National Association of Insurance Commissoners (NAIC)

http://www.naic.org

The mission of the NAIC is to assist state insurance regulators, individually and collectively, in serving the public interest and achieving the following fundamental insurance regulatory goals in a responsive, efficient and cost effective manner, consistent with the wishes of its members: protect the public interest; promote competitive markets; facilitate the fair and equitable treatment of insurance consumers; promote the reliability, solvency and financial solidity of insurance institutions; and support and improve state regulation of insurance.

The NAIC also provides links to State Insurance Department web sites *(http://www.naic.org/state_web_map.htm)*.

The National Association of Managed Care Regulators (NAMCR)

http://www.namcr.org

Includes both regulator members and associate industry members. Established in 1975, NAMCR provides expertise and a forum for discussion to state regulators and managed care companies about current issues facing managed care. NAMCR has also provided expertise to the National Association of Insurance Commissioners (NAIC) in preparation of NAIC Model Acts used by many states.

National Association of State Medicaid Directors (NASMD)

http://www.nasmd.org

Promotes effective Medicaid policy and program administration; works with the federal government on issues through technical advisory groups. Conducts forums on policy and technical issues.

National Committee for Quality Assurance (NCQA)

http://www.ncqa.org

The National Committee for Quality Assurance (NCQA) is a private, not-for-profit organization dedicated to assessing and reporting on the quality of managed care plans. Their efforts are organized around two activities, accreditation and performance measurement, which are complementary strategies for producing information to guide choice.

National Institute for Health Care Management Research and Educational Foundation (NIHCM Foundation)

http://www.nihcm.org

A nonprofit, nonpartisan group that conducts research on health care issues. The Foundation disseminates research findings and analysis and holds forums and briefings for policy makers, the health care industry, consumers, the government, and the media to increase understanding of issues affecting the health care system.

National Quality Forum (NQF)

http://www.qualityforum.org

A not-for-profit membership organization created to develop and implement a national strategy for health care quality measurement and reporting, Prompted by the impact of health care quality on patient outcomes, workforce productivity, and health care costs. NQF has broad participation from all parts of the health care system, including national, state, regional, and local groups representing consumers, public and private purchasers, employers, health care professionals, provider organizations.,health plans, accrediting bodies, labor unions, supporting industries, and organizations.

National Society of Certified Healthcare Business Consultants (NSCHBC)

http://www.ichbc.org

The NSCHBC is a national organization dedicated to serving the needs of consultants who provide ethical, confidential and professional advice to the healthcare industry. Membership by successful completion of certification examination only.

Professional Association of Health Care Office Management (PAHCOM)

http://www.pahcom.com

Supports office managers of small group and solo medical practices. Operates certification program for healthcare office managers.

U.S. Food and Drug Administration (USFDA)

http://www.fda.gov

A department of the U.S. Department of Health and Human Services, the Food and Drug Administration provides information regarding health, medicine and nutrition. Their MedWatch Safety Information and Adverse Event Reporting Program serves both healthcare professionals and the public. MedWatch provides clinical information about safety issues involving medical products, including prescription and over-the-counter drugs, biologics, dietary supplements, and medical devices *(http://www.fda.gov/medwatch)*.

Plan Index

HMO

Aetna Better Health of Michigan Detroit, MI, 404

Aetna Better Health of West Virginia Charleston, WV, 818

Aetna Health of Arizona Hartford, CT, 18

Aetna Health of California Hartford, CT, 58

Aetna Health of Colorado Hartford, CT, 149

Aetna Health of Connecticut Hartford, CT, 170

Aetna Health of Delaware Hartford, CT, 185

Aetna Health of District of Columbia Hartford, CT, 192

Aetna Health of Florida Hartford, CT, 198

Aetna Health of Georgia Hartford, CT, 234

Aetna Health of Illinois Hartford, CT, 267

Aetna Health of Indiana Hartford, CT, 291

Aetna Health of Kansas Hartford, CT, 324, 325

Aetna Health of Kentucky Hartford, CT, 340

Aetna Health of Maine Hartford, CT, 363

Aetna Health of Maryland Hartford, CT, 371

Aetna Health of Massachusetts Hartford, CT, 386

Aetna Health of Michigan Hartford, CT, 405

Aetna Health of Missouri Hartford, CT, 458

Aetna Health of Nevada Hartford, CT, 497

Aetna Health of New Jersey Hartford, CT, 517

Aetna Health of New York Hartford, CT, 543

Aetna Health of North Carolina Hartford, CT, 585

Aetna Health of Ohio Hartford, CT, 603

Aetna Health of Oklahoma Hartford, CT, 627

Aetna Health of Pennsylvania Hartford, CT, 658

Aetna Health of Tennessee Hartford, CT, 720

Aetna Health of Texas Hartford, CT, 733

Aetna Health of Virginia Hartford, CT, 792

Aetna Student Health Hartford, CT, 173

Affinity Health Plan Bronx, NY, 544

Alameda Alliance for Health Alameda, CA, 59

Allegiance Life & Health Insurance Company Missoula, MT, 453

Alliant Health Plans Dalton, GA, 235

Allied Pacific IPA Alhambra, CA, 62

AlohaCare Honolulu, HI, 250

Altius Health Plans of Utah Sandy, UT, 774

American Specialty Health San Diego, CA, 63

Amerigroup Georgia Atlanta, GA, 236

Amerigroup Iowa Clive, IA, 312

Amerigroup Maryland Hanover, MD, 373

Amerigroup Nevada Las Vegas, NV, 498

Amerigroup Tennessee Nashville, TN, 721

Amerigroup Texas Grand Prairie, TX, 737

AmeriHealth New Jersey Cranbury, NJ, 518

AmeriHealth Pennsylvania Philadelphia, PA, 660

Anthem Blue Cross & Blue Shield of Colorado Denver, CO, 151

Anthem Blue Cross & Blue Shield of Connecticut Wallingford, CT, 174

Anthem Blue Cross & Blue Shield of Georgia Atlanta, GA, 237

Anthem Blue Cross & Blue Shield of Indiana Lafayette, IN, 293

Anthem Blue Cross & Blue Shield of Kentucky Lexington, KY, 341

Anthem Blue Cross & Blue Shield of Maine South Portland, ME, 364

Anthem Blue Cross & Blue Shield of Missouri St Louis, MO, 460

Anthem Blue Cross & Blue Shield of Nevada Las Vegas, NV, 499

Anthem Blue Cross & Blue Shield of New Hampshire Manchester, NH, 511

Anthem Blue Cross & Blue Shield of Virginia Richmond, VA, 793

Anthem Blue Cross & Blue Shield of Wisconsin Milwaukee, WI, 830

Anthem Blue Cross of California Los Angeles, CA, 64

Anthem, Inc. Indianapolis, IN, 294

Atlanticare Health Plans Egg Harbor Township, NJ, 519

Aultcare Corporation Canton, OH, 605

Avera Health Plans Sioux Falls, SD, 713

AvMed Gainesville Gainesville, FL, 202

AvMed Jacksonville Jacksonville, FL, 203

AvMed Orlando Orlando, FL, 204

AvMed Tampa Bay Tampa, FL, 206

Baptist Health Plan Lexington, KY, 342

Blue Care Network of Michigan Southfield, MI, 407, 408

Blue Cross & Blue Shield of Arizona Phoenix, AZ, 22

Blue Cross & Blue Shield of Illinois Chicago, IL, 268

Blue Cross & Blue Shield of Massachusetts Boston, MA, 389

Blue Cross & Blue Shield of Minnesota St. Paul, MN, 440

Blue Cross & Blue Shield of Montana Helena, MT, 478

Blue Cross & Blue Shield of New Mexico Albuquerque, NM, 532

Blue Cross & Blue Shield of Oklahoma Tulsa, OK, 629

Blue Cross & Blue Shield of Rhode Island Providence, RI, 697

Blue Cross & Blue Shield of South Carolina Columbia, SC, 705

Blue Cross & Blue Shield of Texas Richardson, TX, 740

Blue Cross & Blue Shield of Wyoming Cheyenne, WY, 856

Blue Cross and Blue Shield of Alabama Birmingham, AL, 4

Blue Cross and Blue Shield of Kansas Topeka, KS, 327

Blue Cross and Blue Shield of Louisiana Baton Rouge, LA, 353

Blue Cross Blue Shield of Georgia Atlanta, GA, 238

Blue Cross Blue Shield of North Carolina Durham, NC, 586

Blue Cross of Idaho Health Service, Inc. Meridian, ID, 259

Blue Shield of California San Francisco, CA, 66

BlueCross BlueShield of Western New York Buffalo, NY, 546

BlueShield of Northeastern New York Latham, NY, 547

Brand New Day HMO Westminster, CA, 67

BridgeSpan Health Salt Like City, UT, 775

Bright Health Alabama Minneapolis, MN, 5

Bright Health Colorado Minneapolis, MN, 155

CalOptima Orange, CA, 71

Capital BlueCross Harrisburg, PA, 662

Capital Health Plan Tallahassee, FL, 207

Care1st Health Plan Arizona Phoenix, AZ, 23

Care1st Health Plan California Monterey Park, CA, 73

CareCentrix Hartford, CT, 175

CareCentrix: Arizona Phoenix, AZ, 24

CareCentrix: Florida Tampa, FL, 208

CareCentrix: Kansas Overland Park, KS, 328

CareCentrix: New York Melville, NY, 548

CareFirst Blue Cross & Blue Shield of Virginia Owings Mills, MD, 794

CareFirst BlueCross BlueShield Baltimore, MD, 375

CDPHP: Capital District Physicians' Health Plan Albany, NY, 550

CenCal Health Santa Barbara, CA, 76

Centene Corporation St. Louis, MO, 462

Central California Alliance for Health Scotts Valley, CA, 77

Children's Mercy Integrated Care Solutions Kansas City, MO, 463

Chinese Community Health Plan San Francisco, CA, 79

Cigna HealthCare of Arizona Bloomfield, CT, 25

Cigna HealthCare of Colorado Denver, CO, 156

Cigna HealthCare of Florida Bloomfield, CT, 210

Cigna HealthCare of Oklahoma Bloomfield, CT, 630

Cigna HealthCare of Tennessee Bloomfield, CT, 631

Cigna HealthCare of Texas Bloomfield, CT, 742

Cigna Medical Group Phoenix, AZ, 26

Colorado Access Aurora, CO, 157

Colorado Choice Health Plans Alamosa, CO, 158

Colorado Health Partnerships Colorado Springs, CO, 159

Community First Health Plans San Antonio, TX, 743

Community Health Group Chula Vista, CA, 83

Community Health Options Lewiston, ME, 365

CompBenefits Corporation Roswell, GA, 239

ConnectiCare Farmington, CT, 178

Contra Costa Health Services Martinez, CA, 85

Coventry Health & Life Ins. Co. of Tennessee Memphis, TN, 726

Coventry Health Care of Alaska Bethesda, MD, 13

Coventry Health Care of California Orange, CA, 86

Coventry Health Care of Colorado Bethesda, MD, 160

Coventry Health Care of Connecticut Bethesda, MD, 179

Coventry Health Care of Florida Sunrise, FL, 211

Coventry Health Care of Georgia Atlanta, GA, 240

Coventry Health Care of Hawaii Bethesda, MD, 252

Coventry Health Care of Illinois Champaign, IL, 273

Coventry Health Care of Indiana Bethesda, MD, 297

Coventry Health Care of Iowa Urbandale, IA, 313

Coventry Health Care of Kansas Wichita, KS, 329

Coventry Health Care of Louisiana Baton Rouge, LA, 354

Coventry Health Care of Maine Bethesda, MD, 366

Coventry Health Care of Michigan Detroit, MI, 412

Coventry Health Care of Minnesota Bethesda, MD, 441

Coventry Health Care of Missouri St. Louis, MO, 464

Coventry Health Care of Montana Bethesda, MD, 479

Coventry Health Care of Nebraska Omaha, NE, 488

Coventry Health Care of Nevada Bethesda, MD, 501

Coventry Health Care of New Hampshire Manchester, NH, 512

Coventry Health Care of New Jersey Trenton, NJ, 521

Coventry Health Care of New Mexico Bethesda, MD, 533

Coventry Health Care of New York Bethesda, MD, 551

Coventry Health Care of North Dakota Bismarck, ND, 597

Coventry Health Care of Rhode Island Bethesda, MD, 698

Coventry Health Care of Texas Irving, TX, 746

Coventry Health Care of the Carolinas Charlotte, NC, 587

Coventry Health Care of Vermont Bethesda, MD, 790

Coventry Health Care of Washington Bethesda, MD, 809

Coventry Health Care of Wisconsin Waukesha, WI, 835

Coventry Health Care, Inc. Bethesda, MD, 376

CoventryCares of Kentucky Louisville, KY, 344

Cox Healthplans Springfield, MO, 465

DakotaCare Sioux Falls, SD, 714

Denver Health Medical Plan Denver, CO, 162

Emi Health Murray, UT, 776

Empire BlueCross BlueShield Brooklyn, NY, 558

Excellus BlueCross BlueShield Rochester, NY, 559

FirstCarolinaCare Pinehurst, NC, 591

Florida Blue Jacksonville, FL, 213

Florida Health Care Plans Holly Hill, FL, 214

Frazier Insurance Agency Little Rock, AR, 51

Gateway Health Pittsburgh, PA, 665

Geisinger Health Plan Danville, PA, 666

Golden Rule Insurance Indianapolis, IN, 300

Group Health Cooperative of Eau Claire Altoona, WI, 839

Group Health Cooperative of South Central Wisconsin Madison, WI, 840

Group Health Insurance New York, NY, 562

Guardian Life Insurance Company of America New York, NY, 563

Gundersen Lutheran Health Plan Onalaska, WI, 841

HAP-Health Alliance Plan: Flint Flint, MI, 417

Harvard Pilgrim Health Care Connecticut Hartford, CT, 180

Harvard Pilgrim Health Care New Hampshire Manchester, NH, 513

Hawaii Medical Service Association Honolulu, HI, 254

hawk-i Healthy and Well Kids in Iowa , IA, 315

HCSC Insurance Services Company Chicago, IL, 276

HCSC Insurance Services Company Helena, MT, 481

HCSC Insurance Services Company Albuquerque, NM, 535

HCSC Insurance Services Company Tulsa, OK, 634

HCSC Insurance Services Company Richardson, TX, 750

Health Alliance Urbana, IL, 277

Health Alliance Plan Detroit, MI, 420

Health Care Service Corporation Chicago, IL, 279

Health Choice Arizona Phoenix, AZ, 29

Health Net, Inc. Woodland Hills, CA, 101

Health New England Springfield, MA, 393

Health Plan of Nevada Las Vegas, NV, 502

Health Plan of San Joaquin French Camp, CA, 102

Health Plan of San Mateo South San Francisco, CA, 103

Health Tradition Onalaska, WI, 842

HealthPartners Bloomington, MN, 443

Healthy Indiana Plan , IN, 301

Heart of America Health Plan Rugby, ND, 598

Hennepin Health Minneapolis, MN, 444

Highmark BCBS Delaware Pittsburgh, PA, 187

Highmark Blue Cross Blue Shield Pittsburgh, PA, 669

Horizon Blue Cross Blue Shield of New Jersey Newark, NJ, 523

Humana Employers Health Plan of Georgia, Inc. Atlanta, GA, 242

Humana Health Insurance Company of Florida, Inc. Doral, FL, 221

Humana Health Insurance of Alabama Huntsville, AL, 7

Humana Health Insurance of Alaska Vancouver, WA, 14

Humana Health Insurance of Arizona Phoenix, AZ, 30

Humana Health Insurance of Arkansas Little Rock, AR, 53

Humana Health Insurance of California Irvine, CA, 105

Humana Health Insurance of Colorado Colorado Springs, CO, 163

Humana Health Insurance of Connecticut Mahwah, NJ, 181

Humana Health Insurance of Delaware Mechanicsburg, PA, 188

Humana Health Insurance of Hawaii Honolulu, HI, 255

Humana Health Insurance of Idaho Meridian, ID, 261

Humana Health Insurance of Illinois Oak Brook, IL, 280

Humana Health Insurance of Indiana Indianapolis, IN, 302

Humana Health Insurance of Iowa Bettendorf, IA, 316

Medicare

GHI Medicare Plan New York, NY, 561

HAP-Health Alliance Plan: Senior Medicare Plan Detroit, MI, 418
Health Alliance Medicare Urbana, IL, 278
Health Alliance Medicare Detroit, MI, 419
Health First Health Plans Rockledge, FL, 216
Health First Medicare Plans Rockledge, FL, 217
Health Partners Plans Philadelphia, PA, 667
HealthSun Coconut Grove, FL, 219
HealthSun Health Plans Coconut Grove, FL, 220
Humana Medicare Lexington, KY, 347

Independent Health Medicare Plan Buffalo, NY, 568
InnovaCare Health Fort Lee, NJ, 691
InStil Health Columbia, SC, 709
Inter Valley Health Plan Pomona, CA, 106

Medica HealthCare Plans, Inc Miami, FL, 119
MediGold Columbus, OH, 612
Meridian Health Plan of Illinois Chicago, IL, 282
MetroPlus Health Plan New York, NY, 574
Molina Healthcare Long Beach, CA, 120
Molina Healthcare of California Long Beach, CA, 121
Molina Healthcare of Florida Miami, FL, 225
Molina Healthcare of Illinois Oak Brook, IL, 283
Molina Healthcare of Michigan Troy, MI, 423
Molina Healthcare of New Mexico Albuquerque, NM, 537
Molina Healthcare of New York North Syracuse, NY, 575
Molina Healthcare of Ohio Columbus, OH, 613
Molina Healthcare of South Carolina North Charleston, SC, 710
Molina Healthcare of Texas Irving, TX, 757
Molina Healthcare of Utah Midvale, UT, 779
Molina Healthcare of Virgina Glen Allen, VA, 799
Molina Healthcare of Washington Bothell, WA, 814
Molina Healthcare of Wisconsin Milwaukee, WI, 846
Molina Medicaid Solutions Long Beach, CA, 122
Molina Medicaid Solutions Boise, ID, 262
Molina Medicaid Solutions Baton Rouge, LA, 357
Molina Medicaid Solutions Augusta, ME, 369
Molina Medicaid Solutions Trenton, NJ, 527
Molina Medicaid Solutions Charleston, WV, 824

Paramount Elite Medicare Plan Maumee, OH, 617
PMC Medicare Choice San Juan, PR, 694
Presbyterian Medicare Advantage Plans Albuquerque, NM, 540
Prime Time Health Medicare Plan Canton, OH, 619
PriorityHealth Medicare Plans Grand Rapids, MI, 427

Quality Health Plans of New York Ronkonkoma, NY, 579

SilverScript Phoenix, AZ, 42
Soundpath Health Federal Way, WA, 815
Sterling Insurance Austin, TX, 763
SummaCare Medicare Advantage Plan Akron, OH, 621

Texas HealthSpring Houston, TX, 765
Tufts Health Medicare Plan Watertown, MA, 400

UnitedHealth Group Minneapolis, MN, 450

Universal American Medicare Plans White Plains, NY, 584

Vantage Medicare Advantage Monroe, LA, 362

WellCare Health Plans Tampa, FL, 233

Multiple

Aetna Inc. Hartford, CT, 171
AlphaCare Brooklyn, NY, 545
Altius Health Plans Sandy, UT, 773
American Family Insurance Madison, WI, 829
Ameritas Lincoln, NE, 486
Arizona Foundation for Medical Care Phoenix, AZ, 20
Arkansas Blue Cross Blue Shield Little Rock, AR, 49
Assurant Employee Benefits Wisconsin Brookfield, WI, 832
Asuris Northwest Health , WA, 807
Avesis: Arizona Phoenix, AZ, 21

Beta Health Association, Inc. Denver, CO, 153
Blue Cross & Blue Shield of Tennessee Chattanooga, TN, 723
Blue Cross Blue Shield of Michigan Detroit, MI, 409
BlueChoice Health Plan of South Carolina Columbia, SC, 706
BlueCross BlueShield of Puerto Rico San Juan, PR, 688

ChiroSource, Inc. Clayton, CA, 80
Cigna Corporation Bloomfield, CT, 176
Cigna HealthCare of California Bloomfield, CT, 81
Community Health Plan of Washington Seattle, WA, 808
CommunityCare Tulsa, OK, 632
Consumers Direct Insurance Services (CDIS) Dallas, TX, 745

Dean Health Plan Madison, WI, 836

eHealthInsurance Services, Inc. Mountain View, CA, 93
EPIC Pharmacy Network Mechanicsville, VA, 797

Fallon Health Worcester, MA, 391
Fidelis Care Rego Park, NY, 560
First Medical Health Plan Guaynabo, PR, 689

Golden West Dental & Vision Camarillo, CA, 97

Harvard Pilgrim Health Care Maine Portland, ME, 367
Harvard Pilgrim Health Care Massachusetts Wellesley, MA, 392
Health Net Federal Services Rancho Cordova, CA, 99
Health Net Insurance Van Nuys, CA, 100
HealthAmerica Harrisburg, PA, 668
Healthfirst New York, NY, 564
HealthLink HMO St. Louis, MO, 470
Hometown Health Plan Reno, NV, 503

Kaiser Permanente Mid-Atlantic Rockville, MD, 380
Kaiser Permanente Southern California San Diego, CA, 109
KelseyCare Advantage Pearland, TX, 754

Magnolia Health Jackson, MS, 456
Martin's Point HealthCare Portland, ME, 368
Medical Card System (MCS) San Juan, PR, 692
Mercy Care Plan/Mercy Care Advantage Phoenix, AZ, 35
Meritain Health Amherst, NY, 573

MHNet Behavioral Health Austin, TX, 756

Mid America Health Greenwood, IN, 303

Mid-Atlantic Behavioral Health Newark, DE, 189

MMM Holdings San Juan, PR, 693

Moda Health Alaska Anchorage, AK, 15

Moda Health Oregon Portland, OR, 648

MVP Health Care Schenectady, NY, 576

Nova Healthcare Administrators Williamsville, NY, 577

Ohio State University Health Plan Inc. Columbus, OH, 615

Optum Complex Medical Conditions Eden Prairie, MN, 448

Pacific Foundation for Medical Care Santa Rosa, CA, 125

PacificSource Health Plans Springfield, OR, 649

Piedmont Community Health Plan Lynchburg, VA, 801

Preferred Care Partners Miami, FL, 228

Preferred Mental Health Management Wichita, KS, 335

Primary Health Medical Group Garden City, ID, 263

Providence Health Plan Portland, OR, 651

QualCare Piscataway, NJ, 528

Regence BlueCross BlueShield of Oregon Portland, OR, 652

Regence BlueCross BlueShield of Utah Portland, OR, 783

Regence BlueShield of Idaho Lewiston, ID, 264

Samaritan Health Plan Operations Corvallis, OR, 653

Scott & White Health Plan Temple, TX, 760

Security Health Plan of Wisconsin Marshfield, WI, 850

Spectera Eyecare Networks Columbia, MD, 382

Sun Life Financial Kansas City, MO, 475

Taylor Benefits San Jose, CA, 138

TexanPlus Medicare Advantage HMO Austin, TX, 764

The Dental Care Plus Group Cincinnati, OH, 623

Trillium Community Health Plan Eugene, OR, 654

Tufts Health Plan Watertown, MA, 401

Tufts Health Plan: Rhode Island Providence, RI, 702

UCare Minneapolis, MN, 449

UniCare West Virginia Charleston, WV, 826

Unity Health Insurance Sauk City, WI, 853

UPMC Health Plan Altoona, PA, 683

Valley Preferred Allentown, PA, 686

Wellmark Blue Cross & Blue Shield of South Dakota Sioux Falls, SD, 719

Wisconsin Physician's Service Madison, WI, 854

PPO

Aetna Health of Alabama Hartford, CT, 1

Aetna Health of Alaska Hartford, CT, 12

Aetna Health of Arkansas Hartford, CT, 48

Aetna Health of California Hartford, CT, 58

Aetna Health of Colorado Hartford, CT, 149

Aetna Health of Connecticut Hartford, CT, 170

Aetna Health of Delaware Hartford, CT, 185

Aetna Health of District of Columbia Hartford, CT, 192

Aetna Health of Florida Hartford, CT, 198

Aetna Health of Georgia Hartford, CT, 234

Aetna Health of Hawaii Hartford, CT, 249

Aetna Health of Idaho Hartford, CT, 258

Aetna Health of Illinois Hartford, CT, 267

Aetna Health of Indiana Hartford, CT, 291

Aetna Health of Iowa Hartford, CT, 311

Aetna Health of Kansas Hartford, CT, 324, 325

Aetna Health of Kentucky Hartford, CT, 340

Aetna Health of Louisiana Hartford, CT, 352

Aetna Health of Maine Hartford, CT, 363

Aetna Health of Maryland Hartford, CT, 371

Aetna Health of Massachusetts Hartford, CT, 386

Aetna Health of Michigan Hartford, CT, 405

Aetna Health of Minnesota Hartford, CT, 437

Aetna Health of Mississippi Hartford, CT, 452

Aetna Health of Missouri Hartford, CT, 458

Aetna Health of Montana Hartford, CT, 477

Aetna Health of Nevada Hartford, CT, 497

Aetna Health of New Jersey Hartford, CT, 517

Aetna Health of New York Hartford, CT, 543

Aetna Health of North Carolina Hartford, CT, 585

Aetna Health of North Dakota Hartford, CT, 596

Aetna Health of Ohio Hartford, CT, 603

Aetna Health of Oklahoma Hartford, CT, 627

Aetna Health of Oregon Hartford, CT, 638

Aetna Health of Pennsylvania Hartford, CT, 658

Aetna Health of Rhode Island Hartford, CT, 696

Aetna Health of South Carolina Hartford, CT, 704

Aetna Health of Tennessee Hartford, CT, 720

Aetna Health of Texas Hartford, CT, 733

Aetna Health of Utah Hartford, CT, 772

Aetna Health of Vermont Hartford, CT, 788

Aetna Health of Virginia Hartford, CT, 792

Aetna Health of Washington Hartford, CT, 805

Aetna Health of West Virginia Hartford, CT, 819

Aetna Health of Wisconsin Hartford, CT, 828

Aetna Health of Wyoming Hartford, CT, 855

Aetna Student Health Hartford, CT, 173

Alliance Regional Health Network Amarillo, TX, 734

Alliant Health Plans Dalton, GA, 235

Altius Health Plans of Utah Sandy, UT, 774

American Health Care Alliance Kansas City, MO, 459

American Health Network Indianapolis, IN, 292

American National Insurance Company Galveston, TX, 735

American Postal Workers Union (APWU) Health Plan Glen Burnie, MD, 372

American PPO Irving, TX, 736

Americas PPO Bloomington, MN, 438

AmeriHealth New Jersey Cranbury, NJ, 518

AmeriHealth Pennsylvania Philadelphia, PA, 660

Anthem Blue Cross & Blue Shield of Colorado Denver, CO, 151

Anthem Blue Cross & Blue Shield of Connecticut Wallingford, CT, 174

Anthem Blue Cross & Blue Shield of Georgia Atlanta, GA, 237

Anthem Blue Cross & Blue Shield of Indiana Lafayette, IN, 293

Anthem Blue Cross & Blue Shield of Kentucky Lexington, KY, 341

Anthem Blue Cross & Blue Shield of Maine South Portland, ME, 364

Vision

Personnel Index

A

Abelman, David Dentaquest, 390

Abraham, Karen Blue Cross & Blue Shield of Arizona, 22

Abrahamson, April Colorado Access, 157

Adams, Derek HAP-Health Alliance Plan: Flint, 417

Adams, Derek Health Alliance Medicare, 419

Adams, Derek Health Alliance Plan, 420

Adams, Derick W. HAP-Health Alliance Plan: Senior Medicare Plan, 418

Adams, Gregory A. Kaiser Permanente Mid-Atlantic, 380

Adams, Gregory A. Kaiser Permanente Northwest, 645

Adams, Joann Florida Health Care Plans, 214

Adams, Lavdena, MD AmeriHealth Caritas District of Columbia, 193

Adler, Jeremy Blue Cross & Blue Shield of Arizona, 22

Aga, Dr. Donald KelseyCare Advantage, 754

Agpaoa, Ronda Taylor Benefits, 138

Albert, Stephanie Delta Dental of Minnesota, 442

Aliabadi, Karen Delta Dental of Washington, 810

Allen, Ashley Health New England, 393

Allen, Calvin HealthPartners, 443

Allen, Kirk Ascension At Home, 2, 295, 326, 406, 628, 738, 831

Allen, Robert W. Intermountain Healthcare, 778

Allford, Allan Delta Dental of Arizona, 27

Almquist, Stacia Sun Life Financial, 475

Altman, Maya Health Plan of San Mateo, 103

Altmann, Lynn Medica, 446

Altmann, Lynn Medica with CHI Health, 491

Altmann, Lynn Medica: Nebraska, 492

Altmann, Lynn Medica: North Dakota, 600

Alvarez, Diana Health Choice Arizona, 29

Alvarez, Nico Liberty Dental Plan of Florida, 223

Alvarez, Nico Liberty Dental Plan of Illinois, 281

Alvarez, Nico Liberty Dental Plan of Nevada, 505

Alvarez, Nico Liberty Dental Plan of New York, 570

Ambrose, David CenCal Health, 76

Amstutz, Karen Magellan Health, 31

Amstutz, Karen Magellan Healthcare, 32

Amstutz, Karen Magellan Complete Care of Florida, 224

Anand, Tej CareCentrix: Arizona, 24

Anand, Tej CareCentrix, 175

Anand, Tej CareCentrix: Florida, 208

Anand, Tej CareCentrix: Kansas, 328

Anand, Tej CareCentrix: New York, 548

Anderl, Richard Mutual of Omaha Dental Insurance, 494

Anderl, Richard Mutual of Omaha Health Plans, 495

Andersen, Lori Santa Clara Family Health Foundations Inc, 132

Anderson, David Delta Dental of Minnesota, 442

Anderson, David W. BlueCross BlueShield of Western New York, 546

Anderson, David W. BlueShield of Northeastern New York, 547

Anderson, Deborah Network Health Plan of Wisconsin, 847

Anderson, Joel Essence Healthcare, 468

Anderson, John Concentra, 744

Anderson, Kraig Moda Health Alaska, 15

Anderson, Mark Delta Dental of Arizona, 27

Anderson, William Assurant Employee Benefits Wisconsin, 832

Anglin, Scott Amerigroup Florida, 199

Ann Tournoux, Mary Health Alliance Medicare, 419

Anthony, William P., MD CHN PPO, 520

Aponte Amador, Jos, Medical Card System (MCS), 692

Arakelian, Ronald, MD Stanislaus Foundation for Medical Care, 136

Armenti, Steve CHN PPO, 520

Armstrong, Cathleen HealthSCOPE Benefits, 52

Arnold-Miller, Erica Colorado Health Partnerships, 159

Arrington Jr, Robyn James, MD Total Health Care, 429

Ash-Jackson, Linda, MD Hometown Health Plan, 503

Asher, Drew WellCare Health Plans, 233

Ashley, Jennine Opticare of Utah, 780

Atkins, C. Richard Blue Cross and Blue Shield of Louisiana, 353

Atkins, Meera CoreSource, 272

Auburn, Steve Trustmark Companies, 288

Aug, Matt Cox Healthplans, 465

Austen, Karla A. MVP Health Care, 576

Avery, Alan Kern Family Health Care, 110

Ayala, Jose Valley Baptist Health Plan, 771

Ayers, Kay AvMed, 200

Ayers, Kay AvMed Ft. Lauderdale, 201

Ayers, Kay AvMed Gainesville, 202

Ayers, Kay AvMed Jacksonville, 203

Ayers, Kay AvMed Orlando, 204

Ayers, Kay AvMed Pembroke Pines, 205

Ayers, Kay AvMed Tampa Bay, 206

B

Baackes, John L.A. Care Health Plan, 111, 112

Bacon, Cindy Island Group Administration, Inc., 569

Bacus, Lisa Cigna Medical Group, 26

Bacus, Lisa Texas HealthSpring, 765

Bahsin, Aman Alameda Alliance for Health, 59

Bahsin, Aman Alameda Medi-Cal Plan, 60

Bailey, Todd Health Plans, Inc., 394

Baird, Mark Medica, 446

Baird, Mark Medica with CHI Health, 491

Baird, Mark Medica: Nebraska, 492

Baird, Mark Medica: North Dakota, 600

Baker, G. Steven Public Employees Health Program, 782

Balladares, Victoria Contra Costa Health Services, 85

Ballard, Jeff Delta Dental of Tennessee, 727

Banatino Jr., Thomas Coventry Health Care of Alaska, 13

Bank, Julie MagnaCare, 572

Barasch, Richard A Universal American Medicare Plans, 584

Barasch, Richard A TexanPlus Medicare Advantage HMO, 764

Barker, Dave SIHO Insurance Services, 308

Barlow, Jeff D. Molina Medicaid Solutions, 122

Barlow, Jeff D. Molina Healthcare of Florida, 225

Barlow, Jeff D. Molina Medicaid Solutions, 262

Barlow, Jeff D. Molina Healthcare of Illinois, 283

Barlow, Jeff D. Molina Medicaid Solutions, 357, 369

Barlow, Jeff D. Molina Healthcare of Michigan, 423

Barlow, Jeff D. Molina Medicaid Solutions, 527

Barlow, Jeff D. Molina Healthcare of New Mexico, 537

Barlow, Jeff D. Molina Healthcare of New York, 575

Barlow, Jeff D. Molina Healthcare of Ohio, 613

Barlow, Jeff D. Molina Healthcare of South Carolina, 710

Barlow, Jeff D. Molina Healthcare of Texas, 757

Barlow, Jeff D. Molina Healthcare of Utah, 779

Barlow, Jeff D. Molina Healthcare of Virgina, 799

Barlow, Jeff D. Molina Healthcare of Washington, 814

Barlow, Jeff D. Molina Medicaid Solutions, 824

Barlow, Jeff D. Molina Healthcare of Wisconsin, 846

Barnett, Curtis Arkansas Blue Cross Blue Shield, 49

Barney, Erin Blue Cross & Blue Shield of Texas, 740

Barth, Anthony S. Delta Dental of California, 87

Barth, Tony Delta Dental of Delaware, 186

Barth, Tony Delta Dental of the District of Columbia, 194

Barth, Tony Delta Dental Insurance Company, 241

Barth, Tony Delta Dental of New York, 553

Barth, Tony Delta Dental of Pennsylvania, 663

Bartlett, Mark Blue Care Network of Michigan, 408

Bartlett, Mark R. Blue Care Network of Michigan, 407

Bartlett, Mark R. Blue Cross Blue Shield of Michigan, 409

Bartlett, Tom HealthSCOPE Benefits, 52

Bartsh, Geoff Medica, 446

Bartsh, Geoff Medica with CHI Health, 491

Bartsh, Geoff Medica: Nebraska, 492

Bartsh, Geoff Medica: North Dakota, 600

Barwig, Mark P EPIC Pharmacy Network, 797

Bass, Stephan, MD GEMCare Health Plan, 96

Batra, Romilla SCAN Health Plan, 134

Batteer, Cathy UPMC Health Plan, 683

Bauer, Jennifer Delta Dental of Kansas, 330

Bauer, Michele, MD Group Health Cooperative of Eau Claire, 839

Bayer, Terry Molina Healthcare, 120

Bayer, Terry Molina Medicaid Solutions, 122

Bayer, Terry Molina Healthcare of Florida, 225

Bayer, Terry Molina Medicaid Solutions, 262

Bayer, Terry Molina Healthcare of Illinois, 283

Bayer, Terry Molina Medicaid Solutions, 357, 369

Bayer, Terry Molina Healthcare of Michigan, 423

Bayer, Terry Molina Medicaid Solutions, 527

Bayer, Terry Molina Healthcare of New Mexico, 537

Bayer, Terry Molina Healthcare of New York, 575

Bayer, Terry Molina Healthcare of Ohio, 613

Bayer, Terry Molina Healthcare of South Carolina, 710

Bayer, Terry Molina Healthcare of Texas, 757

Bayer, Terry Molina Healthcare of Utah, 779

Bayer, Terry Molina Healthcare of Virgina, 799

Bayer, Terry Molina Healthcare of Washington, 814

Bayer, Terry Molina Medicaid Solutions, 824

Bayer, Terry Molina Healthcare of Wisconsin, 846

Bea, Javon R. MercyHealth System, 845

Beagan, Kevin Minuteman Health, 397

Beasley, Tim HealthSCOPE Benefits, 52

Beaver, Cindy Crescent Health Solutions, 588

Becker, Jon Delta Dental of Minnesota, 442

Beckett, Darrell Blue Cross & Blue Shield of Texas, 740

Beckman, Jill Blue Cross Blue Shield of Kansas City, 461

Beed, Margaret, MD Health Plan of San Mateo, 103

Begay, Sandra Presbyterian Health Plan, 539

Bell, Carla The Health Plan of the Ohio Valley/Mountaineer Region, 624

Bellah, Ann Pueblo Health Care, 166

Bennett, John D, MD CDPHP: Capital District Physicians' Health Plan, 550

Bennett, John D. CDPHP Medicare Plan, 549

Bensing, Gary Passport Health Plan, 348

Bentley, Brad AvMed Pembroke Pines, 205

Bentley, Danny Davis Vision, 552

Berardo, Joseph, Jr MagnaCare, 572

Berg, Brad Delta Dental of Washington, 810

Berge, Frank Dencap Dental Plans, 414

Berge, Leanne Community Health Plan of Washington, 808

Bermel, John J. Healthfirst, 564

Bernard, Ken Health New England, 393

Bernard, Milton, DDS Quality Plan Administrators, 195

Bernards, Vicki Wisconsin Physician's Service, 854

Berry, Peter CareFirst Blue Cross & Blue Shield of Virginia, 794

Bertolini, Mark Aetna Health of Alabama, 1

Bertolini, Mark Aetna Health of Alaska, 12

Bertolini, Mark Aetna Health of Arizona, 18

Bertolini, Mark Aetna Health of Arkansas, 48

Bertolini, Mark Aetna Health of California, 58

Bertolini, Mark Aetna Health of Colorado, 149

Bertolini, Mark Aetna Health of Connecticut, 170

Bertolini, Mark Aetna Inc., 171

Bertolini, Mark Aetna Medicare, 172

Bertolini, Mark Aetna Health of Delaware, 185

Bertolini, Mark Aetna Health of District of Columbia, 192

Bertolini, Mark Aetna Health of Florida, 198

Bertolini, Mark Aetna Health of Georgia, 234

Bertolini, Mark Aetna Health of Hawaii, 249

Bertolini, Mark Aetna Health of Idaho, 258

Bertolini, Mark Aetna Health of Illinois, 267

Bertolini, Mark Aetna Health of Indiana, 291

Bertolini, Mark Aetna Health of Iowa, 311

Bertolini, Mark Aetna Health of Kansas, 324, 325

Bertolini, Mark Aetna Health of Kentucky, 340

Bertolini, Mark Aetna Health of Louisiana, 352

Bertolini, Mark Aetna Health of Maine, 363

Bertolini, Mark Aetna Health of Maryland, 371

Bertolini, Mark Aetna Health of Massachusetts, 386

Bertolini, Mark Aetna Health of Michigan, 405

Bertolini, Mark Aetna Health of Minnesota, 437

Bertolini, Mark Aetna Health of Mississippi, 452

Bertolini, Mark Aetna Health of Missouri, 458

Bertolini, Mark Aetna Health of Montana, 477

Bertolini, Mark Aetna Health of Nevada, 497

Bertolini, Mark Aetna Health of New Jersey, 517

Bertolini, Mark Aetna Health of New York, 543

Bertolini, Mark Aetna Health of North Carolina, 585

Broussard, Bruce Humana Health Insurance of Massachusetts, 395

Broussard, Bruce Humana Health Insurance of Minnesota, 445

Broussard, Bruce Humana Health Insurance of Missouri, 471

Broussard, Bruce Humana Health Insurance of Montana, 482

Broussard, Bruce Humana Health Insurance of Nebraska, 490

Broussard, Bruce Humana Health Insurance of Nevada, 504

Broussard, Bruce Humana Health Insurance of New Hampshire, 514

Broussard, Bruce Humana Health Insurance of New Jersey, 525

Broussard, Bruce Humana Health Insurance of New Mexico, 536

Broussard, Bruce Humana Health Insurance of New York, 566

Broussard, Bruce Humana Health Insurance of North Dakota, 599

Broussard, Bruce Humana Health Insurance of Oklahoma, 635

Broussard, Bruce Humana Health Insurance of Oregon, 644

Broussard, Bruce Humana Health Insurance of Pennsylvania, 671

Broussard, Bruce Humana Health Insurance of Puerto Rico, 690

Broussard, Bruce Humana Health Insurance of Rhode Island, 700

Broussard, Bruce Humana Health Insurance of South Carolina, 708

Broussard, Bruce Humana Health Insurance of South Dakota, 717

Broussard, Bruce Humana Health Insurance of Utah, 777

Broussard, Bruce Humana Health Insurance of Virginia, 798

Broussard, Bruce Humana Health Insurance of Washington, 812

Broussard, Bruce Humana Health Insurance of Wyoming, 858

Broussard, Bruce D. Humana Health Insurance of Alaska, 14

Broussard, Bruce D. Humana Health Insurance of Arizona, 30

Broussard, Bruce D. Humana Health Insurance of Colorado, 163

Broussard, Bruce D. CompBenefits Corporation, 239

Broussard, Bruce D. Humana Health Insurance of Illinois, 280

Broussard, Bruce D. Humana Health Insurance of Indiana, 302

Broussard, Bruce D. Humana Health Insurance of Iowa, 316

Broussard, Bruce D. Humana Inc., 346

Broussard, Bruce D. Humana Health Insurance of Michigan, 421

Broussard, Bruce D. Humana Health Insurance of Mississippi, 455

Broussard, Bruce D. Humana Health Insurance of North Carolina, 592

Broussard, Bruce D. Humana Health Insurance of Ohio, 609

Broussard, Bruce D. Humana Health Insurance of Tennessee, 730

Broussard, Bruce D. Humana Health Insurance of Texas, 753

Broussard, Bruce D. Humana Health Insurance of West Virginia, 823

Broussard, Bruce D. Humana Health Insurance of Wisconsin, 843

Brown, David Wellmark Blue Cross Blue Shield, 322

Brown, David Wellmark Blue Cross & Blue Shield of South Dakota, 719

Brown, Diane Trinity Health of Alabama, zzz

9

Brown, Jim Humana Health Insurance of California, 105

Brown, Jim Script Care, Ltd., 761

Brown, Sue Ann Davis Vision, 552

Brown, Susan E. Minuteman Health, 397

Brown Jr., John E. Blue Cross and Blue Shield of Louisiana, 353

Browne, Julie Government Employees Health Association (GEHA), 469

Brumbaugh, Brian Preferred Healthcare System, 677

Brusuelas, Mary, RN, BSN Central California Alliance for Health, 77

Bryan, John First Health, 94

Bryan, John Cofinity, 410

Bryan, Tab Script Care, Ltd., 761

Bryant, Phil HealthPartners, 729

Bryd, Michael Sharp Health Plan, 135

Buchert, Greg Care1st Cal MediConnect Plan, 72

Buchert, Greg Care1st Health Plan California, 73

Buchert, Greg Care1st Medicare, 74

Buck, Eric E. Preferred Health Care, 676

Budden, Joan Priority Health, 426

Budden, Joan PriorityHealth Medicare Plans, 427

Buggle, Janet QualCare, 528

Bunker, Jonathan W Health Plan of Nevada, 502

Buran, Gregory Network Health Plan of Wisconsin, 847

Burch, Vicki HealthPartners, 729

Burdick, Ken Easy Choice Health Plan, 92

Burdick, Ken WellCare Health Plans, 233

Burgin, Meryl CareFirst Blue Cross & Blue Shield of Virginia, 794

Burke, Jonathan Valley Preferred, 686

Burke, Richard P. Fallon Health, zzz

391

Burman, Bill Denver Health Medical Plan, 162

Burnett, Brian Presbyterian Health Plan, 539

Burnett, Brian Presbyterian Medicare Advantage Plans, 540

Burnett, David Neighborhood Health Plan of Rhode Island, 701

Burnett, Peg Denver Health Medical Plan, 162

Burrell, Chet CareFirst BlueCross BlueShield, 375

Burthay, Darcy Ascension At Home, 2, 295, 326, 406, 628, 738, 831

Burzynski, Mark Blue Cross & Blue Shield of Montana, 478

Busch, David BlueCross BlueShield of Western New York, 546

Busch, David BlueShield of Northeastern New York, 547

Bush, Stephen Scott & White Health Plan, 760

Butcher, Jeff Health Choice Arizona, 29

Butler, Martha Essence Healthcare, 468

Butts, Susan Cox Healthplans, 465

C

Cabanis, Clara Behavioral Healthcare, 152

Cagan, Laird, MD Boulder Valley Individual Practice Association, 154

Cahill, Maureen A. Anthem Blue Cross & Blue Shield of Georgia, 237

Cahill, Maureen A. Blue Cross Blue Shield of Georgia, 238

Cahill, Maureen A. BlueCross BlueShield Association, 269

Cahill, Maureen A. Anthem Blue Cross & Blue Shield of Indiana, 293

Cahill, Maureen A. Anthem Blue Cross & Blue Shield of Kentucky, 341

Cahill, Maureen A. Anthem Blue Cross & Blue Shield of Maine, 364

Cahill, Maureen A. Anthem Blue Cross & Blue Shield of Missouri, 460

Cahill, Maureen A. Anthem Blue Cross & Blue Shield of Nevada, 499

Cahill, Maureen A. Anthem Blue Cross & Blue Shield of New Hampshire, 511

Cahill, Maureen A. Empire BlueCross BlueShield, 558

Cahill, Maureen A. Anthem Blue Cross & Blue Shield of Ohio, 604

Cahill, Maureen A. Anthem Blue Cross & Blue Shield of Wisconsin, 830

Calandro, Michele Blue Cross and Blue Shield of Louisiana, 353

Caldwell, Joe Alliant Health Plans, 235

Callender, David L. UTMB HealthCare Systems, 770

Camerlinck, Bryan Blue Cross and Blue Shield of Louisiana, 353

Campanella, Gary, MBA On Lok Lifeways, 123

Campbell, Craig Wisconsin Physician's Service, 854

Campbell, Gemma Trinity Health of Alabama, 9

Campbell, Joe Emi Health, 776

Campos, Alina, MD Leon Medical Centers Health Plan, 222

Canales, Joe Seton Healthcare Family, 762

Cantor, Michael CareCentrix: Arizona, 24

Constantine, Timothy J. United Concordia of New York, 581

Constantine, Timothy J. United Concordia of North Carolina, 594

Constantine, Timothy J. United Concordia of Oregon, 655

Constantine, Timothy J. United Concordia Dental, 680

Constantine, Timothy J. United Concordia of Pennsylvania, 681

Constantine, Timothy J. United Concordia of Texas, 767

Constantine, Timothy J. United Concordia of Virginia, 802

Constantine, Timothy J. United Concordia of Washington, 816

Convington, Richard Behavioral Health Systems, 3

Cook, Anthony A. The Dental Care Plus Group, 623

Cook, Jan Minuteman Health, 397

Cook, Stephanie Dean Health Plan, 836

Cooner, Danny Behavioral Health Systems, 3

Cooney, Kathy HealthPartners, 443

Coons, Margaret M. Horizon Blue Cross Blue Shield of New Jersey, 523

Cooper, Annalisa NIA Magellan, 36

Cooper, Richard Arkansas Blue Cross Blue Shield, 49

Cooper, Rob, MD Ohio State University Health Plan Inc., 615

Corbin, Andrew Blue Cross and Blue Shield of Kansas, 327

Corbin, Andrew C. Advance Insurance Company of Kansas, 323

Cordani, David Cigna Medical Group, 26

Cordani, David Texas HealthSpring, 765

Cordani, David M. Cigna HealthCare of Arizona, 25

Cordani, David M. Cigna HealthCare of California, 81

Cordani, David M. Cigna HealthCare of Colorado, 156

Cordani, David M. Cigna Corporation, 176

Cordani, David M. Cigna-HealthSpring Medicare, 177

Cordani, David M. Cigna HealthCare of Florida, 210

Cordani, David M. Cigna HealthSpring CarePlan of Illinois, 270

Cordani, David M. Cigna HealthCare of Oklahoma, 630

Cordier, Susan Care1st Health Plan Arizona, 23

Cordina, David M. Cigna HealthCare of Tennessee, 631

Cosgriff, Jeff UnitedHealthcare of South Dakota, 718

Cosgriff, John Oxford Health Plans, 182

Cosgriff, John UnitedHealthcare of Connecticut, 184

Cosgriff, John UnitedHealthcare Community Plan Delaware, 191

Cosgriff, John UnitedHealthcare of the District of Columbia, 197

Cosgriff, John Neighborhood Health Partnership, 226

Cosgriff, John UnitedHealthcare of Florida, 231

Cosgriff, John UnitedHealthcare of South Florida, 232

Cosgriff, John UnitedHealthcare of Georgia, 248

Cosgriff, John UnitedHealthcare of Hawaii, 257

Cosgriff, John UnitedHealthcare of Idaho, 266

Cosgriff, John UnitedHealthcare of Illinois, 290

Cosgriff, John UnitedHealthcare of Indiana, 310

Cosgriff, John UnitedHealthcare of Iowa, 321

Cosgriff, John UnitedHealthcare of Kansas, 339

Cosgriff, John UnitedHealthcare of Kentucky, 351

Cosgriff, John UnitedHealthcare of Louisiana, 360

Cosgriff, John UnitedHealthcare of Maine, 370

Cosgriff, John UnitedHealthcare of Maryland, 385

Cosgriff, John UnitedHealthcare of Massachusetts, 403

Cosgriff, John UnitedHealthcare Great Lakes Health Plan, 434

Cosgriff, John UnitedHealthcare of Minnesota, 451

Cosgriff, John UnitedHealthcare of Mississippi, 457

Cosgriff, John UnitedHealthcare of Missouri, 476

Cosgriff, John UnitedHealthcare of Montana, 485

Cosgriff, John UnitedHealthcare of Nebraska, 496

Cosgriff, John UnitedHealthcare of Nevada, 509

Cosgriff, John UnitedHealthcare of New Hampshire, 516

Cosgriff, John UnitedHealthcare of New Jersey, 530

Cosgriff, John UnitedHealthcare of New Mexico, zzz 542

Cosgriff, John UnitedHealthcare of New York, 582

Cosgriff, John UnitedHealthcare of North Carolina, 595

Cosgriff, John UnitedHealthcare of North Dakota, 602

Cosgriff, John UnitedHealthcare of Ohio, 626

Cosgriff, John UnitedHealthcare of Oklahoma, 637

Cosgriff, John UnitedHealthcare of Oregon, 656

Cosgriff, John UnitedHealthcare of Pennsylvania, 682

Cosgriff, John UnitedHealthcare of Puerto Rico, 695

Cosgriff, John UnitedHealthcare of Rhode Island, 703

Cosgriff, John UnitedHealthcare of South Carolina, 712

Cosgriff, John UnitedHealthcare of Tennessee, 732

Cosgriff, John UnitedHealthcare of Texas, 768

Cosgriff, John UnitedHealthcare of Utah, 786

Cosgriff, John UnitedHealthcare of Vermont, 791

Cosgriff, John UnitedHealthcare of Virginia, 803

Cosgriff, John UnitedHealthcare of Washington, 817

Cosgriff, John UnitedHealthcare of West Virginia, 827

Cosgriff, John UnitedHealthcare of Wisconsin, 852

Cotton, Jon Meridian Health Plan, 422

Cotton, Michael Providence Health Plan, 651

Couch, Don Colorado Access, 157

Couch, Donald HealthSmart, 751

Courneya, Patrick, MD Kaiser Permanente, 107

Cox, Karen ProviDRs Care Network, 337

Crane, Gary Fidelis Care, 560

Crawford, Mark Alliance Regional Health Network, 734

Crenshaw, Jenn Amerigroup Florida, 199

Crimminger, Tricia Select Health of South Carolina, 711

Crockett, Gary CalOptima, 71

Croom, Olivia Dentaquest, 390

Cropp, Michael W, MD Independent Health, 567

Cropp, Michael W, MD Independent Health Medicare Plan, 568

Croswell, Thomas A. Tufts Health Plan, 401

Crowley, Daniel D. Western Dental Services, 147

Crowley, Paul Medica, 446

Crowsell, Thomas A. Tufts Health Medicare Plan, 400

Cuda, John MetroPlus Health Plan, 574

Cummings, Melissa Blue Cross & Blue Shield of Rhode Island, 697

Cummings, Scott Care1st Health Plan Arizona, 23

Cunningham, Kristen HCSC Insurance Services Company, 276, 481, 535, 634, 750

Cunningham, Terrence J. AmeriHealth Caritas District of Columbia, 193

Curcio, Trina L. Vale-U-Health, 685

Currier, Cecile CONCERN: Employee Assistance Program, 84

Cusick, Lauren Blue Cross & Blue Shield of Oklahoma, 629

Custer, Dr. Timothy DenteMax, 415

Czyzewski, Sharon UPMC Health Plan, 683

Gallagher, Michael P. AvMed Gainesville, 202

Gallagher, Michael P. AvMed Jacksonville, 203

Gallagher, Michael P. AvMed Orlando, 204

Gallagher, Michael P. AvMed Pembroke Pines, 205

Gallagher, Michael P. AvMed Tampa Bay, 206

Gallina, John Anthem, Inc., 294

Galt, Frederick B. CDPHP Medicare Plan, 549

Galt, Frederick B. CDPHP: Capital District Physicians' Health Plan, 550

Galvin, Eric ConnectiCare, 178

Gannon, Christopher R Blue Cross & Blue Shield of Vermont, 789

Garcia, Richard Easy Choice Health Plan, 92

Gardner, Deana Crescent Health Solutions, 588

Garland, Andrew Blue Cross & Blue Shield of Vermont, 789

Garrett, Andrea DenteMax, 415

Garrigues, Brad Providence Health Plan, 651

Garza, Jesus Seton Healthcare Family, 762

Garzelli, Lisa Foundation f. Medical Care f. Kern & Santa Barbara Counties, 95

Gaspar, Gary Avera Health Plans, 713

Gaulstrand, Paul Spectera Eyecare Networks, 382

Geesaman, Brian AmeriHealth Caritas District of Columbia, 193

Gellert, Jay Health Net, Inc., 101

Genord, Michael, MD HAP-Health Alliance Plan: Flint, 417

Genord, Michael, MD HAP-Health Alliance Plan: Senior Medicare Plan, 418

Genord, Michael, MD Health Alliance Medicare, 419

Genord, Michael, MD Health Alliance Plan, 420

Gentile, James Fallon Health, 391

George, Don Blue Cross & Blue Shield of Vermont, 789

George, William S. Health Partners Plans, 667

Geraghty, Patrick Florida Blue, 213

Gerbus, Dave Delta Dental of Colorado, 161

Gering, Stanley A. Arizona Foundation for Medical Care, 20

Gessel, Barbara Mercy Health Network, 318

Gessells, Tom Ohio State University Health Plan Inc., 615

Ghaly, Christina, M.D. Health Services Los Angeles County, 104

Ghanayem, Darren WellCare Health Plans, 233

Gianturco, Laurie, MD Health New England, 393

Giasi, Steve Affinity Health Plan, 544

Gibboney, Liz Partnership HealthPlan of California, 127

Giblin, John Blue Cross & Blue Shield of Tennessee, 723

Gibson, Sandy Blue Cross & Blue Shield of Arizona, 22

Gielis, Bridget QualCare, 528

Giese, Alexis, MD Colorado Access, 157

Gieseman, Greg Community First Health Plans, 743

Giesler, Scott eHealthInsurance Services, Inc., 93

Gilfillan, Richard Trinity Health, 430

Gilfillan, Richard J. Trinity Health of Florida, 229

Gilfillan, Richard J. Trinity Health of Georgia, 246

Gilfillan, Richard J. Trinity Health of Idaho, 265

Gilfillan, Richard J. Trinity Health of Illinois, 287

Gilfillan, Richard J. Trinity Health of Indiana, 309

Gilfillan, Richard J. Trinity Health of Iowa, 320

Gilfillan, Richard J. Trinity Health of Maryland, 383

Gilfillan, Richard J. Trinity Health of Massachusetts, 399

Gilfillan, Richard J. Trinity Health of Michigan, 431

Gilfillan, Richard J. Trinity Health of New Jersey, 529

Gilfillan, Richard J. Trinity Health of New York, 580

Gilfillan, Richard J. Trinity Health of Ohio, 625

Gilfillan, Richard J. Trinity Health of Pennsylvania, 679

Gilfillian, Richard J. Trinity Health of Delaware, 190

Gill, Laura Avesis: Arizona, 21

Gille, Larry Prevea Health Network, 849

Gilligan, Patrick Blue Cross & Blue Shield of Massachusetts, 389

Gilliland, Robert Florida Health Care Plans, 214

Gladden, John Delta Dental of Oklahoma, 633

Glossy, Bernard Delta Dental of Illinois, 274

Gluckman, Robert Providence Health Plan, 651

Goddard, Kevin Blue Cross & Blue Shield of Vermont, 789

Godley, Patrick Contra Costa Health Services, 85

Goheen, Charles Harvard Pilgrim Health Care Connecticut, 180

Goheen, Charles Harvard Pilgrim Health Care Maine, 367

Goheen, Charles Harvard Pilgrim Health Care Massachusetts, 392

Goheen, Charles Harvard Pilgrim Health Care New Hampshire, 513

Gold, Michael A. Hawaii Medical Service Association, 254

Gold, Stephen J CVS CareMark, 699

Golden, Scott Anthem Blue Cross & Blue Shield of Virginia, 793

Goldstein, Craig CHN PPO, 520

Golovan, Kathy Medical Mutual, 610

Gonick, Denise MVP Health Care, 576

Gonzalez, Orlando MMM Holdings, 693

Gonzalez, Orlando, Esq. PMC Medicare Choice, 694

Goodman, Lowell Kaiser Permanente Southern California, 109

Gootee, Robert Moda Health Alaska, 15

Gootee, Robert Moda Health Oregon, 648

Gordon, Mark Behavioral Health Systems, 3

Goren, Richard Liberty Dental Plan of Florida, 223

Goren, Richard Liberty Dental Plan of Illinois, 281

Goren, Richard Liberty Dental Plan of Nevada, 505

Goren, Richard Liberty Dental Plan of New York, 570

Goren, Rick Liberty Dental Plan of Texas, 755

Gormley, Kate San Francisco Health Plan, 131

Gorsuch, Kirsten Oxford Health Plans, 182

Gorsuch, Kirsten UnitedHealthcare of Connecticut, 184

Gorsuch, Kirsten UnitedHealthcare Community Plan Delaware, 191

Gorsuch, Kirsten UnitedHealthcare of the District of Columbia, 197

Gorsuch, Kirsten Neighborhood Health Partnership, 226

Gorsuch, Kirsten UnitedHealthcare of Florida, 231

Gorsuch, Kirsten UnitedHealthcare of South Florida, 232

Gorsuch, Kirsten UnitedHealthcare of Georgia, 248

Gorsuch, Kirsten UnitedHealthcare of Hawaii, 257

Gorsuch, Kirsten UnitedHealthcare of Idaho, 266

Gorsuch, Kirsten UnitedHealthcare of Illinois, 290

Gorsuch, Kirsten UnitedHealthcare of Indiana, 310

Gorsuch, Kirsten UnitedHealthcare of Iowa, 321

Gorsuch, Kirsten UnitedHealthcare of Kansas, 339

Gorsuch, Kirsten UnitedHealthcare of Kentucky, 351

Gorsuch, Kirsten UnitedHealthcare of Louisiana, 360

Gorsuch, Kirsten UnitedHealthcare of Maine, 370

Gorsuch, Kirsten UnitedHealthcare of Maryland, 385

Gorsuch, Kirsten UnitedHealthcare of Massachusetts, 403

Gorsuch, Kirsten UnitedHealthcare Great Lakes Health Plan, 434

Gorsuch, Kirsten UnitedHealthcare of Minnesota, 451

Gorsuch, Kirsten UnitedHealthcare of Mississippi, 457

H

Huval, Tim Humana Health Insurance of Kansas, 332

Huval, Tim Humana Medicare, 347

Huval, Tim Humana Health Insurance of Louisiana, 356

Huval, Tim Humana Health Insurance of Massachusetts, 395

Huval, Tim Humana Health Insurance of Michigan, 421

Huval, Tim Humana Health Insurance of Minnesota, 445

Huval, Tim Humana Health Insurance of Mississippi, 455

Huval, Tim Humana Health Insurance of Missouri, 471

Huval, Tim Humana Health Insurance of Montana, 482

Huval, Tim Humana Health Insurance of Nebraska, 490

Huval, Tim Humana Health Insurance of Nevada, 504

Huval, Tim Humana Health Insurance of New Hampshire, 514

Huval, Tim Humana Health Insurance of New Jersey, 525

Huval, Tim Humana Health Insurance of New Mexico, 536

Huval, Tim Humana Health Insurance of New York, 566

Huval, Tim Humana Health Insurance of North Carolina, 592

Huval, Tim Humana Health Insurance of North Dakota, 599

Huval, Tim Humana Health Insurance of Ohio, 609

Huval, Tim Humana Health Insurance of Oklahoma, 635

Huval, Tim Humana Health Insurance of Oregon, 644

Huval, Tim Humana Health Insurance of Pennsylvania, 671

Huval, Tim Humana Health Insurance of Puerto Rico, 690

Huval, Tim Humana Health Insurance of Rhode Island, 700

Huval, Tim Humana Health Insurance of South Carolina, 708

Huval, Tim Humana Health Insurance of South Dakota, 717

Huval, Tim Humana Health Insurance of Tennessee, 730

Huval, Tim Humana Health Insurance of Texas, 753

Huval, Tim Humana Health Insurance of Utah, 777

Huval, Tim Humana Health Insurance of Virginia, 798

Huval, Tim Humana Health Insurance of Washington, 812

Huval, Tim Humana Health Insurance of West Virginia, 823

Huval, Tim Humana Health Insurance of Wisconsin, 843

Huval, Tim Humana Health Insurance of Wyoming, 858

I

Iannelli, Lee Ann CHN PPO, 520

Ianniello, Cara CHN PPO, 520

Ignagni, Karen M. EmblemHealth, 556

Ignagni, Karen M. EmblemHealth Enhanced Care Plus (HARP), 557

Ignagni, Karen M. GHI Medicare Plan, 561

Ignagni, Karen M. Group Health Insurance, 562

Ingrum, Jeff Scott & White Health Plan, 760

Isaacs, Richard Kaiser Permanente Mid-Atlantic, 380

Isaacs, Richard S. Kaiser Permanente Georgia, 243

Isaacs, Richard S. Kaiser Permanente Hawaii, 256

Iturriria, Louis Kern Family Health Care, 110

J

Jablonski, Dawn MVP Health Care, 576

Jackson, Amy Avesis: Arizona, 21

Jackson, Laura Wellmark Blue Cross & Blue Shield of South Dakota, 719

Jacobetti, Lorrie Prevea Health Network, 849

Jacobs, Danny O. UTMB HealthCare Systems, 770

Jacobs, Kim UPMC Health Plan, 683

Jacobs, Seth, Esq Blue Shield of California, 66

Jacobson, Jim Medica, 446

Jacobson, Jim Medica with CHI Health, 491

Jacobson, Jim Medica: Nebraska, 492

Jacobson, Jim Medica: North Dakota, 600

Jaconette, Paul CenCal Health, 76

Jain, Sachin H. CareMore Health Plan, 75

James, Marcus Arkansas Blue Cross Blue Shield, 49

Januska, Jeff CenCal Health, 76

Jarboe, David CarePlus Health Plans, 209

Jardine, Edie NIA Magellan, 36

Jardine, Edie National Imaging Associates, 447

Javier Artau Feliciano, Francisco First Medical Health Plan, 689

Jenkins, Mary Beth UPMC Health Plan, 683

Jenkins, Sheila Network Health Plan of Wisconsin, 847

Jennings, Julie American Specialty Health, 63

Jeppesen, David Blue Cross of Idaho Health Service, Inc., 259

Jernigan, J. Michael Select Health of South Carolina, 711

Jhaveri, Vishu J., MD Blue Cross & Blue Shield of Arizona, 22

Johns, Nathan New Mexico Health Connections, 538

Johns, Wendell L. CareFirst BlueCross BlueShield, 375

Johnson, Bruce, MD Pueblo Health Care, 166

Johnson, Karen M. Easy Choice Health Plan, 92

Johnson, Mark Independent Health, 567

Johnson, Mark Independent Health Medicare Plan, 568

Johnson, Pamela MK Children's Mercy Integrated Care Solutions, 463

Johnson, Steven P. Health First Health Plans, 216

Johnson, Steven P. Health First Medicare Plans, 217

Johnson, Steven P., Jr UPMC Susquehanna, 684

Johnson, Thad Oxford Health Plans, 182

Johnson, Thad UnitedHealthcare of Connecticut, 184

Johnson, Thad UnitedHealthcare Community Plan Delaware, 191

Johnson, Thad UnitedHealthcare of the District of Columbia, 197

Johnson, Thad Neighborhood Health Partnership, 226

Johnson, Thad UnitedHealthcare of Florida, 231

Johnson, Thad UnitedHealthcare of South Florida, 232

Johnson, Thad UnitedHealthcare of Georgia, 248

Johnson, Thad UnitedHealthcare of Hawaii, 257

Johnson, Thad UnitedHealthcare of Idaho, 266

Johnson, Thad UnitedHealthcare of Illinois, 290

Johnson, Thad UnitedHealthcare of Indiana, 310

Johnson, Thad UnitedHealthcare of Iowa, 321

Johnson, Thad UnitedHealthcare of Kansas, 339

Johnson, Thad UnitedHealthcare of Kentucky, 351

Johnson, Thad UnitedHealthcare of Louisiana, 360

Johnson, Thad UnitedHealthcare of Maine, 370

Johnson, Thad UnitedHealthcare of Maryland, 385

Johnson, Thad UnitedHealthcare of Massachusetts, 403

Johnson, Thad UnitedHealthcare Great Lakes Health Plan, 434

Johnson, Thad UnitedHealthcare of Minnesota, 451

Johnson, Thad UnitedHealthcare of Mississippi, 457

Johnson, Thad UnitedHealthcare of Missouri, 476

Johnson, Thad UnitedHealthcare of Montana, 485

Johnson, Thad UnitedHealthcare of Nebraska, 496

Johnson, Thad UnitedHealthcare of Nevada, 509

Johnson, Thad UnitedHealthcare of New Hampshire, 516

Johnson, Thad UnitedHealthcare of New Jersey, 530

Johnson, Thad UnitedHealthcare of New Mexico, 542

Johnson, **Thad** UnitedHealthcare of New York, 582
Johnson, **Thad** UnitedHealthcare of North Carolina, 595
Johnson, **Thad** UnitedHealthcare of North Dakota, 602
Johnson, **Thad** UnitedHealthcare of Ohio, 626
Johnson, **Thad** UnitedHealthcare of Oklahoma, 637
Johnson, **Thad** UnitedHealthcare of Oregon, 656
Johnson, **Thad** UnitedHealthcare of Pennsylvania, 682
Johnson, **Thad** UnitedHealthcare of Puerto Rico, 695
Johnson, **Thad** UnitedHealthcare of Rhode Island, 703
Johnson, **Thad** UnitedHealthcare of South Carolina, 712
Johnson, **Thad** UnitedHealthcare of South Dakota, 718
Johnson, **Thad** UnitedHealthcare of Tennessee, 732
Johnson, **Thad** UnitedHealthcare of Texas, 768
Johnson, **Thad** UnitedHealthcare of Utah, 786
Johnson, **Thad** UnitedHealthcare of Vermont, 791
Johnson, **Thad** UnitedHealthcare of Virginia, 803
Johnson, **Thad** UnitedHealthcare of Washington, 817
Johnson, **Thad** UnitedHealthcare of West Virginia, 827
Johnson, **Thad** UnitedHealthcare of Wisconsin, 852
Johnson, **William** Moda Health Alaska, 15
Johnson, **William, MD** Moda Health Oregon, 648
Jones, **Bobby** CareSource Ohio, 606
Jones, **David** Delta Dental of Oklahoma, 633
Jones, **Linza** Scott & White Health Plan, 760
Jones, **Mary Anne** Priority Health, 426
Jones, **Mary Anne** PriorityHealth Medicare Plans, 427
Jones, **Nicole** Cigna Medical Group, 26
Jones, **Nicole** Texas HealthSpring, 765
Jones, **Rich** DakotaCare, 714
Jones, **Richard** Essence Healthcare, 468
Jones, **Scott** Delta Dental of South Dakota, 715
Jos, **Orellana, Juan** Molina Healthcare of New York, 575
Joseph Bell, **Jill** Passport Health Plan, 348
Joyce, **Christopher** InnovaCare Health, 691
Joyce, **Kevin** QualCare, 528
Joyner, **J David** CVS CareMark, 699
Judy, **Steve** Primary Health Medical Group, 263
Julian, **Marcus** Dean Health Plan, 836
Jurkovic, **Goran** Delta Dental of New Mexico, 534

K

Kaercher, **David** Blue Cross Blue Shield of Kansas City, 461
Kaiser, **Kelley C.** Samaritan Health Plan Operations, 653
Kanagal, **Nandini** Arizona Foundation for Medical Care, 20
Kandalaft, **Kevin** UnitedHealthcare of Northern California, 141
Kandalaft, **Kevin** UnitedHealthcare of Southern California, 142
Kane, **Brain** Humana Health Insurance of Utah, 777
Kane, **Brian** Humana Health Insurance of Alabama, 7
Kane, **Brian** Humana Health Insurance of Alaska, 14
Kane, **Brian** Humana Health Insurance of Arizona, 30
Kane, **Brian** Humana Health Insurance of Colorado, 163
Kane, **Brian** Humana Health Insurance of Connecticut, 181
Kane, **Brian** Humana Health Insurance of Delaware, 188
Kane, **Brian** Humana Health Insurance Company of Florida, Inc., 221
Kane, **Brian** CompBenefits Corporation, 239
Kane, **Brian** Humana Employers Health Plan of Georgia, Inc., 242

Kane, **Brian** Humana Health Insurance of Hawaii, 255
Kane, **Brian** Humana Health Insurance of Idaho, 261
Kane, **Brian** Humana Health Insurance of Illinois, 280
Kane, **Brian** Humana Health Insurance of Indiana, 302
Kane, **Brian** Humana Health Insurance of Iowa, 316
Kane, **Brian** Humana Health Insurance of Kansas, 332
Kane, **Brian** Humana Inc., 346
Kane, **Brian** Humana Medicare, 347
Kane, **Brian** Humana Health Insurance of Louisiana, 356
Kane, **Brian** Humana Health Insurance of Massachusetts, 395
Kane, **Brian** Humana Health Insurance of Michigan, 421
Kane, **Brian** Humana Health Insurance of Minnesota, 445
Kane, **Brian** Humana Health Insurance of Mississippi, 455
Kane, **Brian** Humana Health Insurance of Missouri, 471
Kane, **Brian** Humana Health Insurance of Montana, 482
Kane, **Brian** Humana Health Insurance of Nebraska, 490
Kane, **Brian** Humana Health Insurance of Nevada, 504
Kane, **Brian** Humana Health Insurance of New Hampshire, 514
Kane, **Brian** Humana Health Insurance of New Jersey, 525
Kane, **Brian** Humana Health Insurance of New Mexico, 536
Kane, **Brian** Humana Health Insurance of New York, 566
Kane, **Brian** Humana Health Insurance of North Carolina, 592
Kane, **Brian** Humana Health Insurance of North Dakota, 599
Kane, **Brian** Humana Health Insurance of Ohio, 609
Kane, **Brian** Humana Health Insurance of Oklahoma, 635
Kane, **Brian** Humana Health Insurance of Oregon, 644
Kane, **Brian** Humana Health Insurance of Pennsylvania, 671
Kane, **Brian** Humana Health Insurance of Puerto Rico, 690
Kane, **Brian** Humana Health Insurance of Rhode Island, 700
Kane, **Brian** Humana Health Insurance of South Carolina, 708
Kane, **Brian** Humana Health Insurance of South Dakota, 717
Kane, **Brian** Humana Health Insurance of Tennessee, 730
Kane, **Brian** Humana Health Insurance of Texas, 753
Kane, **Brian** Humana Health Insurance of Virginia, 798
Kane, **Brian** Humana Health Insurance of Washington, 812
Kane, **Brian** Humana Health Insurance of West Virginia, 823
Kane, **Brian** Humana Health Insurance of Wisconsin, 843
Kane, **Brian** Humana Health Insurance of Wyoming, 858
Kane, **Sean** Healthfirst, 564
Kao, **John** Alignment Health Plan, 61
Kapic, **Maja** Liberty Dental Plan of Florida, 223
Kapic, **Maja** Liberty Dental Plan of Illinois, 281
Kapic, **Maja** Liberty Dental Plan of Nevada, 505
Kapic, **Maja** Liberty Dental Plan of New York, 570
Kaplan, **Alan** Island Group Administration, Inc., 569
Kaplan, **Lynn** Island Group Administration, Inc., 569
Karl, **Nick** Peoples Health, 358
Karsten, **Wendy** Care N' Care, 741
Kasdagly, **Dino** L.A. Care Health Plan, 111, 112
Kastner, **Rick** Blue Cross Blue Shield of Kansas City, 461
Kasuba, **Paul, MD** Tufts Health Plan, 401
Kasuba, **Pual, MD** Tufts Health Medicare Plan, 400
Kates, **Peter B** Univera Healthcare, 583
Katich, **Wanda** Northeast Georgia Health Partners, 244
Katz, **Mitchell, M.D.** Health Services Los Angeles County, 104
Kaye, **Michel** PTPN, 130

LeClaire, **Brian** Humana Health Insurance of Montana, 482

LeClaire, **Brian** Humana Health Insurance of Nebraska, 490

LeClaire, **Brian** Humana Health Insurance of Nevada, 504

LeClaire, **Brian** Humana Health Insurance of New Hampshire, 514

LeClaire, **Brian** Humana Health Insurance of New Jersey, 525

LeClaire, **Brian** Humana Health Insurance of New Mexico, 536

LeClaire, **Brian** Humana Health Insurance of New York, 566

LeClaire, **Brian** Humana Health Insurance of North Carolina, 592

LeClaire, **Brian** Humana Health Insurance of North Dakota, 599

LeClaire, **Brian** Humana Health Insurance of Ohio, 609

LeClaire, **Brian** Humana Health Insurance of Oklahoma, zzz 635

LeClaire, **Brian** Humana Health Insurance of Oregon, 644

LeClaire, **Brian** Humana Health Insurance of Pennsylvania, 671

LeClaire, **Brian** Humana Health Insurance of Puerto Rico, 690

LeClaire, **Brian** Humana Health Insurance of Rhode Island, 700

LeClaire, **Brian** Humana Health Insurance of South Carolina, 708

LeClaire, **Brian** Humana Health Insurance of South Dakota, 717

LeClaire, **Brian** Humana Health Insurance of Tennessee, 730

LeClaire, **Brian** Humana Health Insurance of Texas, 753

LeClaire, **Brian** Humana Health Insurance of Utah, 777

LeClaire, **Brian** Humana Health Insurance of Virginia, 798

LeClaire, **Brian** Humana Health Insurance of Washington, 812

LeClaire, **Brian** Humana Health Insurance of West Virginia, 823

LeClaire, **Brian** Humana Health Insurance of Wisconsin, 843

LeClaire, **Brian** Humana Health Insurance of Wyoming, 858

Lederberg, **Michele** Blue Cross & Blue Shield of Rhode Island, 697

Lederman, **Alan** Community Health Plan of Washington, 808

Lee, **Lawrence (Larry)** UCare, 449

Lee, **Yolanda** Chinese Community Health Plan, 79

Leeth, **Sarah** Delta Dental of Minnesota, 442

Lennay, **Mark** WellCare Health Plans, 233

Lenth, **Gary** Unity Health Insurance, 853

Lentine, **Joe, Jr** Dencap Dental Plans, 414

Leonard, **Beth A.** EmblemHealth, 556

Leonard, **Beth A.** EmblemHealth Enhanced Care Plus (HARP), 557

Leonard, **Beth A.** GHI Medicare Plan, 561

Leonard, **Beth A.** Group Health Insurance, 562

Leong, **Darryl** CenCal Health, 76

LePan, **Karl R.** Physicians Health Plan of Northern Indiana, 305

Lerner, **Cheryl, MD** Delta Dental of Colorado, 161

Levandoski, **Anne** Upper Peninsula Health Plan, 436

Levin, **Matthew** Alameda Alliance for Health, 59

Levin, **Matthew** Alameda Medi-Cal Plan, 60

Lewis, **Jennifer** Spectera Eyecare Networks, 382

Lewis, **Kevin** Community Health Options, 365

Lewis-Clapper, **Caskie** Magellan Health, 31

Lewis-Clapper, **Caskie** Magellan Healthcare, 32

Lewis-Clapper, **Caskie** Magellan Complete Care of Florida, 224

Li, **Grace, MHA** On Lok Lifeways, 123

Liang, **Janet** Kaiser Permanente Northern California, 108

Lightfoot, **Dan, MD** Pacific Foundation for Medical Care, 125

Lightner, **Debra M.** EmblemHealth, 556

Lightner, **Debra M.** EmblemHealth Enhanced Care Plus (HARP), 557

Lightner, **Debra M.** GHI Medicare Plan, 561

Lightner, **Debra M.** Group Health Insurance, 562

Likness, **Clark** Avera Health Plans, 713

Lindgren, **Charles A.** Dimension Health, 212

Lindquist, **Tom** Medica, 446

Lindquist, **Tom** Medica with CHI Health, 491

Lindquist, **Tom** Medica: Nebraska, 492

Lindquist, **Tom** Medica: North Dakota, 600

Lingafelter, **Lynn** Deaconess Health Plans, 298

Listi, **Daniel** Valley Baptist Health Plan, 771

Little, **Jason** Baptist Health Services Group, 722

Littman, **Harvey** Capital BlueCross, 662

Liu, **Johanna** Santa Clara Family Health Foundations Inc, 132

Livesay, **Craig** Delta Dental of Arizona, 27

Livingston, **Carliedane** Opticare of Utah, 780

Livingston, **David** Prominence Health Plan, 508

Lloyd, **S. David, MD** Care N' Care, 741

Lo, **Eric** Delta Dental of Washington, 810

Loepp, **Daniel** Blue Care Network of Michigan, 408

Loepp, **Daniel J.** Blue Care Network of Michigan, 407

Loepp, **Daniel J.** Blue Cross Blue Shield of Michigan, 409

Loftis, **R. Chet** Public Employees Health Program, 782

Longendyke, **Rob** Medica, 446

Longendyke, **Rob** Medica with CHI Health, 491

Longendyke, **Rob** Medica: Nebraska, 492

Longendyke, **Rob** Medica: North Dakota, 600

Longworth, **Maria** CHN PPO, 520

Loochtan, **Scott** Consumers Direct Insurance Services (CDIS), 745

Lopez, **David** Parkland Community Health Plan, 759

Lopez, **Esteban** Blue Cross & Blue Shield of Texas, 740

Lopez, **Jose** Mid America Health, 303

Lopez Duarte, **Milori** Vision Plan of America, 145

Lopez Jr., **Edward** Delta Dental of New Mexico, 534

Lopez-Fernandez, **Orlando, Jr.** Medica HealthCare Plans, Inc, 119

Lorhan, **Michael** Physicians Plus Insurance Corporation, 848

Louie, **Deena** San Francisco Health Plan, 131

Lovell, **Stephanie** Blue Cross & Blue Shield of Massachusetts, 389

Lowell, **Randy** LifeMap, 646

Lowther, **Ryan** Emi Health, 776

Lubben, **Thomas** HCSC Insurance Services Company, 276, 481, 535, 634, 750

Lucero-Ali, **Cynthia** Delta Dental of New Mexico, 534

Luchetta, **Thomas** Superior Vision, 137

Lucia, **Frank L.** Dean Health Plan, 836

Luddyÿ, **Tom** Physicians Plus Insurance Corporation, 848

Luna, **Richard** Medical Card System (MCS), 692

Lundquist, **Thomas** Optima Health Plan, 800

Lunsford, **Jeanie** CareOregon Health Plan, 641

Luther, **John** Western Dental Services, 147

Luxenberg, **Jay, MD** On Lok Lifeways, 123

Lyman, **Justin** Trillium Community Health Plan, 654

Lynch, **Karen** Aetna Inc., 171

Lynch, **Karen S.** Coventry Health Care of Alaska, 13

Lynch, **Karen S.** Coventry Health Care of Colorado, 160

Lynch, **Karen S.** Aetna Health of Connecticut, 170

Lynch, **Karen S.** Aetna Student Health, 173

Lynch, **Karen S.** Coventry Health Care of Florida, 211

Lynch, **Karen S.** Coventry Health Care of Georgia, 240

Lynch, **Karen S.** Coventry Health Care of Hawaii, 252

McCarthy, Meg Coventry Health Care of Louisiana, 354
McCarthy, Meg Coventry Health Care of Maine, 366
McCarthy, Meg Coventry Health Care, Inc., 376
McCarthy, Meg Aetna Better Health of Michigan, 404
McCarthy, Meg Coventry Health Care of Michigan, 412
McCarthy, Meg Coventry Health Care of Minnesota, 441
McCarthy, Meg Coventry Health Care of Missouri, 464
McCarthy, Meg Coventry Health Care of Montana, 479
McCarthy, Meg Coventry Health Care of Nebraska, 488
McCarthy, Meg Coventry Health Care of Nevada, 501
McCarthy, Meg Coventry Health Care of New Hampshire, 512
McCarthy, Meg Coventry Health Care of New Jersey, 521
McCarthy, Meg Coventry Health Care of New Mexico, 533
McCarthy, Meg Coventry Health Care of New York, 551
McCarthy, Meg Coventry Health Care of the Carolinas, 587
McCarthy, Meg Coventry Health Care of North Dakota, 597
McCarthy, Meg Coventry Health Care of Rhode Island, 698
McCarthy, Meg Coventry Health & Life Ins. Co. of Tennessee, 726
McCarthy, Meg Coventry Health Care of Texas, 746
McCarthy, Meg MHNet Behavioral Health, 756
McCarthy, Meg Altius Health Plans of Utah, 774
McCarthy, Meg Coventry Health Care of Vermont, 790
McCarthy, Meg Coventry Health Care of Washington, 809
McCarthy, Meg Aetna Better Health of West Virginia, 818
McCarthy, Meg Coventry Health Care of Wisconsin, 835
McCay, Alan Central California Alliance for Health, 77
McClelland, Patricia Santa Clara Family Health Foundations Inc, 132
McClure, Elizabeth Mid America Health, 303
McClure, Nance HealthPartners, 443
McConathy, Chris Golden West Dental & Vision, 97
McCook, Rick One Call Care Management, 227
McCormick, Mark Neighborhood Health Plan, 398
McCorriston, William C. Hawaii Medical Assurance Association, 253
McCoy, Dan Blue Cross & Blue Shield of Texas, 740
McCoy, Shawn Deaconess Health Plans, 298
McCulley, Daniel Midlands Choice, 493
McCurry, Michael Mercy Clinic Missouri, 474
McDaniel, Marie Devon Health Services, 664
McDonald, Glen Superior Vision, 137
McFadden, Darin Group Health Cooperative of Eau Claire, 839
McFarland, Patti Partnership HealthPlan of California, 127
McGuire, Marilee Community Health Plan of Washington, 808
McGuire, Michael Delta Dental of Minnesota, 442
McKoy, Phil Oxford Health Plans, 182
McKoy, Phil UnitedHealthcare of Connecticut, 184
McKoy, Phil UnitedHealthcare Community Plan Delaware, 191
McKoy, Phil UnitedHealthcare of the District of Columbia, 197
McKoy, Phil Neighborhood Health Partnership, 226
McKoy, Phil UnitedHealthcare of Florida, 231
McKoy, Phil UnitedHealthcare of South Florida, 232
McKoy, Phil UnitedHealthcare of Georgia, 248
McKoy, Phil UnitedHealthcare of Hawaii, 257
McKoy, Phil UnitedHealthcare of Idaho, 266
McKoy, Phil UnitedHealthcare of Illinois, 290
McKoy, Phil UnitedHealthcare of Indiana, 310
McKoy, Phil UnitedHealthcare of Iowa, 321

McKoy, Phil UnitedHealthcare of Kansas, 339
McKoy, Phil UnitedHealthcare of Kentucky, 351
McKoy, Phil UnitedHealthcare of Louisiana, 360
McKoy, Phil UnitedHealthcare of Maine, 370
McKoy, Phil UnitedHealthcare of Maryland, 385
McKoy, Phil UnitedHealthcare of Massachusetts, 403
McKoy, Phil UnitedHealthcare Great Lakes Health Plan, 434
McKoy, Phil UnitedHealthcare of Minnesota, 451
McKoy, Phil UnitedHealthcare of Mississippi, 457
McKoy, Phil UnitedHealthcare of Missouri, 476
McKoy, Phil UnitedHealthcare of Montana, 485
McKoy, Phil UnitedHealthcare of Nebraska, 496
McKoy, Phil UnitedHealthcare of Nevada, 509
McKoy, Phil UnitedHealthcare of New Hampshire, 516
McKoy, Phil UnitedHealthcare of New Jersey, 530
McKoy, Phil UnitedHealthcare of New Mexico, 542
McKoy, Phil UnitedHealthcare of New York, 582
McKoy, Phil UnitedHealthcare of North Carolina, 595
McKoy, Phil UnitedHealthcare of North Dakota, 602
McKoy, Phil UnitedHealthcare of Ohio, 626
McKoy, Phil UnitedHealthcare of Oklahoma, 637
McKoy, Phil UnitedHealthcare of Oregon, 656
McKoy, Phil UnitedHealthcare of Pennsylvania, 682
McKoy, Phil UnitedHealthcare of Puerto Rico, 695
McKoy, Phil UnitedHealthcare of Rhode Island, 703
McKoy, Phil UnitedHealthcare of South Carolina, 712
McKoy, Phil UnitedHealthcare of South Dakota, 718
McKoy, Phil UnitedHealthcare of Tennessee, 732
McKoy, Phil UnitedHealthcare of Texas, 768
McKoy, Phil UnitedHealthcare of Utah, 786
McKoy, Phil UnitedHealthcare of Vermont, 791
McKoy, Phil UnitedHealthcare of Virginia, 803
McKoy, Phil UnitedHealthcare of Washington, 817
McKoy, Phil UnitedHealthcare of West Virginia, 827
McKoy, Phil UnitedHealthcare of Wisconsin, 852
McManus, Jim Blue Cross & Blue Shield of Minnesota, 440
McMinn, Kathleen Superior Vision, 137
McNeil, Michael, MD QualCare, 528
McNeilly, Steven Northeast Georgia Health Partners, 244
McPhetres, Joyce Community Health Options, 365
McQuaide, Jay Blue Cross & Blue Shield of Massachusetts, 389
Meaney, Frank Neighborhood Health Plan of Rhode Island, 701
Mech, Ann B. CareFirst BlueCross BlueShield, 375
Meeks, Connie, MD Arkansas Blue Cross Blue Shield, 49
Meffert, Walt Davis Vision, 552
Mehelic, Phil American Health Care Alliance, 459
Meier, John Paramount Elite Medicare Plan, 617
Meier, John Paramount Health Care, 618
Mejorado, Alma Colorado Health Partnerships, 159
Merkel, F.G. (Chip) United Concordia of Arizona, 44
Merlo, Kristin Delta Dental of Washington, 810
Merlo, Larry J CVS CareMark, 699
Merlo, Larry J. SilverScript, 42
Mertinson, Jay Wisconsin Physician's Service, 854
Mertz, Laura J. Valley Preferred, 686
Messina, Elizabeth A. Blue Cross & Blue Shield of Arizona, 22

N

Neumann, Paul G. Trinity Health of Florida, 229
Neumann, Paul G. Trinity Health of Georgia, 246
Neumann, Paul G. Trinity Health of Idaho, 265
Neumann, Paul G. Trinity Health of Illinois, 287
Neumann, Paul G. Trinity Health of Indiana, 309
Neumann, Paul G. Trinity Health of Iowa, 320
Neumann, Paul G. Trinity Health of Maryland, 383
Neumann, Paul G. Trinity Health of Massachusetts, 399
Neumann, Paul G. Trinity Health, 430
Neumann, Paul G. Trinity Health of Michigan, 431
Neumann, Paul G. Trinity Health of New Jersey, 529
Neumann, Paul G. Trinity Health of New York, 580
Neumann, Paul G. Trinity Health of Ohio, 625
Neumann, Paul G. Trinity Health of Pennsylvania, 679
Newby, Sandra Virginia Health Network, 804
Newman, Kermit Lakeside Community Healthcare Network, 113
Newton, Angie Health Partners of Kansas, 331
Newton, Cecil San Francisco Health Plan, 131
Newton, Dean Delta Dental of Kansas, 330
Newton, Keith Concentra, 744
Nguyen, Paul Community First Health Plans, 743
Nicholas, Jonathan Moda Health Alaska, 15
Nicholas, Jonathan Moda Health Oregon, 648
Nicholson, Jennifer Northeast Georgia Health Partners, 244
Nicklaus, Dave eHealthInsurance Services, Inc., 93
Nieri, Phil Health Choice Arizona, 29
Nightingale, Tom Blue Cross Blue Shield of Kansas City, 461
Nolan, David C. On Lok Lifeways, 123
Norton, Deborah A. Harvard Pilgrim Health Care Connecticut, 180
Norton, Deborah A. Harvard Pilgrim Health Care Maine, 367
Norton, Deborah A. Harvard Pilgrim Health Care Massachusetts, 392
Norton, Deborah A. Harvard Pilgrim Health Care New Hampshire, 513
Nuzzi, Rosemarie Island Group Administration, Inc., 569

O

O 'Drobinak, Jim Medical Card System (MCS), 692
O'Brien, Kevin Optum Complex Medical Conditions, 448
O'Connor, Richard Harvard Pilgrim Health Care Connecticut, 180
O'Connor, Richard Harvard Pilgrim Health Care Maine, 367
O'Connor, Richard Harvard Pilgrim Health Care Massachusetts, 392
O'Connor, Richard Harvard Pilgrim Health Care New Hampshire, 513
O'Hollaren, Janet Kaiser Permanente Northwest, 645
O'Toole Mahoney, Mary Tufts Health Plan, 401
Odom, Lisa Cox Healthplans, 465
Oestreich, Kathleen University Care Advantage, 46
Oestreich, Kathleen University Family Care Health Plan, 47
Oliva, Lucy Liberty Health Advantage HMO, 571
Ollech, Brian Network Health Plan of Wisconsin, 847
Olsen, Frank Quality Health Plans of New York, 579
Olson, Fred, MD Blue Cross & Blue Shield of Montana, 478
Onorati, Annette Preferred Care Partners, 228
Orellana, Juan Jos, Molina Healthcare, 120
Orellana, Juan Jos, Molina Medicaid Solutions, 122
Orellana, Juan Jos, Molina Healthcare of Florida, 225
Orellana, Juan Jos, Molina Medicaid Solutions, 262
Orellana, Juan Jos, Molina Healthcare of Illinois, 283

Orellana, Juan Jos, Molina Medicaid Solutions, 357, 369
Orellana, Juan Jos, Molina Healthcare of Michigan, 423
Orellana, Juan Jos, Molina Medicaid Solutions, 527
Orellana, Juan Jos, Molina Healthcare of New Mexico, 537
Orellana, Juan Jos, Molina Healthcare of Ohio, 613
Orellana, Juan Jos, Molina Healthcare of South Carolina, 710
Orellana, Juan Jos, Molina Healthcare of Texas, 757
Orellana, Juan Jos, Molina Healthcare of Utah, 779
Orellana, Juan Jos, Molina Healthcare of Virgina, 799
Orellana, Juan Jos, Molina Healthcare of Washington, 814
Orellana, Juan Jos, Molina Medicaid Solutions, 824
Orellana, Juan Jos, Molina Healthcare of Wisconsin, 846
Ortego, Janice Peoples Health, 358
Osorio, Rosemary Dimension Health, 212
Ostrowski, Lynne Preferred Health Care, 676

P

Pack, Kent Children's Mercy Integrated Care Solutions, 463
Page, Erin Universal American Medicare Plans, 584
Page, Erin TexanPlus Medicare Advantage HMO, 764
Palmateer, Michael EmblemHealth, 556
Palmateer, Michael EmblemHealth Enhanced Care Plus (HARP), 557
Palmateer, Michael Group Health Insurance, 562
Palmateer, Michael . GHI Medicare Plan, 561
Palmer, Cynthia Colorado Choice Health Plans, 158
Palmer, Eric Cigna Medical Group, 26
Palmer, Rob Wisconsin Physician's Service, 854
Palumbo, Fara M. Blue Cross Blue Shield of North Carolina, 586
Pando, Roberto Medical Card System (MCS), 692
Panneton, Kirk BlueShield of Northeastern New York, 547
Pardis, Payam Access Dental Services, 57
Parietti, Daniel M. AlphaCare, 545
Park, Ben, MD American Health Network, 292
Parker, Barrie CenCal Health, 76
Parks, Douglas BlueCross BlueShield of Western New York, 546
Parr, Chris Health Plans, Inc., 394
Parrott, Chris Total Dental Administrators, 43
Parton, Ron Dean Health Plan, 836
Pass, Kathy Pacific Foundation for Medical Care, 125
Patel, Nilesh Delta Dental of California, 87
Patel, Nilesh Delta Dental of Delaware, 186
Patel, Nilesh Delta Dental of the District of Columbia, 194
Patel, Nilesh Delta Dental Insurance Company, 241
Patel, Nilesh Delta Dental of New York, 553
Patel, Nilesh Delta Dental of Pennsylvania, 663
Patterson, M.D., William M. Behavioral Health Systems, 3
Paulson, Trisha Prevea Health Network, 849
Pawenski, Pamela J. Univera Healthcare, 583
Paz, Harold, MD Aetna Inc., 171
Paz, Harold L. Coventry Health Care of Alaska, 13
Paz, Harold L. Coventry Health Care of Colorado, 160
Paz, Harold L., MD Aetna Health of Connecticut, 170
Paz, Harold L. Aetna Student Health, 173
Paz, Harold L. Coventry Health Care of Florida, 211
Paz, Harold L. Coventry Health Care of Georgia, 240
Paz, Harold L. Coventry Health Care of Hawaii, 252

Putnam, Jeff UnitedHealthcare of North Dakota, 602
Putnam, Jeff UnitedHealthcare of Ohio, 626
Putnam, Jeff UnitedHealthcare of Oklahoma, 637
Putnam, Jeff UnitedHealthcare of Oregon, 656
Putnam, Jeff UnitedHealthcare of Pennsylvania, 682
Putnam, Jeff UnitedHealthcare of Puerto Rico, 695
Putnam, Jeff UnitedHealthcare of Rhode Island, 703
Putnam, Jeff UnitedHealthcare of South Carolina, 712
Putnam, Jeff UnitedHealthcare of South Dakota, 718
Putnam, Jeff UnitedHealthcare of Tennessee, 732
Putnam, Jeff UnitedHealthcare of Texas, 768
Putnam, Jeff UnitedHealthcare of Utah, 786
Putnam, Jeff UnitedHealthcare of Vermont, 791
Putnam, Jeff UnitedHealthcare of Virginia, 803
Putnam, Jeff UnitedHealthcare of Washington, 817
Putnam, Jeff UnitedHealthcare of West Virginia, 827
Putnam, Jeff UnitedHealthcare of Wisconsin, 852
Pyle, David Managed HealthCare Northwest, 647

Q

Quinlan, Ann Dominion Dental Services, 796
Quivers, Eric Security Health Plan of Wisconsin, 850

R

Raffio, Thomas Northeast Delta Dental, 515
Rai, Ashok, M.D. Prevea Health Network, 849
Rajkumar, Rahul CareFirst Blue Cross & Blue Shield of Virginia, 794
Ramirez, David CareMore Health Plan, 75
Ramos, Candance Children's Mercy Integrated Care Solutions, 463
Ramseier, Mike Anthem Blue Cross & Blue Shield of Colorado, 151
Randolph, Jack Paramount Care of Michigan, 424
Randolph, John C Paramount Elite Medicare Plan, 617
Randolph, John C Paramount Health Care, 618
Rank, Brian HealthPartners, 443
Ransom, Penny Network Health Plan of Wisconsin, 847
Rashti, Dana Neighborhood Health Plan, 398
Rausch, Jay Dominion Dental Services, 796
Rawlins, Wayne ConnectiCare, 178
Ray, Todd Blue Cross & Blue Shield of Tennessee, 723
Razi, Nazneen HCSC Insurance Services Company, 276, 481, 535, 634, 750
Reavis, Jay Delta Dental of Arkansas, 50
Recore, Joan Health Plans, Inc., 394
Rector, Drew Health First Health Plans, 216
Rector, Drew Health First Medicare Plans, 217
Reed, Amanda Alliant Health Plans, 235
Reed, Philip J Colorado Access, 157
Reese, Dennis J Physicians Health Plan of Mid-Michigan, 425
Reid, Chantay CareOregon Health Plan, 641
Reitan, Colleen HCSC Insurance Services Company, 276
Reitan, Colleen Health Care Service Corporation, 279
Reitan, Colleen HCSC Insurance Services Company, 481, 535, 634, 750
Renfro, Larry UnitedHealth Group, 450
Renwick-Espinosa, Kate VSP Vision Care, 146
Repp, James M. AvMed, 200
Repp, James M. AvMed Ft. Lauderdale, 201
Repp, James M. AvMed Gainesville, 202

Repp, James M. AvMed Jacksonville, 203
Repp, James M. AvMed Orlando, 204
Repp, James M. AvMed Pembroke Pines, 205
Repp, James M. AvMed Tampa Bay, 206
Reppert, Joe Health Link PPO, 454
Rex, John UnitedHealth Group, 450
Rhoades, Tonya GEMCare Health Plan, 96
Rhode, Deb Prevea Health Network, 849
Rice-Johnson, Deborah L. Highmark BCBS Delaware, 187
Rice-Johnson, Deborah L. Highmark Blue Cross Blue Shield, 669
Rice-Johnson, Deborah L. Highmark Blue Shield, 670
Rice-Johnson, Deborah L. Highmark BCBS West Virginia, 822
Rich, Tracy L. Guardian Life Insurance Company of America, 563
Richardson, Robin Moda Health Alaska, 15
Richman, Keith S, MD Lakeside Community Healthcare Network, 113
Riner, Kathryn Northeast Georgia Health Partners, 244
Ring, Cynthia Harvard Pilgrim Health Care Connecticut, 180
Ring, Cynthia Harvard Pilgrim Health Care Maine, 367
Ring, Cynthia Harvard Pilgrim Health Care Massachusetts, 392
Ring, Cynthia Harvard Pilgrim Health Care New Hampshire, 513
Ringel, Steve CareSource West Virginia, 820
Riojas, Gil Alameda Alliance for Health, 59
Riojas, Gil Alameda Medi-Cal Plan, 60
Ritz, Bob Mercy Health Network, 318
Rivera, Ixel Medical Card System (MCS), 692
Roach, Susan, MD Boulder Valley Individual Practice Association, 154
Robart, Jason Blue Cross & Blue Shield of Massachusetts, 389
Robert, Adrian Affinity Health Plan, 544
Roberts, Beth Harvard Pilgrim Health Care Connecticut, 180
Roberts, Beth Harvard Pilgrim Health Care Maine, 367
Roberts, Beth Harvard Pilgrim Health Care Massachusetts, 392
Roberts, Beth Harvard Pilgrim Health Care New Hampshire, 513
Roberts, Jonathan C. CVS CareMark, 699
Roberts, Paul Colorado Choice Health Plans, 158
Robertson, Jeff Santa Clara Family Health Foundations Inc, 132
Robertson, Michelle L. Seton Healthcare Family, 762
Robinson, Ron Health Plan of San Mateo, 103
Robinson, Tamera Delta Dental of Minnesota, 442
Robinson-Beale, Rhonda, MD Blue Cross of Idaho Health Service, Inc., 259
Rodenz, Hillary Vale-U-Health, 685
Rodgers, John Independent Health, 567
Rodgers, John Independent Health Medicare Plan, 568
Rodriguez, Navarra, MD EmblemHealth, 556
Rodriguez, Navarra, MD EmblemHealth Enhanced Care Plus (HARP), 557
Rogers, Phyllis Delta Dental of Arkansas, 50
Rogers, Raymond Montana Health Co-Op, 483
Rogers, Raymond Mountain Health Co-Op, 484
Rogersl, Stephanie Scott & White Health Plan, 760
Rohr, Jan Rocky Mountain Health Plans, 167
Rolfing, Kyle Bright Health Alabama, 5
Rolfing, Kyle Bright Health Colorado, 155
Rollow, Brad VIVA Health, 11
Roman, Judith L. AmeriHealth Pennsylvania, 660
Romero, Jay EPIC Pharmacy Network, 797
Roos, John T. Blue Cross Blue Shield of North Carolina, 586
Rose, Carlotta InStil Health, 709

T

Walters, Betty Virginia Health Network, 804

Walters, Laurel Rocky Mountain Health Plans, 167

Wang, Pat Healthfirst, 564

Ward, Karen Blue Cross & Blue Shield of Tennessee, 723

Warner, Venus Galaxy Health Network, 749

Warwick, Rex Blue Cross of Idaho Health Service, Inc., 259

Wathen, Cheryl Deaconess Health Plans, 298

Watson, Chris One Call Care Management, 227

Watts, Brian California Dental Network, 69

Wear, Lisa J Initial Group, 731

Weaver, Jois J. Vale-U-Health, 685

Webb, Traci Central California Alliance for Health, 77

Wecker, Allan Health Services Los Angeles County, 104

Weeks, John Delta Dental of Kentucky, 345

Wehr, Ann O. AvMed, 200

Wehr, Ann O. AvMed Ft. Lauderdale, 201

Wehr, Ann O. AvMed Jacksonville, 203

Wehr, Ann O. AvMed Orlando, 204

Wehr, Ann O., MD, FACP AvMed Pembroke Pines, 205

Wehr, Ann O. AvMed Tampa Bay, 206

Weider, Drigan, MD Boulder Valley Individual Practice Association, 154

Weinper, Michael PTPN, 130

Weir, David UPMC Health Plan, 683

Weis, Brian Alliance Regional Health Network, 734

Welch, Jonathan, MD Medical Center Healthnet Plan, 396

Wendling, Mark Valley Preferred, 686

Wenk, Philip A. Delta Dental of Tennessee, 727

Werksman, Diane Value Behavioral Health of Pennsylvania, 687

West, Emily Fallon Health, 391

Wheeler, Brian Community First Health Plans, 743

Wheeler, Danny HealthPartners, 729

Wheeler, Robert R Blue Cross & Blue Shield of Vermont, 789

White, Joseph Molina Healthcare, 120

White, Joseph W. Molina Medicaid Solutions, 122

White, Joseph W. Molina Healthcare of Florida, 225

White, Joseph W. Molina Medicaid Solutions, 262

White, Joseph W. Molina Healthcare of Illinois, 283

White, Joseph W. Molina Medicaid Solutions, 357, 369

White, Joseph W. Molina Healthcare of Michigan, 423

White, Joseph W. Molina Medicaid Solutions, 527

White, Joseph W. Molina Healthcare of New Mexico, 537

White, Joseph W. Molina Healthcare of New York, 575

White, Joseph W. Molina Healthcare of Ohio, 613

White, Joseph W. Molina Healthcare of South Carolina, 710

White, Joseph W. Molina Healthcare of Texas, 757

White, Joseph W. Molina Healthcare of Utah, 779

White, Joseph W. Molina Healthcare of Virginia, 799

White, Joseph W. Molina Healthcare of Washington, 814

White, Joseph W. Molina Medicaid Solutions, 824

White, Joseph W. Molina Healthcare of Wisconsin, 846

White, Michael Providence Health Plan, 651

White, Robert American Specialty Health, 63

Whited, Amy Kaiser Permanente Northern Colorado, 164

Whited, Amy Kaiser Permanente Southern Colorado, 165

Whitford, Don Priority Health, 426

Whitley, Kim R. Samaritan Health Plan Operations, 653

Whittle, Brenda Neighborhood Health Plan of Rhode Island, 701

Wichmann, David UnitedHealthcare of Connecticut, 184

Wichmann, David UnitedHealthcare of the District of Columbia, 197

Wichmann, David Neighborhood Health Partnership, 226

Wichmann, David UnitedHealthcare of Florida, 231

Wichmann, David UnitedHealthcare of South Florida, 232

Wichmann, David UnitedHealthcare of Georgia, 248

Wichmann, David UnitedHealthcare of Hawaii, 257

Wichmann, David UnitedHealthcare of Idaho, 266

Wichmann, David UnitedHealthcare of Illinois, 290

Wichmann, David UnitedHealthcare of Indiana, 310

Wichmann, David UnitedHealthcare of Iowa, 321

Wichmann, David UnitedHealthcare of Kansas, 339

Wichmann, David UnitedHealthcare of Kentucky, 351

Wichmann, David UnitedHealthcare of Louisiana, 360

Wichmann, David UnitedHealthcare of Maine, 370

Wichmann, David UnitedHealthcare of Maryland, 385

Wichmann, David UnitedHealthcare of Massachusetts, 403

Wichmann, David UnitedHealthcare Great Lakes Health Plan, 434

Wichmann, David UnitedHealthcare of Michigan, 435

Wichmann, David UnitedHealth Group, 450

Wichmann, David UnitedHealthcare of Minnesota, 451

Wichmann, David UnitedHealthcare of Mississippi, 457

Wichmann, David UnitedHealthcare of Missouri, 476

Wichmann, David UnitedHealthcare of Montana, 485

Wichmann, David UnitedHealthcare of Nebraska, 496

Wichmann, David UnitedHealthcare of Nevada, 509

Wichmann, David UnitedHealthcare of New Hampshire, 516

Wichmann, David UnitedHealthcare of New Jersey, 530

Wichmann, David UnitedHealthcare of New Mexico, 542

Wichmann, David UnitedHealthcare of New York, 582

Wichmann, David UnitedHealthcare of North Carolina, 595

Wichmann, David UnitedHealthcare of North Dakota, 602

Wichmann, David UnitedHealthcare of Ohio, 626

Wichmann, David UnitedHealthcare of Oklahoma, 637

Wichmann, David UnitedHealthcare of Oregon, 656

Wichmann, David UnitedHealthcare of Pennsylvania, 682

Wichmann, David UnitedHealthcare of Puerto Rico, 695

Wichmann, David UnitedHealthcare of Rhode Island, 703

Wichmann, David UnitedHealthcare of South Carolina, 712

Wichmann, David UnitedHealthcare of South Dakota, 718

Wichmann, David UnitedHealthcare of Tennessee, 732

Wichmann, David UnitedHealthcare of Texas, 768

Wichmann, David UnitedHealthcare of Utah, 786

Wichmann, David UnitedHealthcare of Vermont, 791

Wichmann, David UnitedHealthcare of Virginia, 803

Wichmann, David UnitedHealthcare of Washington, 817

Wichmann, David UnitedHealthcare of West Virginia, 827

Wichmann, David S. Oxford Health Plans, 182

Wichmann, David S. UnitedHealthcare of Wisconsin, 852

Wilenkin, Anita Affinity Health Plan, 544

Wilkinson, Jeff Total Dental Administrators, 43

Wilkinson, Scott LifeMap, 646

Williams, Amy Trillium Community Health Plan, 654

Williams, David Devon Health Services, 664

Williams, Richard AllCare Health, 639

Membership Enrollment Index

1,900,000	LifeWise, 813	418,000	Health Plan of Nevada, 502
1,800,000	Wellmark Blue Cross & Blue Shield of South Dakota, 719	413,795	CalOptima, 71
1,700,000	Dental Health Alliance, 467	400,000	CDPHP Medicare Plan, 549
1,700,000	Medica, 446	400,000	Preferred Mental Health Management, 335
1,600,000	Medica: North Dakota, 600	400,000	Presbyterian Health Plan, 539
1,500,000	Blue Cross & Blue Shield of Arizona, 22	390,000	Dental Alternatives Insurance Services, 88
1,500,000	Excellus BlueCross BlueShield, 559	390,000	SVS Vision, 428
1,500,000	OSF Healthcare, 285	383,000	Health Alliance Medicare, 419
1,500,000	Univera Healthcare, 583	380,000	The Health Plan of the Ohio Valley/Mountaineer Region, 624
1,326,000	MagnaCare, 572	370,000	Ohio Health Choice, 614
1,300,000	Blue Cross and Blue Shield of Louisiana, 353	367,000	Blue Cross & Blue Shield of New Mexico, 532
1,100,000	CoreSource, 272	365,000	Independent Health, 567
1,018,589	Tufts Health Plan: Rhode Island, 702	350,000	CDPHP: Capital District Physicians' Health Plan, 550
1,000,000	CareSource Indiana, 296	345,000	Cigna-HealthSpring, 725
1,000,000	CareSource Kentucky, 343	340,000	AvMed, 200
1,000,000	CareSource Ohio, 606	340,000	AvMed Ft. Lauderdale, 201
1,000,000	CareSource West Virginia, 820	340,000	AvMed Gainesville, 202
1,000,000	Delta Dental of Oklahoma, 633	340,000	AvMed Jacksonville, 203
1,000,000	HealthSmart, 751	340,000	AvMed Orlando, 204
975,000	CHN PPO, 520	340,000	AvMed Pembroke Pines, 205
950,000	Blue Cross & Blue Shield of South Carolina, 705	340,000	AvMed Tampa Bay, 206
942,000	American Health Care Alliance, 459	338,000	Pacific Health Alliance, 126
900,000	Anthem Blue Cross & Blue Shield of Indiana, 293	332,128	MetroPlus Health Plan, 574
857,252	L.A. Care Health Plan, 112	330,000	Select Health of South Carolina, 711
807,000	Blue Care Network of Michigan, 407	326,000	Colorado Health Partnerships, 159
800,000	Moda Health Alaska, 15	325,000	Mercy Care Plan/Mercy Care Advantage, 35
750,000	Intermountain Healthcare, 778	320,000	Care1st Health Plan California, 73
750,000	Meridian Health Plan, 422	316,000	Preferred Network Access, 286
750,000	Meridian Health Plan of Illinois, 282	315,440	Western Dental Services, 147
750,000	QualCare, 528	300,000	Community Health Plan of Washington, 808
737,411	Tufts Health Plan, 401	300,000	Medical Card System (MCS), 692
717,000	Blue Cross & Blue Shield of Nebraska, 487	300,000	The Dental Care Plus Group, 623
700,000	MVP Health Care, 576	275,000	PacificSource Health Plans, 649, 650
670,000	MedCost, 593	265,000	AmeriHealth New Jersey, 518
650,000	HAP-Health Alliance Plan: Flint, 417	265,000	AmeriHealth Pennsylvania, 660
650,000	Health Alliance Plan, 420	263,200	Health Partners Plans, 667
625,000	Fidelis Care, 560	255,494	Health Alliance Medicare, 278
615,000	Midlands Choice, 493	250,000	Araz Group, 387
614,350	Kaiser Permanente Mid-Atlantic, 380	250,000	Blue Cross & Blue Shield of Montana, 478
600,000	Blue Cross & Blue Shield of Oklahoma, 629	250,000	CareOregon Health Plan, 641
600,000	Blue Cross & Blue Shield of Rhode Island, 697	250,000	Lakeside Community Healthcare Network, 113
596,220	Priority Health, 426	250,000	Santa Clara Family Health Foundations Inc, 132
563,000	Blue Cross of Idaho Health Service, Inc., 259	247,881	Dean Health Plan, 836
560,000	Partnership HealthPlan of California, 127	240,890	Medical Center Healthnet Plan, 396
555,405	BlueCross BlueShield of Western New York, 546	236,962	Rocky Mountain Health Plans, 167
540,000	Geisinger Health Plan, 666	210,000	Central California Alliance for Health, 77
518,000	Health Choice LLC, 728	210,000	Nova Healthcare Administrators, 577
502,000	Behavioral Health Systems, 3	205,677	Guardian Life Insurance Company of America, 563
500,000	Aultcare Corporation, 605	205,000	American Postal Workers Union (APWU) Health Plan, 372
500,000	CommunityCare, 632	205,000	BlueChoice Health Plan of South Carolina, 706
500,000	HealthSCOPE Benefits, 52	200,000	Care Plus Dental Plans, 833
475,000	Trustmark Companies, 288	200,000	Health New England, 393
467,000	Horizon NJ Health, 524	200,000	Initial Group, 731
430,000	Neighborhood Health Plan, 398	200,000	Scott & White Health Plan, 760
430,000	Optima Health Plan, 800	193,498	BlueShield of Northeastern New York, 547
423,244	Baptist Health Services Group, 722	190,000	Neighborhood Health Plan of Rhode Island, 701

187,000	Paramount Care of Michigan, 424		92,000	Western Health Advantage, 148
187,000	Paramount Elite Medicare Plan, 617		90,000	BEST Life and Health Insurance Co., 65
187,000	Paramount Health Care, 618		90,000	Dental Health Services of California, 90
187,000	Security Health Plan of Wisconsin, 850		90,000	Gundersen Lutheran Health Plan, 841
185,000	Priority Partners Health Plans, 381		90,000	Quality Plan Administrators, 195
180,000	Blue Cross & Blue Shield of Vermont, 789		90,000	Total Health Care, 429
180,000	First Medical Health Plan, 689		90,000	Unity Health Insurance, 853
177,854	Public Employees Health Program, 782		90,000	VIVA Health, 11
175,000	Arizona Foundation for Medical Care, 20		88,366	Virginia Health Network, 804
175,000	CenCal Health, 76		87,740	Health Plan of San Mateo, 103
175,000	Wisconsin Physician's Service, 854		87,000	First Choice of the Midwest, 716
174,309	Valley Preferred, 686		86,000	University Health Plans, 787
170,000	Passport Health Plan, 348		80,000	Alliance Regional Health Network, 734
155,070	Health Link PPO, 454		80,000	First Choice Health, 480
154,162	Aetna Health of New York, 543		80,000	Group Health Cooperative of South Central Wisconsin, 840
152,000	ProviDRs Care Network, 337		80,000	UniCare West Virginia, 826
150,000	Atlanticare Health Plans, 519		75,000	Group Health Cooperative of Eau Claire, 839
150,000	ChiroCare of Wisconsin, 834		71,000	Asuris Northwest Health, 807
150,000	Landmark Healthplan of California, 114		70,000	AlohaCare, 250
150,000	Nevada Preferred Healthcare Providers, 506		70,000	Martin's Point HealthCare, 368
150,000	Opticare of Utah, 780		68,942	Physicians Health Plan of Mid-Michigan, 425
148,000	Altius Health Plans, 773		68,000	Secure Health PPO Newtork, 245
147,000	UCare, 449		66,000	North Alabama Managed Care Inc, 8
146,000	Community Health Group, 83		63,000	Avera Health Plans, 713
144,000	Medical Mutual Services, 611		60,000	Boulder Valley Individual Practice Association, 154
140,000	Alameda Alliance for Health, 59		60,000	Essence Healthcare, 468
140,000	Contra Costa Health Services, 85		55,000	MediGold, 612
136,472	Baptist Health Plan, 342		55,000	San Francisco Health Plan, 131
134,837	Affinity Health Plan, 544		54,418	Mutual of Omaha Health Plans, 495
134,000	Advance Insurance Company of Kansas, 323		54,000	AllCare Health, 639
130,000	Employers Dental Services, 28		53,000	GHI Medicare Plan, 561
130,000	Golden Dental Plans, 416		53,000	PMC Medicare Choice, 694
130,000	Managed Health Services, 844		52,000	Island Group Administration, Inc., 569
128,272	SCAN Health Plan, 134		52,000	Ohio State University Health Plan Inc., 615
126,000	MMM Holdings, 693		50,715	Maricopa Health Plan, 34
125,000	Capital Health Plan, 207		50,000	Care1st Health Plan Arizona, 23
125,000	Managed HealthCare Northwest, 647		50,000	Peoples Health, 358
125,000	Premier Access Insurance/Access Dental, 128		50,000	Sanford Health Plan, 319
123,880	Access Dental Services, 57		50,000	Vantage Health Plan, 361
120,000	Horizon Health Corporation, 752		49,976	Children's Mercy Integrated Care Solutions, 463
120,000	Sant, Community Physicians, 133		49,000	Sharp Health Plan, 135
119,712	Prevea Health Network, 849		48,477	HealthPartners, 729
118,600	DakotaCare, 714		47,000	Upper Peninsula Health Plan, 436
118,000	Network Health Plan of Wisconsin, 847		45,000	Health Choice of Alabama, 6
115,000	Health Choice Arizona, 29		45,000	Medical Associates, 317
112,000	Physicians Plus Insurance Corporation, 848		45,000	Preferred Care Partners, 228
111,000	CarePlus Health Plans, 209		44,000	Sterling Insurance, 763
110,000	Community First Health Plans, 743		42,000	TexanPlus Medicare Advantage HMO, 764
110,000	Preferred Health Plan, Inc., 349		40,000	Crescent Health Solutions, 588
109,000	Health Plan of San Joaquin, 102		34,000	Health Tradition, 842
108,000	Neighborhood Health Partnership, 226		33,000	South Central Preferred Health Network, 678
101,000	UPMC Health Plan, 683		32,000	Hometown Health Plan, 503
100,000	Blue Cross & Blue Shield of Wyoming, 856		30,000	InStil Health, 709
100,000	OhioHealth Group, 616		30,000	Piedmont Community Health Plan, 801
97,000	Kern Family Health Care, 110		27,000	Leon Medical Centers Health Plan, 222
95,000	Health Partners of Kansas, 331		26,000	SummaCare Medicare Advantage Plan, 621

Primary Care Physician Index

4,300	Cigna-HealthSpring, 725
4,300	Health New England, 393
4,200	Universal American Medicare Plans, 584
4,000	Alameda Alliance for Health, 59
4,000	Alameda Medi-Cal Plan, 60
4,000	Baptist Health Services Group, 722
4,000	NovaSys Health, 55
4,000	Prominence Health Plan, 508
4,000	The Health Plan of the Ohio Valley/Mountaineer Region, 624
3,800	Altius Health Plans, 773
3,800	Blue Cross & Blue Shield of Texas, 740
3,780	Phoenix Health Plan, 38
3,600	Trinity Health, 430
3,555	L.A. Care Health Plan, 112
3,532	Anthem Blue Cross & Blue Shield of Indiana, 293
3,500	Aultcare Corporation, 605
3,500	CalOptima, 71
3,500	Emi Health, 776
3,500	Geisinger Health Plan, 666
3,500	PCC Preferred Chiropractic Care, 334
3,500	PTPN, 130
3,500	UniCare West Virginia, 826
3,434	Blue Cross & Blue Shield of South Carolina, 705
3,322	Blue Cross & Blue Shield of New Mexico, 532
3,300	Premera Blue Cross Blue Shield of Alaska, 16
3,300	Trilogy Health Insurance, 851
3,250	Ohio State University Health Plan Inc., 615
3,200	Delta Dental of Colorado, 161
3,200	Golden Dental Plans, 416
3,100	Physicians Health Plan of Mid-Michigan, 425
3,000	Health Alliance Medicare, 278
3,000	Medical Center Healthnet Plan, 396
3,000	Parkland Community Health Plan, 759
2,855	Healthplex, 565
2,800	Neighborhood Health Plan, 398
2,691	Aetna Health of New York, 543
2,643	Rocky Mountain Health Plans, 167
2,500	Community Health Plan of Washington, 808
2,490	Blue Cross & Blue Shield of Tennessee, 723
2,300	San Francisco Health Plan, 131
2,200	AlohaCare, 250
2,000	Access Dental Services, 57
1,923	First Health, 94
1,900	Blue Cross & Blue Shield of Montana, 478
1,900	Crescent Health Solutions, 588
1,900	Paramount Care of Michigan, 424
1,900	Paramount Elite Medicare Plan, 617
1,900	Paramount Health Care, 618
1,900	Preferred Health Care, 676
1,750	University Health Plans, 787
1,700	Western Dental Services, 147
1,631	Blue Cross of Idaho Health Service, Inc., 259
1,611	Blue Cross & Blue Shield of Arizona, 22
1,602	Prevea Health Network, 849
1,590	Central California Alliance for Health, 77
1,551	Blue Cross & Blue Shield of Oklahoma, 629

1,500	AllCare Health, 639
1,500	Bright Health Alabama, 5
1,500	Dean Health Plan, 836
1,500	Delta Dental of Oklahoma, 633
1,500	Health Link PPO, 454
1,500	Preferred Care Partners, 228
1,400	Affinity Health Plan, 544
1,400	EPIC Pharmacy Network, 797
1,400	Health Choice LLC, 728
1,400	Highmark BCBS West Virginia, 822
1,400	Medica with CHI Health, 491
1,400	Trinity Health of Idaho, 265
1,340	Employers Dental Services, 28
1,282	Neighborhood Health Partnership, 226
1,228	Managed HealthCare Northwest, 647
1,200	Elderplan, 555
1,200	Leon Medical Centers Health Plan, 222
1,200	Sant, Community Physicians, 133
1,161	Inter Valley Health Plan, 106
1,125	Independent Health, 567
1,121	Kaiser Permanente Northern Colorado, 164
1,121	Kaiser Permanente Southern Colorado, 165
1,100	Kaiser Permanente Mid-Atlantic, 380
1,090	UPMC Susquehanna, 684
1,050	MediGold, 612
1,000	Alliance Regional Health Network, 734
1,000	Cox Healthplans, 465
1,000	Dental Health Services of California, 90
1,000	Health Partners of Kansas, 331
1,000	Premier Access Insurance/Access Dental, 41, 128, 507, 781
1,000	Scott & White Health Plan, 760
983	Santa Clara Family Health Foundations Inc, 132
980	First Choice Health, 480, 643, 811
979	Delta Dental of New Mexico, 534
962	Blue Cross and Blue Shield of Louisiana, 353
950	CareOregon Health Plan, 641
950	Secure Health PPO Newtork, 245
908	Unity Health Insurance, 853
900	HAP-Health Alliance Plan: Flint, 417
900	HAP-Health Alliance Plan: Senior Medicare Plan, 418
900	Neighborhood Health Plan of Rhode Island, 701
900	Trinity Health of Connecticut, 183
880	Kaiser Permanente Northwest, 645
850	Gundersen Lutheran Health Plan, 841
825	DakotaCare, 714
800	Allied Pacific IPA, 62
800	Health Tradition, 842
778	Valley Preferred, 686
764	Baptist Health Plan, 342
750	Dentaquest, 390
750	Northeast Georgia Health Partners, 244
700	Mercy Clinic Arkansas, 54
700	Mercy Clinic Kansas, 333
700	Mercy Clinic Missouri, 474
700	Mercy Clinic Oklahoma, 636
700	OSF Healthcare, 285

Referral/Specialty Physician Index

2017 Title List
Visit www.GreyHouse.com for Product Information, Table of Contents, and Sample Pages.

General Reference
An African Biographical Dictionary
America's College Museums
American Environmental Leaders: From Colonial Times to the Present
Encyclopedia of African-American Writing
Encyclopedia of Constitutional Amendments
An Encyclopedia of Human Rights in the United States
Encyclopedia of Invasions & Conquests
Encyclopedia of Prisoners of War & Internment
Encyclopedia of Religion & Law in America
Encyclopedia of Rural America
Encyclopedia of the Continental Congress
Encyclopedia of the United States Cabinet, 1789-2010
Encyclopedia of War Journalism
Encyclopedia of Warrior Peoples & Fighting Groups
The Environmental Debate: A Documentary History
The Evolution Wars: A Guide to the Debates
From Suffrage to the Senate: America's Political Women
Gun Debate: An Encyclopedia of Gun Control & Gun Rights
Political Corruption in America
Privacy Rights in the Digital Era
The Religious Right: A Reference Handbook
Speakers of the House of Representatives, 1789-2009
This is Who We Were: 1880-1900
This is Who We Were: A Companion to the 1940 Census
This is Who We Were: In the 1900s
This is Who We Were: In the 1910s
This is Who We Were: In the 1920s
This is Who We Were: In the 1940s
This is Who We Were: In the 1950s
This is Who We Were: In the 1960s
This is Who We Were: In the 1970s
This is Who We Were: In the 1980s
This is Who We Were: In the 1990s
U.S. Land & Natural Resource Policy
The Value of a Dollar 1600-1865: Colonial Era to the Civil War
The Value of a Dollar: 1860-2014
Working Americans 1770-1869 Vol. IX: Revolutionary War to the Civil War
Working Americans 1880-1999 Vol. I: The Working Class
Working Americans 1880-1999 Vol. II: The Middle Class
Working Americans 1880-1999 Vol. III: The Upper Class
Working Americans 1880-1999 Vol. IV: Their Children
Working Americans 1880-2015 Vol. V: Americans At War
Working Americans 1880-2005 Vol. VI: Women at Work
Working Americans 1880-2006 Vol. VII: Social Movements
Working Americans 1880-2007 Vol. VIII: Immigrants
Working Americans 1880-2009 Vol. X: Sports & Recreation
Working Americans 1880-2010 Vol. XI: Inventors & Entrepreneurs
Working Americans 1880-2011 Vol. XII: Our History through Music
Working Americans 1880-2012 Vol. XIII: Education & Educators
Working Americans 1880-2016 Vol. XIV: Industry Through the Ages
World Cultural Leaders of the 20th & 21st Centuries

Education Information
Charter School Movement
Comparative Guide to American Elementary & Secondary Schools
Complete Learning Disabilities Directory
Educators Resource Directory
Special Education: Policy and Curriculum Development

Health Information
Comparative Guide to American Hospitals
Complete Directory for Pediatric Disorders
Complete Directory for People with Chronic Illness
Complete Directory for People with Disabilities
Complete Mental Health Directory
Diabetes in America: Analysis of an Epidemic
Directory of Health Care Group Purchasing Organizations
HMO/PPO Directory
Medical Device Market Place
Older Americans Information Directory

Business Information
Complete Television, Radio & Cable Industry Directory
Directory of Business Information Resources
Directory of Mail Order Catalogs

Directory of Venture Capital & Private Equity Firms
Environmental Resource Handbook
Food & Beverage Market Place
Grey House Homeland Security Directory
Grey House Performing Arts Directory
Grey House Safety & Security Directory
Hudson's Washington News Media Contacts Directory
New York State Directory
Sports Market Place Directory

Statistics & Demographics
American Tally
America's Top-Rated Cities
America's Top-Rated Smaller Cities
Ancestry & Ethnicity in America
The Asian Databook
Comparative Guide to American Suburbs
The Hispanic Databook
Profiles of America
"Profiles of" Series – State Handbooks
Weather America

Financial Ratings Series
TheStreet Ratings' Guide to Bond & Money Market Mutual Funds
TheStreet Ratings' Guide to Common Stocks
TheStreet Ratings' Guide to Exchange-Traded Funds
TheStreet Ratings' Guide to Stock Mutual Funds
TheStreet Ratings' Ultimate Guided Tour of Stock Investing
Weiss Ratings' Consumer Guides
Weiss Ratings' Financial Literary Basic Guides
Weiss Ratings' Guide to Banks
Weiss Ratings' Guide to Credit Unions
Weiss Ratings' Guide to Health Insurers
Weiss Ratings' Guide to Life & Annuity Insurers
Weiss Ratings' Guide to Property & Casualty Insurers

Bowker's Books In Print® Titles
American Book Publishing Record® Annual
American Book Publishing Record® Monthly
Books In Print®
Books In Print® Supplement
Books Out Loud™
Bowker's Complete Video Directory™
Children's Books In Print®
El-Hi Textbooks & Serials In Print®
Forthcoming Books®
Law Books & Serials In Print™
Medical & Health Care Books In Print™
Publishers, Distributors & Wholesalers of the US™
Subject Guide to Books In Print®
Subject Guide to Children's Books In Print®

Canadian General Reference
Associations Canada
Canadian Almanac & Directory
Canadian Environmental Resource Guide
Canadian Parliamentary Guide
Canadian Venture Capital & Private Equity Firms
Financial Post Directory of Directors
Financial Services Canada
Governments Canada
Health Guide Canada
The History of Canada
Libraries Canada
Major Canadian Cities

2017 Title List

Visit www.SalemPress.com for Product Information, Table of Contents, and Sample Pages.

Science, Careers & Mathematics

Ancient Creatures
Applied Science
Applied Science: Engineering & Mathematics
Applied Science: Science & Medicine
Applied Science: Technology
Biomes and Ecosystems
Careers in The Arts: Fine, Performing & Visual
Careers in Building Construction
Careers in Business
Careers in Chemistry
Careers in Communications & Media
Careers in Environment & Conservation
Careers in Financial Services
Careers in Healthcare
Careers in Hospitality & Tourism
Careers in Human Services
Careers in Law, Criminal Justice & Emergency Services
Careers in Manufacturing
Careers in Overseas Jobs
Careers in Physics
Careers in Sales, Insurance & Real Estate
Careers in Science & Engineering
Careers in Sports & Fitness
Careers in Technology Services & Repair
Computer Technology Innovators
Contemporary Biographies in Business
Contemporary Biographies in Chemistry
Contemporary Biographies in Communications & Media
Contemporary Biographies in Environment & Conservation
Contemporary Biographies in Healthcare
Contemporary Biographies in Hospitality & Tourism
Contemporary Biographies in Law & Criminal Justice
Contemporary Biographies in Physics
Earth Science
Earth Science: Earth Materials & Resources
Earth Science: Earth's Surface and History
Earth Science: Physics & Chemistry of the Earth
Earth Science: Weather, Water & Atmosphere
Encyclopedia of Energy
Encyclopedia of Environmental Issues
Encyclopedia of Environmental Issues: Atmosphere and Air Pollution
Encyclopedia of Environmental Issues: Ecology and Ecosystems
Encyclopedia of Environmental Issues: Energy and Energy Use
Encyclopedia of Environmental Issues: Policy and Activism
Encyclopedia of Environmental Issues: Preservation/Wilderness Issues
Encyclopedia of Environmental Issues: Water and Water Pollution
Encyclopedia of Global Resources
Encyclopedia of Global Warming
Encyclopedia of Mathematics & Society
Encyclopedia of Mathematics & Society: Engineering, Tech, Medicine
Encyclopedia of Mathematics & Society: Great Mathematicians
Encyclopedia of Mathematics & Society: Math & Social Sciences
Encyclopedia of Mathematics & Society: Math Development/Concepts
Encyclopedia of Mathematics & Society: Math in Culture & Society
Encyclopedia of Mathematics & Society: Space, Science, Environment
Encyclopedia of the Ancient World
Forensic Science
Geography Basics
Internet Innovators
Inventions and Inventors
Magill's Encyclopedia of Science: Animal Life
Magill's Encyclopedia of Science: Plant life
Notable Natural Disasters
Principles of Astronomy
Principles of Biology
Principles of Chemistry
Principles of Physical Science
Principles of Physics
Principles of Research Methods
Principles of Sustainability
Science and Scientists
Solar System
Solar System: Great Astronomers
Solar System: Study of the Universe
Solar System: The Inner Planets
Solar System: The Moon and Other Small Bodies
Solar System: The Outer Planets
Solar System: The Sun and Other Stars
World Geography

Literature

American Ethnic Writers
Classics of Science Fiction & Fantasy Literature
Critical Approaches: Feminist
Critical Approaches: Multicultural
Critical Approaches: Moral
Critical Approaches: Psychological
Critical Insights: Authors
Critical Insights: Film
Critical Insights: Literary Collection Bundles
Critical Insights: Themes
Critical Insights: Works
Critical Survey of Drama
Critical Survey of Graphic Novels: Heroes & Super Heroes
Critical Survey of Graphic Novels: History, Theme & Technique
Critical Survey of Graphic Novels: Independents/Underground Classics
Critical Survey of Graphic Novels: Manga
Critical Survey of Long Fiction
Critical Survey of Mystery & Detective Fiction
Critical Survey of Mythology and Folklore: Heroes and Heroines
Critical Survey of Mythology and Folklore: Love, Sexuality & Desire
Critical Survey of Mythology and Folklore: World Mythology
Critical Survey of Poetry
Critical Survey of Poetry: American Poets
Critical Survey of Poetry: British, Irish & Commonwealth Poets
Critical Survey of Poetry: Cumulative Index
Critical Survey of Poetry: European Poets
Critical Survey of Poetry: Topical Essays
Critical Survey of Poetry: World Poets
Critical Survey of Science Fiction & Fantasy
Critical Survey of Shakespeare's Plays
Critical Survey of Shakespeare's Sonnets
Critical Survey of Short Fiction
Critical Survey of Short Fiction: American Writers
Critical Survey of Short Fiction: British, Irish, Commonwealth Writers
Critical Survey of Short Fiction: Cumulative Index
Critical Survey of Short Fiction: European Writers
Critical Survey of Short Fiction: Topical Essays
Critical Survey of Short Fiction: World Writers
Critical Survey of World Literature
Critical Survey of Young Adult Literature
Cyclopedia of Literary Characters
Cyclopedia of Literary Places
Holocaust Literature
Introduction to Literary Context: American Poetry of the 20th Century
Introduction to Literary Context: American Post-Modernist Novels
Introduction to Literary Context: American Short Fiction
Introduction to Literary Context: English Literature
Introduction to Literary Context: Plays
Introduction to Literary Context: World Literature
Magill's Literary Annual 2015
Magill's Survey of American Literature
Magill's Survey of World Literature
Masterplots
Masterplots II: African American Literature
Masterplots II: American Fiction Series
Masterplots II: British & Commonwealth Fiction Series
Masterplots II: Christian Literature
Masterplots II: Drama Series
Masterplots II: Juvenile & Young Adult Literature, Supplement
Masterplots II: Nonfiction Series
Masterplots II: Poetry Series
Masterplots II: Short Story Series
Masterplots II: Women's Literature Series
Notable African American Writers
Notable American Novelists
Notable Playwrights
Notable Poets
Recommended Reading: 600 Classics Reviewed
Short Story Writers

Grey House Publishing | Salem Press | H.W. Wilson | 4919 Route, 22 PO Box 56, Amenia NY 12501-0056

2017 Title List

Visit **www.SalemPress.com** for Product Information, Table of Contents, and Sample Pages.

History and Social Science

The 2000s in America
50 States
African American History
Agriculture in History
American First Ladies
American Heroes
American Indian Culture
American Indian History
American Indian Tribes
American Presidents
American Villains
America's Historic Sites
Ancient Greece
The Bill of Rights
The Civil Rights Movement
The Cold War
Countries, Peoples & Cultures
Countries, Peoples & Cultures: Central & South America
Countries, Peoples & Cultures: Central, South & Southeast Asia
Countries, Peoples & Cultures: East & South Africa
Countries, Peoples & Cultures: East Asia & the Pacific
Countries, Peoples & Cultures: Eastern Europe
Countries, Peoples & Cultures: Middle East & North Africa
Countries, Peoples & Cultures: North America & the Caribbean
Countries, Peoples & Cultures: West & Central Africa
Countries, Peoples & Cultures: Western Europe
Defining Documents: American Revolution
Defining Documents: American West
Defining Documents: Ancient World
Defining Documents: Civil Rights
Defining Documents: Civil War
Defining Documents: Court Cases
Defining Documents: Dissent & Protest
Defining Documents: Emergence of Modern America
Defining Documents: Exploration & Colonial America
Defining Documents: Immigration & Immigrant Communities
Defining Documents: Manifest Destiny
Defining Documents: Middle Ages
Defining Documents: Nationalism & Populism
Defining Documents: Native Americans
Defining Documents: Postwar 1940s
Defining Documents: Reconstruction
Defining Documents: Renaissance & Early Modern Era
Defining Documents: 1920s
Defining Documents: 1930s
Defining Documents: 1950s
Defining Documents: 1960s
Defining Documents: 1970s
Defining Documents: The 17th Century
Defining Documents: The 18th Century
Defining Documents: Vietnam War
Defining Documents: Women
Defining Documents: World War I
Defining Documents: World War II
The Eighties in America
Encyclopedia of American Immigration
Encyclopedia of Flight
Encyclopedia of the Ancient World
Fashion Innovators
The Fifties in America
The Forties in America
Great Athletes
Great Athletes: Baseball
Great Athletes: Basketball
Great Athletes: Boxing & Soccer
Great Athletes: Cumulative Index
Great Athletes: Football
Great Athletes: Golf & Tennis
Great Athletes: Olympics
Great Athletes: Racing & Individual Sports
Great Events from History: 17th Century
Great Events from History: 18th Century
Great Events from History: 19th Century
Great Events from History: 20th Century (1901-1940)
Great Events from History: 20th Century (1941-1970)

Great Events from History: 20th Century (1971-2000)
Great Events from History: 21st Century (2000-2016)
Great Events from History: African American History
Great Events from History: Cumulative Indexes
Great Events from History: LGBTG
Great Events from History: Middle Ages
Great Events from History: Modern Scandals
Great Events from History: Renaissance & Early Modern Era
Great Lives from History: 17th Century
Great Lives from History: 18th Century
Great Lives from History: 19th Century
Great Lives from History: 20th Century
Great Lives from History: 21st Century (2000-2016)
Great Lives from History: American Women
Great Lives from History: Ancient World
Great Lives from History: Asian & Pacific Islander Americans
Great Lives from History: Cumulative Indexes
Great Lives from History: Incredibly Wealthy
Great Lives from History: Inventors & Inventions
Great Lives from History: Jewish Americans
Great Lives from History: Latinos
Great Lives from History: Notorious Lives
Great Lives from History: Renaissance & Early Modern Era
Great Lives from History: Scientists & Science
Historical Encyclopedia of American Business
Issues in U.S. Immigration
Magill's Guide to Military History
Milestone Documents in African American History
Milestone Documents in American History
Milestone Documents in World History
Milestone Documents of American Leaders
Milestone Documents of World Religions
Music Innovators
Musicians & Composers 20th Century
The Nineties in America
The Seventies in America
The Sixties in America
Survey of American Industry and Careers
The Thirties in America
The Twenties in America
United States at War
U.S. Court Cases
U.S. Government Leaders
U.S. Laws, Acts, and Treaties
U.S. Legal System
U.S. Supreme Court
Weapons and Warfare
World Conflicts: Asia and the Middle East

Health

Addictions & Substance Abuse
Adolescent Health & Wellness
Cancer
Complementary & Alternative Medicine
Community & Family Health
Genetics & Inherited Conditions
Health Issues
Infectious Diseases & Conditions
Magill's Medical Guide
Nutrition
Nursing
Psychology & Behavioral Health
Psychology Basics

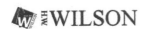

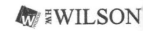

2017 Title List

Visit **www.HWWilsonInPrint.com** for Product Information, Table of Contents and Sample Pages

Current Biography
Current Biography Cumulative Index 1946-2013
Current Biography Monthly Magazine
Current Biography Yearbook: 2003
Current Biography Yearbook: 2004
Current Biography Yearbook: 2005
Current Biography Yearbook: 2006
Current Biography Yearbook: 2007
Current Biography Yearbook: 2008
Current Biography Yearbook: 2009
Current Biography Yearbook: 2010
Current Biography Yearbook: 2011
Current Biography Yearbook: 2012
Current Biography Yearbook: 2013
Current Biography Yearbook: 2014
Current Biography Yearbook: 2015
Current Biography Yearbook: 2016

Core Collections
Children's Core Collection
Fiction Core Collection
Graphic Novels Core Collection
Middle & Junior High School Core
Public Library Core Collection: Nonfiction
Senior High Core Collection
Young Adult Fiction Core Collection

The Reference Shelf
Aging in America
American Military Presence Overseas
The Arab Spring
The Brain
The Business of Food
Campaign Trends & Election Law
Conspiracy Theories
The Digital Age
Dinosaurs
Embracing New Paradigms in Education
Faith & Science
Families: Traditional and New Structures
The Future of U.S. Economic Relations: Mexico, Cuba, and Venezuela
Global Climate Change
Graphic Novels and Comic Books
Guns in America
Immigration
Immigration in the U.S.
Internet Abuses & Privacy Rights
Internet Safety
LGBTQ in the 21st Century
Marijuana Reform
The News and its Future
The Paranormal
Politics of the Ocean
Prescription Drug Abuse
Racial Tension in a "Postracial" Age
Reality Television
Representative American Speeches: 2008-2009
Representative American Speeches: 2009-2010
Representative American Speeches: 2010-2011
Representative American Speeches: 2011-2012
Representative American Speeches: 2012-2013
Representative American Speeches: 2013-2014
Representative American Speeches: 2014-2015
Representative American Speeches: 2015-2016
Representative American Speeches: 2016-2017
Rethinking Work
Revisiting Gender
Robotics
Russia
Social Networking
Social Services for the Poor
Space Exploration & Development
Sports in America

The Supreme Court
The Transformation of American Cities
U.S. Infrastructure
U.S. National Debate Topic: Educational Reform
U.S. National Debate Topic: Surveillance
U.S. National Debate Topic: The Ocean
U.S. National Debate Topic: Transportation Infrastructure
Whistleblowers

Readers' Guide
Abridged Readers' Guide to Periodical Literature
Readers' Guide to Periodical Literature

Indexes
Index to Legal Periodicals & Books
Short Story Index
Book Review Digest

Sears List
Sears List of Subject Headings
Sears: Lista de Encabezamientos de Materia

Facts About Series
Facts About American Immigration
Facts About China
Facts About the 20th Century
Facts About the Presidents
Facts About the World's Languages

Nobel Prize Winners
Nobel Prize Winners: 1901-1986
Nobel Prize Winners: 1987-1991
Nobel Prize Winners: 1992-1996
Nobel Prize Winners: 1997-2001

World Authors
World Authors: 1995-2000
World Authors: 2000-2005

Famous First Facts
Famous First Facts
Famous First Facts About American Politics
Famous First Facts About Sports
Famous First Facts About the Environment
Famous First Facts: International Edition

American Book of Days
The American Book of Days
The International Book of Days

Monographs
American Reformers
The Barnhart Dictionary of Etymology
Celebrate the World
Guide to the Ancient World
Indexing from A to Z
The Poetry Break
Radical Change: Books for Youth in a Digital Age

Wilson Chronology
Wilson Chronology of Asia and the Pacific
Wilson Chronology of Human Rights
Wilson Chronology of Ideas
Wilson Chronology of the Arts
Wilson Chronology of the World's Religions
Wilson Chronology of Women's Achievements

Grey House Publishing | Salem Press | H.W. Wilson | 4919 Route, 22 PO Box 56, Amenia NY 12501-0056